Acta Neurochirurgica
Supplements

Editor: H.-J. Reulen
Assistant Editor: H.-J. Steiger

Brain Edema X

Proceedings of the Tenth International Symposium,
San Diego, California, October 20–23, 1996

Edited by
H. E. James, L. F. Marshall,
H.-J. Reulen, A. Baethmann,
A. Marmarou, U. Ito, J. T. Hoff,
T. Kuroiwa, Z. Czernicki

Acta Neurochirurgica
Supplement 70

SpringerWienNewYork

Hector E. James, M.D.
Pediatric Neurosurgery, San Diego, CA, U.S.A.

Lawrence F. Marshall, M.D.
Division of Neurological Surgery, San Diego Medical Center,
University of California, San Diego, CA, U.S.A.

Hans J. Reulen, Prof. Dr.
Institut für Neurochirurgie, Klinikum Grosshadern, Ludwig-
Maximilians-Universität, München, Federal Republic of Germany

Alexander Baethmann, Prof. Dr.
Institut für Chirurgische Forschung, Klinikum Grosshadern, Ludwig-
Maximilians-Universität, München, Federal Republic of Germany

Anthony Marmarou, Ph.D.
Neurological Surgery, Virginia Commonwealth University,
Richmond, VA, U.S.A.

Umeo Ito, M.D.
Department of Neurosurgery, Musashino Red Cross Hospital,
Tokyo, Japan

Julian T. Hoff, M.D.
Taubmann Health Care Center, The University of Michigan,
Ann Arbor, MI, U.S.A.

Toshihiko Kuroiwa, M.D.
Department of Neuropathology, Tokyo Medical and Dental
University, Medical Research Institute, Tokyo, Japan

Zbigniew Czernicki, M.D., Ph.D.
Department of Neurosurgery, Medical Resarch Center, Polish
Academy of Sciences, Warsaw, Poland

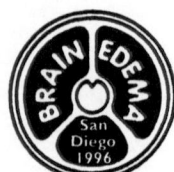

Proceedings of the Tenth International Brain Edema Symposium
Cellular Injury and Brain Edema 1996

Honorary Member: I. Klatzo. *Organizing Committee*: H. E. James, A. Marmarou, L. F. Marshall. *Advisory Board*: A. Baethmann, Z. Czernicki, J. T. Hoff, K. A. Hossmann, U. Ito, H. E. James, T. Kuroiwa, A. Marmarou, H. J. Reulen. *Critical Care Consultant*: P. M. Kochanek. *Coordinating Office:* H. E. James

Graphic design: Ecke Bonk

Printed on acid-free and chlorine free bleached paper
SPIN: 10570170

With 121 partly coloured Figures

Library of Congress Cataloging-in-Publication Data

Brain edema X : proceedings of the tenth international symposium, San
Diego, California, October 20-23, 1996 / edited by H.E. James ...
[et al.].
      p. cm. -- (Acta neurochirurgica. Supplement, ISSN 0065-1419
; 70)
    "Papers presented at the Tenth International Symposium on Brain
Edema"--Pref.
    Includes bibliographical references and index.
    1. Cerebral edema--Congresses. I. James, H. E.
II. International Symposium on Brain Edema (10th : 1996 : San Diego,
Calif.) III. Series.
    [DNLM: 1. Brain Edema--etiology--congresses. 2. Brain Edema--
-physiopathology--congresses. 3. Brain Edema--therapy--congresses.
W1 AC8661 no.70 1997 / WL 348 B81442 1997]
RC394.E3B726 1997
616.8--dc21
DNLM/DLC
for Library of Congress   97-39789
                                                            CIP

ISSN 0065-1419

ISBN-13: 978-3-7091-7418-0   e-ISBN-13: 978-3-7091-6837-0
DOI: 10.1007/978-3-7091-6837-0

Preface

This volume is a compilation of papers presented at the Tenth International Symposium on Brain Edema held on October 20–23, 1996, in San Diego, California. This follows the sequence of meetings that was initiated 31 years ago in the First International Symposium held in Vienna. Subsequent symposiums were held in Mainz, Montreal, Berlin, Groningen, Tokyo, Baltimore, Bern, and Tokyo (Yokohama).

A considerable number of papers was chosen from over 100 papers that were received. The organizers wish to thank the Advisory Committee for the excellent work done in selection of the papers. We also wish to thank all the persons who contributed to the success of the Tenth International Symposium, especially the staff who worked behind the scenes.

These papers were reviewed, edited, approved or disapproved by the Editorial Board. Those manuscripts that were felt not pertinent to this publication were not accepted by the Editorial Board. Therefore, the excellent quality of those that are in the book are a reflection of the authors' dedication and work and that of those of the Editorial Board in their review process.

For the reader's convenience, the papers are structured according to the various disease processes which are associated with the primary topic: hypertension, hydrocephalus, infection, ischemia, tumor, etc. We do hope that the reader will enjoy the articles and that they will provide an impetus and insight for future work.

The Advisory Board, as in the past meetings, has felt that for this manuscript to be of value, the written record of the meeting should be quickly available and be relatively inexpensive. In order to come close to such an ideal, the manuscripts were to be delivered at the time of the meeting and must adhere strictly to prepared guidelines. We wish to compliment the authors, the Editorial Board, and all those who enabled us to meet this deadline. We also wish to acknowledge our gratitude to Springer-Verlag, Vienna, for the technical aid and for their prompt publication of this volume.

As in the past, brain edema and disturbance of metabolism arising from acute insults of any etiology, remain the central issue of research. The supportive role of biochemically activated mediators, changes in blood brain barrier, spread of the edema process, always elicit great scientific as well as clinical interest. Therapeutic interventions can only be effectively directed to these problems once the understanding of the underlying biochemical disturbances, disturbances in cerebral perfusion and parallel events, are mastered. This theme has been the essence of all the Brain Edema Meetings. This volume provides a comprehensive survey of the state of the art of this topic as of October 1996.

The Eleventh International Symposium on Brain Edema will be held in England in 1999. This will be the final meeting of the century, and we hope that the 1996 and 1999 meetings will set the pace for the next century.

The Editors

Contents

Section II – Trauma

Section III – Cellular Swelling and Injury

Section IV – Neoplasms

Section V – Therapy

Section VI – Molecular Mechanisms

Section VII – Blood Brain Barrier

Section VIII – Thermal Effects

Listed in Current Contents

Acta Neurochir (1997) [Suppl] 70: 1–3
© Springer-Verlag 1997

Glutamate Uptake and Na,K-ATPase Activity in Rat Astrocyte Cultures Exposed to Ischemia

D. B. Stanimirovic, R. Ball, and **J. P. Durkin**

Institute for Biological Sciences, National Research Council of Canada, Ottawa, Canada

Summary

In this study we demonstrate the stimulation of both glutamate uptake and Na,K-ATPase activity in rat astrocyte cultures in response to a sublethal ischemic insult *in vitro*. To measure sodium pump activity and glutamate uptake, ^{3}H-glutamate and ^{86}Rb were simultaneously added to the cultures in the presence or absence of 2 mM ouabain. Na,K-ATPase activity was defined as ouabain-sensitive ^{86}Rb uptake. Cell death was assessed by exclusion of the vital dye, calcein-AM from cells. Concomitant transient increases (2–3 fold above control levels) in both Na,K-ATPase and glutamate transporter activities were observed in astrocytes after 2–4 hours of ischemia. By contrast, 24 hours of ischemia caused a profound loss of both activities which paralleled significant cell death. The addition of 5 mM glucose to the cells after 4 hours of ischemia prevented the loss of sodium pump activity and glutamate uptake, and rescued astrocytes from the lethal effects of 24 hours of ischemia.

Keywords: Cerebral ischemia; glutamate uptake; astrocyte Na,K-ATPase; cell culture.

Introduction

Under physiological conditions, the postsynaptic excitatory actions of glutamate are rapidly terminated by high affinity glutamate uptake into presynaptic terminals or neighboring glial cells [2, 5, 6]. In astrocytes, high affinity glutamate transport is an electrogenic process by which glutamate is co-transported with $2Na^+$ into cells in exchange for K^+ and OH^- (or HCO_3^-) [2, 5]. The energy-dependent sodium pump (Na,K-ATPase) generates an electrochemical sodium gradient which is utilized by the transporter to drive the uptake of glutamate [2, 4].

In this study we demonstrate that a sublethal ischemic insult stimulates both sodium pump activity and glutamate uptake in rat cortical astrocytes, whereas a profound inhibition of both parallels the death of cells under lethal ischemic conditions.

Materials and Methods

Cell Culture

Primary cultures of rat cortical type I astrocytes were obtained by the modified differential adhesion method [9]. The cortices of 2–4 days old Sprague-Dawley rats were dissociated by the combination of mechanical disruption and enzymatic digestion [9]. Primary mixed glial cultures were initiated in medium DMEM containing 4.5 g/l glucose, 2 mM glutamine, 10% fetal bovine serum and 25 µg/ml gentamycin at 37°C in an atmosphere of 7% CO_2 in air. After 7–10 days, loosely attached cells (mainly progenitor cells and macrophages) were removed by repeated shaking of the cultures in an orbital shaker [9]. The firmly attached cells were propagated to yield cultures in which > 95% of cells were glial fibrillary acidic protein (GFAP) and S100-positive and consisted almost exclusively of "flat" (type I) astrocytes.

Simulated in vitro Ischemia

Astrocyte cultures were subjected to a combination of glucose-free Krebs solution [(in mM) 119 NaCl, 4.7 KCl, 1.2 KH_2PO_4, 25 $NaHCO_3$, 2.5 $CaCl_2$, 1 $MgCl_2$] and hypoxia (< 2% O_2) in a Forma Scientific anaerobic chamber Model 1024, equipped with a humidified, temperature-controlled incubator with direct access from within the chamber. All experimental manipulations and biochemical assays (i.e., ^{86}Rb and ^{3}H-glutamate uptake) were carried out within the chamber. Reoxygenation was initiated by exposing cells to ambient air after various times of ischemia.

Cell Viability

Cell death was determined by exclusion of the vital dye, calcein-AM (CA-AM) from damaged cells. The intensity of cell labeling following a 30 min exposure of cells to 5 µM CA-AM was quantified using CytoFluor 2350 (Millipore) microplate reader.

Na/K-ATPase/Glutamate Uptake Assay

^{86}Rb and ^{3}H-glutamate uptake experiments were conducted on astrocytes grown in 24 well plates essentially as described by Dong *et al.* [3] and Volterra *et al.* [13] respectively. Briefly, experiments were initiated by the addition of 2.5 µCi/ml of ^{86}Rb and 0.5 µCi/ml of L-[2,3-^{3}H] glutamic acid to the same cultures, in the absence or presence of the selective inhibitor of Na,K-ATPase, ouabain (2 mM), and uptake of both labels was measured after 15 min (linear part of uptake) at room temperature. The reaction was stopped by rapidly washing the cells 3 times with ice-cold PBS. Cells were then lysed in 0.1% Triton X-100, and the ^{86}Rb and ^{3}H-glutamate content of the lysates determined by dual-label scintillation counting with energy windows set at 008–110 and 136–222 for ^{3}H and ^{86}Rb, respectively. Uptake results were corrected for spillover (< 4%) between the channels, and expressed as cpm/min/mg protein. Sodium pump (Na,K-ATPase) activity was defined as the ouabain-sensitive component of total ^{86}Rb uptake. Protein content was determined in aliquots of the lysates by the method of Lowry *et al.* [8].

Results and Discussion

The exposure of astrocytes to simulated *in vitro* ischemia resulted in a transient and, in most cases, concomitant increase in both sodium pump and glutamate transporter activities (Table 1). Ischemia caused a 1.5–2.5 fold increase in both activities within 1–4 hours, and this was followed by a progressive decline in activity over the next 24 hours (Table 1). The phase of decline closely paralleled a loss in cell viability in that 4 hours of ischemia decreased CA-AM staining of astrocytes by about 15% (Table 1)? while 24 hours of ischemia resulted in majority (60–70%) of cells excluding the vital dye (Table 1). These results indicated that the collapse of sodium pump and glutamate transporter activities detected in astrocyte cultures at 24 hours of ischemia coincided with significant ischemia-induced cell death. By contrast, the increase in both ouabain-sensitive potassium influx and ^{3}H-glutamate uptake activity observed after 1–4 hours of ischemia were accompanied by only small changes in cell viability and appeared to represent the principal functional/metabolic effect of the ischemic insult on astrocytes in culture.

The mechanism(s) by which sublethal ischemia up-regulates Na,K-ATPase and glutamate transporter activities in astrocytes is unclear. One possible explanation is that the enzyme/transporter activities passively respond to changes in ionic gradients effected by ischemia. For example, Na,K-ATPase can readily be activated by ischemia-induced increases in $[Na^+]_i$ caused by the activation of the sodium-proton exchanger [1] in its attempt to compensate for intracellular acidosis [1, 7]. Consistent with this hypothesis is the observed ability of the Na^+/H^+ exchanger inhibitor, 5-(N,N-dimethyl)-amiloride (DMA; 0.5–5 µM), to partly attenuate the stimulation of sodium pump activity induced by ischemia (Fig. 1). It has recently been suggested that the glutamate-induced increase in oxygen consumption in neonatal rat astrocytes [10] is due to the activation of Na,K-ATPase caused by Na^+ transport *via* the high-affinity glutamate transporter [10]. Alternatively, glutamate transporter activity can be modulated in a manner independent of Na,K-ATPase by signal-transduction pathways/molecules (e.g., protein kinases, proteases, $[Ca^{2+}]_i$, etc.) affected by ischemia. The possibility of enhanced *de novo* synthe-

Table 1. *Effects of Simulated in vitro Ischemia and Reoxygenation on Na,K-ATPase Activity, ^{3}H-Glutamate Uptake and Cell Viability in Rat Cortical Astrocyte Cultures*

		Na,K-ATPase (cpm/mg protein/min)	^{3}H-Glutamate (cpm/mg protein/min)	CA-AM (fluorescence units)
Control		1562 ± 114	4068 ± 464	3754 ± 279
Ischemia	1 hr	3999 ± 353[a]	5449 + 380[a]	4800 + 386
	2 hrs	3877 ± 277[a]	6071 ± 460[a]	3786 ± 147
	4 hrs	2488 ± 214[a]	6513 ± 553[a]	3282 ± 255
	+ Reox., 20 hrs	695 ± 53[a–c]	4635 ± 236[b, c]	4677 ± 230
	24 hrs	494 ± 45[a]	1323 ± 126[a]	1542 ± 147[a]
	+ 5 mM glu at 4 hrs	2347 ± 120[a, c]	6055 ± 813[a, c]	2762 ± 297[a, h]
	48 hrs	not detected	520 ± 43[a]	965 ± 63[a]
	+ 5 mM glu at 24 hrs	378 ± 12[a, c]	1072 ± 47[a, c]	1943 ± 155[a, b]

Cells were exposed to the simulated *in vitro* 'ischemia' and then subjected to either 20 hours of reoxygenation or to the addition of 5 mM glucose (glu) under hypoxia. Na,K-ATPase activity and ^{3}H-glutamate uptake were then measured for 15 min as described in Material and Methods. Cell viability was quantified at the indicated times by the exclusion of the vital dye, CA-AM, as described in Materials and Methods. The results are expressed as mean ± S.E.M. of six repcate wells. The data are representative of the results of 3 separate experiments.
[a] Indicates significant difference (P < 0.01, ANOVA) from the corresponding control.
[b] Indicates significant difference (P < 0.01, ANOVA) from the 4 hour ischemia alone.
[c] Indicates significant difference (P < 0.01, ANOVA) from 24 hours 'ischemia' alone.

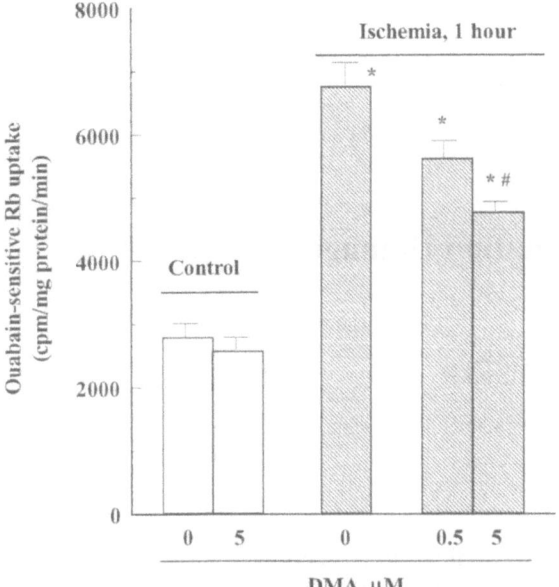

Fig. 1. The effect of the Na⁺-H⁺ exchanger inhibitor, DMA, on the ischemia-induced increase in sodium-pump activity. The indicated concentrations of DMA were added to control cultures or to cultures cells subjected to 1 hour of ischemia, and sodium pump activity was measured as ouabain-sensitive uptake of ^{86}Rb, as described in Materials and Methods. Each value represents the mean ± S.E.M. of six replicate dishes in one of two experiments yielding similar results. Asterisks indicate significant differences ($p < 0.01$; ANOVA) compared to the corresponding control; # indicates significant difference as compared to ischemia alone

sis and increased expression of the enzyme/transporter molecules cannot be excluded since protein synthesis in astrocytes is not largely affected by ischemia [5].

The importance of maintaining glycolysis under ischemia-like conditions for astrocyte survival was further substantiated by the observation that adding glucose to ischemic cultures protected the cells from death and prevented the loss of essential functions, even in the absence of oxygen (Table 1). Thus, when glucose levels were restored after 4 hours of ischemia, both Na,K-ATPase and glutamate transporter activities remained elevated over the subsequent 20 hours (Table 1) and cell viability was preserved at levels observed after 4 hours of ischemia (Table 1).

In contrast to the above, cells exposed to 4 hours of ischemia followed by 20 hours of reoxygenation exhibited a profound 55% decrease in Na,K-ATPase activity relative to control cultures, whereas glutamate uptake was maintained at control values (Table 1). This selective inhibition of sodium pump activity may be due to free radicals and/or arachidonic acid, both shown to be released during ischemia/reoxygenation [6] and to cause a protracted inhibition of the Na,K-ATPase in tissues and cells [6, 12, 13]. Inhibition of Na,K-ATPase activity by ouabain or ischemia has been shown to cause cell swelling *in vitro* and brain edema *in vivo* (reviewed in [6]).

References

1. Aronson PS (1985) Kinetic properties of the plasma membrane Na⁺-H⁺ exchanger. Ann Rev Physiol 47: 545–560
2. Danbolt N (1994) The high affinity uptake system for excitatory amino acids in the brain. Prog Neurobiol 44: 377–396
3. Dong J, Delamere NA, and Coca-Prados M (1994) Inhibition of Na⁺-K⁺-ATPase activates Na⁺-K⁺-2Cl⁻ cotransporter activity in cultured ciliary epithelium. Am J Physiol 266: C198–C205
4. Kanner B (1993) Glutamate transporters from brain: A novel neurotransmitter transporter familly. FEBS Lett 325: 95–99
5. Landis DMD (1994) The early reactions of non-neuronal cells to brain injury. Ann Rev Neurosci 17: 133–151
6. Lees GJ (1991) Inhibition of sodium-potassium-ATPase: a potentially ubiquitous mechanism contributing to central nervous system neuropathology. Brain Res Rev 16: 283–300
7. Longuemare MC, Swanson, RA (1995) Excitatory amino acid release from astrocytes during energy failure by reversal of sodium-dependent uptake. J Neurosci Res 40: 379–386
8. Lowry OH, Rosebrough NU, Farr AL, Randall RJ (1951) Protein measurement with the folin phenol reagent. J Biol Chem 193: 265–275
9. McCarthy KD, de Vellis J (1980) Preparation of separate astroglial and oligodendroglial cell cultures from rat cerebral tissue. J Cell Biol 85: 890–902
10. Pellerin L, Magistretti PJ (1994) Glutamate uptake into astrocytes stimulates aerobic glycolysis: a mechanism coupling neuronal activity to glucose utilization. Proc Natl Acad Sci USA 91: 10625–10629
11. Rothman SM, Olney JW (1986) Glutamate and the pathophysiology of hypoxic-ischemic brain damage. Ann Neurol 19: 105–111
12. Stanimirovic DB, Wong J, Ball R, Durkin JP (1995) Free radical-induced endothelial membrane dysfunction at the site of blood brain barrier: relationship between lipid peroxidation, Na,K-ATPase activity and ^{51}Cr release. Neurochem Res 20: 1417–1427
13. Volterra A, Trotti D, Tromba C, Floridi S, Racagni G (1994) Glutamate uptake inhibition by oxygen free radicals in rat cortical astrocytes. J Neurosci 14: 2924–2932

Correspondence: Dr. Danica Stanimirovic, Cellular Neurobiology Group, Institute for Biological Sciences, National Research Council of Canada, Montreal Road Campus, Bldg. M-54, Ottawa, ONT, Canada, K1A 0R6, Canada.

Acta Neurochir (1997) [Suppl] 70: 4–7

The Role of Calcium Ion in Anoxia/Reoxygenation Damage of Cultured Brain Capillary Endothelial Cells

K. Ikeda[1], T. Nagashima[1], S. Wu[1], M. Yamaguchi[2], and N. Tamaki[1]

[1] Department of Neurosurgery and [2] Faculty of Health Science, Kobe University School of Medicine, Kobe, Japan

Summary

Capillary endothelial cells are critical targets in both ischemia and reperfusion of the brain. Arachidonic acids and oxygen free radicals have been shown to cause disruption of blood-brain barrier (BBB) by destruction of capillary endothelial cell membrane. However, the exact mechanism of BBB breakdown by cerebral ischemia/reperfusion remains undetermined.

The aim of the present study is to clarify the mechanism of intracellular calcium ion ($[Ca^{2+}]_i$) change in brain capillary endothelial cells under anoxia/reoxygenation. Brains capillary endothelial cells were isolated from ten male Sprague-Dawley rats by a two step enzymatic process. $[Ca^{2+}]_i$ was measured by means of a confocal laser scanning microscope using Indo 1-A/M as a calcium indicator. The endothelial cells were subjected to anoxia and reoxygenization under different conditions.

$[Ca^{2+}]_i$ increased gradually during anoxia and slightly decreased after reoxygenation.

Indomethacin and SOD suppressed the elevation of $[Ca^{2+}]_i$ during anoxia. N^G-nitro-L-arginine methyl ester and catalase moderately supressed the elevation, however nifedipine did not supress it at all. In this model, rapid $[Ca^{2+}]_i$ change was not observed during the reoxygenation phase.

The results indicate that the anoxia induced elevation of $[Ca^{2+}]_i$ in the brain capillary endothelial cells depends on superoxide and peroxynitrite generation.

Keywords: Blood-brain barrier; endothelium; calcium ion; laser scanning confocal microscopy.

Introduction

The specialized functions of the cerebral microvascular endothelial cell are the formation of the blood-brain barrier (BBB) which isolate the brain from toxic substances in the plasma, the facilitation of transport of essential nutrients, and ion homeostasis. The endothelial cells are critical targets in both ischemia and reperfusion of the brain. Reperfusion of the ischemic brain produces a biphasic change with early and transient increase of permeability followed by a delayed, persistent disruption of BBB. Arachidonic acids and oxy-gen free radicals have been shown to cause disruption of BBB by destruction of capillary endothelial cell membrane. However, the exact mechanism of BBB breakdown by cerebral ischemia/reperfusion remain undetermined.

An increase of $[Ca^{2+}]_i$ resulting from energy deficiency has been reported by several authors as a cause of cell damage during ischemia/reperfusion. The increased $[Ca^{2+}]_i$ in capillary endothelial cells produces a variety of vasoregulatory substances including prostaglandins, leukotriencs, nitic oxide, and endothelin. The mechanism of increase of $[Ca^{2+}]_i$ caused by anoxia has been revealed to be different in various tissues such as the cardiac myocyte, the white matter and the gray matter. Little is known about the mechanism of regulation of $[Ca^{2+}]_i$ in brain capillary endothelial cells at ischemia. In this study we investigated the mechanism of the increase of $[Ca^{2+}]_i$ under anoxia and reoxygenation conditions.

Materials and Methods

1. Preparation of Endothelial Cells

Brains capillary endothelial cells were isolated from ten male, Sprague-Dawley rats (300–350 g) by two step enzymatic treatment. In brief, brain tissues were incubated at 37°C in 20 ml of a medium containing 0.5% dispase for 3 hours. It was then suspended in 80 ml of a medium containing 13% dextran. The microvessels were separated from the brain tissue by centrifugation at 5,800 g for 10 minutes and treated with 1 mg/ml collagenase/dispase for 6 hours. The pellet of cells was layered over 50% Percoll gradients and centrifuged at 26,000 g for 50 minutes. The second band containing mainly endothelial cells was removed and seeded onto a collagen-coated dish. The cells were cultured in Dulbecco's medium containing 10% fetal bovine serum on collagen coated plastic dishes and maintained at 37°C in a humidified incubator with an atmosphere of 95% air and 5% CO_2. Two weeks after seeding, a plaque of homogeneous cells showed a characteristic cobblestone pattern. Identification as capillary endothelium was accomplished by the presence of Factor VIII-related antigen. Cultures from second to fifth passages were used in this study.

2. Calcium Assay

The cultured cells on the glass bottom dishes coated with collagen were washed with PB S twice and loaded in PBS(+) containing 2 μM Indo-1-AM for 30 min at room temperature. Indo-1-AM was removed and 0.2 ml of buffers were add to make thin-film-like buffer. $[Ca^{2+}]_i$ was measured by means of a confocal laser scanning microscope (Meridian ACAS 570).

3. Anoxia-Reoxygenation

A small anoxic chamber was constructed on the microscope stage for real time measurement of $[Ca^{2+}]_i$. The endothelial cells were subjected to 90 min anoxia with 95% N_2 / 5% CO_2 and reoxygenized with room air. The change of $[Ca^{2+}]_i$ during anoxia and reoxygenation was monitored in Ca^{2+} free-PBS, PBS(+), PBS(+) with superoxide dismutase (SOD, 1000, 100 U/ml), indomethacin (100 μM), catalase (1000 U/ml), N^G-nitro-L-arginine methyl ester (L-NAME, 1 mM) or nifedipine (10 μM). The change in $[Ca^{2+}]_i$ was expressed as the % of the basal level of $[Ca^{2+}]_i$.

Results

(1) After the initiation of anoxia, $[Ca^{2+}]_i$ increased gradually up to 30% of the basal level. During reoxygenation, $[Ca^{2+}]_i$ kept the same level or decreased slightly (Figs. 1a, 2a). The peak value was about one fourth of the $[Ca^{2+}]_i$ elevation induced by a receptor agonist thrombin.

(2) When the extracellular fluid was changed to PBS(–), the elevation of $[Ca^{2+}]_i$ was partially suppressed. The result indicated that the source of elevated $[Ca^{2+}]_i$ was both extracellular and intracellular.

(3) SOD (1000 U/ml) and indomethacin (100 μM) inhibited the increase of $[Ca^{2+}]_i$. Catalase (1000 U/ml) and L-NAME (1 mM) suppressed it mildly. Nifedipine did not inhibit the elevation of $[Ca^{2+}]_i$ (Figs. 1b, 2b).

Discussion

Injury to the endothelium is a major consequence of ischemia/reperfusion injury, causing edema formation due to BBB disruption. Several factors such as toxic agents, loss of ATP activity and ATP-resupply, oxygen lack, superoxide, peroxynitrite, pH-change, calcium ion, arachidonic acid, cAMP or other messengers affect the injury of endothelial cells in anoxia and reoxygenation. However, the mechanism of BBB disruption in ischemia is not well understood. Sustained increases in $[Ca^{2+}]_i$ can lead to the activation of enzymes such as phospholipase, proteases, and endonucleases and can result in mitochondrial dysfunction, cytoskeltal dysfunction, and DNA degeneration [11]. The mechanism

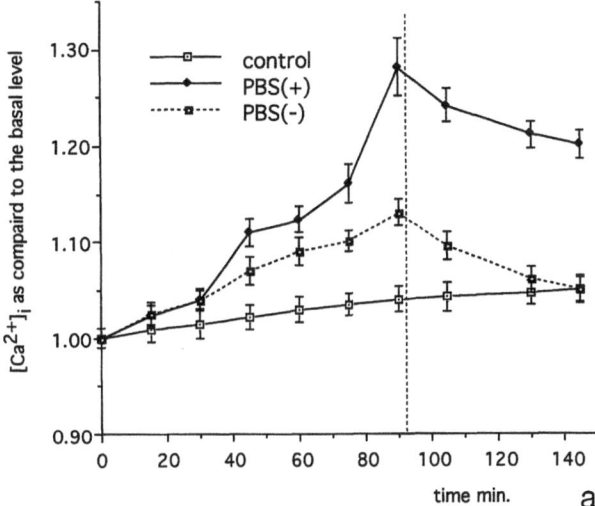

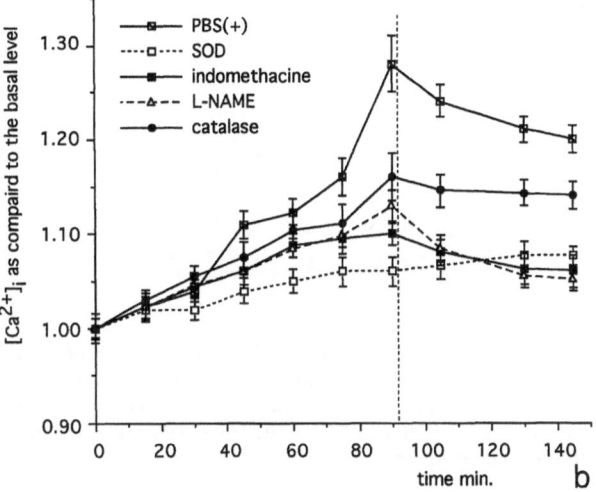

Fig. 1. (a) $[Ca^{2+}]_i$ is expressed as compared to the basal level. Endothelial cells were subjected to 90 min anoxia and then reoxygenized in PBS(–) and PBS(+). Control cells did not subjected to anoxia. (b) Effects of drugs on time course of $[Ca^{2+}]_i$ of endothelial cells subjected to 90 min anoxia and then reoxygenized

of cell injury caused by Ca^{2+} increase may involve calcium-activated phospholipases. Ca^{2+} increase in endothelium is known to increase superoxide production.

The increase of $[Ca^{2+}]_i$ in brain capillary endothelial cells can occurs by several mechanisms [1]; Ca^{2+} influxes from extra cellular space via a receptor mediated channel, a calcium leak channel, a stretch-activated channel [12] or Na^+/Ca^{2+} exchanger. In studies of CNS white matter and CNS axons, Na^+/Ca^{2+} exchanger have an important role in $[Ca^{2+}]_i$ increase in anoxic injury [13, 14].

Loss in Ca^{2+} ATPase activity causes dysfunction of the efflux-mechanism, and Ca^{2+} release from intracellular store is activated by the generation of IP_3. Many

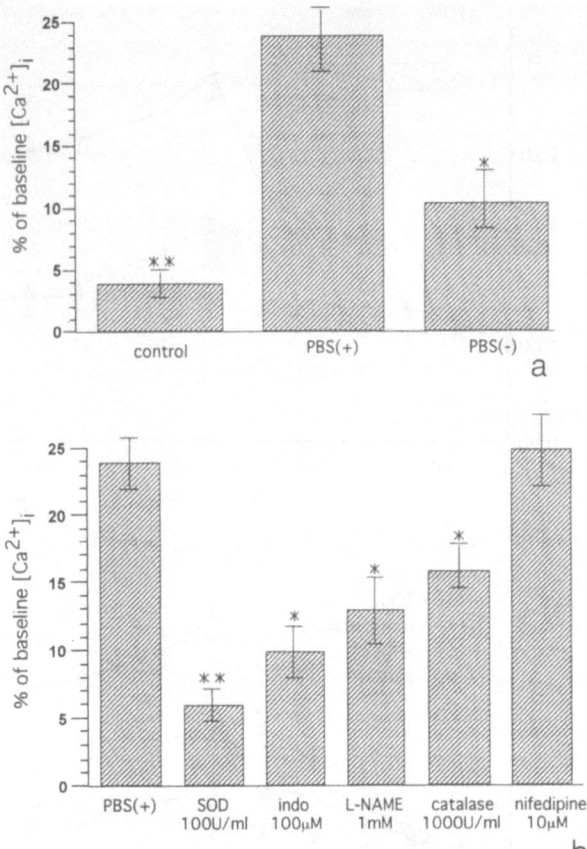

Fig. 2 (a, b). Increase (%) in [Ca²⁺]ᵢ after anoxia was monitored by fluorescence ratio with Indo-1. Endothelial cells were subjected to 90 min anoxia in the presence or absence of drugs. The values were compared at 90 min anoxia. * $P < 0.01$, ** $P < 0.05$, difference from PBS(+). *Indo* Indomethacine

oxide, and toxic substances [7] and release arachidonic acid (AA) from membranes by phospholipase. AA is converted to prostaglandin by cyclooxygenase [8]. AA and oxygen free radicals cause BBB breakdown through destruction of endothelial cells. Superoxide is produced in a conversion process of PG-G2 to PG-H2 and the other free radicals are generated in a metabolism of AA. Superoxide is also produced by xanthine oxidase pathway [9]. Superoxide induced cell injury by peroxidation of DNA and cell membrane [10]. In our study, SOD inhibited an increase of [Ca²⁺]ᵢ in anoxia but catalase showed little suppression. Indomethacin reduced the increase of [Ca²⁺]ᵢ but this effect was milder than that of SOD. Thus generation of superoxide in metabolism of AA may have a role in [Ca²⁺]ᵢ increase.

Nitric oxide(NO·) is one of the endothelium-derived relaxing factors (EDRF), and is produced in endothelial cells [6]. Although nitric oxide improves blood flow during anoxia by an promoting vascular dilatation, peroxynitrite (ONOO⁻) which is a product of the reaction between superoxide and NO· is a highly toxic free radical [3]. Recently it has been reported that a relatively small increase in the rate of superoxide and NO· production may great increase ONOO⁻ formation to potentially cytotoxic levels [3].

In our study, L-NAME reduced the increase of [Ca²⁺]ᵢ in anoxia. This result indicates that peroxynitrite may have a role in endothelial injury under anoxic conditions.

investigators believe that increases of [Ca²⁺]ᵢ in an energy-depleted state is due to influx. In our study the increase of [Ca²⁺]ᵢ in anoxia observed in PBS(+) was suppressed in some degrees in PBS(−). The results indicate that an increase of [Ca²⁺]ᵢ by anoxic stress is caused not only by influx of Ca²⁺ but also by activation of Ca²⁺ release from intracellular calcium stocks or by dysfunction of ATP-dependent Ca²⁺ pump.

Reperfusion injuries of various endothelial cells in relation to [Ca²⁺]ᵢ have been examined by many investigators. There is a report of renal epithelial cells in which a dramatic increase in [Ca²⁺]ᵢ was induced after reoxygenation [5] on the other hand, [Ca²⁺]ᵢ recovery after reoxygenation was reported in a study of umbilical endothelial cells [2]. In our study [Ca²⁺]ᵢ levels were elevated or were decreasing after 90 min anoxia. Tissue difference or severity of the anoxic condition may contribute to these differences.

Brain endothelial cells produce vasoregulatory substances such as endothelin, prostaglandins and nitric

References

1. Adams DJ, Barakeh J, Laskey R, Breemen CV (1989) Ion channels and regulation of intracellular calcium in vascular endothelial cells. FASEB J 3: 2389–2400
2. Arnould T, Michiels C, Alexandre I, Remacle J (1992) Effect of hypoxia upon intracellular calcium concentration of human endothelial cells. J Cell Physiol 152: 215–221
3. Beckman JS, Beckman TW, Chen J, Marshall PA, Freeman BA (1990) Apparent hydroxyl radical production by peroxynitrite: Implications for endothelial injury from nitric oxide and superoxide. Proc Nat Acad Sci 87: 1620–1624
4. Espinoza MI, Parer JT (1991) Mechanisms of asphyxial brain damage, and possible pharmacologic interventions, in the fetus. Am J Obstet Gynecol 164: 1582–1591
5. Greene EL, Paller MS (1994) Calcium and free radicals in hypoxia/reoxygenation injury of renal epithelial cells. Am J Physiol 266: F13–F20
6. Hampl V, Cornfield DN, Cowan NJ, Archer SL (1995) Hypoxia potentiales nitric oxide synthesis and transiently increases cytosolic calcium levels in pulmonary artery endothelial cells. Eur Respir J 8: 515–522
7. Hsu CY, Liu TH, Xu J, Hogan EL, Chao J, Sun G, Tai HH, Beckman JS, Freeman BA (1989) Arachidonic acid and its metabolites in cerebral ischemia. Ann NY Acad Sci 559: 282–295

8. Ikeda M, Busto R, Yoshida S, Santiso M, Martinrz E, Ginsberg MD (1988) Cerebral phosphoinositide, triacylglycerol and energy metabolism during severe hypoxia and recovery. Brain Res 459: 344–350

9. Kvietys PR, Inauen W, Bacon BR, Grisham MB (1989) Xanthine oxidase-induced injury to endothelium: role of intracellular iron and hydroxyl radical. Am J Physiol 257: H1640–H1646

10. McGowan JE, McGowan JC, Mishra OP, Papadopoulos DM (1994) Effect of cyclooxygenase inhibition on brain cell membrane lipid peroxidation during hypoxia in newborn piglets. Biol Neonate 66: 367–375

11. Orrenius S, Ankarcrona M, Nicotera P (1996) Mechanisms of calcium-related cell death. Adv Neurol 71: 137–151

12. Popp R, Hoyer J, Meyer J, Galla HJ, Gogelein H (1992) Stretch-activated non-selective cation channels in the antiluminal membrane of porcine cerebral capillaries. J Physiol 454: 435–449

13. Stys PK, Waxman SG, Ransom BR (1992) Ionic mechanism of anoxic injury in mammalian CNS white matter: role of Na^+ channels and Na^+-Ca^{2+} exchanger. J Neurosci 12: 430–439

14. Waxman SG, Black JA, Ransom BR, Stys PK (1994) Anoxic injury of rat optic nerve: ultrastuctual evidence for coupling between Na^+ influx and Ca^{2+}-mediated injury in myelinated CNS axons. Brain Res 644: 197–204

Correspondence: Tatsuya Nagashima, M.D., Department of Neurosurgery, Kobe University School of Medicine, Kobe, Japan.

Acta Neurochir (1997) [Suppl] 70: 8–11
© Springer-Verlag 1997

Hypoxia Modulates Free Radical Formation in Brain Microvascular Endothelium

A. Strasser, D. Stanimirovic, N. Kawai, R. M. McCarron, and **M. Spatz**

Stroke Banch NINDS, National Institutes of Health, Bethesda, MD, U.S.A.

Summary

Although free radical species (ROS; i.e., $\cdot O_2^-$, $\cdot OH$, H_2O_2) among other mediators, may be involved in altering the blood-brain barrier (BBB), little is known about the endogenous ability of cerebromicrovascular endothelium to generate ROS. This study examines the capacity of rat endothelial cells (RBEC) to produce ROS in normoxia and hypoxia/reoxygenation. Cultured RBEC were exposed to an oxygen-depleted atmosphere (containing 95% N2 and 5% CO_2) for 4 hr at 37°C and air (10 min) at room temperature to simulate "ischemia/reperfusion". Nitroblue tetrazolium (NBT) reduction [formation of nitroblue formazan (NBF)] served as a marker for the production of ROS. The release of lactate dehydrogenase (LDH) and [³H]arachidonic acid (AA) was used to assess cellular integrity. RBEC exposed to hypoxia/reoxygenation produced up to 59% greater NBF formation than controls without affecting the LDH or AA release. The production of ROS was calcium-dependent and not affected by AA or its metabolites. The findings indicate that the RBEC can produce superoxide dismutase (SOD)-inhibitable ROS which are augmented by hypoxia/reoxygenation. It is suggested that *in vivo* cerebromicrovascular endothelium may contribute to the formation of ROS and play a role in ischemic brain edema.

Keywords: Cerebral hypoxia; free radical formation; microvascular endothelium; blood-brain barrier.

Introduction

Release or overproduction of various substances (i.e., polyunsaturated fatty acids, neurotransmitters, peptides and nitric oxide) originating from dysfunctional cellular membranes and/or cytosolic compartments have been implicated in altering blood-brain barrier (BBB) permeability and in the formation of brain edema in ischemia and/or trauma [2–6, 9, 11]. Some of these compounds may be derived from either the cellular components of the brain or blood. In the last decade, a number of studies demonstrated that exogenous arachidonic acid (AA) and enzymatically generated reactive species ROS; ($\cdot O_2^-$, $\cdot OH$, H_2O_2) among other mediators can alter BBB permeability, induce tissue injury and edema in the brain [3, 4, 6]. These agents were also shown to change the cellular integrity of cultured endothelium from either cerebromicrovessels or peripheral vasculature [8, 13–15]. However, relatively little information is available regarding the endogenous capability of cerebromicrovascular endothelium to generate ROS in response to hypoxia/reoxygenation which could potentially contribute to the formation of brain edema in ischemia and/or trauma. This report demonstrates that mild hypoxia/reoxygenation induces an augmented production of ROS in RBEC without affecting the cellular integrity.

Materials and Methods

Endothelial cell cultures: Preparation, growth, and propagation of brain capillary and microvascular cells from adult rats (RBEC) were similar to that described by Spatz *et al.* [l2] The purity of RBEC was > 95% as reported previously. To simulate "ischemia/reperfusion" in an *in vitro* model, the RBEC grown to confluency in Petri dishes (35 mm) were exposed to oxygen-depleted atmosphere (containing 95% N_2 and 5% CO_2) for 4 hr at 37°C and air (10 min) at room temperature. Nitroblue tetrazolium (NBT) reduction [formation of nitroblue formazan (NBF) served as a marker for the production of oxygen-derived ROS [1]. The incubation medium contained NBT (1 mg/ml), gelatin (0.1 mg/ml) in phosphate-buffered saline (PBS) supplemented by the tested substances indicated below. Cell membrane integrity was assessed by measuring the release of lactate dehydrogenase (LDH) activity using a commercially available assay kit (Sigma Co., St. Louis, MO) and [³H] arachidonic acid (AA) as well as cellular viability by trypan blue exclusion in similarly prepared cultures treated the same way but without NBT. The release of LDH and AA was calculated and expressed as the percent of total release. The ATP content was determined in separate groups of RBEC exposed to hypoxia/reoxygenation [7]. The cellular protein content was assayed by the Bio-Rad Detergent Compatible protein assay kit (Bio Rad Laboratories, CA).

Table 1. *The Effects of SOD on Nitro-Blue Tetrazolium Reduction in Cultured Rat Cerebromicrovascular Endothelial Cells*

Treatment	NBF (nmol/mg protein)		
	Total	+ 200 U SOD	SOD-inhibitable
Normoxia	57.42 ± 1.21	26.87 ± 0.98	30.55 ± 1.56
Hypoxia/reoxygenation	91.05 ± 4.32[a]	36.95 ± 1.34[a]	54.10 ± 4.52[a]

Data represent NBF (nitro-blue formazan) formation and are expressed as means ± SE of three replicate cultures and are representative of the results obtained from 3–5 separate experiments.
[a] Indicates significant differences (ANOVA, $p < 0.01$) from control value.

Statistics: Each type of experiment was performed in triplicate with at least three independent determinations using separate RBEC cultures. Results were statistically analyzed using the one-way analysis of variance (ANOVA) followed by Fisher's protected least-squares difference test (F-PLSD).

Results

RBEC exposed to hypoxia/reoxygenation contained significantly less ATP than those maintained under normoxia (12.8 ± 0.4 nmol/mg protein and 15.5 ± 0.7 nmol/mg protein, respectively; $p < 0.01$). Both conditions led to variably reduced levels of NBT. However, hypoxia/reoxygenation always induced greater production of NBF (38–59%) than normoxia in these cells

Table 2. *The Effects of Various Inhibitors on Nitro-Blue Tetrazolium Reduction in Cultured Rat Cerebromicrovascular Endothelial Cells*

Treatment	NBF (% of control)
Normoxia	
Control	100 0 ± 3 8
+ 10 μM dexamethasone	107 9 ± 6 3
+ 100 μM ASA	84.6 ± 8.8
+ 200 U SOD	26.6 ± 5.3[a]
Hypoxia/reoxygenation	
Control	100.0 ± 5.4
+ 10 μM dexamethasone	100.1 ± 7.1
+ 100 μM ASA	114.9 ± 3.6[b]
+ 200 U SOD	17.9 ± 7.0 [b]

Data represent NBF (nitro-blue formazan) formation and are expressed as a percent of response observed in cultures incubated under either normoxic or hypoxic conditions without additions. Values for control normoxic and hypoxic cultures were 55.6 ± 2.1 and 76.6 ± 4.1 nmol/mg protein respectively. Results were calculated from means ± SE of three replicate cultures and are representative of the results obtained from 3–5 separate experiments.
[a] Indicates significant differences (ANOVA, $p < 0.01$) from control normoxic values.
[b] Indicates significant differences (ANOVA, $p < 0.01$) from control hypoxic values.

without affecting LDH release [1.21 ± 0.05% vs. 0.98 ± 0.2% (control) or AA [1.23 ± 0.36 vs. 1.71 ± 0.46% (control)]. Table 1 demonstrates that about 59% of the total NBF formation was inhibitable in the presence of superoxide dismutase [(SOD-inhibitable) i.e., $\cdot O_2^-$] in hypoxia/reoxygenation as compared to 53% in controls. However, overall 70% of NBF stimulated by hypoxia/reoxygenation was inhibited by SOD. RBEC incubated in Ca^{2+}-free medium or in the presence of verapamil (Ca^{2+} channel blocker) exhibited significantly less NBF formation in hypoxia/reoxygenation (42% and 18% of control, respectively) than in normoxia (70% and 43% of control, respectively) (Fig. 1). Neither dexamethasone (inhibitor of phospholipase A_2 and cyclooxygenase II nor acetylsalicylic acid (inhibitor of cyclooxygenase I) had any effect on NBF formation (Table 2).

Discussion

The findings indicate that RBEC have the capacity to produce SOD-inhibitable ROS which are augmented by mild hypoxia-reoxygenation as indicated by reduced ATP. These results also strongly suggest that the increased ROS formation induced by ischemia/reoxygenation did not obviously affect cellular membrane integrity because neither the release of LDH and AA nor the uptake of trypan blue was greater than that observed in normoxia. In addition, the data indicate that the production of ROS is Ca^{2+}-dependent since their formation was reduced in RBEC exposed to Ca^{2+}-free medium or incubated in the presence of verapamil.

It is generally known that brain and peripheral small and large vessels as well as the cultured endothelium-derived vessels are rich in antioxidant enzymes (i.e., xanthine dehydrogenase, SOD, glutathione peroxidase, catalase) [14]. Thus, the observed augmented formation of NBF in RBEC induced by hypoxia/reoxygenation strongly suggest an existing imbalance between the oxidative and antioxidative processes.

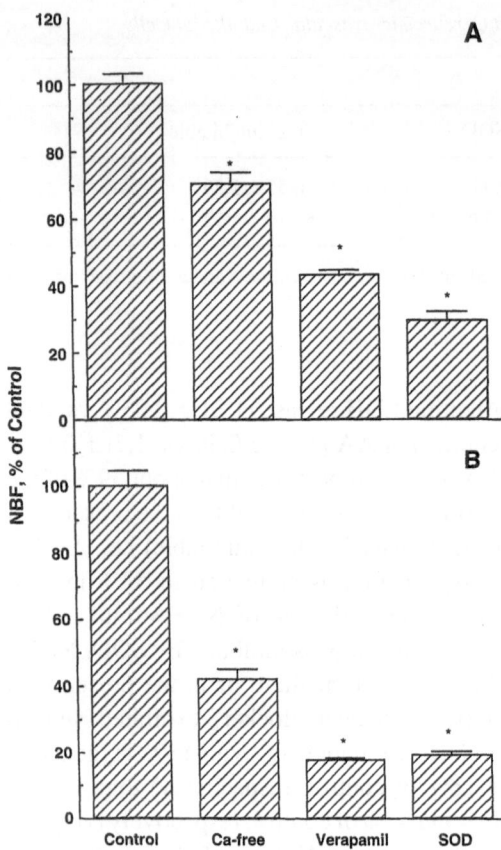

Fig. 1. Data represent NBF (nitro-blue formazan) formation and are expressed as a percent of response observed in control cultures incubated without additions under conditions of either normoxia (A) or hypoxia/reoxygenation (B). Values for control normoxic and hypoxic cultures were 94.6 ± 3.1 and 129.0 ± 1.8 nmol/mg protein, respectively. Results were calculated from means $\pm$ SE of three replicate cultures and are representative of the results obtained from 3–5 separate experiments. * Indicates significant differences (ANOVA, $p < 0.01$) from control values

endothelium from injury. Thus, the ability of SOD to reduce the production of ROS in normoxic and hypoxic RBEC implicate the superoxide anion radical $\cdot O_2^-$ formation during this event.

Based on the results of this study, it appears that mild hypoxia/reoxygenation induces an overproduction of ROS which are not deleterious to the RBEC. However, one should keep in mind that the formed $\cdot O_2^-$ may be toxic alone, or as suggested by Beckman *et al.* [2], may react with NO to form a peroxynitrite anion ($ONOO^-$), which by decomposition, generates a more toxic oxidant with reactivity similar to $\cdot OH$. All the above-mentioned molecules diffuse easily and therefore, may potentially not only adversely affect the function of the endothelium itself but adjacent cells as well.

In conclusion, these studies demonstrate that the ability of cultured RBEC to produce ROS (i.e., $\cdot O_2^-$) is increased after mild hypoxiafreoxygenation. It is suggested that *in vivo* the cerebromicrovascular endothelium may contribute to formation of ROS and play a role in ischemic reperfusion (reoxygenation) injury which includes brain edema.

Acknowledgement

The authors wish to thank Ms. Joliet Bembry and Mrs. Nancy Merkel for their excellent technical support and Ms. Devera Schoenberg, M.S. for her expert editorial assistance in the preparation of this manuscript.

References

1. Baehner RL, Boxer LA, Davis J (1976) The biochemical basis of nitroblue tetrazolium reduction in normal human and chronic granulomatous disease polymorphonuclear leukocytes. Blood 48: 309–313
2. Beckman JS, Beckman TW, Chen J, Marshall PA, Freeman BA (1990) Apparent hydroxyl radical production by peroxynitrite: Implications for endothelial injury from nitric oxide and superoxide. Proc Natl Acad Sci USA 87: 1620–1624
3. Chan PH (1989) The role of oxygen radicals in brain injury and edema, Chapter 30. In: Chow CK (ed) Cellular antioxidant defense mechanisms, Vol III. CRC, Boca Raton, Florida, pp 89–109
4. Chan PH, Schmidley JW, Fishman RA, Longar SM (1984) Brain injury, edema, and vascular permeability changes induced by oxygen-derived free radicals. Neurology 34: 315–320
5. Halliwell B (1992) Reactive oxygen species and the central nervous system. J Neurochem 59: 1609–1623
6. Halliwell B (1993) The role of oxygen radicals in human disease, with particular reference to the vascular system. Haemostasis 23 [Suppl 1]: 118–126
7. Lowry OH, Passonneau JV (1972) A flexible system of enzymatic analysis. Academic Press, New York
8. McCarron RM, Uematsu S, Merkel N, Long D, Bembry J, Spatz M (1990) The role of arachidonic acid and oxygen radicals on cerebromicrovascular endothelial permeability. Acta Neurochir (Wien) [Suppl] 51: 61–64

The results also indicate that neither AA nor its metabolites are responsible for the observed overproduction of ROS in hypoxia/reoxygenation since the amount of released AA was similar to that in normoxia. In addition, none of the ROS formed during normoxia or hypoxia/reoxygenation in RBEC were susceptible to dexamethasone or acetylsalicylic acid inhibition. The most likely source for the observed augmented formation of NBF in hypoxia/reperfusion is NO which is produced by endothelium [10]. This substance is known to be induced by hypoxia-reoxygenation. NO has been recognized as the major component of endothelium-derived relaxing factor (EDRF) which participates in controlling vascular tone. The half-life of EDRF and NO is very short (4–50 sec) and can be increased by SOD through scavenging of $\cdot O_2^-$ derived from NO. It has been suggested that SOD protects

9. Menger MD, Lehr H-A, Messmer K (1991) Role of oxygen radicals in the microcirculatory manifestations of postischemic injury. Klin Wochenschr 69: 1050–1055

10. Moncada S, Palmer RM, Higgs EA (1991) Nitric oxide: physiology, pathophysiology, and pharmacology. Pharmacol Rev 43: 109–142

11. Mrsulja BB, Djuric BM, Crejic V, Mrsulja BJ, Abe K, Spatz M, Klatzo I (1980) Biochemistry of experimental ischemic edema. Adv Neurol 28: 217–230

12. Spatz M, Bembry J, Dodson RF, Hervonen H, Murray, MR (1980) Endothelial cell culture derived from isolated cerebral microvessels. Brain Res 191: 577–582

13. Stanimirovic DB, Bertrand N, McCarron R, Uematsu S, Spatz M (1994) Arachidonic acid release and permeability changes induced by endothelins in human cerebromicrovascular endothelium. Acta Neurochir (Wien) [Suppl] 60: 71–75

14. Vercellotti GM, Dolson M, Schorer AE, Moldow CR (1988) Endothelial cell heterogeneity: antioxidant profiles determine vulnerability to oxidant injury. Proc Soc Exp Biol Med 187: 181–189

15. Villacara A, Spatz M, Dodson RF, Corn C, Bembry J (1989) Effect of arachidonic acid on cultured cerebromicrovascular endothelium: permeability, lipid peroxidation and membrane fluidity. Acta Neuropathol (Berl) 78: 310–316

Correspondence: Maria Spatz, M.D., Stroke Branch, NINDS, NIH, 36 Convent DR, MSC 4128, Bethesda, MD 20892-8112, U.S.A.

Acta Neurochir (1997) [Suppl] 70: 12–16
© Springer-Verlag 1997

Increase in Surface Expression of ICAM-1, VCAM-1 and E-Selectin in Human Cerebromicrovascular Endothelial Cells Subjected to Ischemia-Like Insults

D. B. Stanimirovic, J. Wong, A. Shapiro, and **J. P. Durkin**

Institue for Biological Sciences, National Research Council of Canada, Ottawa, Canada

Summary

Secondary ischemic brain injury has been shown to develop as a consequence of inflammation and vasogenic brain edema. In this study we show that inflammatory cytokines and simulated *in vitro* ischemia stimulate the surface expression of intercellular adhesion molecule-1 (ICAM-1), vascular cell adhesion molecule-1 (VCAM-1) and endothelial-leukocyte adhesion molecule-1 (E-selectin) in human cerebromicrovascular endothelial cells (HCEC) in culture. The levels of all three adhesion molecules were dramatically (3 to 10-fold) up-regulated by 4–24 hour exposure to the inflammatory cytokines, IL-1β (10–200 u/ml) or TNFα (50–200 u/ml), and by a 4 hour exposure to "simulated" *in vitro* ischemia, as determined by immunocytochemistry and ELISA. Following 24 hours of subsequent reperfusion, the expression of ICAM-1 and VCAM-1 was maintained at ischemia-induced levels, whereas E-selectin was no longer detectable. Both the cytokine- and ischemia-induced up-regulation of adhesion molecules were completely abolished by the transcriptional inhibitor, actinomycin D (10 μg/ml), and inhibited by the cycloxygenase (COX) inhibitor, indomethacin (300 μM). These findings implicate HCEC in the processes of leukocyte adhesion and recruitment in the brain durin stroke *in vivo*.

Keywords: Cerebral ischemia; intercellular adhesion molecules; cytokines; *in vitro* model.

Introduction

Brain ischemia is accompanied by an acute inflammatory response characterized by leukocyte infiltration and development of brain edema [2, 8]. Neutrophils are usually the first exogenous cells to enter ischemic brain tissue followed by the infiltration of mononuclear phagocytes [7, 8]. Neutrophils contribute to the development of ischemic brain injury by causing capillary plugging, reducing cerebromicrovascular blood flow, increasing microvascular permeability [7, 8], and secreting a variety of injurious chemical mediators including reactive oxygen species, cytokines, and proteases [8].

It is now clear that adhesion of leukocytes to the cerebral endothelium (CEC) is mediated by a receptor-ligand system consisting of the immunoglobulin, integrin, and selectin families of adhesion molecules (for review see [3]) and precedes leukocyte infiltration into the brain. The importance of leukocyte/CEC interactions in regulating inflammatory responses of ischemic brain tissue is supported by the findings that: a) depleting circulating neutrophils reduces infarct volume and edema in a focal model of cerebral ischemia [4]; b) increased leukocyte infiltration in the brain during ischemia/reperfusion is accompanied by increased expression of adhesion molecules in cerebral microvessels [10]; c) administration of antibodies against leukocyte- or endothelium-expressed adhesion molecules to experimental animals before and/or after ischemia decreases infarct size and brain swelling [5, 10] and d) transgenic ICAM-1-deficient mice are less susceptible to brain ischemia-reperfusion injury [13].

Inflammatory cytokines, lipopolysaccharide, and vasoactive peptides have previously been shown to stimulate the expression of ICAM-1, VCAM-1, and E-selectin in HCEC in culture [12, 15]. However, much less is known about the extra- and intracellular processes regulating the induction and expression of adhesion molecules in HCEC during ischemia. In this study we demonstrate increased transcription and surface expression of ICAM-1, VCAM-1 and E-selectin in human HCEC exposed to inflammatory cytokines and simulated *in vitro* ischemia.

Materials and Methods

Cell Culture

HCEC were isolated using a modification [14] of the procedure of Gerhart *et al.* [9]. Briefly, microvessels and capillaries were derived from small samples of human temporal lobe surgically removed for the treatment of idiopathic epilepsy and dissociated by exposure to 1 mg/ml type IV collagenase. Endothelial cell colonies emerging from microvessels at days 4–5 after seeding were isolated using cloning rings (BELLCO Glass, Inc., Vineland, NJ) and 2–3 of these cloned colonies were pooled and further passaged. Passages 3–7 were used for the experiments in this study.

Both primary and propagated HCEC exhibited a "cobblestone" appearance in confluent monolayers typical of microvascular endothelium in culture. More than 95% of the cells expressed Factor VIII-related antigen and high levels of the cerebral endothelium-specific enzymes, γ-glutamyl-transpeptidase and alkaline phosphatase [14].

Simulated in vitro Ischemia

"Ischemia" was induced by subjecting HCEC cultures to a combination of glucose-free Krebs solution containing (in mM) 119 NaCl, 4.7 KCl, 1.2 KH_2PO_4, 25 $NaHCO_3$, 2.5 $CaCl_2$, 1 $MgCl_2$ and hypoxia in a Forma Scientific anaerobic chamber Model 1024. The entire system was purged with 95% N_2 / 5% CO_2 atmosphere. The pO_2 values of the culture media decreased to 2.26 ± 0.3 kPa (2% O_2) after 15 min of incubation in the chamber.

Reperfusion was induced by exposing cells to ambient air (reoxygenation) and adding 5 mM glucose to the cell media after various times of ischemia.

Immunocytochemistry

The expression of ICAM-1, VCAM-1 and E-selectin was assessed in HCEC grown on 10 µg/ml fibronectin-coated glass coverslips as described by Wong *et al.*, 1995 [15]. Briefly, cells were washed in PBS and incubated at room temperature with 2 µg/ml mouse hybridoma monoclonal antibodies (IgG) to human ICAM-1 (clone CD54), VCAM-1 (clone NSO), or E-selectin (clone H18/7) (UBI, Lake Placid, NY) for 40 min in medium M199. Following the

incubation with primary antibody, cells were washed and incubated for 1 hour with a 1:50 dilution of 4 nm colloidal gold particles-conjugated goat anti-mouse IgG antibody (Accurate Chem. Sci. Corp., Westbury, NY). Coverslips were fixed for 30 seconds with 9.25% formaldehyde and 45% acetone, incubated in a silver enhancing solution (IntenSE™, Amersham, Oakville, ONT) for 25 minutes, and counterstained with Giemsa stain.

ELISA

An enzyme-linked immunosorbent assay (ELISA) was performed in HCEC cultures grown in 96-well microtiter plates (5 × 10^4 cells/well) using monoclonal anti-human adhesion molecule antibodies (same as above; 2 µg/ml for 1 hr at 37°C) [12] and 1:500 diluted peroxidase (HRP)-conjugated, goat anti-mouse IgG antibody (45 min at 37°C) [12]. Non-specific binding sites were blocked with a carrier buffer containing 2% BSA. The reaction was developed with HRP substrate 2,2'-azinobis (3 ethylbenzthiazoline-6-sulfonic acid) (Pierce, Rockford, IL) for 10 min and stopped with 1% SDS. The optical density (O.D.) of the developed color was read at 405 nm using a SpectraMAX (Molecular Devices, Menlo Park, CA) microplate reader.

Results and Discussion

A growing body of evidence indicates that neutrophils mediate ischemia/reperfusion-induced microvascular and parenchymal cell dysfunction in a variety of organ systems, including brain [7, 8, 10]. It is generally believed that reperfusion of ischemic tissue results in the formation of pro-inflammatory mediators, such as IL-1 and TNFα, that promote the adherence and

Table 1. *Effects of the Inflammatory Cytokines, TNFα and IL-1β and Simulated in vitro Ischemia on the Expression of Adhesion Molecules in HCEC*

Treatment	ICAM-1	VCAM-1	E-selectin
Basal	0.436 ± 0.021	0.208 ± 0.012	0.011 ± 0.002
TNFα, 50 u/ml	1.634 ± 0.087^a	0.876 ± 0.056^a	not determined
TNFα, 200 u/ml	2.436 ± 0.123^a	1.739 ± 0.082^a	0.258 ± 0.014^a
+ AcD, 10 µg/ml	0.541 ± 0.042^b	0.254 ± 0.013^b	$0.034 \pm 0.002^{a, b}$
+ Indo, 300 µM	$1.592 \pm 0.117^{a, b}$	$0.302 \pm 0.021^{a, b}$	$0.052 \pm 0.004^{a, b}$
IL-1β, 10 u/ml	1.025 ± 0.076^a	1.435 ± 0.100^a	not determined
IL-1β, 200 u/ml	1.852 ± 0.053^a	2.841 ± 0.175^a	$0.092 1 0.006^a$
+ AcD, 10 µg/ml	$0.421 + 0.021^b$	0.179 ± 0.014^b	0.015 ± 0.001^b
+ Indo, 300 µM	$0.898 \pm 0.037^{a, b}$	$0.267 + 0.021^b$	$0.021 \pm 0.002^{a, b}$
Ischemia, 4 hrs	0.815 ± 0.046^a	0.613 ± 0.039^a	$0.074 + 0.004^a$
+ AcD, 10 µg/ml	$0.342 + 0.027^b$	0.213 ± 0.015^b	0.014 ± 0.002^b
+ Indo, 300 µM	$0.390 + 0.012^b$	0.173 ± 0.011^b	$0.034 \pm 0.002^{a, b}$

HCEC were treated with the indicated concentrations of TNFα and IL-1β for 24 hours, or were exposed to 4 hours of simulated ischemia *in vitro* (see Materials and Methods), in the absence or presence of actinomycin D (AcD) or indomethacin (Indo). The levels of ICAM-1, VCAM-1, and E-selectin were determined by ELISA as described in Materials and Methods. At these concentrations, neither AcD nor Indo affected basal levels of adhesion molecule expression (data not shown). The results are expressed in O.D. units read at 405 nm and represent the mean ± S.E.M. of six replicate wells in one of at least three experiments yielding similar results.

[a] Indicates significant difference (P < 0.01, ANOVA) from the corresponding control.

[b] Indicates significant difference (P < 0.01, ANOVA) from the TNFα, or IL-1β or 4 hour "ischemia" alone.

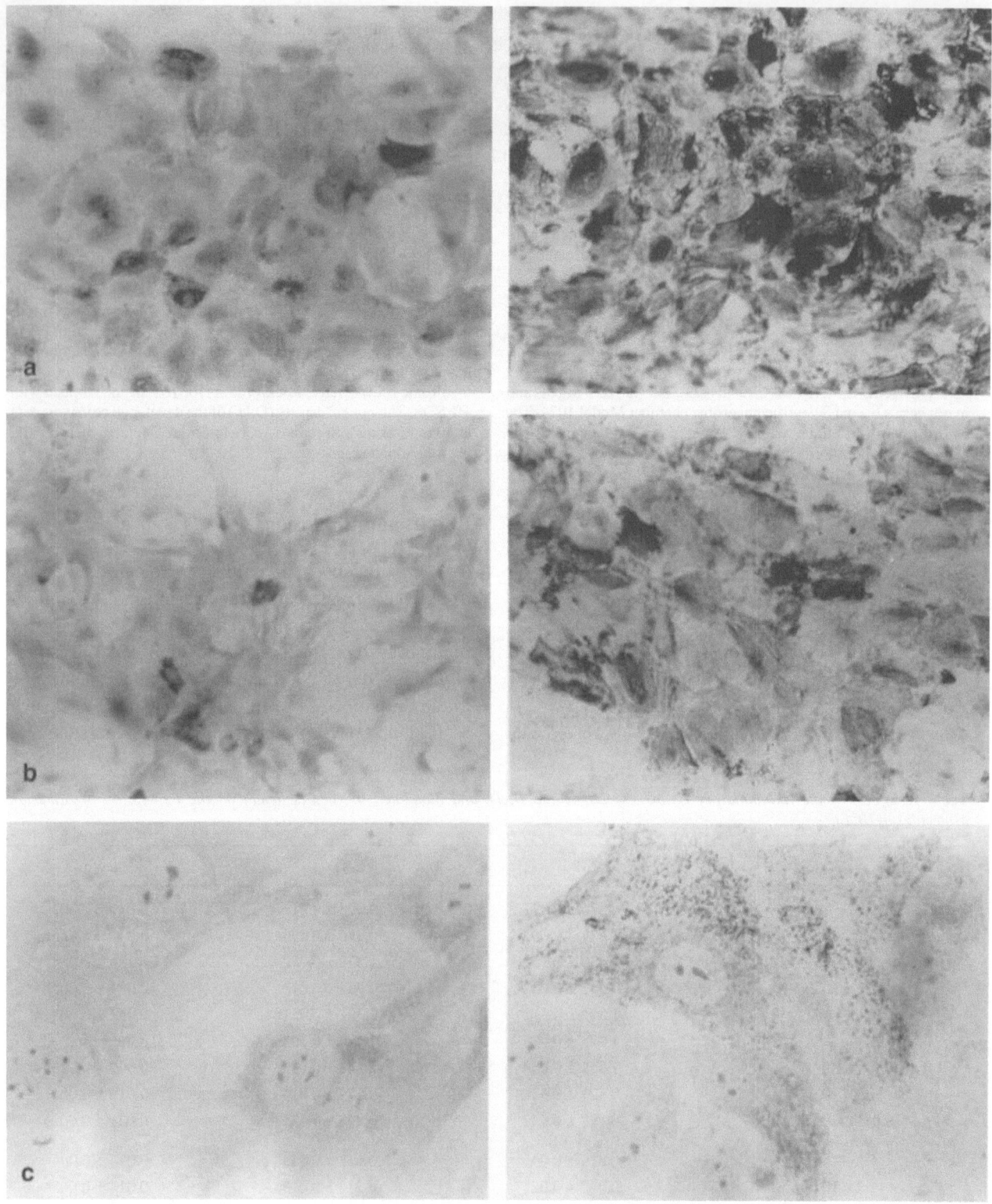

Fig 1. Effects of simulated *in vitro* ischemia on the surface expression of ICAM-1, VCAM-1 and E-selectin by HCEC in culture. Left side panels show bright field micrographs of control HCEC and right side panels those of HCEC exposed to 4 hours of simulated *in vitro* ischemia (hypoxia and glucose- and nutrient-free media). Cultures were stained by immunocytochemical methods for the expression of ICAM-1 (a) (× 20), VCAM-1 (b) (× 40), and E-selectin (c) (× 80) as described in Materials and Methods

emigration of neutrophils from postcapillary venules [7, 8].

In this study we demonstrate that the exposure of HCEC to the inflammatory cytokines, IL-1β (10–200 u/ml) or TNFα (50–200 u/ml), for 4 (data not shown) or 24 hours (Table 1), results in a marked increase in the levels of ICAM-1 and VCAM-1 and induction of E-selectin expression (Table 1). This cytokine-induced increase in the expression of adhesion molecules was abolished in cells treated with the transcriptional inhibitor, AcD (10 μg/ml) (Table 1), indicating that their up-regulation was transcriptionally controlled. Therefore, inflammatory cytokines and chemokines induced by ischemia in the brain [7, 8] likely facilitate leukocyte penetration into the CNS by up-regulating endothelial adhesion receptors (Table 1) and inducing avid HCEC/neutrophil interactions.

Subjecting HCEC to an ischemic insult in the absence of exogenously added cytokines also resulted in the increased transcription and surface expression of adhesion molecules. This was evident from the ability of 4 hours of simulated *in vitro* ischemia to increase the levels of ICAM-1 (2 fold) and VCAM-1 (3 fold) and to induce the expression of E-selectin (Fig. 1, Table 1) and from the fact that this ischemic induction/up-regulation of adhesion molecules was completely blocked by 10 μg/ml AcD (Table 1). Moreover, at the end of the 24 hour reperfusion period, the levels of ICAM-1 and VCAM-1 were still maintained at ischemia-stimulated levels, whereas E-selectin was no longer detectable (data not shown). None of the above treatments resulted in significant cell death/damage as determined by propidium iodide staining (data not shown).

The exact mechanism(s) by which ischemia activates the transcription of ICAM-1, VCAM-1 and E-selectin in HCEC is not clear. However, a possible mediator of this response may be the nuclear factor κB (NF-κB) which plays an important role in regulating the cytokine-induced transcription of endothelial adhesion molecules [6], and is activated by various factors induced by ischemia, including reactive oxygen species [6]. Alternatively, the stimulation of adhesion molecule expression in HCEC by ischemia may arise from the autocrine effects of IL-1α and/or platelet-activating factor, since both have been shown to stimulate neutrophil adhesion and to be secreted by peripheral endothelial cells exposed to ischemia [1].

Cytokine- and ischemia-induced expression of ICAM-1, VCAM-1, and E-selectin by HCEC was inhibited by the COX inhibitor, indomethacin (Table 1). IL-1β and other cytokines have been shown to induce

prostaglandin production in peripheral endothelial cells [11] whereas ischemia stimulates the release of arachidonic acid from HCEC (unpublished observations). Therefore, the mechanism(s) by which indomethacin suppresses adhesion molecule up-regulation may involve elimination of the autocrine effects of COX-derived prostaglandins on HCEC.

Parenthetically, it has recently been reported that cytokine-inducible enhancer NF-κB is also involved in trancriptional regulation of inducible COX II [6, 11].

In conclusion, these findings implicate HCEC as an important component in processes leading to neutrophil adhesion and infiltration in human brain during inflammatory and ischemic brain disorders.

Acknowledgements

This project is supported by a grant (# ST2718) from the Heart and Stroke Foundation of Ontario. The project is approved by NRC, McGill University, and CHEO's Human Research Ethics Committees. We wish to express our gratitude to Mrs. Rita Ball for her expert technical help with human cerebral endothelial cell cultures and to Dr. Robert Monette for his help with experiments using confocal microscopy.

References

1. Arnould T, Michelis C, Remacle J (1993) Increased PMN adherence on endothelial cells after hypoxia: involvement of PAF, CD18/CD11b, and ICAM-1. Am J Physiol 264: C1102–C1110
2. Barone FC, Hillegass LM, Price WJ, White RF, Feuerstein GZ, Sarau HM, Clark RK, Griswold DE (1991) Polymorphonuclear leukocyte infiltration into cerebral focal ischemic tissue: myeloperoxidase activity assay and histologic verification. J Neurosci Res 29: 336–348
3. Carlos TM, Harlan JM (1994) Leukocyte-endothelial adhesion molecules. Blood 84: 2068–2101
4. Chen H, Chopp M, Bodzin G (1992) Neutropenia reduces the volume of cerebral infarct after transient middle cerebral artery occlusion in the rat. Neurosci Res Commun 11: 93–99
5. Chopp M, Zhan RL, Chen H, Li Y, Jiang N, Rusche R (1994) Postischemic administration of an Mac-1 antibody reduces ischemic cell damage after transient middle cerebral artery occlusion in rats. Stroke 25: 869–876
6. Collins T, Read MA, Neish AS, Whitley MZ, Thanos D, Maniatis T (1995) Transcriptional regulation of endothelial cell adhesion molecules: NF-κB and cytokine-inducible enhancers. FASEB J 9: 899–909
7. del Zoppo GJ (1994) Microvascular changes during cerebral ischemia and reperfusion. Cerebrovasc Brain Metab Rev 6: 47–96
8. Feuerstein GZ, Liu T, Barone FC (1994) Cytokines, inflammation, and brain injury: role of tumor necrosis factor α. Cereb Brain Metab Rev 6: 341–360
9. Gerhart ZD, Broderius AM, Drewes RL (1988) Cultured human and canine endothelial cells from brain microvessels. Brain Res Bull 21: 785–793
10. Matsuo Y, Onodera H, Shiga Y, Nakamura M, Ninomiya M, Kihara T, Kogure K (1994) Correlation between myeloperoxi-

dase-quantified neutrophil accumulation and ischemic brain injury in rat: effects of neutrophil depletion. Stroke 25: 1469–1475

11. Maier JA, Hia T, Maciag T (1990) Cyclo-oxygenase is an immediate early gene induced by interleukin-1 in human endothelial cells. J Biol Chem 265: 10805–10808

12. McCarron RM, Wang L, Stanimirovic DB, Spatz M (1995) Differential regulation of adhesion molecule expression by human cerebrovascular and umbilical vein endothelial cells. Endothelium 2: 339–346

13. Soriano SG, Lipton SA, Wang YF, Xiao M, Springer TA, Gutierrez-Ramos J-C, Hickey PR (1996) Intercellular adhesion molecule-1-deficient mice are less susceptible to cerebral ischemia-reperfusion injury. Ann Neurol 39: 618–624

14. Stanimirovic DB, Morley P, Ball R, Harnel E, Mealing G, Durkin JP (1996) Angiotensin II-induced fluid phase endocytosis in human cerebromicrovascular endothelial cells is regulated by the inositol phosphate signalling pathway. J Cell Physiol

15. Wong D, Dorovini-Zis K (1995) Expression of vascular cell adhesion molecule-1 (VCAM-1) by human brain microvessel endothelial cells in primary culture. Microvasc Res 49: 325–339

Correspondence: Dr. Danica Stanimirovic, Cellular Neurobiology Group, Institue for Biological Sciences, National Research Council of Canada, Montreal Road Campus, Bldg. M-54, Ottawa, ONT, Canada, K1A 0R6.

Acta Neurochir (1997) [Suppl] 70: 17–19

Assessment of the Relationship Between Ischemic Damage and Brain Swelling in Frozen Brain Slices

C. K. Park, S. S. Jun, S. H. Cho, and **J. K. Kang**

Department of Neurosurgery, Catholic University Medical College, Seoul, Korea

Summary

The purpose of the study was to verify a method for the measurement of both cerebral infarction and brain swelling in frozen brain slices for histology. The animals were divided into two groups, sham-operated control (n = 10) and focal cerebral ischemia group (n = 10). Focal cerebral ischemia was produced by permanent occlusion of the left middle cerebral artery. The rats were sacrificed 24 hours postocclusion. The brain was divided into two through the corpus callosum. Each hemisphere was weighed and frozen. Cerebral infarction and brain swelling were each assessed at 8 predetermined coronal planes. The volume of brain swelling was obtained by subtracting the total volume of nonischemic hemisphere from the total volume of the ischemic one.

In the MCA occlusion group, brain infarction and the differences of hemispheric volume and weight between the right and left hemispheres were consistently observed, whereas sham-operated rats demonstrated no brain infarction or significant differences between two hemispheres. There were good correlationships not only between the volumes of brain edema and infarction (p < 0.05) but between the volume of brain edema and the difference in weight (p < 0.01) also.

The results indicate that the measurement of the volume of ischemic brain edema in frozen brain slices may be useful in elusidating relationship with ischemic brain damage.

Keywords: Ischemic damage; brain swelling; pathology; hemispheric weight.

Introduction

Brain swelling caused by brain edema after an ischemic episode remains a major clinical problem [11]. Despite the recent advances in our knowledge of the pathophysiology of brain edema formation, no specific therapy is yet available. Based on the pathophysiology of ischemic brain edema, various pharmacological agents such as NMDA antagonists and oxygen free radical scavengers have been suggested as, anti-ischemic brain edema agent and widely investigated [9, 15]. Although the relationship between the degree of ischemic brain damage and the extent of brain swelling must be elucidated to evaluate a specific antiedema drug in brain ischemia, there has not been a proper experimental model to assess the relationship in a single experimental procedure. Recently a method, in which cerebral infarction and edema were quantified concomittantly by image analysis of frozen brain sections processed for histology, has been used in the assessment of the neuroprotective drugs [3, 4, 9]. This experimental model appeared to demonstrate the relationship between ischemic brain damage and swelling in an identical animal [8], though there had not been any attempt to verify the method using frozen brain slices. The current study attempted to verify this experimental model and establish its suitability in the study of ischemic brain edema.

Materials and Methods

We studied twenty adult male Sprague-Dawley rats weighing 300 to 350g. The animals were divided into two groups: sham-operated control group (n = 10); middle cerebral artery (MCA) occlusion group (n = 10). The animals were anesthetized using halothane and a nitrous oxide-oxygen mixture (70:30%) during the surgical procedure, less than 30min in duration. Spontaneous respiration was maintained by a face mask. Cannulation of the femoral artery was first carried out, and the animals were maintained normothermic by a homeothermic system (Havard Apparatus, Kent, U.K.). The temporal muscle temperature (Therm 2250, Ahlborn Mess- und Regelungstechnik, Germany) was continuously monitored during surgery. The arterial catheter was removed and anesthesia was discontinued immediately after completion of the surgical procedure.

In the MCA occlusion group, the animals underwent the occlusion of the left MCA via a subtemporal approach without removal of the zygomatic arch or temporal muscle. Under high power magnification, the left MCA was coagulated with a micro-bipolar coagulator from the olfactory tract to the most proximal portion of the MCA and divided. In the sham-operated control group, the animals underwent the same surgical procedure except arterial occlusion as in the MCA occlusion group.

Twenty-four hours following MCA occlusion, the rats were sacrificed. The brain was removed from the calvaria immediately after sacrifice, and divided into two pieces through the corpus callosum in a humidified chamber. Each hemisphere was weighed on an electric balance and frozen in a cryostat (–25°C). Coronal sections (20 µm thick) were cut with a cryostat and stained with hematoxylin-eosin. The infarcted area and the extent of brain swelling were readily deliniated. Eight coronal sections which corresponded to planes of the predetermined forebrain were selected among the stained slices, and the volumes of each hemisphere and infarction were computed from the areas of the hemisphere and ischemic damage measured at the different coronal planes and their anteroposterior coordinates, as decribed previously [10]. To measure the volume of brain swelling, the total volume of the nonischemic hemisphere in each brain was subtracted from the total volume of the ischemic one.

For comparision between the two different groups of animals and between the right and left hemispheres of each animal, unpaired and paired two tailed Student's t-test was used respectively. The relationships between brain swelling and infarction and between brain swelling and the difference in hemispheric weight were assessed by linear regression analysis and Pearson's correlation coefficient values.

Adequate oxygenation, normocapnia and nonmothermia were maintained in the both experimental groups throughout surgical procedures.

Results

There were significant differences in the hemispheric volume between the right and left hemispheres not only in the MCA occlusion group ($P < 0.001$, paired t-test) but also in sham-operated group ($P < 0.05$, paired t-test). However as compared to the MCA occlusion group, the sham-operated animals, showed only a small difference (35.3 ± 8.4 vs. 138.3 ± 16.1 mm^3, $P < 0.0001$, unpaired t-test) in hemispheric volume (Table 1).

There was a good correlation both between the volumes of brain swelling and infarction ($r = 0.73$, $P < 0.05$) and between the volume of brain swelling

and the difference in the hemispheric weight ($r = 0.85$, $P < 0.01$) in individual animals with almost every animal close to the overall regression line (Fig. 1).

Discussion

Several clinical [14], experimental [2, 5], and autopsy [7] studies have underscored the importance of brain swelling and herniation as a cause of death in the acute phase of ischemic stroke. The extent of brain swelling depends on the size of infarct. Massive hemispheric swelling usually occurs in multilobar infarction from internal carotid or middle cerebral artery thrombosis [12]. Therefore, it would be desirable to observe changes of brain damage and brain swelling concomittently in an identical brain ischemic experimental animal.

In studies of ischemic brain damage, the coventional histopathalogy or TTC (triphenyltetrazolium chloride) technique has been used [1], while in the studies of brain edema, the drying-weighing method or the microgravimetry technique has been one of the choices [13]. Recently, it has been reported that MRI might be useful in the assessments of ischemic brain damage and edema concomittently in an identical animal [6]. But MRI studies may have some drawbacks, the most important points of which are high cost to set up and maintain facility and faculties and difficulties in quantifying the data especially in small animals.

As compared to sham-operated control group, the MCA-occluded animals demonstrated focal cerebral

Table 1. *Hemispheric Volume and Statistical Analysis* (mm^3, means ± S.E.)

Group	Hemisphere			% of difference
	Left	Right	Difference	
Sham-operated Control (n = 10)	714.3 ± 7.6	679.0 ± 11.6	35.3 ± 8.4	5.0
MCA occlusion (n = 10)	827.1 ± 25.0	688.8 ± 19.3	138.3 ± 16.1	16.7

Control vs. MCAO	difference	$P < 0.0001$	(unpaired t-test)
	right	$P = $ N.S.	(unpaired t-test)
	left	$P < 0.001$	(unpaired t-test)
In control	left vs. right	$P < 0.05$	(paired t-test)
In MCAO	left vs. right	$P < 0.0001$	(paired t-test)

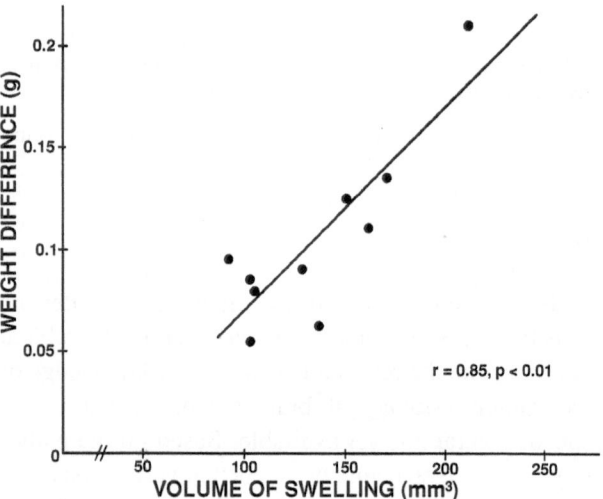

Fig. 1. Scatter diagram of difference in weight (g) between the left and right hemispheres as a function of the volume of brain swelling (mm^3) in MCA-occluded animals. The difference in weight is linearly proportional to the volume of brain swelling. Linear regression analysis yielded $r = 0.85$ ($P < 0.01$)

infarction and significant brain swelling in the ipsilateral hemisphere. Interestingly enough, small amout of brain swelling (5% of the total left hemispheric volume) was also observed even in sham-operated control animals, which might be caused by the sham-operation procedures. For this reason, it is essential to include a sham-operated control group in a study of brain swelling with frozen brain slices. The difference in weight between the right and left hemispheres was directly proportional to the volume of ischemic brain damage ($r = 0.85$, $P < 0.01$).

The present data provides verification that ischemic brain damage and swelling can be assessed concomittently in an identical animal in frozen brain sections processed for histology This implicates that the relationship between ischemic brain damage and swelling could be demonstrated in this experimental model. The method using frozen brain sections appears to be a useful and economical alternative to MRI in the study of ischemic brain edema. The frozen brain section method is a useful tool to evaluate the effect of anti-ischemic agents specifically on ischemic brain edema.

Acknowledgement

The investigations were supported in part by the Catholic Medical Center, Korea, and by Non Directed Research Fund, Korea Research Foundation. We would like to acknowledge the technical assistance of Ms. J. A. Jun and the assistance of Ms. Y. J. Chung in the preparation of the manuscript.

References

1. Bederson JB, Pitts LH, Germano SM, Nishimura MC, Davis RL, Bartowski HM (1986) Evaluation of 2,3,5-triphenyltetrazolium chloride as a stain for detection and quantification of experimental cerebral infarction in rats. Stroke 17: 1304–1308
2. Ivamoto HS, Numoto M, Donaghy RMP (1974) Surgical decompression for cerebral and cerebellar infarcts. Stroke 5: 365–369
3. Jacewicz M, Brint S, Tanabe J, Pulsinelli WA (1990) Continuous nimodipine treatment attenuates cortical infarction in rats subjected to 24 hours of focal cerebral ischemia. J Cereb Blood Flow Metab 10: 89–96
4. Kusumoto K, Mackay KB, McCulloch J (1992) The effect of the kappa-opioid receptor agonist Cl-977 in a rat model of focal cerebral ischemia. Brain Res 576: 147–151
5. Laurent JP, Molinari GF, Moseley JI (1975) Clinicopathological validation of a primate stroke model. Surg Neurol 4: 449–445
6. Minematsu K, Fisher M, Li L, Davis MA, Knapp AG, Cotter RE, McBurney RN, Sotak CH (1993) Effects of a novel NMDA antagonist on experimental stroke rapidly and quantitatively assessed by diffusion-weighted MRI. Neurology 43: 397–403
7. Ng LKY, Nimmannitya J (1970) Massive cerebral infarction with severe brain swelling: a clinicopathological sudy. Stroke 1: 158–163
8. Park CK, McCulloch J, Jung DS, Kang JK, Choi CR (1994) Do N-methyl-D-aspartate antagonists have disproportionately greater effects on brain swelling than on ischemic damage in focal cerebral infarction? Acta Neurochir (Wien) [Suppl] 60: 276–281
9. Park CK, McCulloch J, Kang JK, Choi CR (1994) Pretreatment with a competitive NMDA antagonist D-CPPene attenuates focal cerebral infarction and brain swelling in awake rats. Acta Neurochir (Wien) 127: 220–226
10. Park CK, Nehls DG, Graham DI, Teasdale GM, McCulloch J (1988) The glutamate antagonist MK-801 reduces focal ischaemic brain damage in the rat. Ann Neurol 24: 543–551
11. Rengachary SS (1986) Surgery for acute brain infarction with mass effect. In: Wilkins RH, Rengachary SS (eds) Neurosurgery, 2nd edn. McGraw-Hill, New York, pp 2151–2155
12. Ropper AH, Shafran B (1984) Brain edema after stroke. Clinical syndrome and intracranial pressure. Arch Neurol 41: 26–29
13. Shigeno T, Brock M, Shigend S, Fritschda E, Cervós-Navarro J (1982) The determination of brain water content: microgravimetry versus drying-weighing method. J Neurosurg 57: 99–107
14. Van Trotsenburg L, Vinken PJ (1966) Fatal cerebral infarction simulating an acute expanding lesion. J Neurol Neurosurg Psychiatry 29: 2471
15. Young W, Wojak JC, DeCrescito V (1988) Aminosteroid lipid peroxidation inhibitor reduces ion shifts and edema in the rat middle cerebral artery occlusion model of regional ischemia. Stroke 19: 1013–1019

Correspondence: Dr. C. K. Park, Department of Neurosurgery, Kangnam St. Mary's Hospital, Catholic University Medical College, 505, Banpo-Dong Seocho-ku, Seoul 137-040, Korea.

Acta Neurochir (1997) [Suppl] 70: 20–22
© Springer-Verlag 1997

Brain Edema Associated with Progressive Selective Neuronal Death or Impending Infarction in the Cerebral Cortex

Y. Hakamata[1], S. Hanyu[1], T. Kuroiwa[2], and U. Ito[3]

[1] Department of Neurology, Jichi Medical School, Tochigi, [2] Department of Neuropathology, Medical Research Institute, Tokyo Medical and Dental University, and [3] Department of Neurosurgery, Musashino Red Cross Hospital, Tokyo, Japan

Summary

This study examined the temporal profile of brain edema in the cerebral cortex associated with selective neuronal death or focal infarction after repeated ischemia at an intensity of ischemic insult just under and above the threshold level to induce infarction. The left carotid artery of adult gerbils was twice occluded for 10 min each time with a 5-hr interval between the blockages. In this model, focal infarction developed in coronal sections examined at the chiasmatic level (face A), whereas only selective neuronal death without infarction was found in the coronal section observed at the infundibular level (face B). In each animal, Evans blue (2%) was intravenously injected 1 hr prior to sacrifice as an indicator of blood-brain barrier (BBB) disruption. Brain edema was assessed by gravimetry in samples taken from both faces at 15 min, 5 hr, 12 hr, 24 hr, and 48 hr after the 2nd 10-min ischemia. Evans blue extravasated only in face A, corresponding to focal infarction at 24 and 48 hr after the 2nd 10-min ischemia. The specific gravities of the ischemic cortex of both faces decreased significantly from control at 15 min ($P < 0.05$) and had recovered by 5 hr after ischemia. By 12 hr, the specific gravities of both faces had again decreased significantly from the control values ($P < 0.05$), but did not differ significantly from each other. At 24 and 48 hr, the specific gravities of both faces were significantly lower than the control values ($P < 0.01$), and the specific gravity of face A was markedly lower than that of face B ($P < 0.01$). We concluded that in face B, where only selective neuronal death without infarction occurred only cytotoxic edema develops, whereas in face A, where infarction progresses, vasogenic edema develops in addition to cytotoxic edema.

Keywords: Cerebral ischemia; impending cerebral infarction; selective neuronal loss; brain edema.

Introduction

Cytotoxic edema after an ischemic insult is considered a detrimental sign, and is thought to be due to disruption of the Gibbs-Donann equilibrium by an energetic disturbance of Na/K ATPase activity in cerebral cells. However, a recent investigation using cultured astrocytes and C6 glioma cells indicated that viable astrocytes actively removed H+, glutamate, free radicals, K+, and some of the mediators from the extracellular space, thus acting as a housekeeper of the neuronal environment, and consequently swelled by themselves [10, 12–15, 17, 19, 20].

By changing the duration of intervening intervals of repetitive insults of short ischemia, a single one of which does not cause significant neuronal loss in the cortex, we have developed an ischemic model in which only selective neuronal death progresses reproducibly in the ischemic hemisphere in the gerbil, and established a threshold value of ischemic insults for the transition from progressing selective neuronal death to the development of focal infarction [2, 3, 8, 9].

In the present study, to determine if the findings on cultured astrocytes and C6 glioma cells can be applied to the *in vivo* situation, we compared the temporal profile of brain edema in the cerebral cortex where only selective neuronal death progresses without astrocytic necrosis with that where infarction develops after repeated ischemia at an intensity just under and above the threshold level to develop cerebral infarction at different brain levels.

Materials and Methods

In the present study, we occluded the left carotid artery of adult Mongolian gerbils, anesthetized with 2% halothane, 70% nitrous oxide, and 30% oxygen, twice for 10 minutes each time with a 5-hr interval between the insults. Ischemia-positive animals were selected during the first 10-min ischemia [18]. In this model, following reperfusion, focal infarction develops in the coronal section examined at the chiasmatic level (face A), whereas only selective neuronal death without infarction progresses in the coronal section observed at the infundibular level (face B). One hour prior to decapitation, 2% Evans blue was injected intravenously, 15 min, 5 hr, 12 hr, 24 hr, or 48 hr after the 2nd 10-min ischemia. The brain was then removed and sectioned coronally to expose faces A and B. On each face, we measured the specific gravity of the cortical slice including the middle 1/3 segment between the interhemispheric fissure (IF) and the rhinal fissure (RF). We also performed histological examination of the coronal section of each face just opposite to the area used for the measurement of specific gravity. Statistical evaluation was performed by Student's t-test for unpaired samples.

Results

Evans blue extravasated only in the middle 1/3 cortical segment between the IF and RF of face A, corresponding to the infarcted focus observed histologically in the coronal section just opposite to face A, 24 hr and 48 hr after the 2nd 10-min ischemia (Table 1).

The specific gravities of the ischemic cortex of both faces at 15 min after the 2nd 10-min ischemia had decreased slightly but significantly from the control values (P < 0.05, Table 2). The specific gravity of both faces recovered to near control levels by 5 hr. By 12 hr, however, the specific gravities of both faces were again significantly lower than the control values (P < 0.05), but did not differ significantly from each other. At 24 hr, the specific gravities of both faces were still significantly lower than the control values (P < 0.01), but the specific gravity of face A was now markedly lower than that of face B (P < 0.01) and continued to be so up to 48 hr.

Table 1. *Incidence of Number of Animals with Positive Evans Blue Extravasation in Cerebral Cortex after Repeated Ischemia.* Time after recirculation

	15 min	5 h	12 h	24 h	48 h
Face A	0/6	0/6	0/6	6/6	6/6
Face B	0/6	0/6	0/6	0/6	0/6

Table 2. *Specific Gravity of Cerebral Cortex after Repeated Ischemia*

Time after recirculation	Face A	Face B
Control	1.0494 ± 0.0003	1.0491 ± 0.0003
15 min	1.0467 ± 0.0005[a]	1.0468 ± 0.0005[a]
5 h	1.0488 ± 0.0005	1.0485 ± 0.0006
12 h	1.0474 ± 0.0008[a]	1.0479 ± 0.0003[a]
24 h	1.0380 ± 0.0009[b, c]	1.0428 ± 0.0008[b]
48 h	1.0341 ± 0.0007[b, c]	1.0397 ± 0.0016[b]

Values are mean ± SE (n = 6).
[a] P < 0.05 significantly from control values.
[b] P < 0.01 significantly from control values.
[c] P < 0.01 significantly from values in face B.

Discussion

In the reperfusion ischemia model, cytotoxic brain edema develops first and vasogenic edema then develops later after the start of reperfusion [5, 6, 11]. No study to date has separately examined the temporal profiles of brain edema in the cerebral cortex where only selective neuronal death has progressed and where infarction has developed after reperfusion has begun. In the previous single transient ischemia model, the threshold of ischemic intensity from selective neuronal death to infarction showed considerable variability due to individual differences between animals [4, 7]. By using a repetitive ischemia model with ischemic insults under and above the threshold to induce cerebral infarction, we were able to separately demonstrate the temporal profiles of both brain edemas.

Both of the temporal profiles of brain edema associated with progressive selective neuronal death (face B) and impending infarction (face A) showed a biphasic pattern [16]; the first edema occurred 15 min after the 2nd 10-min ischemia; and the second, at 12 to 24 hr. The first one was very slight, and the Evans blue did not extravasate during this edema, suggesting that the BBB had not been disrupted. We suggest that the main cause of the first brain edema was water movement (bulk flow [1]) associated with an abrupt increase in hydrostatic pressure after the start of reperfusion. By 5 hr after the 2nd 10-min ischemia, the specific gravity recovered to the control level.

In face B, where only selective neuronal death progresses, second brain edema developed up to 12 hr after the 2nd 10-min ischemia and continued to increase up to 48 hr without disruption of the BBB as judged by the absence of Evans blue permeability. Therefore, the brain edema associated with selective neuronal death is cytotoxic edema. In face A, where infarction develops 24 hr after the 2nd 10-min ischemia, the temporal profile of brain edema was similar to that in face B up to 12 hr, after which time the edema became more pronounced than that in face B. At 24 and 48 hr in the infarcted focus, the BBB was disrupted and severe brain edema progressed. Therefore, in face A, cytotoxic edema developed by 12 hr after the 2nd 10-min ischemia and vasogenic edema, at 24 hr, corresponding to the infarcted focus. As the infarction does not develop in face B where only neurons die and astrocytes are viable [9], the cytotoxic edema associated with progressive selective neuronal death is probably due to active swelling of viable astrocytes, as was observed in experiments on cultured cells [10, 12–15, 17, 19, 20].

Conclusion

We conclude that in face B, where only selective neuronal death without necrosis of astrocytes progresses, only cytotoxic edema develops, whereas in face A, where infarction progresses, vasogenic edema develops in addition to cytotoxic edema.

References

1. Fenstermacher JD, Patlack CS (1976) The movement of water and solution in the brain of mammals. In: Pappius HM, Feindel W (eds) Dynamics of brain edema. Springer, Berlin Heidelberg New York, pp 87–94
2. Hanyu S, Ito U, Hakamata Y, Yoshida M (1993) Repeated unilateral carotid occlusion in Mongolian gerbils: quantitative analysis of cortical neuronal loss. Acta Neuropathol (Berl) 86: 16–20
3. Hanyu S, Ito U, Hakamata Y, Yoshida M (1995) Transition from ischemic neuronal necrosis to infarction in repeated ischemia. Brain Res 686: 44–48
4. Ito U, Spatz M, Walker JJ, Klatzo I (1975) Experimental cerebral ischemia in mongolian gerbils. I. Light microscopic observations. Acta Neuropathol (Berl) 32: 209–223
5. Ito U, Go KG, Walker JJ, Spatz M, Klatzo I (1976) Experimental cerebral ischemia in Mongolian gerbils III. Behaviour of the blood-brain barrier. Acta Neuropathol (Berl) 34: 1–6
6. Ito U, Ohno K, Nakamura R, Suganuma F, Inaba Y (1979) Brain edema during ischemia and after restoration of blood flow. Measurement of water, sodium, potassium content and plasma protein permeability. Stroke 10: 542–547
7. Ito U, Yamaguchi T, Tomita H, *et al* (1992) Maturation phenomenon of ischemic injuries observed in Mongolian gerbils: introductory remarks. In: Ito U, Kirino T, Kuroiwa T, Klatzo I (eds) Maturation phenomenon in cerebral ischemia. Springer, Berlin Heidelberg New York Tokyo, pp 1–13
8. Ito U, Hanyu S, Hakamata Y, Yoshida M (1995) Selective neuronal death and focal infarction in repeated ischemia. J Cereb Blood Flow Metab 15 [Suppl 1]: S199
9. Ito U, Hanyu S, Hakamata Y, Nakamura K, Arima K (1997) Ultrastructure of astrocytes associated with selective neuronal death of cerebral cortex after repeated ischemia. Acta Neurochir (Wien) [Suppl] 70: 46–49
10. Juurlink BH, Chen Y, Hertz L (1992) Use of cell cultures to differentiate among effects of various ischemia factors on astrocytic cell volume. Can J Physiol Pharmacol 70: S344–349
11. Katzman R, Clasen R, Klatzo I, Meyer JS, Pappius HM, Waltz AG (1977) Report of Joint Committee for Stroke Resources. IV. Brain edema in stroke [Review]. Stroke 8: 512–540
12. Kempski O, Staub F, Jansen M, Schodel F, Baethmann A (1988) Glial swelling during extracellular acidosis *in vitro*. Stroke 19: 385–392
13. Kempski OS, Volk C (1994) Neuron-glial interaction-during injury and edema of the CNS [Review]. Acta Neurochir [Suppl] 60: 7–11
14. Kimelberg HK, Rutledge E, Goderie S, Charniga C (1995) Astrocytic swelling due to hypotonic or high K+ medium causes inhibition of glutamate and aspartate uptake and increases their release. J Cereb Blood Flow Metab 15: 409–416
15. Kraig RP, Chesler M (1990) Astrocytic acidosis in hyperglycemic and complete ischemia. J Cereb Blood Flow Metab 10: 104–114
16. Kuroiwa T, Ting P, Martinez H, Klatzo I (1985) The biphasic opening of the blood-brain barrier to proteins following temporary middle cerebral artery occlusion. Acta Neuropathol (Berl) 68: 122–129
17. Lomneth R, Gruenstein EI (1989) Energy-dependent cell volume maintenance in UC-11MG human astrocytomas. Am J Physiol 257: C817–C824
18. Ohno K, Ito U, Inaba Y (1984) Regional cerebral blood flow and stroke index after left carotid artery ligation in the conscious gerbil. Brain Res 297: 151–157
19. Staub F, Winkler A, Peters J, Kempski O, Kachel V, Baethmann A (1994) Swelling, acidosis, and irreversible damage of glial cells from exposure to arachidonic acid *in vitro*. J Cereb Blood Flow Metab 14: 1030–1039
20. Walz W, Klimaszewski A, Paterson IA (1993) Glial swelling in ischemia: a hypothesis. Dev Neurosci 15: 216–225

Correspondence: Yoji Hakamata, Ph.D., Laboratory of Experimental Medicine, Jichi Medical School, 3311-1, Minamikawachi-machi, Kawachi-gun, Tochigi, Japan.

Acta Neurochir (1997) [Suppl] 70: 23–26
© Springer-Verlag 1997

Blood Volume and Flow Velocity Through Parenchymal Microvessels in Ischemic Brain Edema of Rats

S. Hatashita[1], A. Tajima[1], H. Ueno[1], S. Ishimaru[2], H. Sato[3], and S. Takahashi[3]

Department of Neurosurgery, [1] Juntendo University Urayasu Hospital and [2] Izunagaoka Hospital, and
[3] Comparative Radiotoxicology, National Institute Radiological Sciences, Japan

Summary

Focal cerebral ischemia was produced in rats with left middle cerebral artery occlusion for 24 hours. Regional CBF was measured by the ^{14}C-iodoantipyrine technique. The distribution of red blood cells (RBC) and plasma in cerebral microvessels was determined by radioluminography using ^{51}Cr-RBC and ^{125}I-bovine serum albumin, respectively. The mean transit times of RBC and plasma, blood volume, and hematocrit were calculated. The water content was measured by specific gravity. The blood flow was reduced to 2% of the control value in the central core, where the brain edema was the most severe. The blood volume decreased to 25% and the mean transit times of RBC and plasma increased about tenfold. In the outer periphery, where CBF was reduced to 39% but brain edema was not induced, the blood volume was decreased to 76% while the mean transit time of RBC was increased 2.1-fold, being greater than the increase in the plasma transit time. These findings indicate that focal ischemia has variable effects on the blood volume and flow velocities of RBC and plasma in the parenchymal microvessels depending on the depth of blood flow and edema. A decrease in blood flow is probably related to a reduction in the flow velocities of RBC and plasma in the surrounding ischemic tissue rather than to decreased number of perfused capillaries in the ischemic core.

Keywords: Brain edema; blood volume; CBF; cerebal ischemia; flow velocity.

Introduction

In the cerebral microvascular network, the capillaries contain both red blood cells (RBC) and plasma or only plasma, and the flow is either continuous or intermittent [3]. Changes in cerebral blood flow are affected by alteration of the flow velocity through the perfused capillaries, variation of the number of perfused capillaries or modulation of the diameter of perfused capillaries. Fenstermacher and co-workers have reported that the alteration in rCBF by hypercapnia or pentobarbital is mainly due to the change in both RBC and plasma flow velocities in the perfused cerebral microvessels [2, 9]. In addition, with hypercapnia, an increment in blood flow is partly related to recruitment capillaries and/or increasing microvessel diameter. The volumes and flow velocities of RBC and plasma through parenchymal microvessels are related, in particular, to the cerebral blood flow.

Occlusion of a major end artery of the brain lowers the regional blood flow to varying degrees in and around the region supplied by the artery, which may cause brain edema depending on the duration and depth of ischemia. We have recently demonstrated that early accumulation of edema fluid contributes to a hydrostatic pressure gradient, which develops soon after the onset of ischemia and is followed by the development of an osmotic pressure gradient [4, 5]. After these pressure gradients dissipate, further accumulation of edema fluid is associated with disruption of the blood-brain barrier to small molecules [6]. On the other hand, it remains unclear how the volumes and flow velocities of RBC and plasma are influenced by the degree of ischemia and edema in brain tissue.

The present experiment was designed to ascertain whether the change in cerebral blood flow is associated with the blood volume and the flow velocities of RBC and plasma in the cerebral hemodymanics in ischemic brain edema. We sought to clarify the relationships among blood flow, blood volume, flow velocities of RBC and plasma, and brain edema in the adjacent cortical gray matter made variably ischemic.

Materials and Methods

Sprague-Dawley rats were anesthetized with ketamine (40 mg/kg) and xylazine (10 mg/kg). Focal cerebral ischemia was induced by occlusion of the left middle cerebral artery (MCA) for 24 hours in 30 rats. Twenty sham operated rats served as controls. The measurements were begun after recovery from anesthesia. Regional cerebral blood flow (rCBF) was measured by the ^{14}C-iodoantipyrine technique. The distribution spaces of RBC and plasma in cerebral microvessels were determined by quantitative radioluminography using ^{51}Cr-RBC (100 µCi) and ^{125}I-bovine serum albumin (50 µCi), previously described elsewhere [7]. The volumes of RBC (Vr) and plasma (Vp) were calculated by each equation. The blood volume (Vb) and the hematocrit (Hctm) in parenchymal microvessels was given by the formula Vb = Vr + Vp and Hctm = 100 (Vr / Vb), respectively. The mean transit time of blood (Tb), RBC (Tr) and plasma (Tp) was calculated as follows: Tb = Vb / rCBF, Tr = Tt (Hctm) / Hcta, and Tp = Tt (1-Hctm) / (1-Hcta), respectively, where Hcta is the hematocrit of arterial blood. They were regarded as indicators of the flow velocities of blood, RBC and plasma. Brain water content was measured by specific gravity method. The inner periphery and outer periphery were identified in the forelimb area of the frontal cortex adjacent to the MCA territory and in the hindlimb area, respectively for histologic analysis. The core was the central area of the parietal cortex. The non-ischemic cortical tissue was area 1 of the frontal cortex.

Results

Regional Cerebral Blood Flow

The blood flow in the control was 185.90 ± 2.56 ml/100 g/min in the frontal cortex and 195.36 ± 2.35 ml/100 g/min in the parietal cortex. In the MCA occlusion animals, the blood flow in the core and that in the inner periphery was markedly reduced to 4.65 ± 0.53 and 11.21 ± 0.79 ml/100 g/min, respectively. In contrast, the outer periphery surrounding the MCA territory showed a moderate reduction in the blood flow, to 73.60 ± 3.35 ml/100 g/min. Furthermore, the blood flow was decreased, to 108.12 ± 4.39 ml/100 g/min, even in the non-ischemic tissue. Thus, a gradient change of flow rates between the ischemic and normal tissues was observed.

Water Content in the Brain Tissue

The water content was markedly increased in the core and the inner periphery. In contrast, there was no significant increase in water content in the outer periphery or in the non-ischemic tissue.

Red Blood Cell and Plasma Volumes

The volumes of RBC and plasma in the rats with MCA occlusion and in the control rats are shown in Fig. 1. The RBC and plasma volume in the cortical gray matter areas of control rats ranged from 2.45 ± 0.23 to 3.22 ± 0.37 µl/g and from 6.51 ± 0.36 to 7.13 ± 0.47 µl/g, respectively (Fig. 2). The volume of plasma was about 2.5-fold and consistently larger than

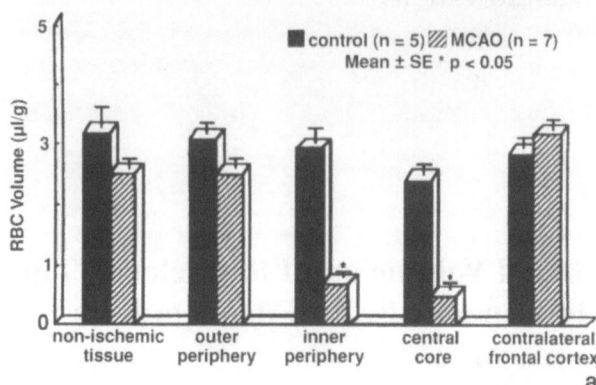

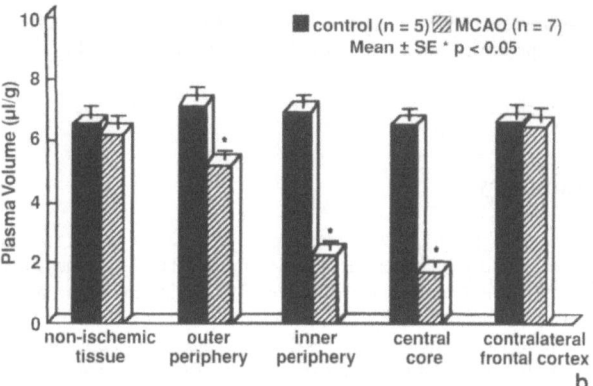

Fig. 1. Changes in the volumes of red blood cells (a) and plasma (b) 24 hours after middle cerebral artery occlusion (MCAO) and sham operation (control). *P* Statistical significance from values with control

that of the RBC. In the MCA occlusion animals, the RBC and plasma volumes in the ischemic core were markedly decreased to 0.50 ± 0.11 and 1.73 ± 0.17 µl/g, respectively. They were similar to those in the inner periphery. In contrast, the plasma volume in the outer periphery was decreased slightly to 5.22 ± 0.26 µl/g, but the RBC volume was 2.55 ± 0.25 µl/g and did not change significantly. In the non-ischemic tissue, the RBC volume was 2.56 ± 0.20 µl/g and the plasma volume was 6.22 ± 0.39 µl/g, which were the same as those in the control.

Blood Volume and Microvascular Hematocrit

In the MCA occlusion animals, a marked reduction in blood volume was observed in the central core and the inner periphery. The average blood volume was 2.23 µl/g in the central core and 2.95 µl/g in the inner periphery, due to the decrease in both RBC and plasma volumes. In contrast, the blood volume in the outer periphery was decreased slightly to 7.77 µl/g and this was related to the decrease in plasma volume. In the

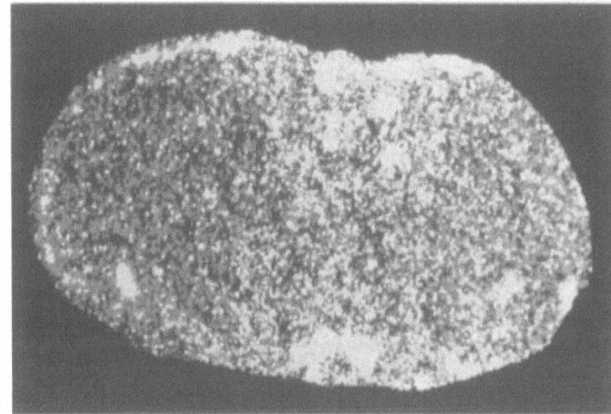

a

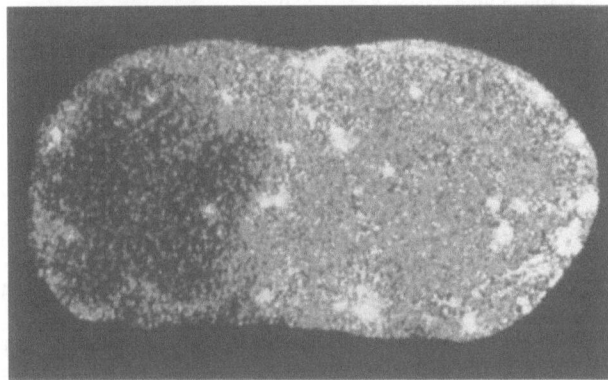

b

Fig. 2. Coronal sections of brain on ^{51}Cr-RBC radioluminogram (a) and ^{125}I-BSA radioluminogram (b) 24 hours after middle cerebral artery occlusion

non-ischemic tissue, the blood volume was 8.78 μl/g, similar to that in the control.

The average microvascular hematocrit was 30% in the cortical gray matter areas of control rats, which value was about 64% of the larger, vessel hematocrit. In the MCA occlusion animals, the microvascular hematocrit was much lower in the ischemic core and the inner periphery. The value was 22% in the central core. In the outer periphery, in contrast, the hematocrit was slightly higher at 33%. The hematocrit in the non-ischemic tissue was 29%, being the same as the control value.

Mean Transit Times of RBC and Plasma

The mean transit times of RBC and plasma through the parenchymal microvessels of control rats ranged from 0.16 to 0.22 second (s) and from 0.37 to 0.43 s, respectively. The transit time of RBCs was consistantly shorter than that of plasma. MCA occlusion markedly lengthened the mean transit times of both RBC and plasma within the ischemic tissue, to 1.36 s and 4.24 s,

respectively. In contrast, the mean transit time of RBC in the outer periphery increased twofold to 0.44 s The increment was more pronounced than that in the plasma transit time, which contrasts with other areas. In the non-ischemic tissue, the mean transit times of RBC and plasma lengthened slightly to 0.30 s and 0.66 s, respectively.

Discussion

We evaluated the RBC and plasma volumes in cerebral microvessels with ^{51}Cr-RBC and ^{125}I-BSA radioluminogram. This new quantitative radioluminography method employs a highly sensitive sensor imaging plate for radionuclides instead of conventional X-ray film [1]. Therefore, this technique can be applied with shorter exposure time and smaller doses of radionuclides when compared with X-ray film autoradiography [7, 8]. We believe that the distribution spaces of ^{51}Cr and ^{125}I in the cerebral microvessels with diameter less than 50 μm can be successfully determined with quantitative radioluminography, to a similar or better extent than with autoradiography.

We have demonstrated that focal ischemia has variable effects on the distributions of RBC and plasma, flow velocities, and blood volume in the parenchymal microvessels depending on the depth of blood flow and edema. There is no simple direct correlation between any of the blood flow, volumes and flow velocities of RBCs and plasma in ischemic brain edema.

In the present study, the blood volume decreased markedly while the mean transit time of blood increased within the ischemic tissue where the blood flow was markedly reduced and brain edema was severe. This reduction of the blood volume, including both RBC and plasma volumes, is probably due to the decrease in the number of perfused microvessels by which capillary retirement appears to occur. Furthermore, the microvascular hematocrit decreased to 22%. This implies only plasma flows in some remaining capillaries. These plasma-containing capillaries could be the result of greater flow resistance. Thus, the large reduction in blood flow is primarily attributed to a reduced perfusion of microvessels compressed by brain edema in addition to lowering of the perfusion pressure.

On the other hand, in the outer peripheral zone surrounding the ischemic tissue where blood flow was moderately reduced but brain edema was not induced, the plasma volume was somewhat decreased whereas RBC volume did not change significantly.

This slight decrease in plasma volume may be related to capillary narrowing or the diminished number of perfused capillaries, or both. This drop in plasma volume, however, is not matched by a decrease in blood flow. The mean transit time of RBC increased 2.1-fold and that of plasma by 1.87-fold. The microvascular hematocrit was 32% and increased slightly. This finding indicates a change in the distribution of plasma and RBC among the population of perfused capillaries. The flow velocity of RBC decelerates faster than that of plasma. The main mechanism of this moderate reduction in blood flow is probably the decreased velocity of blood flow, which is greater for RBC flow than plasma flow.

In the non-ischemic tissue outside the MCA territory, where blood flow was decreased by 42% compared to control and brain edema was not induced, none of the volumes of RBC and plasma, and the microvessel hematocrit showed any significant change. All capillaries were perfused by both RBC and plasma and they seem to be hematic capillaries. The mean transit times of RBC and plasma increased by 36% and 62%, respectively. These findings indicate that the reduction of blood flow is presumably caused by the lowered velocities of RBC and plasma flows and not by a decreased number of perfused parenchymal microvessels.

References

1. Amemiya Y, Miyahara J (1988) Imaging plate illuminates many fields. Nature 336: 89–90
2. Bereczki D, Wei L, Ostuka T, Hans FJ, Acuff V, Patlak C, Fenstermacher J (1993) Hypercapnia slightly raises blood volume and sizably elevates flow velocity in brain microvessels. Am J Physiol 264: H1360–1524
3. Gobel U, Theilen H, Kuschinsky W (1990) Congruence of total and perfused capillary network in rat brains. Circ Res 66: 271–281
4. Hatashita S, Hoff JT (1986) Role of a hydrostatic pressure gradient in the formation of early ischemic brain edema. J Cereb Blood Flow Metab 6: 546–552
5. Hatashita S, Hoff JT, Salamat SM (1988) Ischemic brain edema and the osmotic gradient between blood and brain. J Cereb Blood Flow Metab 8: 552–559
6. Hatashita S, Hoff JT (1990) Brain edema and cerebrovascular permeability during cerebral ischemia in rats. Stroke 21: 582–588
7. Ishimaru S, Hatashita S, Tajima A, Ueno H, Sato H, Takahashi S (1995) New quantitative assessment for regional red blood cell volume through parechmal microvessels in normal rats using radioluminography. J Cereb Blood Flow Metab [Suppl] 15: S637
8. Tajima A, Nakata H, Lin S-Z, Acuff V, Fenstermacher J (1992) Differences and similarities in albumin and red blood cell flows through cerebral microvessels. Am J Physiol 262: H1515–1524
9. Wei L, Ostuka T, Acuff V, Bereczki D, Pettigrew K, Patlak C, Fenstermacher J (1993) The velocities of red cell and plasma flows through parenchymal microvessels of rat brain are decreased by pentobarbital. J Cereb Blood Flow Metab 13: 487–497

Correspondence: Shizuo Hatashita, M.D., Neurosurgery, Juntendo University Urayasu Hospital, 2-1-1 Tomioka, Urayasu 279, Japan.

Acta Neurochir (1997) [Suppl] 70: 27–29
© Springer-Verlag 1997

Hyperglycemia and the Vascular Effects of Cerebral Ischemia

N. Kawai[1], **R. F. Keep**[1], and **A. Lorris Betz**[1, 2]

Department of [1] Surgery (Neurosurgery) and [2] Pediatrics and Neurology, University of Michigan, Ann Arbor, MI, U.S.A.

Summary

Hyperglycemia generally enhances cerebral ischemic injury. Most research has focused on the adverse effect of increased lactate production (acidosis) leading to neuronal injury. The effects of hyperglycemia on another possible primary target, the cerebral microvasculature, is examined in this study. Focal cerebral ischemia was achieved by thread occlusion of the middle cerebral artery (MCA). Preischemic hyperglycemia was induced by intraperitoneal administration of 50% of D-glucose solution. In contrast to normoglycemic controls, glucose-injected rats showed a well demarcated pale infarct after 2 or 4 hours of ischemia reflecting a reduction in cerebral plasma volume (CPV) to 73 ± 9 and $55 \pm 6\%$ of the contralateral hemisphere by 2 and 4 hours respectively. Cerebral blood flow (CBF) measured by laser-Doppler flowmetry indicated that after the initial decline in CBF with MCA occlusion, hyperglycemia led to a further progressive reduction during ischemia. On reperfusion, hyperglycemia resulted in poor restoration of CBF, increased occurrence of hemorrhagic infarction (12 of 12) and a large infarct volume. Hyperglycemia induces progressive cerebrovascular changes during ischemia and affects hemodynamic recovery on reperfusion. These changes may contribute to the adverse effects of hyperglycemia in stroke. A reduction in CPV may be a useful indicator of an increased incidence of hemorrhagic infarction after thrombolytic therapy for ischemic stroke.

Keywords: Ischemia; hyperglycemia; MCA occlusion; cerebral microvasculature.

Introduction

Hyperglycemia generally enhances cerebral ischemic injury [2]. This had usually been attributed to the potentially adverse effects of neuronal acidosis due to increased lactate production [1]. However, the effects of lactate itself in producing brain damage also has been questioned since brain lactate does not correlate with ischemic damage [5].

In our early studies on rat middle cerebral artery (MCA) occlusion, it was noted that hyperglycemic animals had a very well demarcated pale infarct after 4 hours of ischemia in contrast to normoglycemic rats. In this study, we examined whether this apparent differ-

ence was due to cerebrovascular effects of hyperglycemia, including changes in blood volume, and cerebral blood flow during ischemia and reperfusion.

Materials and Methods

Animal Preparations and Experimental Protocols

Adult male Sprague-Dawley rats weighing 250–300 g were used for all experiment. Rats were anesthetized with sodium pentobarbital (50 mg/kg, i.p.). The MCA was occluded using the suture method of Zea Longa *et al.* [9]. Acute hyperglycemia was induced by intraperitoneal administration of 2 ml of 50% D-glucose 20 minutes prior to MCA occlusion. Normoglycemic rats received a similar osmotic load of mannitol. Cerebral plasma volume (CPV) was determined using ^{3}H-inulin after 1, 2 and 4 hours of permanent occlusion and cerebral blood flow (CBF) using ^{14}C-iodoantipyrine after 4 hours of occlusion with and without 2 hours of reperfusion. Furthermore, CBF was continuously measured by laser-Doppler flowmetry (LDF) throughout 2 hours of occlusion followed by 2 hours of reperfusion. Finally, to determine the effects of hyperglycemia on brain injury, brain infarct volume was measured using 2,3,5-triphenyltetrazolium (TTC) after 4 hours of ischemia and 2 hours of reperfusion.

Cerebral Plasma Volume

Twenty µCi of ^{3}H-inulin, a plasma volume marker, was injected into the femoral vein and allowed to circulate for 2 minutes. At the end of the experiment, plasma and both ipsilateral and contralateral cortex from the center of the MCA distribution were sampled. The samples were weighed and counted in a scintillation counter. The CPV was calculated as (dpm / g brain) / (dpm / ml plasma).

Cerebral Blood Flow Measurement

For continuous CBF measurement, an LDF monitor was used. Flow was measured in an ischemic core area located 6 mm lateral to the midline and 1 mm posterior to the bregma. A stable baseline CBF reading was obtained for at least 20 minutes before MCA occlusion. LDF values were averaged over 10-second intervals and recorded every 20 minutes during the occlusion. The CBF values were expressed as percentage of the baseline value.

Absolute CBF values were obtained with 10 µCi of 4-[N-methyl-^{14}C]-iodoantipyrine. Animal preparation was as for the CPV measurement except for the placement of an arterial cannula for blood withdrawal during the 10 second circulation of the isotope. Blood flow was calculated as:

$$Fb / Mb \doteq Qb\ (T) \cdot Fs / Qs\ (T) \cdot Mb$$

where Fb = the brain blood flow; Mb = the brain mass (g); Qb (T) = the quantity of indicator in the tissue at time T; Fs = the rate of blood withdrawal from t = 0 to t = T; Qs (T) = the quantity of indicator present in the withdrawal at time T.

Brain Infarct Volume

The volume of cerebral infarction was quantified using TTC staining. The brains were sectioned coronally at 2-mm intervals. All slices were incubated for 20 minutes in 2% solution of TTC at 37°C. Using a computerized image analysis system (NIH image, version 1.55), the infarct area of each section was determined and the lesion volume was calculated by multiplying by the distance between sections.

Results

In hyperglycemic rats, there was a demarcated infarct after 2 hours of MCA occlusion and a more evident white infarct after 4 hours of occlusion. This was not evident in normoglycemic rats. The cause of this difference appears to be blood volume. In hyperglycemic rats, the CPV of the ischemic tissue progressively declined with time, being $89 \pm 5\%$ of contralateral at 1 hour, but 73 ± 9 and $55 \pm 6\%$ at 2 and 4 hours respectively (Fig. 1). In contrast, there was no significant differences between ipsilateral and contralateral tissue at any time points in normoglycemic rats.

Hyperglycemia was also associated with changes in ischemic CBF. After 20 minutes of MCA occlusion,

laser-Doppler flow was reduced to 16 to 18% of the baseline in normoglycemic and hyperglycemic rats. However, while flow in the normoglycemic rats remained constant over the next two hours, that in the hyperglycemic rats showed a progressive decline over the first hour following occlusion (to 9%; Table 1). The differences in flow between the two groups were significant at the time points between 40 and 120 minutes. During 2 hours of reperfusion following 2 hours of ischemia, blood flow only returned 27 to 45% of baseline in hyperglycemic rats, in contrast to the normoglycemic rats, where flow recovered to 67 to 115% of baseline.

Measurements with ^{14}C-iodoantipyrine indicated a similar pattern. In the contralateral hemisphere, CBF at 4 hours after MCA occlusion was not significantly different between normoglycemic and hyperglycemic rats (58 + 3 and 58 + 5 ml/100 g/min respectively) and although the CBF in the ipsilateral tissue was about half in the hyperglycemic compared to normoglycemic rats (8 ± 2 and 15 ± 3 ml/100 g/min), this did not reach

Table 1. *Cerebral Blood Flow from the Ischemic Core*

	Hyperglycemia (glucose) n = 4	Normoglycemia (mannitol) n = 4
Baseline	100	100
Ischemia (min)		
20	16.3 ± 2.6	18.3 ± 2.8
40	11.8 ± 1.5^a	18.0 ± 1.4
60	$9.0 \pm 1.5^{b,\,c}$	21.9 ± 2.8
80	$8.2 \pm 1.0^{b,\,c}$	18.0 ± 1.9
100	$8.7 \pm 1.5^{b,\,c}$	17.5 ± 2.4
120	$8.3 \pm 1.3^{b,\,c}$	17.7 ± 2.8
Reperfusion (min)		
20	45.0 ± 8.0^a	115.0 ± 24.4
40	39.3 ± 7.0^b	91.4 ± 13.9
60	36.7 ± 5.8^b	97.2 ± 11.5
80	27.0 ± 3.6^b	73.2 ± 12.4
100	27.6 ± 2.7^b	67.0 ± 5.5
120	34.3 ± 4.3^a	80.9 ± 13.7

Measurements were made continuously with laser-Doppler flowmetry throughout 2 hours of MCA occlusion followed by 2 hours of reperfusion and expressed as a percent of baseline (preischemic) value. All values are mean ± SE.
[a, b] Indicate a significant difference (p < 0.05 and p < 0.01 levels respectively) between the two groups.
[c] Indicates a significant difference (p < 0.05) between the value at 20 minutes after MCA occlusion and other time points in glucose-injected rats.

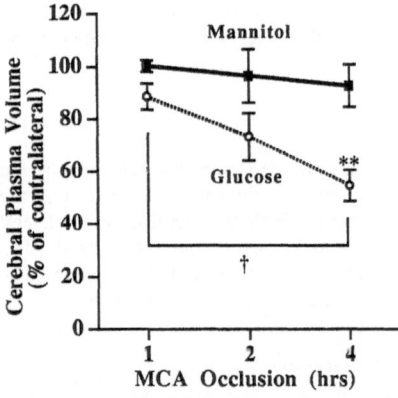

Fig. 1. Cerebral plasma volume in the ischemic core samples from glucose- and mannitol-injected rats. Measurements were made with ^{3}H-inulin after 1, 2 and 4 hours of MCA occlusion and are expressed as a percent of non-ischemic (contralateral) tissue. Values are mean ± S.E.; n = 5–10; ** indicates a significant difference (p < 0.01) between the two groups; † indicates a significant difference (p < 0.05) between the value at one hour and 4 hours occlusion in glucose-injected rats

significance. However, after 4 hours of temporary occlusion and 2 hours of reperfusion, hyperglycemia led to poor reperfusion compared to normoglycemic rats (24 ± 8 and 66 ± 10 ml/100 g/min respectively; $p < 0.01$).

After 4 hours of ischemia and 2 hours of reperfusion, the total TTC lesion volume in the glucose-injected group was 158 ± 38 mm^3, significantly larger than the mannitol-injected group (39 ± 23 mm^3; $p < 0.001$). Hyperglycemia also affected the occurrence of hemorrhagic infarction. Following 4 hours of ischemia and 2 hours reperfusion, all of 12 hyperglycemic rats showed hemorrhagic conversion in the ischemic tissue, whereas only one hemorrhage was observed in 7 normoglycemic rats ($p < 0.01$).

Discussion

The present study indicates that hyperglycemia induces progressive cerebrovascular changes during ischemia and can affect hemodynamic recovery on reperfusion. This may be important in both the understanding and the treatment of ischemic events during ischemia.

A well demarcated pale infarct was observed after 2 or 4 hours of ischemia in hyperglycemic rats. This appears to be due to a decrease in cerebral blood volume in the ischemic tissue as shown in the CPV measurements. As well as changes in cerebral blood volume, the laser-Doppler flow measurements indicate that hyperglycemia also affects CBF during ischemia and during reperfusion. Although marked reductions in CBF during reperfusion have been reported in hyperglycemic animals [4, 8], changes during ischemia have not.

The decline in ischemic CBF in hyperglycemic rats occurred over the first hour of MCA occlusion and, thus, appears to precede the decline in CPV that was only first observed at two hours. This could mean that the change in CBF leads to the change in CPV since well defined CBF thresholds are of critical importance in the development of irreversible ischemic damage [7]. Alternatively, both CBF and cerebral blood volume changes may reflect progressive endothelial damage. Paljärvi et al. [5] examined the effect of acute hyperglycemia on endothelial cells after global ischemia and reperfusion. They reported endothelial swelling and decreased luminal diameter in hyperglycemic rats and postulated that such endothelial swelling

could lead to capillary occlusion and hamper post-ischemic perfusion.

Hyperglycemia at the time of cerebral ischemia increases the risk of hemorrhage on reperfusion [3]. Cerebral hemorrhage has been the major complication for thrombolytic therapy for ischemic stroke and parameters that might be used to indicate the risk of hemorrhage could have major clinical importance. In our studies, the increased risk of hemorrhage on reperfusion in hyperglycemic rats was associated with a marked reduction in CPV during ischemia. It is possible, therefore, that CPV could be a useful predictor of an enhanced risk of hemorrhage in thrombolytic therapy for ischemic stroke.

Acknowledgemets

Supported by grants NS-23870 and NS-34709 from the National Institutes of Health.

References

1. Chopp M, Welch KMA, Tidwell CD, Helpern JA (1988) Global cerebral ischemia and intracellular pH during hyperglycemia and hypoglycemia in cats. Stroke 19: 1383–1387
2. de Courten-Myers G, Myers RE, Schoolfield L (1988) Hyperglycemia enlarges infarct size in cerebrovascular occlusion in cats. Stroke 19: 623–630
3. de Courten-Myers GM, Kleinholz M, Holm P, DeVoe G, Schmitt G, Wagner KR, Myers RE (1992) Hemorrhagic infarct conversion in experimental stroke. Ann Emerg Med 21: 120–126
4. Ginsberg MD, Welsh FA, Budd WW (1980) Deleterious effect of glucose pretreatment on recovery from diffuse cerebral ischemia in the cat. Stroke 11: 347–354
5. Lin B, Busto R, Globus MY-T, Martinez E, Ginsberg MD (1995) Brain temperature modulations during global ischemia fail to influence extracellular lactate levels in rats. Stroke 26: 1634–1638
6. Paljärvi L, Rehncrona S, Söderfeldt B, Olsson Y, Kalimo H (1983) Brain lactic acidosis and ischemic cell damage: quantitative ultrastuctural changes in capillaries of rat cerebral cortex. Acta Neuropathol (Berl) 60: 232–240
7. Tamura A, Asano T, Sano K (1980) Correlation between rCBF and histological changes following temporary middle cerebral artery occlusion. Stroke 11: 487–493
8. Venables GS, Miller SA, Gibson G, Hardy JA, Strong AJ (1985) The effects of hyperglycaemia on changes during reperfusion following focal cerebral ischemia in the cat. J Neurol Neurosurg Psychiatry 48: 663–669
9. Zea Longa E, Weinstein PR, Carlson S, Cummins R (1989) Reversible middle cerebral artery occlusion without craniotomy in rats. Stroke 20: 84–91

Correspondence: Richard F. Keep, Ph.D., Department of Surgery (Neurosurgery), University of Michigan, R5605 Kresge I, Ann Arbor, MI 48109-0532, U.S.A.

Acta Neurochir (1997) [Suppl] 70: 30–33
© Springer-Verlag 1997

The Effect of Non-Competitive N-Methyl-D-Aspartate Receptor Antagonism on Cerebral Oedema and Cerebral Infarct Size in the Aging Ischaemic Brain

M. Davis, R. H. Perry, and **A. D. Mendelow**

Departments of Surgery (Neurosurgery), Medicine (Geriatrics) and Neuropathology, University of Newcastle upon Tyne, England, U.K.

Summary

Although vulnerability to ischemic neuronal injury is enhanced with age, the aging brain may be less amenable to neuroprotection as a result of quantitative and qualitative changes in the NMDA receptor. In addition, the elderly may be less tolerant of adverse effects of neuroprotective drugs and this might ultimately limit therapeutic potential in human stroke. However, antagonism of the excitotoxic effects of glutamate by parenteral administration of the non competitive NMDA antagonist magnesium has been well tolerated and has shown to be neuroprotective in young animal models of stroke and head injury. We therefore evaluated the potential of magnesium chloride to reduce ischemic neuronal injury in aged rodents subjected to permanent occlusion of the middle cerebral artery.

Treatment with magnesium chloride induced hypotension and hyperglycaemia in both adult and aged rats and did not reduce ischemic neuronal injury or cerebral edema. However, despite these adverse haemodynamic and biochemical effects, which may augment cerebral infarct size, ischemic damage was not exacerbated in the treated groups, suggesting that magnesium has the potential to salvage penumbral neurons and that inotropic support and maintenance of normoglycaemia may permit realisation of its neuroprotective potential. This may have important implications for future clinical stroke trials.

Keywords: NMDA receptor; antagonism; ischemia; aging brain.

Introduction

Stroke is predominantly a disease of the elderly and potential neuroprotective strategies should therefore be evaluated in experimental models of a relevant age. Under similar experimental conditions, aged animals have been shown to develop significantly larger cerebral infarcts than adults after proximal occlusion of the left middle cerebral artery [5]. However, despite an age related decline in both the density and function of N-Methyl-D-aspartate (NMDA) receptors [21], competitive antagonists of this receptor have exhibited neuroprotective properties in focal ischaemic lesions of the aged brain [5]. This is thought to be effected via antagonism of the excitotoxic activity of glutamate at the neurotransmitter recognition site on the NMDA receptor, with subsequent inhibition of calcium influx.

Both competitive and noncompetitive glutamate antagonists induce several adverse effects, which include behavioral disturbances, movement disorders and cardiorespiratory depression. This may be of particular importance in the elderly, in whom susceptibility to treatment side effects may be enhanced, with subsequent Limitation of therapeutic potential. Magnesium exerts a voltage dependent blockade of the ion channel on the NMDA receptor and under normal resting membrane potentiale, it prevents calcium influx via this route [13]. As nature's NMDA receptor antagonist, it may limit excitotoxicity in association with fewer adverse side effects, and has been shown to be neuroprotective in young experimental models of head injury [12] and occlusive stroke [9]. We hypothesised that magnesium would be well tolerated in aged animals and that it would reduce focal ischaemic neuronal injury following middle cerebral artery occlusion in the aging brain.

Materials and Methods

The experiments were conducted in accordance with the Animals (Scientific Procedures) Act 1986, in adult (< 17 months) and aged (30 month) male Wistar rats. Anaesthesia was induced by the inhalation of 4% halothane in a mixture of nitrous oxide and oxygen (70/30) and after intubation, was maintained using 1–2% halothane, with reduction to 0.4% subsequent to all surgical procedures. Ventilation was monitored continuously via pulse oximetry and a capnograph. Core temperature was maintained using a heating pad and a rectal thermistor probe. The femoral vessels were cannulated for the monitoring of mean arterial blood pressure, the measurement of arterial blood gases, glucose and haematocrit, and the administration of drugs and fluid. The left middle cerebral artery was exposed via a microcraniectomy according to the technique of Tamura, but with preservation of the zygomatic arch [18], and the vessel was occluded by thermocoagulation using microbipolar diathermy, proximal to the origin of the lenticulostriate branch. Ischemic damage was assessed histologically, with perfusion fixation of the animals 6 hours after left middle cerebral artery occlusion (LMCAO), using 40% formaldehyde / glacial acetic acid / methanol (FAM 1 : 1 : 8). The brains were removed, embedded in paraffin wax, sectioned at 20 μm intervals, stained alternately with hematoxylin and eosin and cresyl fast violet, and analyzed by light microscopy. Those sections corresponding to eight predetermined stereotactic levels were used to map the infarction on line diagrams. The ischemic areas were measured by a video plan image analyzer. The infarct volume was calculated by integrating the ischemic areas at each coronal section over their anteroposterior coordinates. Specific gravity (SG) was measured as an index of brain edema 4 hours post LMCAO, using calibrated gravimetric columns [10]. A coronal slice (from an identical site corresponding to the bregma in each brain) was used to cut paired 1 mm³ cubes of tissue from the cerebral cortex, caudate nucleus, white matter and cerebellar cortex (which acted as a control) of each hemisphere. Samples were allowed to fall in bromobenzene/kerosene columns and the level of descent at one minute was recorded. The SG was calculated using linear regression analysis derived from calibration of the column with potassium sulphate droplets of known specific gravity.

Adult and aged animals were randomly allocated into treated and untreated groups. Treated animals received an intravenous infusion of magnesium chloride (1 mmol.kg⁻¹) 15 minutes prior to LMCAO, followed by an intraperitoneal injection (1 mmol.kg⁻¹), 1 hour after LMCAO, according to a protocol which has been shown to be neuroprotective in young animals [9]. Untreated animals received similar volumes of saline. Data are presented as means with their standard errors and statistical analysis has been conducted using non-parametric Mann Whitney tests.

Results

Mean Arterial Blood Pressure

Treatment with magnesium led to a significant drop in mean arterial blood pressure within 15 minutes of intraperitoneal administration in both age groups. In the histology experiments, the mean values in treated aged rats were 80 ± 2, 80 ± 2 and 82 ± 3 mmHg, compared with 91 ± 3, 92 ± 3, and 94 ± 2 mmHg in their untreated counterparts at 75, 90 and 105 minutes post LMCAO respectively ($p < 0.05$). In adult animals, the mean values were 76 ± 4 and 82 ± 3 mmHg in the treated group, compared with values of 87 ± 2 and 91 ± 2 in untreated animals at 75 and 90 minutes post LMCAO respectively ($p < 0.05$). A similar haemodynamic response was documented in the treated animals of both age groups during the experiments for analysis of specific gravity.

Blood Glucose

Baseline blood glucose levels were similar in all groups, but rose significantly in the treated groups in the histology experiments to 10.3 ± 0.6 mmol.l⁻¹ in aged rats and 10.5 mmol.l⁻¹ in adults, compared with mean values of 6.2 ± 0.7 mmol.l⁻¹, and 6.5 ± 0.5 mmol.l⁻¹ in their untreated counterparts respectively ($p < 0.01$). A similar hyperglycaemic response was documented following the infusion of magnesium in animals in whom cerebral specific gravity was analysed.

Neuropathology

Aging was associated with a significant increase in cerebral infarct size. The mean infarct volume (expressed as a percentage of the total volume of the left hemisphere) was $39.58 \pm 0.94\%$ in aged untreated rats (n = 6), compared with 27.07 ± 3.32 in untreated adults (n = 7, $p < 0.05$). Treatment with magnesium chloride did not reduce the volume of infarction in either age group. The treated aged group (n = 7) had a mean infarct volume of $37.18 \pm 4.64\%$, whilst the mean value in treated adults (n = 6) was $33.58 \pm 4.75\%$ ($p = 0.94$ and $p = 0.35$ for treated versus untreated aged and adult rats respectively).

Cerebral Specific Gravity

Treatment with magnesium chloride had no significant effect on the SG of the cerebral cortex, caudate nucleus or white matter in either age group (Figs. 1 and 2). Treated aged rats had a mean cortical SG of 1.0404 ± 0.0013, compared with 1.0379 ± 0.0011 in the untreated group ($p = 0.31$). Treated and untreated adults had mean values of 1.0411 ± 0.0008 and 1.0396 ± 0.0012 respectively ($p = 0.15$).

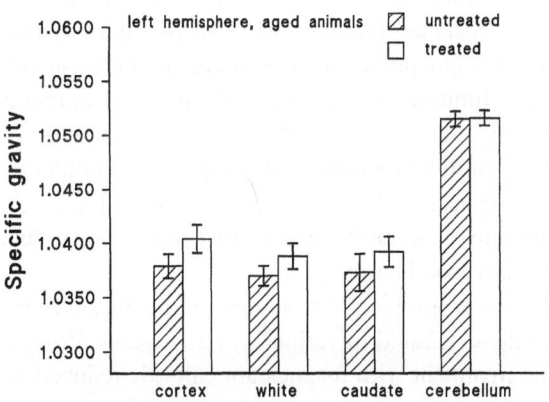

Fig. 1. Bar graph shows the specific gravities of samples from the cerebral cortex, caudate nucleus and white matter in the lesioned left hemisphere of treated (magnesium chloride) and untreated (saline) *aged* rats (no significant difference for treated versus untreated animals)

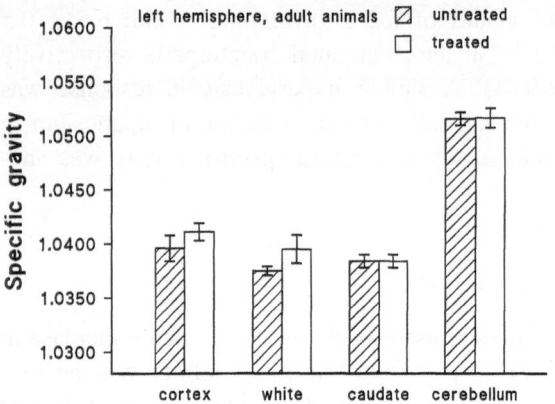

Fig. 2. Bar graph shows the specific gravities of samples from the cerebral cortex, caudate nucleus and white matter in the lesioned left hemisphere of treated (magnesium chloride) and untreated (saline) *adult* rats (no significant difference for treated versus untreated animals)

Discussion

Pre-treatment with magnesium chloride did not confer neuroprotection in either adult or aged animals. The volume of infarcted brain tissue was similar in treated and untreated groups and there was no significant difference in the severity of cerebral oedema. These results were surprising in the light of evidence from both *in vitro* and *in vivo* studies, which has suggested that magnesium may play an important role in limiting the pathogenesis of ischaemic neuronal injury. The magnesium ion is involved in a number of essential cellular processes including glycolysis [8], oxidative phosphorylation [7], protein synthesis, DNA and RNA aggregation [17], and the maintenance of membran integrity [1]. Magnesium also plays an importart role in calcium transport and accumulation [1, 7], and under normal resting membrane potentiale, it acts as nature's NMDA receptor blocker [11, 13]. Magnesium may inhibit presynaptic excitatory amino acid release [14] and can limit the production of glutamate from reductive amination of 2-oxoglutarate, via inhibition of the activity of mitochondrial and synaptosomal glutamate dehydrogenase [10]. Magnesium is also involved in the regulation of smooth muscle tone and may induce cerebral vasodilatation [2, 3].

The neuroprotective potential of magnesium has been demonstrated in various *in vivo* studies. Prophylactic treatment with magnesium chloride reduced focal ischaemic brain damage after MCAO in rats [9], and improved neurological recovery in a fluid percussion model of traumatic brain injury in rodents [12], and in an experimental model of spinal cord ischaemia in rabbits [19]. However, these investigations were conducted in young animals which may explain the leck of haemodynamic changes attributable to drug administration. Infusion of magnesium salts has been associated with cardiodepressant effects [4] and in the current study, magnesium was found to be negatively inotropic in both mature adult and aged rats, suggesting that the ageing myocardium and vasculature are more susceptible to its adverse haemodynamic effects. In experimental stroke and head injury models, hypotension is associated with augmentation of neuronal injury and this would tend to counteract any neuroprotective effect from glutamate receptor antagonism or inhibition of the activity of calcium [16, 17, 20]. The adverse influence of the consequent fall in cerebral perfusion is related to both the severity and duration of ischaemia and hence both aspects of the hypotensive episode are important. The fall in cerebral perfusion is thought to be secondary to loss of cerebral autoregulation, such that cerebral blood flow varies passively with the cerebral perfusion pressure [17, 20].

As well as inducing adverse haemodynamic effects, magnesium may promote hyperglycaemia through suppression of insulin release and this may also exacerbate ischaemic brain damage [6]. The exacerbation of ischaemic neuronal injury is thought to be mediated by anaerobic metabolism of the extra glucose stores, which results in excessive lactic acidosis. In the current study, treated animals had higher blood sugar levels than their untreated counterparts, whilst in Izumi's study in which a neuroprotective effect was demonstrated, magnesium and insulin were administered concurrently to counteract the hyperglycaemic effect. The maintenance of normoglycaemia and normotension in a much younger brain would facilitate the limitation of ischaemic brain damage by magnesium, and may explain the discrepant results.

Although the administration of magnesium did not reduce the volume of cerebral infarction, it may still have conferred a beneficial effect, since despite the cardiodepressant and hyperglycaemic effect, treatment was not associated with enhancement of ischaemic neuronal damage. Inotropic support and maintenance of normoglycemia may therefore be required to realise any neuroprotective potential of magnesium and this may have important implications for future clinical stroke trials.

References

1. Aikawa JK (1981) In: Magnesium: its biological significance. CRC, Boca Raton, pp 21–29

2. Altura BM, Altura BT, Gebrewold A, Ising H, Gunther T (1984) Magnesium-deficient diets and microcirculatory changes *in situ*. Science 223: 1315–1317
3. Altura BT, Altura BM (1981) The role of magnesium in etiology of strokes and cerebrovasospasm. Magnesium 1: 277–291
4. Chaudry IH (1982) Preparation of ATP-MgCl$_2$ and precautions for its use in the study and treatment of shock and ischemia. Am J Physiol 43: R604–R605
5. Davis M, Mendelow AD, Perry RH, Chambers IR, James OFW (1995) Experimental stroke and neuroprotection in the aging rat brain. Stroke 26: 1072–1078
6. Duverger D, MacKenzie ET (1988) The quantification of cerebral infarction following focal ischaemia in the rat: Influence of strain, arterial pressure, blood glucose concentration, and age. J Cereb Blood Flow Metab 8: 449–461
7. Ebel H, Gunther T (1980) Magnesium metabolism: a review. J Clin Chem Clin Biochem 18: 257–270
8. Garfinkel L, Garfinkel D (1985) Magnesium regulation of the glycolytic pathway and the enzymes involved. Magnesium 14: 60–72
9. Izumi (1991) J Cereb Blood Flow Metab 1025
10. Kuo N, Michalik M, Erecinska M (1994) Inhibition of glutamate dehydrogenase in brain mitochondria and synaptosomes by Mg^{++} and polyamines: a possible cause for its low *in vivo* activity. J Neurochem 63: 751–757
11. Mayer ML, Westbrook GL, Guthrie PB (1984) Voltage-dependent block by Mg^{2+} of NMDA responses in spinal cord neurons. Nature 309: 261–263
12. McIntosh TK, Vink R, Weiner M, Faden AI (1987) Alterations in free magnesium, high-energy phosphates and lactate following traumatic brain injury: assessment by nuclear magnetic resonance spectroscopy. J Cereb Blood Flow Metab [Suppl 1]: S620
13. Nowak L, Bregestovski P, Ascher P, Herbelt A, Prochiantz A (1984) Magnesium gates glutamate-activated channels in mouse central neurones. Nature 307: 462–465
14. Rothman SM (1984) Synaptic release of excitatory amino acid neurotransmitter mediates anoxic neuronal death. J Neurosci 4: 1884 1891
15. Rubin H (1976) Magnesium deprivation reproduces the coordinate effects of serum removal or cortisol addition on transport and metabolism in chick embryo fibroblasts. J Cell Physiol 89: 613–626
16. Sundt TM, Waltz AG (1971) Cerebral ischemia and reactive hyperemia: Studies of cortical blood flow and microcirculation before, during and after temporary occlusion of middle cerebral artery of squirrel monkeys. Circ Res 28: 426–431
17. Symon L, Branston NM, Strong AJ (1976) Autoregulation in acute focal ischaemia: an experimental study. Stroke 7: 547–554
18. Tamura A, Graham DI, McCulloch J, Teasdale GM (1981) Focal cerebral ischaemia in the rat: 1. Description of technique and early neuropathological consequences following middle cerebral artery occlusion. J Cereb Blood Flow Metab 1: 53–60
19. Vacanti FX, Adelbert A (1984) Mild hypothermia and magnesium protect against irreversible damage during CNS ischemia. Stroke 15: 695–698
20. Waltz AG (1968) Effect of blood pressure on blood flow in ischaemic and in non-ischaemic cerebral cortex. The phenomena of autoregulation and luxury perfusion. Neurology 18: 613–621
21. Wenk GE, Walker LC, Price DE, Cork LC (1991) Loss of NMDA but not GABA-A binding in the brains of aged rats and monkeys. Neurobiol Aging 12: 93–98

Correspondence: Dr. Michelle Davis, c/o Professor A. D. Mendelow, The Regional Neurosciences Centre, Newcastle General Hospital, Westgate Road, Newcastle upon Tyne, England, U.K.

Acta Neurochir (1997) [Suppl] 70: 34–36
© Springer-Verlag 1997

Effects of Hyperglycemia on Cerebral Blood Flow and Edema Formation After Carotid Artery Occlusion in Fischer 344 Rats

N. Kawai[1], R. F. Keep[2], and A. L. Betz[1,2]

Department of [1] Surgery (Neurosurgery) and [2] Pediatrics and Neurology, University of Michigan, Ann Arbor, MI, U.S.A.

Summary

This study examines whether during bilateral carotid artery occlusion in Fischer 344 rats, hyperglycemia induces cerebrovascular changes that enhance brain edema formation. Preischemic hyperglycemia was induced by intraperitoneal administration of D-glucose solution. Laser-Doppler flowmetry, indicated that after the initial decline in blood flow with carotid occlusion ($36 \pm 4\%$ of preischemic), hyperglycemic but not control rats showed a further progressive decrease to $19 \pm 2\%$ of preischemic at 120 minutes ($p < 0.001$). Brain water content was significantly higher in hyper-compared to normoglycemic rats after both 2 hours of permanent occlusion (3.86 ± 0.05 vs. 3.73 ± 0.03 g/g dry wt.; $p < 0.05$) and 2 hours of temporary occlusion followed by 1 hour of reperfusion (4.01 ± 0.08 vs. 3.71 ± 0.03 g/g dry wt.; $p < 0.05$). The difference in brain edema formation between normo-and hyperglycemic rats appears to primarily reflect the effects of hyperglycemia on CBF. Cerebral plasma volume (CPV) 2 hours after occlusion was also reduced in hyper-compared to normoglycemic rats (3.9 ± 0.9 and 7.2 ± 0.1 μl/g; $p < 0.01$). Thus, hyperglycemia in a model of global ischemia induces a reduction in CPV and progressive decline in CBF. In this model, the decline in CBF is of sufficient magnitude to enhance brain injury as evidenced by edema formation.

Keywords: Hyperglycemia; cerebral blod flow (CBF); brain edema; ischemia.

Introduction

Hyperglycemia has been shown to worsen cerebral injury in several ischemic models. In a rat model of the middle cerebral artery (MCA) occlusion with an intraluminal monofilament, our studies have shown that hyperglycemia induces progressive cerebrovascular changes during ischemia and affects hemodynamic recovery on reperfusion, resulting in a larger infarct area [4]. In this model, however, it is possible that the nylon monofilament used to occlude the MCA might cause endothelial injury and induce thrombus formation, thus trampering the microcirculation during ischemia and reperfusion.

Following bilateral carotid occlusion in Fischer 344 rats, a significant reduction in cerebral blood flow (CBF) was observed in the cerebral cortex [1] and produced subsequent brain edema formation [6]. This model has the advantages of ease of surgical preparation and instituting cerebral recirculation without endothelial injury in the cerebral vasculature. Using this model, we examined whether hyperglycemia induces similar cerebrovascular changes as in MCA occlusion during ischemia and reperfusion. We also determined whether the effects of hyperglycemia are of a magnitude to alter brain edema formation during ischemia and reperfusion.

Materials and Methods

Animal Preparation and Experimental Protocols

Adult male Fischer 344 rats weighing 200–250 g were used for all experiments. Rats were anesthetized for surgery with sodium pentobarbital (50 mg/kg i.p.). Global ischemia was produced by a bilateral occlusion of the common carotid artery. Hyperglycemia was induced 20 minutes prior to the onset of ischemia by intraperitoneal injection of 1.5 ml of 50% D-glucose solution. Normoglycemic rats received D-mannitol solution to simulate this osmotic load. Control animals were subjected to a sham operation and received either glucose or mannitol solution.

Rats were used for two sets of experiment. In experiment one, to examine the effect of hyperglycemia on edema formation, brain water content in each hemisphere was determined after 2 hours of permanent occlusion (p-CCAO) or 2 hours of temporary occlusion followed by 1 hour of reperfusion (t-CCAO). Controls were used to determine the effect of glucose and mannitol solution itself on brain water content after 2 hours of sham operation. In experiment two, to examine the effect of hyperglycemia on cerebral plasma volume (CPV), CPV was measured using ^{3}H-inulin after 2 hours of permanent occlusion. All rats were subjected to continuous measurement of CBF by a laser-Doppler flowmetry (LDF).

Cerebral Blood Flow Measurement

An LDF monitor (Vasamedics, BPM2) equipped with a small caliber probe of 0.7 mm in diameter (Vasamedics, P-433) was used for continuous CBF measurement. Flow was measured in the ischemic core area located 6 mm lateral to the midline and 1 mm posterior to the bregma. A stable baseline CBF reading was obtained for at least 20 minutes before carotid occlusion. CBF was determined immediately after the occlusion (5–7 minutes after occlusion) and then continuously recorded during the experiment. At intervals of 20 minutes, the displayed value of LDF was recorded and expressed as percentage of the baseline value.

Cerebral Plasma Volume

Fifteen μCi of ^{3}H-inulin, a plasma volume marker, was injected into the femoral vein and allowed to circulate for 2 minutes. At the end of experiment, a terminal plasma sample was taken and the rat was killed by decapitation. The cortices were rapidly removed, weighed and digested for scintillation counting. The CPV was calculated as (dpm / g brain) / (dpm / ml plasma).

Brain Water Content

After 2 hours of occlusion with or without 1 hour of reperfusion, rats were killed by decapitation. The brain was removed rapidly and divided into cortex and basal ganglia. These samples were weighed and then dried at 95°C for 24 hours to obtain the dry weight. The brain water content was calculated as (wet weight – dry weight) / dry weight.

Results

Laser-Doppler flow measurements indicated that bilateral occlusion of the carotid arteries produced a rapid fall in the cortical blood flow. After the initial decline (36 ± 4% of preischemic at 5–7 minutes), hyperglycemic rats showed a further progressive decrease to 19 ± 2% of preischemic values at 120 minutes after occlusion (Table 1). In normoglycemic rats, however, the initial decline on occlusion was similar (34 ± 4% of preischemic) and there was no significant change in CBF during ischemia, being 29 ± 2% of preischemic at 120 minutes after occlusion. At time points from 20 minutes to 120 minutes, LDF was significantly lower in hyper-compared to normoglycemic rats ($p < 0.001$).

Brain water contents were not significantly different in sham-operated hyper- and normoglycemic rats (3.68 ± 0.01 and 3.64 ± 0.02 g/g dry wt.). Following p-CCAO, brain water content was significantly higher in hyperglycemic arts (3.86 ± 0.05 g/g dry wt.) compared to normoglycemic rats (3.73 ± 0.03 g/g dry wt.; $p < 0.05$). This was more evident in t-CCAO, being 4.01 ± 0.08 g/g dry wt. in hyperglycemic rats and 3.71 ± 0.03 g/g dry wt. in normoglycemic rats ($p < 0.05$). In order to determine whether the enhanced edema formation in hyperglycemic rats was secondary to the effects of hyperglycemia on CBF, brain water content was compared in hyperand normoglycemic rats where CBF was in the normoglycemic range. There was no significant difference in brain water content between the normo- and hyperglycemic groups in either p-CCAO (3.70 ± 0.04 vs. 3.77 ± 0.04 g/g dry wt.) or t-CCAO (3.72 ± 0.03 vs. 3.81 ± 0.03 g/g/dry wt.).

Table 1. *Laser-Doppler Cerebral Blood Flow*

	min	Hyperglycemia (glucose) n = 40 (hemispheres)	Normoglycemia (mannitol) n = 20 (hemispheres)
Baseline		100	100
Ischemia	5–7	36.0 ± 4.3	33.9 ± 4.4
	20	25.6 ± 1.8[a, b]	35.8 ± 2.8
	40	20.7 ± 1.6[a, c]	32.5 ± 2.5
	60	20.3 ± 1.7[a, c]	34.7 ± 3.1
	80	19.8 ± 1.7[a, c]	32.0 ± 2.3
	100	19.4 ± 1.5[a, c]	30.3 ± 2.1
	120	18.7 ± 1.5[a, c]	28.6 ± 2.2
Reperfusion	10	53.6 ± 7.1	62.8 ± 8.9
	20	58.1 ± 6.9	64.1 ± 6.1
	40	52.3 ± 6.1	61.5 ± 6.9
	60	48.5 ± 5.5	58.6 ± 5.8

Cerebral blood flow in the parietal cortex from glucose- and mannitol-injected Fischer 344 rats. Measurements were made bilaterally with laser-Doppler flowmetry throughout 2 hours of bilateral carotid artey occlusion followed by 1 hour of reperfusion and expressed as a percent of baseline (preischemic) value. All values are means ± SE.
[a] Indicates a significant difference ($p < 0.001$) between the two groups.
[b, c] Indicate a significant difference ($p < 0.01$ and $p < 0.001$ levels respectively) between the values at 5–7 minutes after occlusion and other time points in glucose injected rats.

In glucose-injected hyperglycemic rats, there was a more evident white infarct in brains after 2 hours of permanent carotid artery occlusion compared to normoglycemic rats. The cause of this difference appears to be CPV. In hyperglycemic rats, the CPV (3.9 ± 0.9 µl/g) was significantly lower compared to normoglycemic rats (7.2 ± 0.1 µl/g; p < 0.01).

Discussion

In our previous study with 4 hours of permanent MCA occlusion in the Sprague-Dawley rats [4], we found that hyperglycemia led to a marked reduction in CPV in the ischemic tissue. Hyperglycemia was also associated with lower CBF during ischemia and poor restoration on reperfusion. The present study indicates that hyperglycemia also induces similar cerebrovascular changes during global ischemia achieved by bilateral carotid occlusion in Fischer 344 rats. It, therefore, suggests that the results with MCA occlusion are not due to the use of a foreign object to occlude the cerebrovasculature.

A pale white infarct was evident after 2 hours of carotid artery occlusion in hyperglycemic rats but not in normoglycemic rats. This appears to be due to a decrease in CPV in the ischemic tissue as there is a significant reduction in CPV in hyperglycemic rats (54% of normoglycemia). Hyperglycemia also affects ischemic CBF measured by laser-Doppler flowmetry. After the initial decline in CBF with occlusion, a further progressive reduction in CBF was observed up to 40 minutes after occlusion in hyperglycemic but not in normoglycemic rats. A few studies have addressed the effects of hyperglycemia during ischemia and reperfusion. Although marked reductions in CBF during reperfusion have been reported in most studies [2, 3, 7], changes during ischemia are controversial [5, 7].

In rats with hyperglycemia, there was a marked edema formation in the brain associated with a reduction in CBF below 20% of preischemic values during 2 hours of ischemia. After 2 hours of occlusion, one hour of reperfusion resulted in a more pronounced edema formation in hyperglycemic rats. On the contrary, the mean residual CBF remained above 30% of preischemic values in normoglycemic rats and there was minimal brain edema formation after 2 hours of occlusion. These results may indicate that the factor responsible for edema formation is the degree of reduction in CBF during ischemia and changes in CBF in hyperglycemia may be associated with the damage to the cerebrovasculature (blood-brain barrier). This is also evident in hyperglycemic rats where if the CBF remained within the range found in normoglycemic rats, there was no significant brain edema formation in neither t-CCAO nor p-CCAO.

In conclusion, as in MCA occlusion, hyperglycemia during bilateral carotid artery occlusion in Fischer 344 rats induces a reduction in CPV and progressive decline in CBF. In Fischer 344 rats, this decline in CBF is a of magnitude to cause brain injury as evidenced by edema formation.

Acknowledgement

This work was supported by grants NS-23870 and NS-34709 from the National Institutes of Health.

References

1. Coyle P, Panzenbeck MJ (1990) Collateral development after carotid artery occlusion in Fischer 344 rats. Stroke 21: 316–321
2. Ginsberg MD, Welsh FA, Budd WW (1980) Deleterious effect of glucose pretreatment on recovery from diffuse cerebral ischemia in the cat. Stroke 11: 347–354
3. Kågström E, Smith M-L, Siesjo BK (1983) Recirculation in the rat brain following imcomplete ischemia. J Cereb Blood Flow Metab 3: 183–192
4. Kawai N, Keep RF, Betz AL (inpress) Hyperglycemia and the vascular effects of cerebral ischemia. Stroke
5. Nakai H, Yamamoto YL, Diksic M, Worsley KJ, Takara E (1988) Triple-tracer autoradiography demonstrates effects of hyperglycemia on cerebral blood flow, pH, and glucose utilization in cerebral ischemia of rats. Stroke 19: 764–772
6. Silvia RC, Slizgi GR, Ludens JH, Tang AH (1987) Protection from ischemia-induced cerebral edema in the rat by U-50488H, a kappa opioid receptor agonist. Brain Res 403: 52–57
7. Venables GS, Miller SA, Gibson G, Hardy JA, Strong AJ (1985) The effects of hyperglycaemia on changes during reperfusion following focal cerebral ischemia. J Neurol Neurosurg Psychiatry 48: 663–669

Correspondence: Richard F. Keep, Ph.D., Department of Surgery (Neurosurgery), University of Michigan, R5605 Kresge I, Ann Arbor, MI 48109-0532, U.S.A.

Acta Neurochir (1997) [Suppl] 70: 37–39
© Springer-Verlag 1997

The Mechanism of Free Radical Generation in Brain Capillary Endothelial Cells After Anoxia and Reoxygenation

S. Wu[1], **T. Nagashima**[1], **K. Ikeda**[1], **T. Kondoh**[1], **M. Yamaguchi**[2], and **N. Tamaki**[1]

[1] Department of Neurosurgery and [2] Institute of Health Science, Kobe University School of Medicine, Kobe, Japan

Summary

We studied the mechanism of reoxygenation injury of cerebral microvessels in cultured rat brain capillary endothelial cells (BCECs). BCECs were isolated from rat cerebral cortices by a two step enzymatic treatment. The monolayers of BCECs were subjected to anoxia for 20 minutes followed by reoxygenation for 3 hours. Cell damage was assessed by measuring the leakage of intracellular lactic dehydrogenase (LDH). The control group was anoxia/reoxygenated BCECs without any protective reagents. To study the protective effect of free radical scavengers and antioxidants, superoxide dismutase, catalase, deferoxamine, oxypurinol, indomethacin, or N^G-nitro-L-arginine methyl ester (L-NAME) was applied during anoxia/reoxygenation. Thus 7 experimental conditions were established.

Lactic dehydrogenase (LDH) leaked from reoxygenated BCECs due to cell membrane damage. This leakage was almost totally suppressed by superoxide dismutase, indicating that reoxygenation injury of BCECs is mediated by superoxide generation. The other scavengers and antioxidants partially suppressed LDH leakage. Reduction of Ca^{2+} in the culture medium from 1.6 mM to 0.016 mM also suppressed LDH leakage.

These results indicate that BCECs subjected to anoxia/reoxygenation become potent generators of superoxide anion, which is thought to be responsible for reoxygenation injury. The superoxide generation partially depends on the xanthine oxidase and cyclooxygenase pathways. As L-NAME partially suppressed LDH leakage peroxynitrite may contribute to reoxygenation injury of BCECs. The extracellular Ca^{2+} concentration also plays a critical role in the reoxygenation injury of BCECs.

Keywords: Cerebral anoxia; capillary endothelium; free radical generation; *in vitro* model.

Introduction

Oxygen free radicals are important mediators of brain injury and brain edema in ischemia. Recent experimental studies have demonstrated that oxygen free radicals are generated in postischemic microvessels; however, the mechanism of free radical generation is still poorly understood. Xanthine oxidase (XO) and cyclooxygenase in vascular endothelial cells have been reported to be responsible for free radical generation during anoxia and reoxygenation [4, 7]. However, it has been reported that XO is probably not an important source of free radicals in focal cerebral ischemia [2]. It has also been reported that allopurinol, a XO inhibitor, does not limit the size of cerebral infarction after ischemia and reperfusion in dogs [5]. Moreover, the cyclooxygenase blocker indomethacin does not appear to affect the magnitude of radical generation in reoxygenated human endothelial cells [10]. The role of the XO and cyclooxygenase pathways in reperfusion injury of microvessels is still undetermined.

The sources of free radical generation during reperfusion are multiple and complex and may vary in different species and different tissues. The brain capillary endothelial cells (BCECs) perform unique functions related to the formation of the blood-brain barrier (BBB) and the regulation of cerebral blood flow. Not only can they be the target of oxidant injury, they also can produce free radicals by themselves. Injury to the endothelium is a major consequence of ischemia/reperfusion, causing disruption of the barrier function and edema. The aim of the present study was to clarify the mechanism of free radical generation in reoxygenated BCECs. The LDH leakage from the BCECs was assessed and considered as an index of cellular injury. The role of extracellular Ca^{2+} in reoxygenation injury was also investigated.

Material and Methods

Preparation of Endothelial Cells

BCECs from male Sprague-Dawley rats were isolated by a two step enzymatic treatment and with centrifugation [3]. In brief, 10 brain tissue samples were incubated at 37°C in 20 ml of Dulbecco-MEM (D-MEM) with 0.5% dispase for 3 hours, then suspended in

80 ml of D-MEM containing 13% dextran. The microvessels were separated from the brain tissue by centrifugation at 5800 g for 10 minutes and treated with 1 mg/ml of collagenase/dispase for 6 hours. The cell pellet was layered over a 50% Percoll gradient and centrifugated at 26000 g for 50 minutes The band containing endothelial cells was removed and seeded onto a collagen-coated dish. Two weeks after seeding, homogeneous cells showed a characteristic cobblestone pattern. Identification of capillary endothelium was accomplished immunohistochemically using the immunoreactivity of factor VIII-related antigen.

Experimental Protocol

BCECs were replaced in 24 well dish and the medium was changed to Ca^{2+}-free, glucosefree Dulbecco's phosphate-buffered saline (D-PBS) 2 hours before the study. The cell plates were placed in a airtight chamber under a continuous flow of nilrogen gas with 0.5% CO_2 at 37°C for 20 minutes, followed by reoxygenation for 3 hours. The control group was anoxia/reoxygenated BCECs without any protective reagents. One of the following six reagents was applied to the D-PBS before anoxia/reoxygenation superoxide dismutase (SOD, 2000 U/ml), catalase (CAT, 2000 U/ml), deferoxamine (DFO, 1.0 mM), oxypurinol (1 mM), indomethacin (100 µM), or N^G-nitro-L-arginine methyl ester (L-NAME, 100 µM). Thus 7 experimental conditions were established. In addition, calcium, at three different calcium concentrations (0.016 mM, 0.16 mM, and 1.6 mM), was added to examine the role of extracellular calcium ion.

The anoxia/reoxygenation injury of the BCECs was assessed by the measurement of leakage of intracellular LDH. After anoxia/reoxygenation, LDH leakage was assayed with a spectrophotometer and expressed as a percentage of total LDH (LDH in medium + LDH in cells).

Results

In the absence of anoxia, LDH leakage was $8.2 \pm 1.3\%$ to of the total LDH after 3 hours incubation. With 20 minutes of anoxia followed by 3 hours of reoxygenation, LDH leakage from BCECs significantly increased to $44.8 \pm 3.3\%$ ($p < 0.01$). By the application of

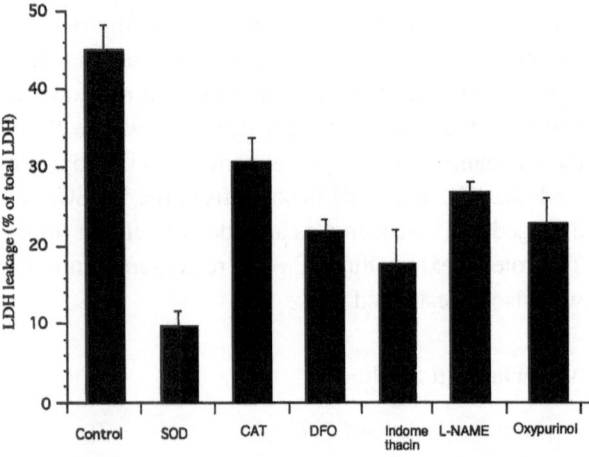

Fig. 1. Effects of antioxidants/scavengers on LDH leakage from the reoxygenated BCECs. Each bar represents mean ± S.E. (n = 4 for each)

SOD, LDM leakage was suppressed to $9.4 \pm 1.6\%$ (Fig. 1). There was no significant difference in LDH leakage between the reoxygenated cells treated with SOD and the normoxic cells. With the application of catalase, the LDH leakage was partially suppressed to $30.6 \pm 3.2\%$ There was a significant difference between the cells treated with SOD and those treated with catalase ($p < 0.0l$). In the presence of high-affinity ferric iron chelator deferoxamine, LDH leakage by reoxygenation was partially suppressed to $21.9 \pm 2.3\%$. By the application of oxypurinol, indomethacin, and L-NAME, LDH leakage was partially suppressed to $23.2 \pm 2.5\%$, $17.5 \pm 1.8\%$, and $26.7 \pm 1.2\%$ respectively (Fig. 1).

The leakage of LDH from reoxygenated BCECs following reoxygenation depended on the Ca^{2+} concentration of the extracellular fluid (Table 1).

Discussion

It has been reported that neither SOD alone nor catalase alone prevented free radical generation under anoxia/reoxygenation in rat pulmonary artery endothelial cells, whereas a combination of these two enzymes was quite effective [8]. Superoxide anion alone is thought to be a minor toxic metabolise. It is likely to exert its deleterious effect toward the very powerful oxidant hydroxyl radical only in the presence of H_2O_2. It has been observed, however, that radical generation was totally quenched by both SOD and catalase alone in studies of human umbilical vein endothelial cells [10], totally quenched by SOD, and 80–90% quenched by catalase in human aortic endothelial cells [9]. The present study showed that LDH leakage was almost totally quenched by SOD alone, and that catalase was less effective than SOD. It is conceivable that only a part of the superoxide generated by anoxia/reoxygenation is converted to hydrogen peroxide. Another part of the superoxide may react with nitric oxide to form the

Table 1. *Effects the Extracellular Ca^{2+} Concentration on the LDH Leakage in Reoxygenated BCECs*

Ca^{2+} concentration (mM)	LDH leakage
0.016	45 ± 4
0.16	53 ± 6[a]
1.6	69 ± 7[b]

Leakage is expressed as % of total LDH. Data are expressed as mean ± SE (n = 4 for each); p < 0.05.
[a] p < 0.01, [b] in comparison with 0.016 mM Ca^{2+}.

peroxynitrite anion which has considerably greater toxicity than the hydroxyl radical [1]. The protective action of SOD may be due in part to preventing the decomposition of nitric oxide by scavenging superoxide, since nitric oxide is unstable and its stability is enhanced by SOD. The capillary endothelial cells contain the inducible form of nitric oxide synthase. Nitric oxide act as an endothelium-derived relaxing factor. L-NAME has been recently characterized as an inhibitor of nitric oxide synthase in the brain [6]. The present study showed that L-NAME can inhibit endothelial cell injury by anoxia/reoxygenation. This suggests that NO may be a factor in reoxygenated injury processes.

The present study showed that the xanthine oxidase blocker oxypurinol did reduce LDH leakage, however, less potently than SOD. We assume that xanthine oxidase is partially responsible for free radical generation. The other source of superoxide generation is related to the arachidonic acid cascade. Cyclooxygenase has been found in vascular endothelial cells, and it has been proposed to be a source of free radical generation. Indomethacin irreversibly acetylates cyclooxygenase and can inhibit superoxide radical formation. The present study suggests that only a part of the superoxide anion is generated by the cyclooxygenase pathway.

Our studies also showed that extracellular Ca^{2+} accelerates BCECs injury in a concentration-dependent manner, indicating that reoxygenation injury of endothelial cells is a calcium dependent phenomenon. The mechanism of calcium ion influx into the endothelial cells should be determined to understand the mechanism of reoxygenation cell injury.

In conclusion, the present study indicates that BCECs subject to short time anoxia followed by reoxygenation become potent generators of superoxide anion, which is mainly responsible for reoxygenation injury. Superoxide generation partially depends on the xanthine oxidase pathway as well as the cyclooxygenase pathway. The reoxygenated BCECs injury may be due to the involvement of the secondary toxic product peroxynitrite. The extracellular Ca^{2+} concentration plays a critical role in the genesis of reoxygenated BCECs damage.

References

1. Beckman JS, Beckman TW, Chen J, Marshall PA, Freeman BA (1990) Apparent hydroxyl radical production by peroxynitrite: implications for endothelial injury from nitrit oxide and superoxide. Proc Natl Acad Sci USA 87: 1620–1624
2. Betz AL, Jeff R, Bean M (1991) Xanthine oxidase is not a major source of free radicals in focal cerebral ischemia Ann J Physiol 260 (Heart Circ Physiol 29): H563–H568
3. Bowman PD, Betz AL, Ar D (1981) Primary culture of capillary endothelium from rat brain. In vitro 17: 353–362
4. Jarasch ED, Bruder G, Heid HW (1986) Significance of xanthine oxidase in capillary, endothelial cells. Acta Physiol Scand 548: 39–46
5. Reimer KA, Jennings RB (1985) Failure of the xanthine oxidase inhibitor allopurinol to limit infarct size after ischemia end reperfusion in dogs. Circulation 71: 1069–1075
6. Knowles RG, Palacios M, Palmer MJ, Moncada S (1990) Kinetic characteristics of nitric oxide synthase from rat brain Biochem J 2651: 207–210
7. McCord JM (1985) Oxygen derived free radicals in post-ischemic tissue injury. Engl J Med 312: 159–163
8. Ratych RE, Chuknyiska RS, Bulkley GB (1987) The primary localization of free radical generation after anoxial reoxygenation in isolated endothelial cells. Surgery 102: 122–131
9. Zweier JL, Broderick R, Kuppusamy P, Thompson-Gorman S, Lutty GA (1994) Determination of the mechanism of free radical generation in human aortic endothelial cells exposed to anoxia and reoxygenation. J Biol Chem 269: 24156–24162
10. Zweier JI, Kuppusamy P, Thompson-Gorman S, Klunk D, Lutty GA (1994) Measurement and characterization of free radical generation in reoxygenated human endothelial cells. Am J Physiol 266 (Cell Physiol 35): C700–C708

Correspondence: Tatsuya Nagashima, M.D., Department of Neurosurgery, Kobe University School of Medicine, 7-5-1, Kusunoki-cho, Chuo-ku, Kobe 650, Japan.

Acta Neurochir (1997) [Suppl] 70: 40–42
© Springer-Verlag 1997

Mannitol Decreases ICP but Does Not Improve Brain-Tissue pO$_2$ in Severely Head-Injured Patients with Intracranial Hypertension

R. Härtl, T. F. Bardt, K. L. Kiening, A. S. Sarrafzadeh, G.-H. Schneider, and **A. W. Unterberg**

Department of Neurosurgery, Virchow Medical Center, Humboldt-University of Berlin, Federal Republic of Germany

Summary

Little is known about the effect of post-traumatic mannitol infusion on cerebral metabolism and oxygenation. The purpose of this study was to investigate the effects of mannitol in comatose patients on PtiO$_2$, PtiCO$_2$ and brain tissue pH using Clark-type electrodes implanted into cerebral white matter. In the neurosurgical intensive care unit PtiO$_2$, PtiCO$_2$, brain tissue pH, arterial blood pressure, intracranial pressure (ICP), cerebral perfusion pressure (CPP) and jugular bulb oxygen saturation (SjvO$_2$) were prospectively studied in eleven patients with severe traumatic brain injury (TBI) during a total of 30 mannitol administrations (125 ml of 20% Mannitol infused over 30 min through a central vein). When the initial ICP before mannitol infusion was below 20 mmHg neither ICP nor any of the other parameters changed significantly during or after mannitol infusion. With a pre-infusion ICP above 20 mmHg a significant effect was seen on ICP (decrease from 23 ± 1 to 16 ± 2 mmHg at 60 min) and CPP (increase from 68 ± 2 to 80 ± 3 mmHg at 120 min). These effects were not reflected in PtiO$_2$ or SjvO$_2$, which were 29 ± 4 mmHg and 61 ± 3%, respectively, at the beginning of mannitol injection and remained unchanged during the observation period. PtiCO$_2$ and brain tissue pH were not affected by mannitol infusion. Future studies should focus on the identification of ICP or CPP thresholds where infusion of mannitol may actually improve O$_2$-supply to the brain.

Keywords: Cerebral oxygenation; head injury; traumatic brain injury; neuromonitoring.

Introduction

Early detection of impending cerebral ischemia in head-injured patients is important to avoid secondary insults to the injured brain [2, 9].

Direct monitoring of cerebral white matter oxygenation (PtiO$_2$) is a promising new technique that has attracted considerable interest over the last several years [6–8, 13, 16]. Mannitol infusion has become a standard in the treatment of brain edema and intracranial hypertension. Little is known, however, about its effect on cerebral metabolism and oxygenation.

The present study was conducted in order to investigate the effect of mannitol infusion directed at lowering elevated intracranial pressure on PtiO$_2$, brain tissue PCO$_2$ (PtiCO$_2$) and pH (ptiH).

Patients and Methods

Eleven severely head-injured patients with a post-resuscitation Glasgow Coma Score (GCS) < 9 were enrolled in this study.*

All patients were monitored in the neurosurgical intensive care unit. The patients were sedated, intubated and mechanically ventilated to maintain an arterial PO$_2$ greater than 100 mmHg and a PaCO$_2$ of approximately 35 mmHg. Space occupying lesions greater than 25 cc were surgically evacuated. Clinical intensive care management followed a standardized protocol:

Intracranial hypertension exceeding 20 mmHg initiated a defined cascade of therapeutic interventions (elevation of head, induction of moderate hypocapnia by hyperventilation to a PaCO$_2$ of 30–35 mmHg, mannitol infusion, barbiturate coma). Regardless of ICP levels, efforts were made to maintain the CPP above 60 mmHg using isotonic fluids and vasopressors. Mean arterial blood pressure (MAP), ICP (intraparenchymal fiberoptic device, Camino Laboratories), arterial oxygen saturation, end-tidal CO$_2$ (EtCO$_2$), jugular bulb oximetry (SjvO$_2$) and PtiO$_2$ were monitored between day one and 12 after insult. SjvO$_2$ was determined using the OXIMETRIX-3 SYSTEM, Abbott Laboratories, North Chicago, Illinois with a No. 5.5 French fiberoptic catheter in a technique described recently [14]. The system was recalibrated using jugular venous blood samples and a co-oximeter every 12 h.

For measuring cerebral white matter PtiO$_2$ a flexible polarographic Clark-type microcatheter (Licox System, GMS mBH, Kiel, Germany) was inserted into the frontal lobe contralateral to the main pathological finding on the initial CT scan. Proper location in the cerebral white matter and exclusion of catheter-induced hemorrhage was ascertained by CT. In six patients a multiparameter sensor (Paratrend 7; Biomedical Sensors, High Wycombe, UK) was used that allowed simultanous measurement of brain-tissue PCO$_2$ (PtiCO$_2$), pH (ptiH), and brain temperature.

---

* Permission was granted by the Local Institutional Ethics Committee. During all surgical procedures and medical interventions greatest care was taken not to interfere with ongoing therapy and to guarantee state-of-the-art treatment.

The multimodal monitoring system digitized the analog signals of all parameters at 0.1 Hz and stored them. CPP was calculated on-line as MAP-ICP by the computer software. A total of 30 mannitol administrations (125 ml of 20% Mannitol infused over 30 min through a central vein) in eleven patients were studied. Ten minute blocks of continuously recorded data were put together and averaged at time points immediately before infusion and 5–15 min, 25–35 min, 55–65 min and 115–125 min after start of infusion. Mannitol data were split into three subgroups according to the sensor used and the initial ICP before infusion (Licox system: ICP < 20 mmHg; n = 9, ICP > 20 mmHg; n = 7). Data obtained with the Paratrend system are presented separately (ICP > 20 mmHg, n = 14).

Results

When the initial ICP before mannitol infusion was below 20 mmHg (15 ± 1 mmHg with a PtiO₂ of 395 mmHg and a of SjvO₂ 692%) neither ICP nor any of the other parameters changed significantly during or after mannitol infusion. In cases where the pre-infusion ICP was above 20 mmHg a significant effect was

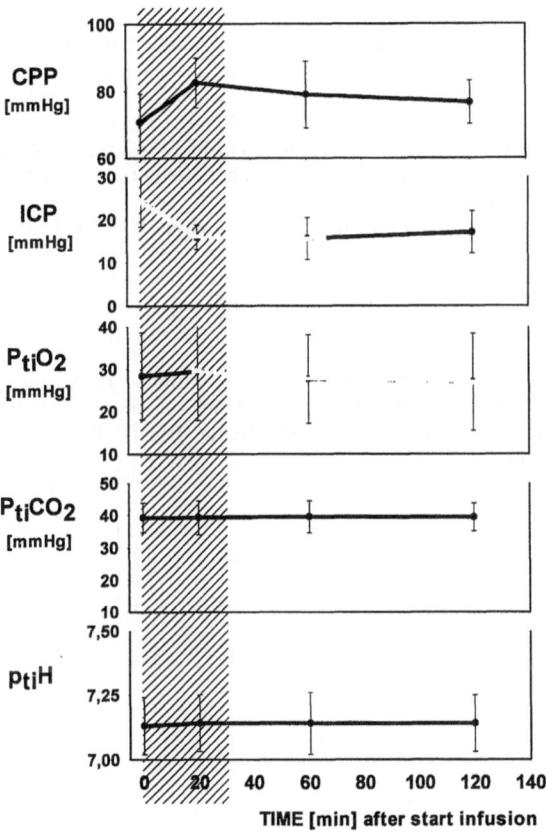

Fig. 1. In six patients a multiparameter sensor (Paratrend 7; Biomedical Sensors, High Wycombe, UK) was used that allowed measurement of brain-tissue PO₂, (PtiO₂), PCO₂ (PtiCO₂) and pH (ptiH). A total of 14 mannitol administrations (125 ml of 20% Mannitol infused over 30 min through a central vein) were studied. While ICP decreased during mannitol infusion from 24 ± 6 to 16 ± 3 and CPP increased from 71 ± 8 to 83 ± 7 mmHg at 20 min after start of infusion, no change was seen in either PtiO₂, PtiCO₂ or ptiH

seen on ICP (maximal decrease from 23 ± 1 to 16 ± 2 mmHg at 60 min) and CPP (maximal increase from 68 ± 2 to 80 ± 3 mmHg at 120 min). However, these effects were not reflected in PtiO₂ or SjvO₂, which were 29 ± 4 mmHg and 61 ± 3%, respectively, at the beginning of mannitol injection and remained unchanged during the observation period (30 ± 5 mmHg and 64 ± 3% at 120 min). Very similar results were obtained when PtO₂, PtiCO₂ and ptiH were measured simultaneously. While ICP decreased during mannitol infusion from 24 ± 6 to 16 ± 3 and CPP increased from 71 ± 8 to 83 ± 7 mmHg at 20 min after start of infusion, no change was seen in either PtiO₂, PtiCO₂ or ptiH (Fig. 1).

Discussion

Aggressive ICP management is considered a cornerstone in the treatment of severely head-injured patients [3]. Administration of mannitol in patients with intracranial hypertension or patients at risk of developing intracranial hypertension has become routine. Two different mechanisms by which mannitol reduces ICP are currently established. Improvement of blood rheology leading to an increased CBF and compensatory cerebral vasoconstriction may cause the early ICP drop observed shortly after infusion [10, 11]. A delayed decrease of ICP following 30 min to 6 h after infusion is attributed to an osmotic gradient produced between plasma and parenchymal cells [1, 4].

Treatment with mannitol yielded several results that have been described previously: The effect of mannitol is most pronounce: with a CPP below 70 mmHg [12] and ICP above 20 mmHg [10, 12, 15]. In the present study, when the initial ICP and CPP were < 20 and > 70 mmHg, respectively, mannitol infusion did not alter these parameters over the course of two hours. In contrast, for an ICP of 23 ± 1 mmHg and a CPP of 68 ± 2 mmHg mannitol caused a reduction of ICP by 30% at 60 min and improved CPP to 80 ± 3 mmHg at 120 min. The ICP change was similar to the one reported by Gaab *et al.* (32% reduction of ICP for 69 min) [5].

An important finding is that neither at initially low (< 20 mmHg) nor at elevated (> 20 mmHg) ICP did mannitol alter cerebral oxygen delivery, PtiCO₂, ptiH or SjvO₂, even though it significantly improved CPP and ICP (Fig. 4). We attribute this to the fact that CPP before mannitol injection was sufficient (> 60 mmHg) to maintain a "normal" PtiO₂, which did not benefit from further CPP elevation. Our results, however, do not permit us to draw conclusions on the effect of mannitol in ptients with *severe* intracranial hypertension (e.g. > 40 mmHg). Conceivably, brain tissue PO$_2$ will then profit from mannitol because CPP is likely to be < 60 mmHg.

Mannitol remains a frequently used drug with potentially harmful side-effects. The present results once again illustrate that critical care management relying only on ICP as a treatment criteria neglects the importance of brain-tissue PO$_2$. Future studies should focus on the identification of ICP or CPP thresholds where infusion of mannitol may actually improve O$_2$-supply to the brain.

Acknowledgement

This work was supported by the Deutsche Forschungsgemeinschaft (DFG) Un 56/7–1.

References

1. Berger S, Schürer L, Härtl R, *et al* (1995) Reduction of posttraumatic intracranial hypertension by hypertonic/hyperoncotic saline/dextran and mannitol. Neurosurgery 37: 98–108
2. Chesnut RM, Marshall SB, Piek J, *et al* (1993) Early and late systemic hypotension as a frequent and fundamental source of cerebral ischemia following severe brain injury in the Traumatic Coma Data Bank. Acta Neurochir (Wien) [Supp] 59: 121–125
3. Eisenberg HM, Frankowski RF, Contant CF, *et al* (1988) High-dose barbiturate control of elevated intracranial pressure in patients with severe head injury. J Neurosurg 69: 15–23
4. Freshman SP, Battistella FD, Matteucci M, *et al* (1993) Hypertonic saline (7.5%) versus mannitol: a comparison for treatment of acute head injuries. J Trauma 35: 344–348
5. Gaab M, Seegers K, Smedema R (1990) A comparative analysis of THAM in traumatic brain edema. Acta Neurochir (Wien) [Suppl] 51: 320–323
6. Härtl R, Bardt T, Kiening K, *et al* (1996) Brain-tissue PO$_2$ during cardiac arrest and cerebral herniation in severely head-injured patients. Cardiovasc Eng
7. Kiening K, Unterberg A, Bardt T, *et al* (1996) Monitoring of cerebral oxygenation in severely head-injured patients: brain tissue PO$_2$ vs. jugular venous oxygen saturation. J Neurosurg
8. Maas A, Fleckenstein W, de Jong D, *et al* (1993) Monitoring cerebral oxygenation: experimental studies and preliminary clinical results of continuous monitoring of cerebrospinal fluid and brain tissue tension. In: Unterberg AW, Schneider G-H, Lanksch W (eds) Monitoring of cerebral blood flow and metabolism in intensiv care. Acta Neurochir (Wien) [Suppl] 59: 50–57
9. Miller JD, Becker DP (1982) Secondary insults to the injured brain. J R Coll Surg Edinb 27: 292–298
10. Muizelaar JP, Lutz HA, Becker DP (1984) Effect of mannitol on ICP and CBF and correlation with pressure autoregulation in severely head-injured patients. J Neurosurg 61: 700–706
11. Muizelaar JP, Wei EP, Kontos HA, *et al* (1983) Mannitol causes compensatory cerebral vasoconstriction and vasodilation in response to blood viscosity changes. J Neurosurg 59: 822–828
12. Rosner M, Coley I (1987) Cerebral perfusion pressure: a hemodynamic mechanism of mannitol and the pre-mannitol hemogram. Neurosurgery 21: 147–156
13. Santbrink H v, Maas A, Avezaat C (1996) Continuous monitoring of partial pressure of brain tissue oxygen in patients with severe head injury. Neurosurgery 38: 21–31
14. Sheinberg M, Kanter MJ, Robertson CS, *et al* (1992) Continuous monitoring of jugular venous oxygen saturation in head-injured patients. J Neurosurg 76: 212–217
15. Takagi H, Saito T, Kitahara T (1983) The mechanism of the ICP reducing effect of mannitol. In: Ishii S, Nagai H, Brock N (eds) Intracranial pressure V. Springer, Berlin Heidelberg New York Tokyo, pp 729–733
16. Unterberg A, Kiening K, Schneider G-H, *et al* (1995) Monitoring of cerebral oxygenation in severe head injury – jugular venous oxygen saturation vs. brain tissue pO$_2$ and near infrared spectroscopy. J Neurotrauma 12: 405

Correspondence: Roger Härtl, M.D., Department of Neurosurgery, Virchow Medical Center, Humboldt University of Berlin, Augustenburger Platz 1, D-13353 Berlin, Federal Republic of Germany.

Acta Neurochir (1997) [Suppl] 70: 43–45
© Springer-Verlag 1997

A Chronological Evaluation of Experimental Brain Infarct by Diffusion-Mapping and Magnetization Transfer Contrast Imaging

Z. Kovács[1], **K. Ikezaki**[1], **M. Takahashi**[2], **J. Kawai**[2], and **M. Fukui**[1]

[1] Neurosurgical Department, Neurological Institute, Faculty of Medicine, Kyushu University, and
[2] Research Department, Diagnostic-Laboratory, Nihon Shering K.K., Japan

Summary

Background and purpose: There is a complex system of evolving physiochemical processes in the ischemic brain. The evaluation of this chain of processes is a major challenge of recent stroke studies. Two magnetic resonance imaging techniques; diffusion-weighted (DW) and magnetization transfer contrast (MTC) imaging were introduced in experimental studies and were shown to have sensitivity for different stages of brain infarct.

Materials and methods: We used a reproducible middle cerebral artery (MCA) occlusion model in rat to examine infarcts of different time courses. Magnetic resonance T_2-weighted (T_2), DW, and MTC imaging were performed 3 h, 1 d, 3 d, 5 d, 7 d, 2 w, 3 w, and 4 w after MCA occlusion. Haematoxylin/eosin (HE) stained sections, which revealed sub regions within infarct lesions, were compared to T_2, DW, diffusion-mapping and MTC-mapping images.

Results: On DW images 3 hours post occlusion lesions were detected as an area with high signal intensity, while T_2 imaging does not raise significant contrast of the lesion at this early stage. Three sub regions of the lesion having different ADCs, are discernible on diffusion-mapping images from 1 day to 7 days. The decrease of MTC effect was measured within the infarct lesion from core to marginal zone, from 7 days to 4 weeks.

Conclusions: Diffusion-mapping imaging may help to examine brain infarction from 3 hours to 5 days. MTC imaging recognizes infarcts 7 days after the onset. Following this stage, MTC-mapping images may provide a quantitative method to assess infarct size.

Keywords: Cerebral infarction; rat; apparent diffusion coefficient; magnetization transfer contrast.

Introduction

Early stage stroke has been widely investigated, while fewer studies have addressed the later stages of cerebral infarction. Ischemic brain parenchyma is recognized on DW images within minutes after injury [5, 6]. In early stage stroke ADCs are able to differentiate core, penumbra, and normal brain, based on water diffusion differences [2, 11]. Nevertheless, DW images could not be used to quantify infarct volume 7 days after MCA occlusion, because there was no uniform signal within the damaged area [3]. Thus, to assess a chronic stage infarction, other MRI methods then those sensitive to water diffusibility are required.

MT imaging works by the interaction of free and temporarily bound (to protein macromolecules) water protons of tissue. Since, different tissues have different macromolecular composition, MT imaging can generate very high tissue contrast that is based on well-defined physiochemical properties [1]. An MRI study of stroke by MT technique revealed that MT effect decreases as the chronicity of infarct increases [10].

The purpose of this study was to compare T_2, DW, diffusion-mapping and MTC-mapping images of the different time course infarctions and to analyze correlating them with histological sections.

Methods

Animal Model

Twenty-seven adult male Wistar rats, weighing 250–300 g were intravenously anaesthetized with 35 mg/kg sodium pentobarbital. Femoral artery and vein catheters were induced for continuous arterial blood pressure and blood gases monitoring. All animals, but the three sham operated (craniectomized but not MCA ligated), underwent complete suture ligation of the MCA, as described previously [7]. The rats were then placed in the MRI unit to perform T_2, DW, and MTC images at different time courses (3 h, 1 d, 3 d, 5 d, 7 d, 2 w, 3 w, 4 w) after MCA occlusion. At the end of MR imaging, the brains were quickly removed from the cranium. Coronal sections were cut from the formaldehyde fixed brains, and stained with HE. MR images were correlated with histological sections at the level of optic chiasm.

Magnetic Resonance Imaging Protocol

Imaging experiments were performed on a 4.7 T animal imager (Omega CSI-II, GE NMR Instrument, Fremont, CA) equipped with self-shielded gradients in combination with a home-made bird-cage coil. T$_2$ (TR/TE = 1500/80 msec) a multislice sequence techniques yielding four 2.5 mm thick transverse images of the brain were used to localize lesions. Diffusion-on images, in the spin echo sequences with motion probe gradients, MTC-on and MTC-off images, in the gradient echo (ORE) sequences (TR/TE = 100/8 msec) with and without preparation pulse, were obtained. The additional pulse to saturate the signal from bound protons, was applied before GRE sequence on MTC-on images. ADC and MTC values were calculated using the following equations;

$$ADC = -1n \ (SI\text{-}DW \ / \ SI\text{-}T_2^*) \ / \ b,$$
$$MTC = 1 - (SI\text{-}MTC \ / \ SI\text{-}T_2^*)$$

where SI means signal intensity and b = 1096 mm^2/sec is the degree of diffusion weighting calculated in our sequence. To obtain diffusion-mapping or MTC-mapping images, the signal intensity in every four voxels were used for calculation. On each image, ADC and MTC values were calculated in four different regions of interest (ROI); three ROIs within the damaged area and one ROI in the contra lateral cortex as reference.

Histological Classification

On histological sections the infarcts were detected as eliptiform areas with reduced stainability of neuropil, localized in the occluded MCA supplying territory. The histological appearance of acute (3 h), subacute (1 d, 3 d, 5 d), and chronic stage infarctions are different. An acute stage lesion appears as an area with slightly pale neuropil, without stratification. Subacute and chronic stage infarctions divide in three regions; core, periphery and marginal zone. The histological features of regions within the lesion are different in subacute and in the chronic stage. The core has pale myelin and vacuolation around neurons in the subacute stage and contains necrotic debris lacking cells in the chronic stage. In the periphery polymorphonuclear leucocytic infiltration and swollen axons are succeeded by vascular elements and lipid phagocytes. In the marginal zone, astrocytes with shrunken or swollen nuclei are followed by fiber-forming astrocytes, microglial phagocytes and degenerated myelin.

Results

The earliest detection of the lesion in our series, was at 3 hours on DW images, at 1 day on T$_2$ images and at 7 days on MTC-on images (Fig. 1).

On DW images ischemic lesions appear as regions with high signal intensity as early as 3 hours after MCA occlusion. In the subacute stage, from 1 day to 5 days, on diffusion-mapping images the signal intensity within lesions is heterogeneous allowing the differentiation of three sub-regions, which correspond to core, periphery and marginal zone on histological sections. The calculated ADCs are lower in core and higher in the periphery of lesions when compared to ADC of the contra lateral cortex. Peak ADCs were measured in the periphery of lesion; the lowest at 1 day, the highest at 3 weeks after MCA occlusion (Fig. 2a).

With MT pulse saturation, lesions demonstrated increase of the signal intensity after 7 days only. The conspicuity of damaged area increased substantially on MTC-mapping images 2, 3 and 4 weeks after MCA occlusion. A gradually decreasing MT effect was

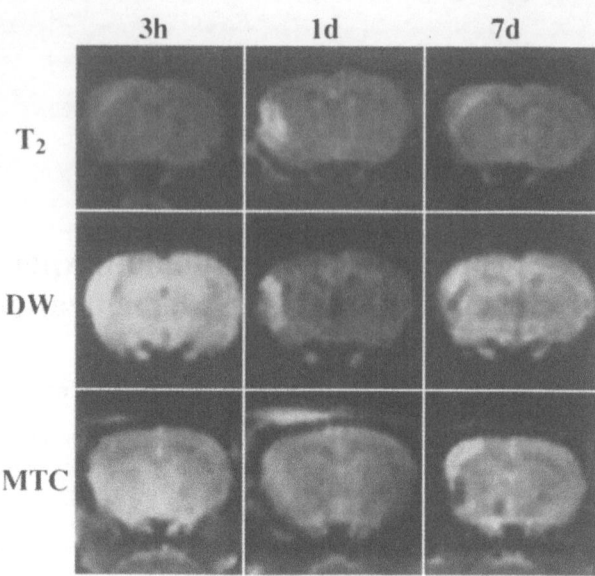

Fig. 1. T$_2$-weighted images (top series), DW-on images (middle series), and MTC-on images (bottom series) of 3 hours, 1 day and 7 days infarctions. The lesion is recognized after 1 day on T$_2$, after 3 hours on DW and after 7 days on MTC-on images

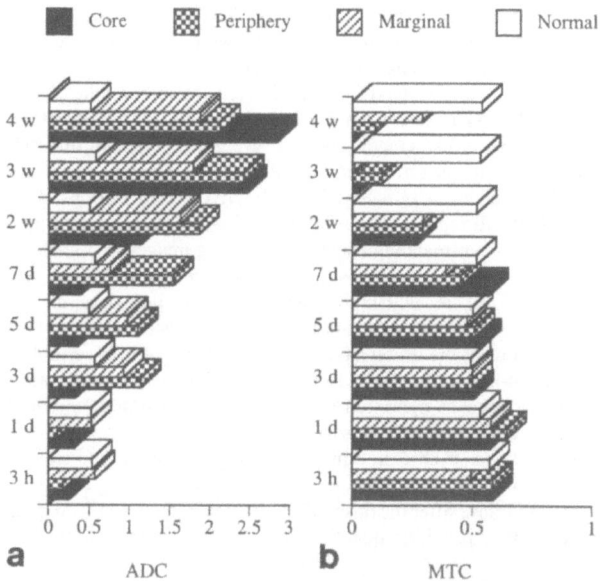

Fig. 2. ADC and MTC values calculated in different ROIs in the subsequent stages of infarct. (a) ADC in core is lower then in the normal brain before 7 days and higher after 7 days. The turning point in periphery is at 1 day. (b) MTC values decrease in the lesion from 7 days and there are different values in sub regions

measured from the core, through the periphery, to the marginal zone of 7-day-old infarcts (Fig. 2b).

Discussion

Three stages of infarct are distinguished based on histological findings; an acute stage (3 h), a subacute stage (1 d, 3 d, 5 d) and a chronic stage (7 d, 2 w, 3 w, 4 w). The acute stage infarct lesions are recognized as regions with slightly decreased stainability of neuropil and blurring of the cytoplasmic boundaries. The 3 hour ischemic lesion on T_2 images with slightly elevated signal intensity has only poor contrast to the normal brain, but it is well distinguished as a homogenous high signal intensity area on DW images. This suggests that the decrease of water diffusibility is one of the earliest pathophysiological modifications after arterial occlusion in brain parenchyma. This finding clearly demonstrates the advantage of DW images in early detection of brain ischemic lesions.

The stratification of subacute stage infarction becomes evident on both HE stained sections and diffusion-mapping images. Although, on T_2 and DW images the damaged area is heterogeneous, the histological sub regions are not discernible. Elevated in periphery, slightly elevated in marginal zone and diminished in core, ADC proved to be susceptible to the pathophysiological changes in subacute stage infarction. The reduction of ADC, in previous studies, was associated with the accumulation of intracellular water (cytotoxic edema) [4], while nonischemic edematous regions (vasogenic edema) has been shown to have elevated ADC [9]. In a rat infarct model, as shown by Menzis *et al.*, ischemic edema develops in the core of lesion from 12 hours to 7 days, while blood brain barrier (BBB) hyper permeability was observed in the periphery after 24 hours to 7 days [8]. This spatial and temporal correlation suggests that ischemic edema (cytotoxic edema) and BBB disruption (vasogenic edema) in infarct are distinguished on diffusion-mapping images by the contrast between core and periphery of ischemic lesions.

The lesions after 7 days, appear as homogenous high signal intensity areas on both T_2 and DW images. Accordingly, diffusion-mapping images do not reflect the histological subdivision of chronic stage infarction and do not enable us to distinguish unfunctional gliotic scar tissue from adjacent functional brain parenchyma. Nevertheless, the histological subdivision of a 7 day infarct is detectable on MTC-mapping images. Furthermore, chronic lesions detected on MTC-mapping images are larger and correlate better with the damaged area identified on histological sections. The analysis of histological sections also revealed that between 5 and 7 days the core of the lesion transforms from a tissue with shrunken ischemic neurons to necrotic debris containing cyst-like regions. MTC images start to recognize infarct around 5 to 7 days, which may suggest that the decrease of MTC effect is related to appearance of tissue necrosis, loss of the cell structure and/or cyst formation. However, the major challenge remains to identify what physiochemical process is detected by MT technique in brain infarction.

References

1. Balaban RS, Ceckler TL (1992) Magnetization transfer contrast in magnetic resonance imaging [Review]. Magn Res Quarterly 8: 116–137
2. Dardzinski BJ, Sotak CH, Fisher M (1993) Apparent diffusion coefficient mapping of experimental focal cerebral ischemia using diffusion-weighted echo-planar imaging. Magn Res Med 30: 318–325
3. Gill R, Sibson NR, Hatfield RH (1995) A comparison of the early development of ischaemic damage following permanent middle cerebral artery occlusion in rats as assessed using magnetic resonance imaging and histology. J Cereb Blood Flow Metab 15: 1–11
4. Hasegawa Y, Fisher M, Latour LL (1994) MRI diffusion mapping of reversible and irreversible ischemic injury in focal brain ischemia. Neurology 44: 1484–1490
5. Hossmann KA, Hoehn-Berlage M (1995) Diffusion and perfusion MR imaging of cerebral ischemia [Review]. Cerebrovasc Brain Metab Rev 7: 187–217
6. Kohno K, Hoehn-Berlage M, Mies G (1995) Relationship between diffusion-weighted MR images, cerebral blood flow, and energy state in experimental brain infarction. Magn Res Imaging 13: 73–80
7. Kovacs Z, Ikezaki K, Samoto K (1996) VEGF and flt expression time kinetics in rat brain infarct. Stroke 27: 1865–1873
8. Menzies SA, Betz AL, Hoff JT (1993) Contributions of ions and albumin to the formation and resolution of ischemic brain edema. J Neurosurg 78: 257–266
9. Pierpaoli C, Righini A, Linfante I (1993) Histopathologic correlates of abnormal water diffusion in cerebral ischemia: diffusion-weighted MR imaging and light and electron microscopic study. Radiology 189: 439–448
10. Prager JM, Rosenblum JD, Huddle DC (1994) The magnetization transfer effect in cerebral infarction. AJNR 15: 1497–1500
11. Takahashi M, Fritz-Zieroth B, Chikugo T (1993) Differentiation of chronic lesions after stroke in stroke-prone spontaneously hypertensive rats using diffusion weighted MRI. Magn Res Med 30: 485–488

Correspondence: Zsombor Kovacs, M.D., Department of Neurosurgery, Neurological Institute, Kyushu University, Faculty of Medicine, Fukuoka 812-82, Japan.

Acta Neurochir (1997) [Suppl] 70: 46–49
© Springer-Verlag 1997

Ultrastructure of Astrocytes Associated with Selective Neuronal Death of Cerebral Cortex After Repeated Ischemia

U. Ito[1], **S. Hanyu**[2], **Y. Hakamata**[2], **M. Nakamura**[3], and **K. Arima**[3]

[1] Department of Neurosurgery, Musashino Red Cross Hospital, Tokyo, [2] Department of Neurology, Jichi Medical School, Tochigi, and [3] Tokyo Institute of Psychiatry, Tokyo, Japan

Summary

Astrocytic swelling after ischemic insult has been considered a sign of parturbed cell viability. Investigations using cultured astrocytes and C6 glioma cells have revealed that viable astrocytes swell, spatially buffering various metabolites which are increased by the metabolic turmoil following ischemic insults. In the present study, we have studied the temporal profile of ultrastructural changes of astrocytes in the cerebral cortex associated with progressive selective neuronal, death where infarction is not induced. We occluded the left carotid artery of the Mongolian gerbil twice for 10 minutes at a 5 hr interval. In this model, following reperfusion, selective neuronal death progresses in the coronal section cut at the infundibular level. The whole brains of the sham operated control and postischemic animals were fixed by transcardiac perfusion of glutaraldehyde fixatives, at 15 min, 5 and 12 hr after the 2nd 10 min ischemia. Ultrathin sections including the 3rd and 5th cortical layers were prepared from the cut surface at the level of infundibulum. Mild swelling of astrocytic processes and perivascular end-feet was observed in the 15 min group. Glycogen granules were not prominent. In the 5 hr group, we found a few necrotic neurons disseminated in the cortex. All astrocytic cell processes were swollen with increased number of glycogen granules, especially marked in the perivascular end-feet. In the 12 hr group, necrotic neurons increased in number, astrocytic swelling was more extensive, and glycogen granules were evident in astrocytes. No cellular destruction was observed. We conclude: 1. Swelling progresses in astrocytes which however still remain viable and this process is associated with selective progression of neuronal death. 2. Glycogen granules increase in the swollen yet viable astrocytic cell processes.

Keywords: Astrocyte; selective neuronal death; cerebral infarction; cytotoxic edema; cerebral ischemia.

Introduction

Astrocytic swelling after ischemic insult had been considered a detrimental sign, due to disruption of the Gibbs-Donan equilibrium of the cell membrane by an energetic disturbance of Na^+/K^+ ATPase activity in the cell membrane. Investigations using cultured astrocytes and C6 glioma cells have revealed that hypoxia as well as ouabaine inhibit Na^+/K^+ ATPase activity but do not effect cell swelling [18, 23], whereas viable astrocytes swell by themselves when various mediators such as lactate, glutamate, K^+ and arachidonic acid are increased in the culture-medium [15, 17, 19, 21, 28, 30]. Therefore, cytotoxic edema occurring after ischemic insult could be considered as a swelling of viable astrocytes and furthermore as a neuronal protective mechanism provided by astrocytes [20, 25] which spatially buffer various mediators increased by the metabolic turmoil following ischemic insults.

Ischemic edema following temporary ischemia has been considered as a cytotoxic edema followed by vasogenic edema [9, 12, 14, 16]. In a single ischemic insult, the transition from selective neuronal death to infarction in the cerebral cortex shows considerable variability [13, 14]; thus, it is usually difficult to evaluate the cytotoxic edema associated with viable or necrotic swelling of astrocytes. By repeating short ischemic insults at various repetitive intervals, a single one of which does not cause significant neuronal loss, we have developed a model to induce selective neuronal death in the cerebral cortex without causing focal infarction. We have found that with an increase in the number of these insults and a shortening of their intervals, the ischemic injury has matured from less intensive to more intensive selective neuronal death, and that it proceeds to cerebral infarction after reaching a critical threshold level of insults [6–8, 10, 11].

In the present study, we have studied the temporal profile of ultrastructural changes in astrocytes of the cerebral cortex using a system in which only selective neuronal death has progressed following repeated ischemia at an intensity just under the threshold level required to induce focal infarction.

Materials and Methods

The left carotid artery of adult Mongolian gerbils was clipped under 2% halothane, 70% nitrous oxide and 30% oxygen anesthesia. Anesthesia was discontinued immediately after the procedure. Using the stroke index score [24], ischemic-positive animals were selected during the first 10 min occlusion. Animals were subjected to an additional second 10 min occlusion with a 5-hr interval after the first 10 min ischemia. In this model, following reperfusion, focal infarction develops in the coronal section cut at the chiasmatic level, while only selective neuronal death without infarction was found in the coronal section cut at the infundibular level [6]. All animals were sacrificed 15 min, 5, 12 hr after the second 10 min ischemia, by transcardiac perfusion with cacodylate buffered glutalaldehyde fixatives for ultrastructural study (3 animals in each group). The fixed brains were cut coronally at the infundibular level. Ultrathin sections including the 3rd~5th cortical layers in the coronal section were prepared from the left ischemic cerebral hemisphere at the mid-point between the interhemispheric and rhinal fissures. Alternative sections were double-stained by uranyl acetate and lead citrate solution, and observed by a JEM-2000EX electron microscope.

Results

Mild swelling of all astrocytic processes and perivascular end-feet was observed in the 15 min group. However, the number of glycogen granules did not increase. Five hours after the last ischemic episode, we found a few degenerating neurons scattered in the cortex. There was moderate swelling of all astrocytic cell processes with increased numbers of glycogen granules (Fig. 1).

These findings were especially conspicuous in the perivascular endfeet. The number of mitochondria increased in the perikarya of the astrocytic cell bodies, which were also swollen and demonstrated increased numbers of glycogen granules (Fig. 1). Twelve hours after the last ischemic episode, necrotic neurons increased in number, whereas astrocytes revealed cytoplasmic swelling and increased numbers of glycogen granules in their processes. No cellular destruction was observed in the astrocytic cell processes and their end-feet. The number of mitochondria was markedly increased in astrocytic perikarya. The number of necrotic neurons was also increased and swelling of astrocytic cell processes was intensified, while glycogen granules decreased in number in animals sacrificed 24 hr after the last ischemic episode. However, even at the latter time period, no cellular destruction was observed in astrocytic cell processes and end-feet.

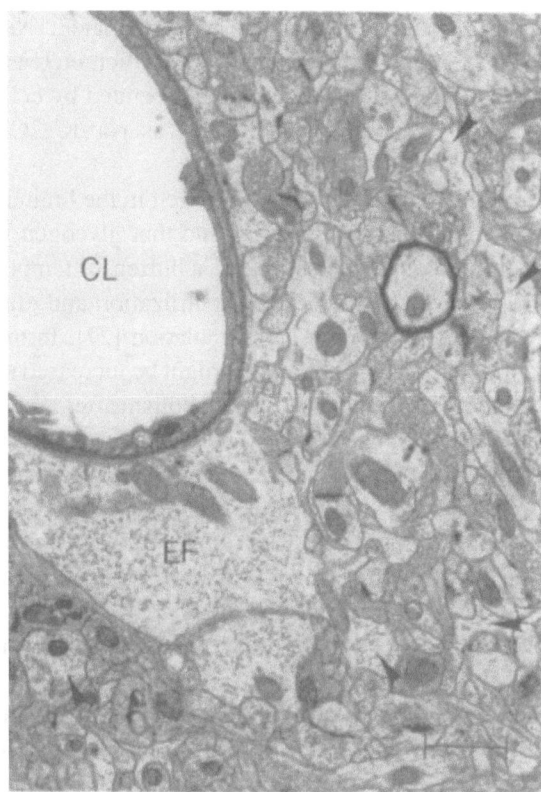

Fig. 1. Capillary of 3rd cortical layer in Facer B, 12-hr after the last ischemic episode. Perivascular astrocytic end-feet (*EF*) and astrocytic cell processes in the neuropil (arrows) are markedly swollen with increased number of glycogen granules. *CL* Capillary lumen

Discussion

Astrocytic swelling after ischemic insult has been ascribed to dysfunction of the Na^+ pump of cell-membrane-bound Na^+/K^+ ATPase due to energy failure. Therefore, it is a detrimental sign of astrocytic viability. In the present study, we have investigated ischemic injury in which selective neuronal death has progressed without infarction, and have found that viable astrocytes swell and contain increased numbers of glycogen granules, without ultrastructural evidence of cytoplasmic destruction.

Based on previous *in vitro* studies, the astrocyte has been considered to swell actively where: 1) accumulating Na^+ and expelling H^+ which increase in the astrocytic cytoplasm by an elevation of lactacidosis and respiratory products, operated by cell-membrane bound ion-channels as Na^+/H^+ antiporter, Na^+/HCO_3^- cotransporter, and Na^+-dependent Cl^-/HCO_3^- exchanger; these ion-channels are especially rich in the end-feet around capillaries; 2) accumulating Na^+ and glutamate which increase at the synapse, operated by cell-membrane bound ion-channels as glutamate/2 Na+ cotransporter; and 3) accumulating K+ which increase extracellarly by neuronal excitation, operated by cell-membrane bound ion-channels such as Na+/K+/2Cl− transporter [15, 17, 19, 21, 28, 30].

It is generally accepted that glycogen in the brain is primarily confined to astrocytes and that glycogen is constantly turning over, serving as a buffer for temporary imbalances between glucose utilization and glucose resupply by the cerebral circulation [27]. In the present study, glycogen granules might be increased as a reaction to perturbed glucose metabolism after reperfusion [29] and/or to astrocytic gluconeogenesis which consumes lactic acid formed in the brain during anaerobic glycolysis [4, 26]. These findings suggest that viable astrocytes swell and carry on a perturbed glycogen metabolism which in turn might be an expression of disturbed glucose utilisation induced by a disrupted mitochondrial electron-conducting energy metabolism [1–3, 22].

The temporal profile of the present ultrastructural report coincides well with measurements of specific gravity and Evans blue permeability [5] in the same model. In the present study, dying neurons in various stages of necrosis are found scattered among viable neurons. All capillaries and astrocytes with their cell processes are apparently viable and without ultrastructural disruption. This diffuse swelling of viable astrocytes corresponds to the cytotoxic edema associated with selective neuronal death but without the induction of the process of infarction.

References

1. Abe K, Aoki M, Kawagoe J, Yoshida T, Hattori A, Kogure K, Itoyama Y (1995) Ischemic delayed neuronal death. A mitochondrial hypothesis. Stroke 26: 1478–1489
2. Allen KL, Almeida A, Bates TE, Clark JB (1995) Changes of respiratory chain activity in mitochondrial and synaptosomal fractions isolated from the gerbil brain after graded ischaemia. J Neurochem 64: 2222–2229
3. Chan P, Li Y, Zheng Z, Hu P, Sarbach SD, Guez D (1993) Neurologic and histologic evaluation of almitrine + raubasine (Duxil) in middle cerebral artery occlusion in cats. Eur J Pharmacol 231: 175–182
4. Dringen R, Schmoll D, Cooar M, Hamprecht B (1993) Incorporation of radioactivity from [14C]lactate into the glycogen of cultured mouse astroglial cells. Evidence for gluconeogenesis in brain cells. Biol Chem Hoppe Seyler 374: 343–347
5. Hakamata Y, Hanyu S, Kuroiwa T, Nakano I, Ito U (1997) Brain edema associated with progressing selective neuronal death or impending infarction in cerebral cortex following repeated ischemia. In: James HE, Baethmann A, Marmarou A, Marshall LF, Reulen HJ (eds) Brain edema X. Acta Neurochir (Wien) [Suppl] 70: 20–22
6. Hanyu S, Hakamata Y, Nakano I, Ito U (in preparation)

7. Hanyu S, Ito U, Hakamata Y, Yoshida M (1993) Repeated unilateral carotid occlusion in Mongolian gerbils: quantitative analysis of cortical neuronal loss. Acta Neuropathol Berl 86: 16–20
8. Hanyu S, Ito U, Hakamata Y, Yoshida M (1995) Transition from ischemic neuronal necrosis to infarction in repeated ischemia. Brain Res 686: 44–48
9. Ito U, Go KG, Walker J Jr, Spatz M, Klatzo I (1976) Experimental cerebral ischemia in Mongolian gerbils III. Behaviour of the blood-brain barrier. Acta Neuropathol Berl 34: 1–6
10. Ito U, Hanyu S, Hakamata Y, Kuroiwa T, Yoshida M (1997) Features and threshold of infarct development in ischemic maturation phenomenon. In: Ito U, Kirino T, Kuroiwa T, Klatzo I (eds) Maturation phenomenon in cerebral ischemia. Springer, Berlin Heidelberg New York Tokyo (in press)
11. Ito U, Hanyu C, Hakamata S, Yoshida M (1995) Selective neuronal death and focal infarction in repeated ischemia. J Cereb Blood Flow Metab 15 [Suppl]: S199
12. Ito U, Ohno K, Nakamura R, Suganuma F, Inaba Y (1979) Brain edema during ischemia and after restoration of blood flow. Measurement of water, sodium, potassium content and plasma protein permeability. Stroke 10: 542–547
13. Ito U, Spatz M, Walker J Jr, Klatzo I (1975) Experimental cerebral ischemia in Mongolian gerbils. I. Light microscopic observations. Acta Neuropathol Berl 32: 209–223
14. Ito U, Yamaguchi T, Tomita H, Tone O, Shishido T, Hayashi H, Yoshida M (1992) Maturation phenomenon of ischemic injuries observed in Mongolian gerbils: introductory remarks. In: Ito U, Kirino T, Kuroiwa T, Klatzo I (eds) Maturation phenomenon in cerebral ischemia. Springer, Berlin Heidelberg New York Tokyo, pp 1–13
15. Juurlink BH, Chen Y, Hertz L (1992) Use of cell cultures to differentiate among effects of various ischemia factors on astrocytic cell volume. Can J Physiol Pharmacol 70: S344–349
16. Katzman R, Clasen R, Klatzo I, Meyer JS, Pappius HM, Waltz AG (1977) Report of Joint Committee for Stroke Resources. IV. Brain edema in stroke. Stroke 8: 512–540
17. Kempski O, Staub F, Jansen M, Schodel F, Baethmann A (1988) Glial swelling during extracellular acidosis *in vitro*. Stroke 19: 385–392
18. Kempski OS, Volk C (1994) Neuron-glial interaction during injury and edema of the CNS. In: Ito U, Kirino T, Kuroiwa T, Klatzo I (eds) Brain edema IX: Proceedings of 9th International Symposium on Brain Edema, Tokyo. Acta Neurochir (Wien) [Suppl] 60: 7–11
19. Kimelberg HK, Rutledge E, Goderie S, Charniga C (1995) Astrocytic swelling due to hypotonic or high K+ medium causes inhibition of glutamate and aspartate uptake and increases their release. J Cereb Blood Flow Metab 15: 409–416
20. Kinoshita A, Yamada K, Kohmura E, Hayakawa T (1990) Effect of astrocyte-derived factors on ischemic brain edema induced by rat MCA occlusion. Apmis 98: 851–857
21. Kraig RP, Chesler M (1990) Astrocytic acidosis in hyperglycemic and complete ischemia. J Cereb Blood Flow Metab 10: 104–114
22. Kuroiwa T, Terakado M, Yamaguchi T, Endo S, Ueki M, Okeda R (1996) The pyramidal cell layer of sector CA1 shows the lowest hippocampal succinate dehydrogenase activity in normal and postischemic gerbils. Neurosci Lett 206: 117–120
23. Lomneth R, Gruenstein EI (1989) Energy-dependent cell volume maintenance in UC-11MG human astrocytomas. Am J Physiol 257: C817–824
24. Ohno K, Ito U, Inaba Y (1984) Regional cerebral blood flow and stroke index after left carotid artery ligation in the conscious gerbil. Brain Res 297: 151–157
25. Rosenberg GA, Aizeman E (1989) Hundred-fold increase in neuronal vulnerability to glutamate toxicity in astrocyte-

poor cultures of rat cerebral cortex. Neurosci Lett 103: 162–168

26. Schmoll D, Fuhrmann E, Gebhardt R, Hamprecht B (1995) Significant amounts of glycogen are synthesized from 3-carbon compounds in astroglial primary cultures from mice with participation of the mitochondrial phosphoenolpyruvate carboxykinase isoenzyme. Eur J Biochem 227: 308–315

27. Sokoloff L (1992) Energy metabolism and effects of energy depletion or exposure to glutamate. Can J Physiol Pharmacol 70: S107–112

28. Staub F, Winkler A, Peters J, Kempski O, Kachel V, Baethmann A (1994) Swelling, acidosis, and irreversible damage of glial cells from exposure to arachidonic acid *in vitro*. J Cereb Blood Flow Metab 14: 1030–1039

29. Swanson RA, Choi DW (1993) Glial glycogen stores affect neuronal survival during glucose deprivation *in vitro*. J Cereb Blood Flow Metab 13: 162–169

30. Walz W, Klimaszewski A, Paterson IA (1993) Glial swelling in ischemia: a hypothesis. Dev Neurosc 15: 216–225

Correspondence: Umeo Ito, M.D., Department of Neurosurgery, Musashino Red Cross Hospital, 1-26-1, Kynan-cho, Musashino-shi, Tokyo 180, Japan.

Acta Neurochir (1997) [Suppl] 70: 50–52
© Springer-Verlag 1997

Heterogenous Distribution of Early Energy Failure in Experimental Focal Ischemia of the Cat Brain

M. Ueki, T. Kuroiwa, H. Ichiki, M. Kobayashi, and **R. Okeda**

Department of Neuropathology, Medical Research Institute, Tokyo Medical and Dental University, Tokyo, Japan

Summary

The distribution of succinate dehydrogenase (SDH) activity and the corresponding changes in specific gravity were studied in cats with experimental focal ischemia. Two hours of tandem occlusion of the middle cerebral artery (MCA) and the conunon carotid artery produced a scattered reduction of SDH activity and corresponding brain edema in the cortex. Recirculation ameliorated the SDH reduction and the scattered pattern disappeared, although the brain edema increased further. Four hours of focal ischemia resulted in diffuse reduction of SDH activity in the MCA-perfused area. The scattered area of SDH reduction after 2 hours of focal cerebral ischemia indicates that the ischemic core is multicentric in the early phase, and that these areas fuse together to form a well demarcated infarction, if the blood flow is not reestablished.

A short period of cerebral ischemia produces multicentric small infarcts in the cortex, which resemble granular atrophy.

Keywords: Ischemia; brain edema; succinate dehydrogenase; heterogenous distribution; energy failure.

Introduction

In experimental focal cerebral ischemia, scattered distribution of neuronal necrosis has been observed [1]. To understand the mechanism of formation of cortical heterogeneous ischemic loci, we employed a feline middle cerebral artery occlusion model using various combinations of ischemia and recirculation time. We investigated succinate dehydrogenase (SDH) activity and specific gravity to clarify the relationship between energy metabolism and brain edema.

Material and Methods

Animal Preparation

Twenty-one cats weighing between 2.5 and 4.3 kg were anesthetized with 30 mg/kg ketamine in conjunction with 0.01 mg/kg atropine intramusculaly. Ketamine was further administered, if necessary. A tracheotomy was performed and the animals were placed on a Harvard respirator. The animals were ventilated with room air, and PaCO$_2$ was kept between 35 and 45 mmHg throughout the experimental period. Catheters were inserted into the right femoral artery and vein for monitoring of blood pressure, sampling of arterial blood gases, and administration of drugs. The left common carotid artery was exposed, and a piece of 3.0 nylon suture was placed around it for later occlusion. The animals were kept normothermic (37–37.5°C) using a feedback heating pad. With the aid of an operating microscope, the horizontal portion of the left middle cerebral artery (MCA) was exposed transorbitally [10].

Induction of Ischemia and Recirculation

Focal transient and permanent ischemia of the MCA region were established by placing and removing a plastic clip on the MCA at the lateral margin of the optic nerve and tightening and loosening of the suture placed around the left common carotid artery simultaneously. Cessation or reestablishment of MCA blood flow was confirmed by direct observation of the MCA using an operating microscopy.

The 21 cats were divided randomly into 6 groups; 1 hour of ischemia (n = 3), 1.5 hours of ischemia (n = 3), 2 hours of ischemia (n = 6), 4 hours of ischemia (n = 3), 2 hours of ischemia with 1 hour of recirculation (n = 3) and 2 hours of ischemia with 3 hours of recirculation (n = 3).

Succinate Dehydrogenase (SDH) Activity Measurement

Details of the methods employed have been reported elsewhere [3–5]. Briefly, the brains were immediately removed and placed in a moist chamber kept at 0°C after sacrifice of the animals. The brain was sliced coronally at the caudal end of the anterior ectosylvian gyrus [9] to obtain serial 3-mm-thick coronal sections. These sections were incubated in 1% 2,3,5-triphenyl tetrazolium chloride (TTC) in Dulbecco's tissue culture medium at 35°C for 6 min. Regional changes in the optical density (OD) of the coronal plane due to the accumulation of formazan produced from TTC by SDH were recorded with a color standard at 1, 3, and 6 min using CCD camera (XC-75/CE, Sony, Tokyo). The formazan content was calculated according to the correlation between regional tissue formazan content and the corresponding OD. The regional SDH activity was calculated from initial the rate of formazan production, expressed as a percentage of the SDH activity on the contralateral side and displayed using grey scale (NIH Image 1.60). Data were analyzed using one-way analysis of variance and Fisher's protected least significant difference procedure for multiple comparisons, and expressed as means ± SD.

Specific Gravity Measurement

Specific gravity of the lesion was measured according to Marmarou *et al.* [6]. Specimens of approximately 1 mm³ were taken from the 3-mm-thick coronal section of the brain, which was a mirror surface of the coronal section employed for the measurement of SDH activity. Regions of interest were carefully matched to investigate the relationship between SDH activity and specific gravity.

Results

There was no significant change in the systemic arterial pressure and arterial gas tension throughout the experiment and between groups.

Figure 1a shows the changes in SDH activity and specific gravity of the parietal cortex after 1, 1.5, 2, 4 hours of permanent MCA occlusion. SDH activity remained within the normal range until 1 hour of MCA occlusion. The reduction of SDH activity began from 1.5 hours of focal cerebral ischemia and deteriorated further to $43 \pm 25\%$ by 4 hours. Changes in the specific gravity of this area of the cortex were related to the changes in SDH activity. At 4 hours of MCA occlusion, the specific gravity was 1.0381 ± 0.0035. Recirculation after 2 hours of MCA occlusion ameliorated the reduction in SDH activity, although the brain edema was exacerbated (Fig. 1b).

At 2 hours of MCA occlusion, various patterns of ischemic foci appeared in the marginal area between the frontal and temporal cortex and dorsal portion of the caudate putamen. Figures 2a, 2b show multiple well-delineated spots of reduced SDH activity about 1–2 mm in diameter which appeared in two of the six animals in the 2-hours MCA occlusion group. No animal with recirculation showed this type of scattered distribution of spotty area. After 4 hours of MCA occlusion, well demarcated reduction of SDH activity was observed in the MCA-perfused area (Fig. 2c).

Discussion

SDH is a mitochondrial respiratory enzyme of the tricarboxylic acid (TCA) cycle, involved in aerobic ATP production. SDH is an index of cellular energy metabolic reserve [5]. The reduction in SDH activity was ameliorated by recirculation, in spite of the further

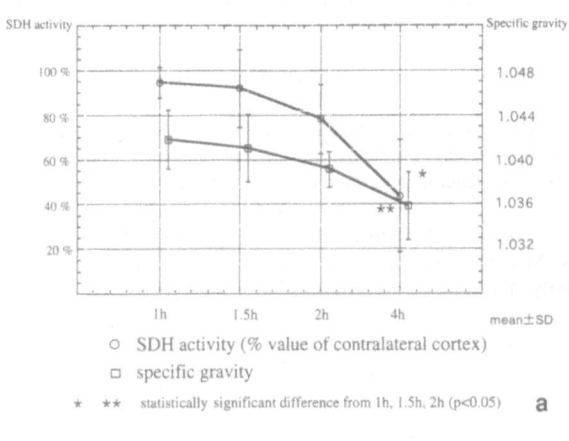
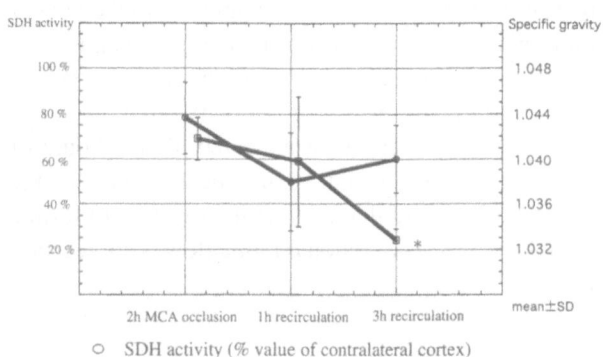

Fig. 1. (a) Changes in SDH activity and specific gravity after permanent MCA occlusion. (b) Changes in SDH activity and specific gravity after 2 hours ischemia with recirculation

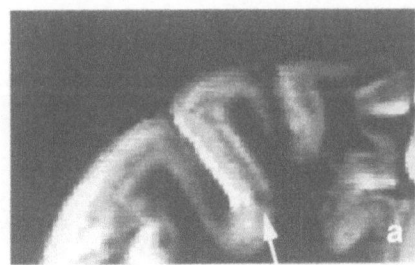
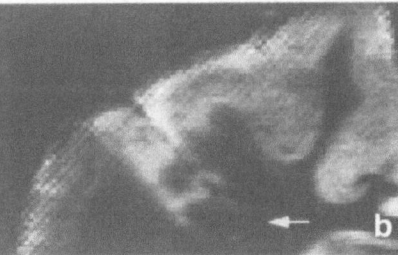
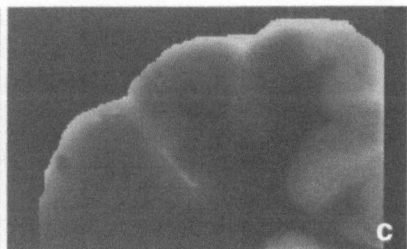

Fig. 2. SDH activity. (a) 2 h ischemia; (b) 2 h ischemia; (c) 4 h ischemia

development of brain edema. This implies that recirculation even after 2 hours of focal cerebral ischemia may be beneficial. In focal cerebral ischemia, the time when intervention is likely to be beneficial is 2–3 hours in rats and 3–4 hours in non-human primates. However, it is highly variable among individuals due to the status of collateral flow, patient age, coexisting metabolic abnormalities, premorbid medical conditions and many other confounding variables [1].

The heterogeneous distribution of the energy metabolism disturbances observed in the present study is basically in line with the results of other investigators, utilizing focal cerebral ischemia. Two hours of middle cerebral artery occlusion with 2 hours of recirculation resulted in scattered spots of neuronal damage in cat [10]. With ischemia, the reduction of regional cerebral blood flow is not homogeneous because of anatomical variations of collateral channels, which produce heterogeneous microcirculation flow, a condition known as patchy non-filling in the ischemic cortex [2, 12]. It has not yet been determined, whether islands of necrosis develop in the unperfused tissue and then coalesce to produce infarct extension [8]. In the ischemic penumbra, however, acidic foci develop, which may lead to recruitment of the ischemic penumbra into the area of infarction [11]. With diffusion-weighted imaging, apparent diffusion coefficient values were heterogenous in the early phase of ischemia [7]. We thus speculate that the spotty foci which appeared after 2 hours of MCA occlusion in our experiment represent the ischemic core, and that these fused together to form a well demarcated infarction if blood flow is not reestablished.

References

1. Fisher M, Takano K (1995) The penumbra, therapeutic time window and acute ischaemic stroke. Baillieres Clin Neurol 4 (2): 279–295
2. Ginsberg MD, Budd WW, Welsh FA (1978) Diffuse cerebral ischemia in the cat. 1. Local blood flow during severe ischemia and recirculation. Ann Neurol 3: 482–492
3. Kuroiwa T, Czernicki Z, Ueki M, Kaneko H, Okeda R (1993) Quantitative imaging of succinic dehydrogenase activity in gerbil brain after unilateral common carotid artery occlusion. J Cereb Blood Flow Metab 13 [Suppl]: 738
4. Kuroiwa T, Ueki M, Chen Q, Suemasu H, Taniguchi I, Okeda R (1994) Biochemical characteristics of brain edema. Acta Neurochir (Wien) [Suppl] 60: 158–161
5. Kuroiwa T, Terakado M, Yamaguchi T, Endo, Ueki M, Okeda R (1996) The pyramidal cell layer of sector CA1 shows the lowest hippocampal succinate dehydrogenase activity in normal and postischemic gerbils. Neurosci Lett 206: 117–120
6. Marmarou A, Tanaka K, Shulman K (1982) An improved gravimetric measure of cerebral edema. J Neurosurg 56: 246–253
7. Reith W, Hasegawa Y, Latour LL (1995) Multislice diffusion mapping for 3-D evolution of cerebral ischemia in a rat stroke model. Neurology 45: 172–177
8. Siesjö BK (1992) Pathoplysiology and treatment of focal cerebral ischemia. Part 1. Pathophysiology. J Neurosurg 77: 169–184
9. Snider RS, Niemer WT (1970) A stereotaxic atlas of the cat brain, 3rd ed. The University of Chicago Press, Chicago
10. Tamura A, Asano T, Sano K (1980) Correlation between rCBF and histological changes following temporary middle cerebral artery occlusion. Stroke 11: 487–493
11. Tomlinson FH, Anderson RE, Meyer FB (1993) Acidic foci within the ischemia penumbra of the New Zealand rabbit. Stroke 24: 2030–2040
12. Welsh FA, Ginsberg MD, Rieder W, Budd WW (1978) Diffuse cerebral ischemia in the cat. 2. Regional metabolites during severe ischemia and recirculation. Ann Neurol 3: 493–501

Correspondence: Masato Ueki, M.D., Department of Neuropathology, Medical Research Institute, Tokyo Medical and Dental University, Yushima 1-5-45, Bunkyo-ku,113 Tokyo, Japan.

Acta Neurochir (1997) [Suppl] 70: 53–55

Leukocyte-Endothelium Interactions in Global Cerebral Ischemia

J. Beck[1], W. Stummer[2], J. Lehmberg[1], A. Baethmann[1], and E. Uhl[2]

[1] Institute for Surgical Research, and [2] Department of Neurosurgery, Grosshadern University Hospital,
Ludwig-Maximilians-University Munich, Federal Republic of Germany

Summary

A closed cranial window was implanted in male Mongolian Gerbils to investigate leukocyte-endothelium interactions (LEI) at the brain surface in global cerebral ischemia (GCI) by intravital fluorescence microscopy. Four days after 15 min of bilateral common carotid artery occlusion the ischemic tissue damage was histologically analysed in selectively vulnerable areas of the brain. The frequency of Rhodamine 6G labeled leukocytes rolling along ("roller") and firmly attached ("sticker") to postcapillary endothelium was assessed before and up to 180 min after GCI. As compared to the sham operated control animals induction of LEI was found in animals with GCI, following a steady increase up to a significant level attained at 60 min (rollers) or at 120 min of reperfusion (sticker), respectively (p < 0.05). In animals with cerebral ischemia histological assessment revealed a significant decrease of viable neurons in the CA 1-sector of hippocampus (neurons/mm² ± SEM: 1308 ± 71 vs. 829 ± 106), in parietal neocortex (727 ± 17 vs. 542 ± 49), and in striatum (547 ± 26 vs. 352 ± 49; p < 0.01), respectively. A significant correlation between the extent of irreversible neuronal damage and the frequency of leukocyte adherence to the endothelium could not be established. Nevertheless a direct correlation between the number of surviving neurons and of rolling leukocytes was observed, which may be suggestive of a protective potential of leukocyte rolling.

Keywords: Leucocyte; endothelium; cerebral ischemia; sticking; rolling.

Introduction

Since the reports of Ames *et al.* [3] on the no-reflow phenomenon after cerebral ischemia a role of leukocyte activation in this process has been considered. As shown in other organs, such as myocardium and skeletal muscle [13], activation of polymorphonuclear leukocytes (PMNLs) may contribute to the reperfusion injury after ischemia. Prior to emigration into the tissue, activated leukocytes may roll along the vessel wall (rollers) and may subsequently become firmly attached to the vascular endothelium (stickers), a phenomenon which is mediated by adhesion molecules [21]. The detrimental potential of leukocyte activation may include enhance-

ment of brain edema and secondary tissue necrosis, for example by a release of proteolytic enzymes and free radicals from these cells [24]. Moreover, it is conceivable that disruption of the blood brain barrier together with impairment of the microcirculation by capillary plugging might be elicited by activation of leukocytes in ischemia. The purpose of the current study was to quantitatively analyse the development of leukocyte-endothelium interactions in the cerebral microcirculation following global cerebral ischemia by fluorescence microscopy. Furthermore, ischemic tissue damage was examined by nerve cell counts in histological brain sections at day 4 following global cerebral ischemia to elucidate a potential correlation between induction of LEI and the extent of irreversible neuronal damage in selectively vulnerable areas of the brain.

Material and Methods

Global cerebral ischemia was induced in Mongolian Gerbils (60–80 g b.w.; n = 12) taking advantage of the incomplete Circulus Willisi, i.e. the anatomical specifity of insufficient anastomotic arterial connections between the carotid arteries and the basilar artery at the basis of the brain [14]. Catheters were inserted under halothane anaesthesia into the tail artery and femoral vein for monitoring arterial blood pressure and for injection of the fluorescent dyes respectively. A closed cranial window of 5 × 5 mm was implanted above the left parietal brain cortex leaving the aura mater intact. Animals were placed on a feedback controlled heating pad to ensure normothermia. To induce complete forebrain ischemia both common carotid arteries were ligated with a 5–0 monofilament thread and reversibly occluded for 15 min. The fluorescent dyes Rhodamine 6G (0.03 µg/kg) and FITC-Dextran (0.7 g/kg) were administered as *in vivo* markers for leukocytes [5] and for contrast enhancement of microvessels. Images of the cerebral microvasculature were obtained with a highly sensitive SIT tubular camera and an epifluorescence microscope, using a 20 × water immersion objective, and recorded by video tape. 100 µm length segments of venules of 15 to 50 µm in diameter were observed for one minute. The animal was placed on a stage with a computer controlled stepping motor for exact identification of regions of interest at any time. The number of leukocytes rolling along the vascular endothelium ("roller") and adhering to the vessel wall ("sticker") (cells / 100 μm × min), respectively were assessed at 40 and 20 min prior to ischemia, and at 5, 20, 40, 60, 90, 120, 180 min of reperfusion. At day 4 after ischemia, animals were intracardially perfused with phosphate-buffered paraformaldehyde (2%; ph 7.4) in deep ether anaesthesia, the brain was subsequently removed, processed and embedded in paraffin. For quantitatively counting of surviving nerve cells 51 μm sections were cut 1.7 mm caudal of the bregma and stained with cresyl violet. Cerebral cortex and the CA1-sector of hippocampus were studied, and the striatum at 0.5mm rostral of the bregma. The surviving neurons meeting well established morphological viability requirements [10] were counted [n/mm²] in these selectively vulnerable regions of the brain using an image analysing program (Optimate 5.1) described by Stummer *et al.* [22].

Results

Leukocyte-Endothelium-Interactions

Under baseline conditions prior to induction of ischemia, the number of leukocytes rolling along and sticking at the vascular endothelium was close to zero in both the experimental and control group. In the control animals the low number of rolling as well as adherent leukocytes remained at the baseline level during the whole observation period. In contrast in animals subjected to 15 min of GCI induction of LEI was found in the postcapillary venules. The quantitative analysis revealed a steady increase of the frequency of rolling leukocytes attaining statistical significance as early as 60 min after ischemia, i.e. 9.44 ± 2.98, (cells/100 ± SEM) as compared to 0.56 ± 0.43 (control; $p < 0.05$ Mann-Whitney-U-test). Leukocyte rolling increased further up to a maximum of 34.33 ± 7.49, at the end of the observation period at 180 min of reperfusion. The number of leukocytes which were firmly attached to the vascular endothelium also rose. This response was significant following 120 min of reperfusion when the number of sticking leukocytes was increased to 2.09 ± 0.96 cells / 100 μm × min as compared to 0 ± 0 in the control group ($p < 0.05$). Again, the maximum of leukocyte sticking was reached at 180 min after ischemia, i.e. 2.33 ± 0.87 ($p < 0.05$).

Nerve Cell Counts

At day 4 after ischemia neuronal damage was severe in the selectively vulnerable areas of the brain [9, 22]. In the CA1-sector of the hippocampus 1308 ± 71 neurons/mm² were counted in the control animals whereas only 829 ± 106 after ischemia ($p < 0.01$; t-test). Global cerebral ischemia also led to a decrease in density of neurons in the parietal neocortex, where only 542 ± 49

neurons/mm² survival compared to 727 ± 17 in the control group or in striatum with 352 ± 49 vs. 547 ± 26 ($p < 0.01$, respectively).

In order to examine whether there was a potential association of the postischemic neuronal loss with the activation of LEI by ischemia regression analysis was performed. The number of rolling leukocytes was statistically significantly correlated with the proportion of surviving nerve cells in both parietal neocortex ($r = 0.90$, $p < 0.01$) and striatum ($r = 0.85$, $p < 0.03$). As to the induction of leukocyte attachment to the venular endothelium after ischemia, however, a significant correlation with the extinction of nerve cells was not observed.

Discussion

Previous studies have emphasized a pathophysiological function of activation of polymorphonuclear leukocytes following cerebral ischemia [2, 10, 14, 16] either based on leukocyte accumulation in the brain which was histologically assessed, on outcome studies with either monoclonal antibodies against adhesion molecules mediating the interaction of PMNLs and endothelium [6, 7], or by using adhesion molecule knock-out animals [8]. In other studies of cerebral ischemia, however, inhibition of leukocyte activation did not result in any therapeutic protection or did not improve respective experimental parameters [1, 4, 11, 18, 23].

The present findings demonstrate that global cerebral ischemia leading to severe injury in various brain regions is associated with activation of leukocyte-endothelium interactions in the cerebral microcirculation during postischemic reperfusion. In order to examine a potential cause-effect relationship of activation of the LEI and the postischemic nerve cell damage, a regression analysis between both parameters was carried out. The result, however, does not support respective conclusions as to the induction of leukocyte sticking. A seemingly paradox relationship emerged with regard to the activation of leukocyte rolling. The results indicate a positive correlation between the activation of leukocyte rolling and the number of surviving neurons in the postischemic brain suggesting a protective role of leukocyte rolling. A protective function of neutrophils is implied also by the results of Schott *et al.* [19] who found an increased mortality from neutrophil depletion in dogs with 10 minutes of global cerebral ischemia. Global cerebral ischemia is associated with the release of inflammatory mediators [17], such as

IL-1 which triggers both activation of PMNLs as well as regenerative processes, such as local formation of nerve growth factor [20]. Thus enhancement of the number of rolling leukocytes following ischemia may be viewed as an indicator of ongoing restorative mechanisms. Yet, in order to further elucidate the phenomenon and its significance additional investigations are required.

Acknowledgment

The excellent technical assistance by Monika Fürst and Claudia Guggenmos is gratefully appreciated. Supported by Deutsche Forschungsgemeinschaft: Uh/62–4.

References

1. Abels C, Röhrich F, Uhl E, Corvin S, Villringer A, Dirnagel U, Baethmann A, Schürer L (1994) Current evidence on a pathophysiological function of leukocyte/endothelial interactions in cerebral ischemia. In: Hartmann A, Yatsu F, Kuschinsky W (eds) Cerebral ischemia and basic mechanisms. Springer, Berlin Heidelberg New York
2. Akopov S, Sercombe R, Seylaz J (1996) Cerebrovascular reactivity: role of endothelium/platelet/leukocyte interactions. Cerebrovasc Brain Metab Rev 8: 11–94
3. Ames A III, Wright RL, Kowada M, Thurston JM, Majano G (1968) The no-reflow phenomenon. Am J Pathol 52: 437–453
4. Aspey BS, Jessimer C, Pereira S, Harrison MJG (1989) Do leukocytes have a role in the cerebral no-reflow phenomenon? J Neurol Neurosurg Psychiatry 52: 526–528
5. Baatz H, Steinbauer M, Harris AG, Krombach F (1995) Kinetics of white blood cell staining by intravascular administration of Rhodamine 6G. Int J Microcirc 15: 85–91
6. Bednar MM, Raymond S, McAuliffe T, Lodge PA, Gross CE (1991) The role of neutrophils and platelets in a rabbit model of thromboembolic stroke. Stroke 22: 44–50
7. Clark WM, Madden KP, Rothlein R, Zivin JA (1991) Reduction of central nervous system ischemic injury in rabbits using leukocyte adhesion antibody treatment. Stroke 22: 877–883
8. Conolly ES, Winfree CJ, Springer TA, Naka Y, Liao H, Yan SD, Stern DM, Solomon RA, Gutierrez-Ramos JC, Pinsky DJ (1996) Cerebral protection in homozygous null ICAM-1 mice after middle cerebral artery occlusion. J Clin Invest 97: 209–216
9. Crain BJ, Westerkam WD, Harrison AH, Nadler JV (1988) Selective neuronal death after transient forebrain ischemia in the Mongolian gerbil: a silver impregnation study. Neuroscience 27: 387–402
10. Del Zoppo GJ, Copeland BR, Harker LA, Waltz TA, Zyroff J, Hanson SR, Battenberg E (1986) Experimental acute thrombotic stroke in baboons. Stroke 17: 1254–1265
11. Dirnagel U, Niwa K, Sixt G, Villringer A (1994) Cortical hypoperfusion after global forebrain ischemia in rats is not caused by microvascular leukocyte plugging. Stroke 25: 1028–1038
12. Eke A, Conger AK (1989) Classifying cells from light microscopic bit features by binary logic. Lab Invest 61: 243–252
13. Engler RL, Schmid-Schönbein GW, Pavelec RS (1983) Leukocyte capillary plugging in myocardial ischemia and reperfusion in the dog. Am J Pathol 111: 98–111
14. Hallenbeck JM, Dutka AJ, Tanishima T, Kochanek PM, Kumaroo KK, Thompson CB, Obrenovitch TP, Contreras TJ (1986) Polymorphonuclear leukocyte accumulation in brain regions with low blood flow during the early postischemic period. Stroke 17: 246–253
15. Levy DE, Brierley JB (1974) Communications between vertebrobasilar and carotid arterial circulations in the gerbil. Exp Neurol 45: 503–508
16. Okada Y, Copeland BR, Mori E, Tung M-M, Thomas WS, del Zoppo GJ (1994) P-selectin and intercellular adhesion molecule-1 expression after focal brain ischemia and reperfusion. Stroke 25: 202–211
17. Saito K, Suyama K, Nishida K, Sei Y, Basile AS (1996) Early increases in TNF-a, IL-6 and IL-1b levels following transient cerebral ischemia in gerbil brain. Neurosci Lett 206: 149–152
18. Schürer L, Grögaard B, Gerdin B, Kempski O, Arfors K-E (1991) Leukocyte depletion does not affect post-ischemic nerve cell damage in the rat. Acta Neurochir (Wien) 111: 54–60
19. Schott RJ, Natale JE, Ressler SW, Burney RE, D'Alecy LG (1989) Neutrophil depletion fails to improve neurologic outcome after cardiac arrest in dogs. Ann Emerg Med 18: 517–522
20. Spranger M, Lindholm D, Brandtlow C, Heuman R, Gnahn H, Nager-Noe M, Thoenen H (1990) Regulation of nerve groth factor (NGF) synthesis in the rat central nervous system: comparison between the effects of interleukin-1 and various growth factors in astrocyte cultures and in vivo. Eur J Neurosci 2: 69–76
21. Springer TA (1990) Adhesion receptors of the immune system. Nature 346: 425–434
22. Stummer W, Weber DVM, Tranmer B, Baethmann A, Kempski O (1994) Reduced mortality and brain damage after locomotor activity in gerbil forebrain ischemia. Stroke 25: 1862–1869
23. Takeshima R, Kirsch JR, Koehler RC, Gomoll AW, Traystmann RJ (1992) Monoclonal leukocyte antibody does not decrease the injury of transient focal cerebral ischemia in cats. Stroke 23: 247–252
24. Weiss SJ (1989) Tissue destruction neutrophils. N Engl J Med 320: 365–376

Correspondence: Eberhard Uhl, M.D., Department of Neurosurgery, Grosshadern University Hospital, Ludwig-Maximilian University of Munich, Marchioninistr. 15, D-81366 Munich, Federal Republic of Germany.

Acta Neurochir (1997) [Suppl] 70: 56–58
© Springer-Verlag 1997

Selective Impairments of Mitochondrial Respiratory Chain Activity During Aging and Ischemic Brain Damage

M. Davis, T. Whitely, D. M. Turnbull, and A. D. Mendelow

Departments of Surgery (Neurosurgery), Medicine (Geriatrics) and Neurology, University of Newcastle upon Tyne, England, U.K.

Summary

Cumulative oxidative damage to mitochondrial deoxyribonucleic acid (DNA) with subsequent defects in oxidative phosphorylation may reduce the capacity of the aging brain to cope with metabolic stress. This may contribute to the age related increase in cerebral infarct size that has been documented following permanent middle cerebral artery occlusion (MCAO) in the rat. This hypothesis was evaluated by assessing mitochondrial respiratory chain complex activity in both ischemic and non ischemic brain tissue of adult (10 month) and aged (28 month) male Wistar rats, six hours after occlusion of the left middle cerebral artery. Aging was associated with a significant decline in cerebral mitochondrial function with impairment of the activities of complexes I, II and IV. The individual respiratory chain complexes also exhibited selective vulnerability to a focal cerebral ischemic lesion, with significant impairment of complex I activity in the lesioned hemisphere of both age groups. The age related decline in complex I activity may be important in the enhanced susceptibility of the aging brain to ischemic neuronal damage.

Keywords: Aging brain; respiratory chain; cerebral ischemia; impaired mitochondria.

Introduction

Mitochondria are ubiquitous intracellular organelles, which are predominantly involved in the generation of energy for subsequent cellular consumption. Structural and functional decline in brain mitochondria may contribute to the impairments of cerebral function that have been documented in association with aging.

Such oxidative damage to mitochondrial DNA and the subsequent defects in oxidative phosphorylation might also be implicated in the pathogenesis of ischemic neuronal damage, and may thereby contribute to the age related increase in cerebral infarct volume that has been documented in a rodent model of focal cerebral ischemia [4].

Mitochondrial function can be assessed by analysis of the activities of the individual respiratory chain complexes that form the electron transport chain, and are responsible for the coupling of oxidative phosphorylation to energy production. The respiratory chain comprises four multicomponent complexes including complex I (NADH: ubiquinone oxidoreductase), complex II (succinate: ubiquinone oxidoreductase), complex III (ubiquinol: cytochrome c oxidoreductase) and complex IV (cytochrome c oxidase), which act as a series of electron carriers of graded redox mid-point potentials that can undergo alternative oxidation and reduction. As electrons pass down the chain, protons are pumped across the mitochondrial inner membrane from the matrix, resulting in the generation of an electrochemical proton gradient or proton motive force. This gradient is subsequently utilised in the production of high energy phosphates.

We hypothesised that age related impairments of respiratory chain complex activity would reduce the capacity of the aging brain to cope with metabolic stress and might thereby render it vulnerable to ischemic neuronal injury.

Materials and Methods

The experiments were conducted in accordance with the Animals (Scientific Procedures) Act 1986, in adult (10 month) and aged (28 month) male Wistar rats. Anaesthesia was induced by the inhalation of 4% halothane in a mixture of nitrous oxide and oxygen (70/30) and after intubation, was maintained using 1–2% halothane, with reduction to 0.4% subsequent to all surgical procedures. Ventilation was monitored continuously via pulse oximetry and a capnograph. Core temperature was maintained using a heating pad and a rectal thermistor probe. The femoral vessels were cannulated for the monitoring of mean arterial blood pressure, the measurement of arterial blood gases, glucose and haematocrit, and the administration of fluid. The left middle cerebral artery was exposed via a microcraniectomy according to the technique of Tamura, but with preservation of the zygomatic arch [15], and the vessel was occluded by thermocoagulation using microbipolar diathermy, proximal to the origin of the lenticulostriate branch. After 6 hours, the animals were decapitated, the brains were rapidly removed, and the hemispheres were placed individually in ice cold isolation medium C (300 mM mannitol, 5 mM Hepes, 0.1 mM ethylene glycol-bis (amino ethylether) N,N,N',N'-tetra-acetic acid (EGTA), 5 mg.ml^{-1} BSA). The brain was homogenised, and underwent a series of centrifugations, resuspension, homogenisation and recentrifugation to promote the removal of synaptosomes and yield a mitochondrial pellet. The mitochondria were washed in medium D (250 mM sucrose/0.5 mM Tris-HCl), recentrifuged and resuspended to yield a concentration of 15–25 mg.ml^{-1}.

The protein concentration of mitochondrial fractions was determined by a modification of the Lowry method [12]. All respiratory chain complex assays were conducted at 30°C in a final volume of 1.0 ml, using a spectrophotometer.

Data are presented as means with their standard errors and statistical analysis has been conducted using Student's t test.

Results

All physiological variables were similar in both age groups. Complex I activity was lower in ischemic brain, with mean values of 91.1 ± 8.8 and 126.7 ± 14 nmol.min.$^{-1}$ mg protein^{-1} in the left and right hemispheres respectively ($p < 0.05$, n = 13). Complex I activity also declined with aging. The mean activity in aged rats (n = 7) was 97.4 ± 15 compared with 160.9 ± 18 nmol.min.$^{-1}$ mg protein^{-1} in adults (n = 6, $p < 0.05$). The activities of complexes II and IV were not significantly impaired in ischemic brain, but both declined with aging. The mean activity of complex II in aged rat brain was 222.1 ± 34 nmol.min.$^{-1}$ mg protein^{-1}, compared with 371.1 ± 39 nmol.min.$^{-1}$ mg protein^{-1} in adults ($p < 0.05$), whilst mean values for complex IV were 3.32 ± 0.52 and 5.41 ± 0.46 K.sec.$^{-1}$ mg protein^{-1} respectively ($p < 0.05$). Complex III and citrate synthase activities were not affected by aging or ischemia.

Discussion

Aging was associated with significant impairment of the activities of complexes I, II and IV. The documented decline in enzyme activities is unlikely to be secondary to a quantitative change in mitochondria, since the mitochondrial enrichment of samples (as reflected by citrate synthase activity) was similar between groups. Citrate synthase is entirely encoded by nuclear DNA which has inherent protective mechanisms against oxidative damage and is therefore relatively resistant to recurrent mutation. The structure and subsequent function of citrate synthase should therefore be preserved during aging, and as the enzyme is remarkably stable, its activity is used as a marker of mitochondrial enrichment in tissue samples. In the current study, the enzyme activities were similar in all groups, suggesting that the tissue samples were equally enriched with mitochondria. The decline in complex activity in aged brain is therefore likely to represent a significant deterioration in mitochondrial function and may result from cumulative oxidative damage to DNA, protein and lipids. Mitochondria are particularly vulnerable to oxidative damage, since during normal metabolism, they constitute and are subsequently exposed to the greatest source of intracellular oxidants. Free radical production increases during normal aging [10, 14] and as mitochondrial DNA possesses limited repair mechanisms and lacks protective histones [1], mutations may accumulate, leading to a 10 fold higher frequency of mutation in mitochondrial than nuclear DNA [10, 17]. The enhanced vulnerability of mitochondrial DNA to mutation may also be secondary to frequent replication. Unlike the nucleus, the mitochondrial genome in post-mitotic cells such as neurons, continues to replicate every 24.4 days [5, 9], culminating in more than 40 recurrent cycles in a 3 year old rat and in excess of 1000 replications in an octogenarian human. Furthermore, with the exception of a small segment involved in replication, its compact supercoiled structure is comprised entirely of coding sequences, rendering most mutational changes potentially injurious to subsequent function [8, 17]. Single point mutations and deletions within mitochondrial DNA therefore increase with age, promoting the production of defective mitochondrial respiratory chain complexes. The polypeptides most likely to be deranged will be those that are predominantly encoded by mitochondrial rather than nuclear DNA. The mitochondrial genome incorporates 11320 base pairs to encode thirteen proteins, seven of which form subunits of complex I [2, 17]. The numbers of mitochondrial base pairs involved in encoding respiratory chain complexes are 6338, 1140 and 3003 for complexes I, II and IV respectively [3]. A random mutation in the mitochondrial genome is therefore most likely to involve the coding sequences for complex I, but may also potentially affect those for complexes II and IV. Similarly, age associated increases in mitochondrial mutations might be reflected preferentially as age related structural and subsequent functional impairments of these complexes I, II and IV, as found in the current investigations. This might also explain the preservation of the activity of complex III with aging, since this protein is entirely encoded by nuclear DNA [3].

Complex I activity was significantly impaired in the ischaemic hemisphere, but the activities of complexes II, III and IV were unaffected. The decline in complex I activity may enhance free radical production during cerebral ischemia. Inhibition of complex I by rotenone or by MPP⁺, a toxic metabolise of the drug MPTP, has been associated with enhanced mitochondrial production of superoxide *in vitro* [7, 16]. This is thought to be secondary to the channelling of electrons down the transport chain via complex II, which generates about four times as much superoxide as their transfer via complex I [13]. Superoxide could mediate toxicity by promoting the formation of hydroxyl radicals via the Fenton reaction, or via the generation of hydroperoxyl radicals (HO_2) which is favoured by an acidotic environment. Complex I deficiency has been associated with lactic acidosis, as is found in severe ischaemia, and protenation of superoxide to HO_2 radicals has been reported to increase 100 fold in association with a fall in the pH of the mitochondrial matrix from 8 to 6 [3]. Although mitochondria produce large amounts of superoxide during normal aerobic metabolism, the free radicals do not usually penetrate the inner mitochondrial membrane because they are rapidly converted to hydrogen peroxide by the antioxidant enzyme superoxide dismutase [6]. However, the enhanced production of superoxide combined with inhibition of the activity of SOD during ischemia renders the inherent antioxidant mechanism ineffective.

As complex I activity deteriorates with age, this deleterious effect of ischemia may be enhanced in aged neurons. This may lead to a reduced capacity in the aging brain to cope with metabolic stress, and contribute to the subsequent enhancement of neuronal injury associated with a focal cerebral ischaemic lesion.

References

1. Ames BN, Shigenaga MK, Hagen TM (1995) Mitochondrial decay in aging. Biochim Biophys Acta 1271: 165–170
2. Anderson S, Bankier AT, Barrell BG, De Bruijn MMHL, Coulson AR, Droiun J, Eperon IC, Nierlich DP, Roe BA, Sanger F, Schreier PH, Smith AJH, Staden R, Young IG (1981) Sequence and organization of the human mitochondrial genome. Nature 290: 457–465
3. Cortopassi G, Wang E (1995) Modelling the effects of agerelated mtDNA mutation accumulation; Complex I deficiency, superoxide and cell death. Biochim Biophys Acta 1271: 171–176
4. Davis M, Mendelow AD, Perry RH, Chambers IR, James OFW (1995) Experimental stroke and neuroprotection in the aging rat brain. Stroke 26: 1072–1078
5. Gross NJ, Getz GS, Rabinowitz M (1969) Apparent turnover of mitochondrial deoxyribonucleic acid and mitochondrial phospholipids in the tissues of the rat. J Biol Chem 244 (6): 1552–1562
6. Halliwell B (1989) Superoxide, iron, vascular endothelium and reperfusion injury. Free Radic Res Commun 5: 315–318
7. Hasegawa E, Takeshige K, Oishi T, Murai Y, Minikami S (1990) 1-methyl-4-phenylpyridinium (MPP⁺) induces NADH-dependent superoxide formation and enhances NADH-dependent lipid peroxidation in bovine heart submitochondrial particles. Biochem Biophys Res Commun 170(3): 1049–1055
8. Linnane AW, Marzuki S, Ozawa T, Tanaka M (1989) Mitochondrial DNA mutations as an important contributor to aging and degenerative diseases. Lancet 1: 642–645
9. Menzies RA, Gold PH (1971) The turnover of mitochondria in a variety of tissues of young, adult and aged rats. J Biol Chem 246: 2425–2429
10. Miquel J (1991) An integrated theory of aging as the result of mitochondrial-DNA mutation in differentiated cells. Arch Gerontol Geriatr 12: 99–117
11. Ozawa T (1995) Mechanism of somatic mitochondrial DNA mutations associated with age and diseases. Biochim Biophys Acta 1271: 177–189
12. Peterson GL (1977) A simplification of the protein assay method of Lowry *et al.* which is more generally applicable. Anal Biochem 83(2): 346–356
13. Pryor WA (1982) Superoxide radical and hydrogen peroxide in mitochondria. In: Free radicals in biology. Academic Press, New York, pp 65–90
14. Sohal RS, Sohal BH (1991) Hydrogen peroxide release by mitochondria increases during aging. Mech Ageing Dev 57: 187–202
15. Tamura A, Graham DI, McCulloch J, Teasdale GM (1981) Focal cerebral ischaemia in the rat: 1. Description of technique and early neuropathological consequences following middle cerebral artery occlusion. J Cereb Blood Flow Metab 1: 53–60
16. Turrens JK, Boveris A (1980) Generation of the superoxide anion by the NADH dehydrogenase of bovine heart mitochondria. Biochem J 191 (2): 421–427
17. Wallace DC (1992) Mitochondrial genetics: a paradigm for aging and deqenerative diseases? Science 256: 628–632

Corrspondence: Dr. Michelle Davis, c/o Professor A. D. Mendelow, The Regional Neuroscience Centre, Newcastle General Hospital, Westgate Road, Newcastle upon Tyne, England, U.K.

Acta Neurochir (1997) [Suppl] 70: 59–61
© Springer-Verlag 1997

Regional Differences in the Cerebrovascular Reserve Following Acute Global Ischemia in Rabbits

W. Sapieja, N. Kuridze, and **Z. Czernicki**

Department of Neurosurgery, Medical Research Centre, Polish Academy of Sciences, Warsaw, Poland

Summary

The changes of the blood flow velocity in different cerebral arteries under normal and postischemic conditions were investigated in order to evaluate cerebrovascular reserve capacity after the brain ischemia. The experiments were carried out in rabbits. Administration of acetazolamide (Diamox) of 20 mg/kg was performed in all experimental animals and the blood flow velocity in the middle cerebral artery (MCA) and the basilar artery (BA) was measured using the transcranial Doppler sonography. In the control group of animals the intravenous administration of Diamox caused significant increase of the blood flow velocity in the MCA and the BA. In the second group of animals subjected to the acute global ischemia (occlusion of two vessels + hypotension) of 10 min duration prior to the Diamox administration, no increase of the blood flow velocity in the MCA was observed parallel with an increase in the BA. In some animals there was a decrease in the blood flow velocity in MCA. This could be a consequence of stealing phenomenon, as an increase of cerebral blood flow in the posterior fossa compartment, at the cost of the supratentorial circulation. Identification of the areas damaged after the brain ischemia was performed by the 2,3,5-triphenyltetrazoliumchloride (TTC) staining technique. This revealed more pronounced ischemic lesions in the cerebral cortex in comparison to the region of the basal ganglia.

Keywords: Cerebral ischemia; acetazolamide; regional cerebrovascular reactivity.

Introduction

Acetazolamide (Diamox) – the inhibitor of the carbon oxide anhydrase is widely used in treatment of cerebral circulation insufficiency in order to assess the cerebrovascular reserve capacity [3]. In normal conditions intravenous administration of acetazolamide (20 mg/kg) in animals and humans enhances brain blood flow velocity and causes the decrease of peripheral resistance [1, 4, 6]. In this experiments acetolamide was used to evaluate the vasomotor reactivity in different areas of the cerebrovascular system (middle cerebral and basilar arteries) in the control group of rabbits [5] and the group of animals subjected to 10 min of acute global ischemia [5].

Materials and Methods

Experiments were carried out on rabbits of both sexes weighting 3.0 to 3.5 kg. The animals were anaesthetized intravenously with urethane – 10 mg/kg and α-chloralose – 80 mg/kg. Tacheotomy and cannulation of left femoral artery and vein for the arterial and venous pressure monitoring, blood sampling and drug administration was performed in all animals. Another catheter was introduced into the right common carotid artery for blood withdrawing during ischemia and a loose ligature was placed around the left common carotid artery, so it could be tightened if necessary. During the surgical preparation – xylocaine (Astra-R, Sweden) was used for local analgesia. Mera-PIAP (Poland) pressure transducers with MCK4011 (TEMED-Poland) electromanometers and a computer system was used for blood pressure monitoring. After surgical preparation animals were paralyzed with pavulon (Organon) at a dose of 0.2 mg/kg and artificially ventilated. During the experiments the animals were under general anesthesia inhaling nitrous oxide and oxygen in a ratio 2:1. Continuous $P_{Et}CO_2$ monitoring in expired air (Datex Capnograph), and periodic blood gas analysis (CIBA Blood Gas Analyzer) were performed for evaluation of the ventilation conditions and blood pH changes under normal, ischemic and postischemic conditions. The animals were placed in sphinx position with a head immobilized in a stereotaxic apparatus. The blood flow velocity (BFV) in middle cerebral artery (MCA) and basilar artery (BA) was monitored and recorded during the experiments using Transcranial Doppler (TCD) Sonography apparatus (Medasonics). BFV in the investigated vessels was measured by a PW-2MHz TCD probe which was applied either to the right eyeball of the experimental animal for the MCA investigation, or to the back part of the skull for the BA investigation. During ischemia both carotid arteries were ligated for 10 min and systemic arterial blood pressure (SAP) was controlled at 50 mmHg by withdrawal of heparinized blood to a dextran contained reservoir. This blood was reinfused after ischemia to reestablish SAP to the baseline values. In the control group of experimental animals the BFV changes in both investigated cerebral arteries were recorded before and after intravenous administration of acetazolamide (20 mg/kg). In the group subjected to ischemia – BFV changes were measured before ischemia, after restoring initial SAP, before and after injection of the appropriate amount of acetazolamide. TTC staining was applied to 3 mm brain slices to visualize the damaged areas after ischemia.

Brain sections were placed into 35°C. Doublet tissue culture medium for 10 min and afterwards stained with 2% TTC for 10 min, at 37°C.

Results

In the first group (control) of experimental animals intravenous administration of acetazolamide caused an expected increase of BFV in both investigated arteries. The increase of mean BFV in MCA was 10% higher than in the BA (Fig. 1) and these differences were statistically significant.

In the second group of experimental animals subjected to 10 min acute global ischemia different responses to acetazolamide were observed. In the MCA following the SAP restoration, no increase of BFV after drug administration was observed moreover, in some animals [3] a decrease of BFV in comparison to its pre-ischemic values was seen (Fig. 2). However, the changes of BFV after acetazolamide administration in postischemic BA were similar to that obtained in the control group. The differences between these last values were statistically insignificant (Fig. 3).

After each experiment identification of damaged areas following ischemia was performed by the succylate dehydrogenase staining technique with TTC. This revealed "patchy" ischemic lesion areas in neocortex in comparison to almost undamaged basal ganglia, after 10 min of acute global ischemia.

Discussion

The changes of cerebrovascular reserve following cerebral blood supply insufficiency in experimental animals was previously studied [2]. The usefulness of the acetazolamide test in determining the alterations in cerebrovascular reserve including situations with slight reduction of CBF, was demonstrated. In the present study investigation of the influence of short duration global ischemia on vascular reserve in various areas of cerebrovascular system, revealed different degrees of vasomotor disturbances in MCA and BA. The vasodilatatory effect of 10 min ischemia was virtually abolished after acetazolamide administration in the MCA, while in the BA reactions remain unchanged. Such different reactions of these vessels on various hemodynamic alterations has been reported by

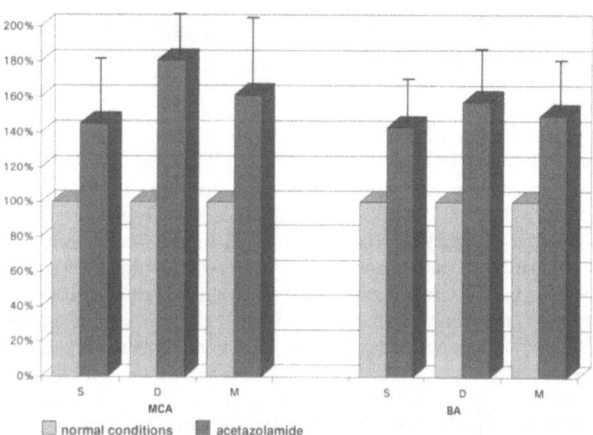

Fig. 1. Blood flow velocity (*BFV*) changes in the middle cerebral artery (*MCA*) and the basilar artery (*BA*) after acetazolamide administration in control group of experimental animals. *S* Systolic blood flow velocity, *D* diastolic blood flow velocity, *M* mean blood flow velocity

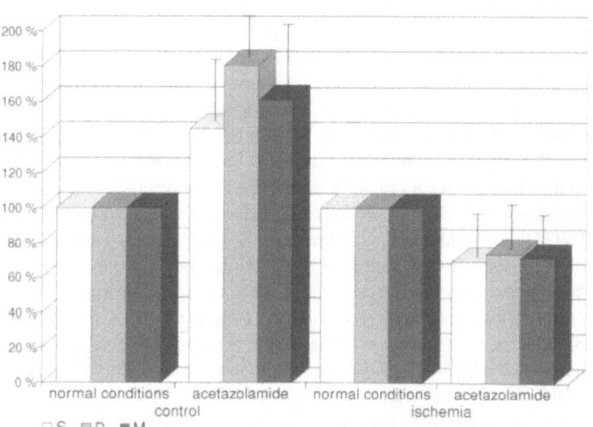

Fig. 2. Blood flow velocity (*BFV*) changes in the middle cerebral artery (*MCA*) after acetazolamide administration in control group of experimental animals and following 10 min global ischemia. *S* Systolic blood flow velocity, *D* diastolic blood flow velocity, *M* mean blood flow velocity

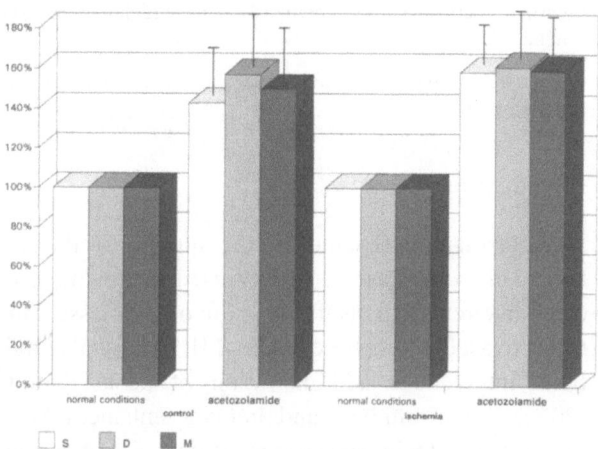

Fig. 3. Blood flow velocity (*BFV*) changes in the basilar artery (*BA*) after acetazolamide administration in control group of experimental animals and following 10 min global ischemia. *S* Systolic blood flow velocity, *D* diastolic blood flow velocity, *M* mean blood flow velocity

others [5]. The mechanism of such vessel reactivity disturbances remains unclear. This phenomenon might be either due to different sensitivity to ischemia of various areas of the brain tissue, or may be caused by the way the cerebral vessels behave in the various areas of the brain.

References

1. Czernicki Z, Kuroiwa T, Ohno K, Endo S, Ito U (1994) Effect of acetazolamide on early ischemic cerebral edema in gerbils. Acta Neurochir (Wien) 60: 329–331
2. Czernicki Z, Suzuki R, Nakagawa K, Hirakawa K, Endo S (1996) Acetazolamide produced blood flow velocity changes measured by laser doppler in gerbils with reduced CBF. Acta Neurochir (Wien) 138: 81–83
3. Piepgras A, Schmiedek P, Leinsinger G, Haberl RL, Kirsch CM, Einhäupl KM (1990) A simple test to assess cerebrovascular reserve capacity using transcranial Doppler sonography and acetazolamide. Stroke 21 (9): 1306–1311
4. Regli F, Yamaguchi T, Waltz AG (1971) Effect of acetazolamide on cerebral ischemia and infarction after experimental occlusion of middle cerebral artery. Stroke 2: 456–460
5. Stepinska G, Czernicki Z, Berdyga J, Jurkiewicz J (1995) Transcranial Doppler sonography in experimental cushing response. Acta Neurochir (Wien) 133: 80–82
6. Sorteberg W, Lindegaard KF, Rootwelt K, Dahl A, Nyberg-Hansen R, Russel D, Nornes H (1989) Effect of acetazolamide on cerebral artery blood velocity and regional cerebral blood flow in normal subject. Acta Neurochir (Wien) 97: 139–145

Correspondence: Dr. Wojcech Sapieja, Department of Neurosurgery, Medical Research Centre, Polish Academy of Sciences, Barska st 22, 02-315 Warsaw, Poland.

Acta Neurochir (1997) [Suppl] 70: 62–64
© Springer-Verlag 1997

Edema Formation Exacerbates Neurological and Histological Outcomes After Focal Cerebral Ischemia in CuZn-Superoxide Dismutase Gene Knockout Mutant Mice

T. Kondo[1, 2], A. G. Reaume[4], T.-T. Huang[3], K. Murakami[1, 2], E. Carlson[3], S. Chen[1, 2], R. W. Scott[4], C. J. Epstein[3], and P. H. Chan[1, 2]

Departments of [1] Neurological Surgery, [2] Neurology, and [3] Pediatrics, University of California, School of Medicine, San Francisco, CA, and [4] Cephalon, Inc., West Chester, PA, U.S.A.

Summary

In a variety of studies, CuZn-superoxide dismutase (CuZn-SOD) has been shown to protect against ischemic brain injury. A possible role for CuZn-SOD-related modulation of neuronal viability has been suggested by the finding that CuZn-SOD inhibits brain edema formation following various kinds of neurological insults. We have evaluated the role of CuZn-SOD on brain edema formation following focal cerebral ischemia in mice bearing a disruption of the CuZn-SOD gene (Sod1). Homozygous mutants (Sod1$^{-/-}$) had no detectable CuZn-SOD activity and heterozygous mutants (Sod1$^{+/-}$) showed a 50% decrease compared to wild-type mice. Sod1$^{-/-}$ mice showed a high level of blood-brain barrier (BBB) disruption shortly after 1 hr of middle cerebral artery occlusion and 100% mortality at 24 hr following ischemia. Sod1$^{+/-}$ mice showed a moderate level of BBB disruption and 30% mortality. The Sod1$^{+/-}$ animals had increased infarct volume and brain swelling, accompanying exacerbated neurological deficits at 24 hr following ischemia. These results indicate the important role of superoxide anions in the development of brain edema after focal cerebral ischemia and suggest the possibility that brain edema formation may contribute to the exacerbation of ischemic brain injury and neurological deficits in knockout mutant mice.

Introduction

Oxygen free radicals, superoxide anion (O_2^-) in particular, are involved in the pathogenesis of a variety of central nervous system (CNS) disorders, including cerebral ischemia and reperfusion [3]. One of the manifestations of oxygen free radical-mediated CNS damage following cerebral ischemia is the formation of brain edema, which plays a key role in the outcome of post-ischemic neurological deficits and in the development of infarction. To investigate the role of O_2^- in the formation of brain edema, we used knockout mutant mice, with the deletion of the CuZn-superoxide dismutase (CuZn-SOD) gene (Sod1), that showed a 50% decrease in the levels of CuZn-SOD activity in heterozygous (Sod1$^{+/-}$) mice, and a trace of activity in homozygous (Sod1$^{-/-}$) mice, compared to wild type (Wt) mice [8]. These mice were subjected to middle cerebral artery (MCA) occlusion; blood-brain barrier (BBB) disruption, neurological deficits and histological findings were evaluated following reperfusion.

Materials and Methods

Wt, Sod1$^{+/-}$ and Sod1$^{-/-}$ animals were derived from the founder stock previously described [8]. They were bred on a CD-1 mouse background. The knockout mutants were identified by qualitative demonstration of CuZn-SOD using nondenaturing gel electrophoresis followed by nitroblue tetrazolium staining [5]. There were no observable phenotypic differences between the knockout mutants and Wt normal littermates [8].

Animals were subjected to 1 hr of MCA occlusion using a method of suture monofilament insertion [11]. To evaluate BBB disruption, Evans blue dye extravasation was measured following ischemia. After the intravenous injection of Evans blue at the end of ischemia, the animals were killed by transcardiac saline perfusion at 2 hr following the injection. The brains were removed, and both ischemic and non-ischemic hemispheres were respectively homogenized. Evans blue concentration in the ischemic and non-ischemic hemispheres was individually measured by a spectrophotometric method [4] at 610 nm wave length.

For neurological and histological assessments, another set of animals was maintained for 24 hr after ischemia. Prior to killing these animals and removing the ischemic brains, their neurological deficits were evaluated as previously described [11]. The brains were sectioned and stained with cresyl violet, then infarct size and hemisphere enlargement were measured using an image analysis system [9].

Results

At 2 hr following 1 hr of MCA occlusion, no Evans blue leakage occurred in the entire brain of Wt mice (Fig. 1A). In contrast, the Evans blue extravasation was observed slightly in the center of the ischemic region in the Sod-1$^{+/-}$ mice, and was much more intensified and extended to the entire ischemic region in Sod1$^{-/-}$ mice (Fig. 1A). A quantitative assay of Evans blue revealed a low background basal level of Evans blue extravasation in the non-ischemic hemisphere. As illustrated in Fig. 1B, the amount of Evans blue leakage was not increased in the ischemic hemisphere of the Wt mice (0.03 ± 0.04 µg/hemisphere), compared to the non-ischemic hemisphere. The amount of Evans blue leakage was moderately increased in the ischemic hemisphere of the Sod1$^{+/-}$ mice (0.59 ± 0.22 µg/hemisphere), and was significantly increased in the Sod1$^{-/-}$ animals (1.96 ± 0.51 µg/hemisphere; $p < 0.01$; Fig. 1B).

Since knockout mutant mice showed higher mortality than Wt mice (Wt, 11%; Sod1$^{+/-}$, 36%; Sod1$^{-/-}$, 100%), neurological and histological findings were only assessed in the surviving animals at 24 hr following ischemia. Neurological deficits were significantly exacerbated in the surviving Sod1$^{+/-}$ mice, compared to the Wt mice (Wt, 1.3 ± 0.3; Sod1$^{+/-}$, 2.0 ± 0.2; $p < 0.05$; Fig. 2A). Histological analysis showed that the total

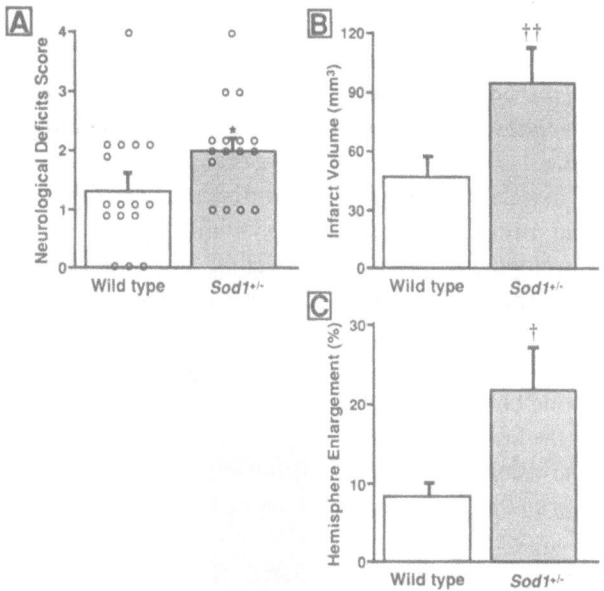

Fig. 2. Neurological and histological evaluation in mutant mice at 24 hr of reperfusion following ischemia. (A) Neurological deficits score of 0–4 (*0* no observable neurological deficit; *1* failure to extend right forepaw; *2* circling to the right; *3* falling to the right; *4* unable to walk spontaneously) was evaluated in Wt (n = 16) and Sod1$^{+/-}$ (n = 16) mice. Each circle represents individual animal, and data shows mean ± SEM of neurological deficits. * Indicates a significant increase of neurological deficits, compared to Wt mice ($p < 0.05$; Mann-Whitney U-test). Infarct volume (B) and hemisphere enlargement (C) in Wt (n = 6) and Sod1$^{+/-}$ (n = 6). Infarct volume was calculated by total accumulation of infarcted areas. Hemisphere enlargement was calculated as [(ischemic hemisphere volume – non-ischemic hemisphere volume) / non-ischemic hemisphere volume] × 100 (%). †, †† Indicate a significant increase of infarct volume or hemisphere enlargement, compared to Wt mice († $p < 0.05$, †† $p < 0.01$; Student's t-test)

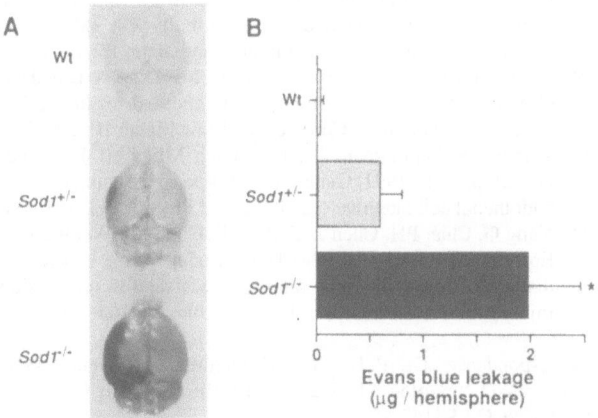

Fig. 1. Evans blue extravasation in mutant mice at 2 hr of reperfusion following ischemia. (A) Representative photographs of Evans blue extravasation in the brains of Wt, Sod1$^{+/-}$ and Sod1$^{-/-}$ mice. The dark stained area indicates Evans blue extravasation. (B) Quantitative assay of Evans blue in the ischemic hemisphere of Wt (n = 8), Sod1$^{+/-}$ (n = 5) and Sod1$^{-/-}$ (n = 5) mice. Values are mean ± SEM of the increase of Evans blue leakage in the ischemic hemisphere (ischemic hemisphere value – non-ischemic hemisphere value). * A significant increase of Evans blue leakage, compared to Wt mice ($p < 0.05$; analysis of variance followed by Fisher's protected least square difference)

infarct volume in Sod1$^{+/-}$ mice was significantly increased to 101.2 ± 15.5 mm^3, compared to 47.2 ± 5.4 mm^3 in Wt mice ($p < 0.01$; Fig. 2B). The brain hemispheres were also increased to 22.7 ± 4.6% in Sod1$^{+/-}$ mice compared to 8.9 ± 1.6% in the Wt mice ($p < 0.05$; Fig. 2C).

Discussion

Target disruption of the Sod1 gene results in the loss of CuZn-SOD activity, although no phenotypic differences are seen in normal physiological conditions [8]. We present data that formation of brain edema and infarction are exacerbated in Sod1 knockout mutant mice after focal cerebral ischemia. These data also include the exacerbation of mortality and neurological deficits, which correlate with the formation of brain edema and infarction. Since the regularly produced O_2^-, under normal physiological conditions, is not capable of affecting the normal tissue, these findings are consistent with the hypothesis that an increased amount of O_2^-, after focal cerebral ischemia, mediates these phenomena in the knockout mutant mice.

In ischemic brain injury, brain edema is an important factor for the acute phase of mortality, because of the development of fatal brain swelling and herniation. In the present study, BBB disruption was confirmed at 2 hr after ischemia in knockout mutant mice by Evans blue leakage into the brain. Evans blue binds to circulating blood serum albumin which is usually increased in the brain after several hours following ischemia [7]. Our results indicate that BBB disruption occurs unusually early in knockout mutant mice. In addition, at 24 hr after ischemia, $Sod1^{+/-}$ mice showed severe brain swelling, which was correlated with the neurological deficit. Thus, early BBB discruption and severe brain edema formation may primarily cause the exacerbation of mortality and of the neurological deficits in knockout mutant mice.

The generation of O_2^- and its role in brain edema formation have received experimental support from a variety of sources. Part of the manifestations of ischemic brain edema is due to O_2^- production of endothelial cells attributable to their high level of xanthine oxidase activity [2, 10]. We have demonstrated early BBB disruption in mutant mice, suggesting that endothelial cells are sensitive to ischemic injury because of the lack of O_2^- detoxification in the mutants. Recent evidence has shown that O_2^- rapidly reacts with nitric oxide to form pro-oxidant peroxynitrite [6], which can further generate hydroxy radicals by self-decomposition [1]. This pathway most likely explains the endothelial vulnerability of knockout mutants, since endothelial cells are an abundant source of nitric oxide due to their constitutive nitric oxide synthase. These highly toxic oxygen free radicals could be noxious to endothelial cells and cause early BBB disruption in mutant mice. From these findings, we conclude that endogenous CuZn-SOD is an important factor of protection against post-ischemic brain edema, resulting in a better neurological outcome after focal cerebral ischemia.

Acknowledgments

This work was supported by NIH grants NS 14543, NS25372 and AG08938. We thank L. F. Reola and B. E. Calagui for their expert technical assistance, and C. Christensen for her editorial assistance.

References

1. Beckman JS, Beckman TW, Chen J, Marshall PA, Freeman BA (1990) Apparent hydroxyl radical production by peroxynitrite: implications for endothelial injury from nitric oxide and superoxide. Proc Natl Acad Sci USA 87: 1620–1624
2. Betz AL (1985) Identification of hypoxanthine transport and xanthine oxidase activity in brain capillaries. J Neurochem 44: 574–579
3. Chan PH (1996) Role of oxidants in ischemic brain damage. Stroke 27: 1124–1129
4. Chan PH, Yang GY, Chen SF, Carlson E, Epstein CJ (1991) Cold-induced brain edema and infarction are reduced in transgenic mice overexpressing CuZn–superoxide dismutase. Ann Neurol 29: 482–486
5. Epstein CJ, Avraham KB, Lovett M, Smith S, Elroy SO, Rotman G, Bry C, Groner Y (1987) Transgenic mice with increased Cu/Zn-superoxide dismutase activity: animal model of dosage effects in Down syndrome. Proc Natl Acad Sci USA 84: 8044–8048
6. Huie RE, Padmaja S (1993) The reaction of NO with superoxide. Free Radic Res Commun 18: 195–199
7. Menzies SA, Betz AL, Hoff JT (1993) Contributions of ions and albumin to the formation and resolution of ischemic brain edema. J Neurosurg 78: 257–266
8. Reaume AG, Elliott JL, Hoffman EK, Kowall NW, Ferrante RJ, Siwek DF, Wilcox IM, Flood DG, Beal MF, Brown RHJ, Scott RW, Snider WD (1996) Motor neurons in Cu/Zn superoxide dismutase-deficient mice develop normally but exhibit enhanced cell death after axonal injury. Nat Genet 13: 43–47
9. Swanson RA, Morton MT, Tsao-Wu G, Savalos RA, Davidson C, Sharp FR (1990) A semiautomated method for measuring brain infarct volume. J Cereb Blood Flow Metab 10: 290–293
10. Terada LS, Willingham IR, Rosandich ME, Leff JA, Kindt GW, Repine JE (1991) Generation of superoxide anion by brain endothelial cell xanthine oxidase. J Cell Physiol 148: 191–196
11. Yang G, Chan PH, Chen J, Carlson E, Chen SF, Weinstein P, Epstein CJ, Kamii H (1994) Human copper-zinc superoxide dismutase transgenic mice are highly resistant to reperfusion injury after focal cerebral ischemia. Stroke 25: 165–170

Correspondence: Dr. P. H. Chan, Departments of Neurological Surgery and Neurology, University of California, Box 0651, San Francisco, CA 94143, U.S.A.

Acta Neurochir (1997) [Suppl] 70: 65–67

Therapeutic Dose and Timing of Administration of RNA Synthesis Inhibitors for Preventing Cerebral Vasospasm after Subarachnoid Hemorrhage

T. Mima, M. G. Mostafa, and **K. Mori**

Department of Neurosurgery, Kochi Medical School, Nankoku, Japan

Summary

A RNA synthesis inhibitor, dactinomycin, intended to suppress induction of vasoconstrictor peptide endothelin, prevented cerebral vasospasm almost completely in the dog subarachnoid hemorrhage (SAM) model [8]. Since endothelin receptor antagonists have not shown so potent effect as dactinomycin in animal SAH models, we aimed clinical use of dactinomycin for improvement of final outcomes of severe SAH patients now suffering vasospasm. Before clinical application, we examined therapeutic dose and timing of administration of dactinomycin in animal models.

In the dog two-hemorrhage model, dactinomycin treatment (0.01 mg/kg i.v. for 5 days) started at 6 hours after the second blood injection on Day 2 prevented vasospasm, but that started on Day 3 did not. Low dose of dactinomycin (0.003 mg/kg i.v. for 5 days) rather aggravated vasospasm even though the treatment started on Day 0. In the rat vasospasm model, high dose of dactinomycin (0.03 mg/kg i.p. for 3 days) or relatively low dose of doxorubicin (0.6 mg/kg i.p. once) prevented vasospasm even though the treatment started on Day 4.

The present study suggests that RNA synthesis inhibitors, such as dactinomycin and doxorubicin, may aufficiently prevent or ameliorate cerebral vasospasm in severe SAH patients.

Keywords: Cerebral vasospasm; subarachnoid hemorrhage; endothelin; dactinomycin; doxorubicin.

Introduction

A RNA synthesis inhibitor, dactinomycin, aimed to suppress de novo synthesis of vasoconstrictor peptide endothelin [5, 10], prevented cerebral vasospasm almost completely in the dog subarachnoid hemorrhage (SAM) model [8]. Although not a few antagonists of endothelin receptors have been innovated and examined on preventing cerebral vasospasm in the animal models, they were not so potent as dactinomycin, showing only moderate prevention of cerebral vasospasm [2–4, 6, 9]. Considering the fact that a number of severe SAH patients result in severe disability or death due to cerebral vasospasm, administration of dactino-

mycin, which has been clinically used as an anti-cancer drug for long time, may be most practical and useful treatment to improve the final outcomes of severe SAH patients now suffering cerebral vasospasm.

Shigeno and colleagues [8] have examined only the effect of clinically standard dose of dactinomycin for anti-cancer therapy, 0.01 mg/kg intravenous injection (i.v.) for 5 days, starting immediately after the first blood injection on Day 0. Therefore, before clinical trial of dactinomycin, we asked three questions: 1) Up to when the drug administration can be delayed after the onset of SAH? 2) What is the optimal dose of dactinomycin for prevention of vasospasm? 3) Is there other RNA synthesis inhibitor which has more potent effect than dactinomycin?

Materials and Methods

All the following animal experiments were conducted according to the guideline for the care and use of animals in the physiological sciences as approved by the Physiological Society of Japan. For the dog two-hemorrhage model [1, 8], we used adult male Beagle dogs weighing 9–15 kg and conducted the same method previously described [8]. The dogs were anesthetized with intravenous pentobarbital sodium (30 mg/kg), intubated, and usually allowed to breath spontaneously. The right vertebral artery was cannulated for basilar artery angiography. On Day 0, following control angiography autologous blood (0.5 mg/kg) was injected into the cisterna magna after removal of the same amount of cerebrospinal fluid. On Day 2, the animals received another injection of blood. The caliber of the basilar artery was measured on the angiograms at three locations: close to the basilar tip, at the midpoint, and close to the vertebrobasilar junction. Changes in the total of these three measurements were expressed as a percentage of the total of the three corresponding calibers on the control angiograms.

For the rat vasospasm model, we used male Wistar rats weighing 300–400 g and slightly modified the method previously described [7]. Under anesthesia of intraperitoneal pentobarbital sodium (50 mg/kg), 10 mm segments of the right proximal femoral artery was exposed in the inguinal region, and 0.1 ml of autologous blood, taken from the femoral vein, was applied inside of a Silastic cuff

(Dow-Corning Corporation) surrounding the right femoral artery on Day 0. The left femoral artery was used as control. On Day 4 or 7, the animals were perfusion-fixed via intracardial infusion with 200 ml of 4% paraformaldehyde and 1% glutaraldehyde in phosphate buffer. Each femoral artery was cross-sectioned at three locations: close to the proximal end, at the midpoint, and close to the distal end. Under microscope, the caliber at the major and the minor axis of each cross-section was measured and changes in the sum of the calibers of the right femoral artery were expressed as a percentage of that of the left femoral artery.

Experiment 1: To test the effect of delayed administration of dactinomycin in the dog two-hemorrhage model, we injected clinically standard dose of dactinomycin, 0.01 mg/kg i.v. for consecutive 5 days according to 4 protocols: no treatment (n = 16); starting immediately after the first blood injection on Day 0 (n = 16); starting at 6 hours after the second blood injection on Day 2 (n = 3); and starting on Day 3 (n = 3). At the same time, to examine the effect of one third lower dose of dactinomycin, we injected 0.003 mg/kg dactinomycin for 5 days starting immediately after the first blood injection on Day 0 (n = 3).

Experiment 2: First, we examined the time course of the vasospasm in the rat vasospasm model, sacrificing the animals on Day 4 (n = 7), and Day 7 (n = 9). Then, we tested the effect of delayed administration of standard dose (0.01 mg/kg i.p. for 5 days) and high dose (0.03 mg/kg i.p. for 3 days) of dactinomycin in this model, measuring the severity of vasospasm on Day 7. Experimental protocols were as follows: no treatment (n = 6); 0.01 mg/kg intraperitoneal injection (i.p.) for 5 days starting on Day 0 (n = 4); 0.01 mg/kg i.p. for 5 days starting on Day 1 (n = 4); 0.03 mg/kg i.p. for 3 days starting on Day 0 (n = 4), 0.03 mg/kg i.p. for 3 days starting on Day 1 (n = 4); and 0.03 mg/kg i.p. for 3 days starting on Day 4 (n = 5).

Experiment 3: In the rat vasospasm model, we tested the effect of doxorubicin, one of the most common anti-cancer drug belonging to the same anthracyclin group as dactinomycin. Clinically standard single dose of doxorubicin, 0.6 mg/kg, was injected intraperitoneally only once on Day 4, and the severity of vasospasm was measured on Day 7 (n = 4). To compare the effect with that of dactinomycin in the same protocol, high dose of dactinomycin (0.03 mg/kg) was injected intraperitoneally only once on Day 4 (n = 7).

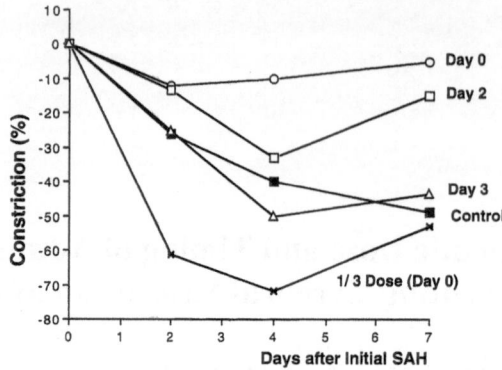

Fig. 1. Timing and dose response of dactinomycin in the canine two-hemorrhage model. With intravenous injection of 0.01 mg/kg dactinomycin for 5 days, cerebral vasospasm was prevented when the treatment started immediately after the initial SAH on Day 0 or at 6 hours after the second SAH on Day 2. However, the treatment started on Day 3 showed no effect. Low dose of dactinomycin (0.003 mg/kg i.v. for 5 days) rather aggravated vasospasm even though started on Day 0

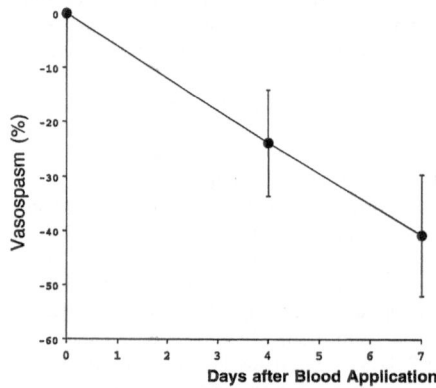

Fig. 2. Time course of vasospasm in the rat vasospasm model

Results

In Experiment 1, cerebral vasospasm was prevented when the treatment started at 6 hours after the second blood injection on Day 2, however, the treatment started on Day 3 revealed no prevention (Fig. 1). Low dose of dactinomycin (0.003 mg/kg i.v. for 5 days) rather aggravated vasospasm even though the treatment started immediately after the first blood injection on Day 0.

In Experiment 2, the natural course of vasospasm indicated 24% and 41% of vasoconstriction on Day 4 and Day 7, respectively (Fig. 2). Our results are consistent with the previous report [7], and similar to the time course of vasospasm in the dog two-hemorrhage model [1, 8]. Standard dose of dactinomycin, when started on Day 0 but not on Day 1, prevented vasospasm completely. In contrast, high dose of dactinomycin prevented vasospasm even though the treatment started on Day 1 or Day 4. Interestingly, in most cases

treated with high dose of dactinomycin, the vasospastic arteries were moderately dilated compared to controls.

In Experiment 3, even single injection of 0.03 mg/kg dactinomycin moderately prevented vasospasm, and 0.6 mg/kg doxorubicin dramatically prevented vasospasm and dilated vasospastic arteries.

Discussion

Shigeno and colleagues [8] reported that clinically standard dose of doxorubicin (0.01 mg/kg i.v. for 5 days) prevented cerebral vasospasm almost completely in the dog two-hemorrhage model, however, the present study indicated that delayed administration of dactinomycin after the onset of SAH significantly diminish potency of the effect.

The dog two-hemorrhage model [1] has been estimated as one of the most severe animal model for cerebral vasospasm, but the method of injecting blood twice on different days perplexes interpretation of the results to define optimal timing of the drug administration. Therefore, we also used the rat vasospasm model [9], causing vasospasm with single blood application. Together with the results in the dog and rat models, we may conclude that the delay of dactinomycin treatment should be within 24 hours with standard dose and within 4 days with high dose of dactinomycin after the onset of SAH.

The total dose of 0.03 mg/kg dactinomycin for 3 days is about twice higher than standard total dose and still within the limitation of clinical use. However, dactinomycin, a drug against Wilms' tumor and chorioepithelioma, is not so commonly used as doxorubicin which is usually a first choice for treating leukemia and other many types of neoplasm. Furthermore, the total dose of 0.6 mg/kg doxorubicin administered only once is rather low for anti-cancer treatment and showed the more potent effect on cerebral vasospasm.

In conclusion, doxorubicin may be more suitable for clinical application to rescue severe SAH patients suffering cerebral vasospasm.

References

1. Chyatte D, Rusch N, Sundt TM Jr (1983) Prevention of chronic experimental cerebral vasospasm with ibuprofen and high-dose methylpredonisolone. J Neurosurg 59: 925–932
2. Foley P, Caner H, Kassell N, Lee K, Weir B, Young W (1994) Reversal of subarachnoid hemorrhage induced vasoconstriction with an endothelin receptor antagonist. Neurosurgery 34: 108–113
3. Itoh S, Sasaki T, Ide K, Ishikawa K, Nishikibe M, Yano M (1993) A novel endothelin ET(A) receptor antagonist, BQ485, and its preventive effect on experimental cerebral vasospasm in dogs. Biochem Biophys Res Commun 195: 969–975
4. Itoh S, Sasaki T, Asai A, Kuchino Y (1994) Prevention of delayed vasospasm by an endothelin ET(A) receptor antagonist, BQ-123: change of ET(A) receptor mRNA expression in a canine subarachnoid hemorrhage model. J Neurosurg 81: 759–764
5. Mima T, Yanagisawa M, Shigeno T, Saito A, Goto K, Takakura K, Masaki (1989) Endothelin acts in feline and canine cerebral arteries from the adventitial side. Stroke 20: 1553–1556
6. Nirei H, Hamada K, Shoubo M, Sogabe K, Notsu Y, Ono T (1993) An endothelin ETA receptor antagonist, FR139317, ameliorates cerebral vasospasm in dogs. Life Sci 52: 1869–1874
7. Okada T, Harada T, Bark D, Mayberg M (1990) A rat femoral artery model for vasospasm. Neurosurgery 27: 349–356
8. Shigeno T, Mima T, Yanagisawa M, Saito A, Goto K, Yamashita K, Takenouchi T, Matsunra N, Yamasaki Y, Yamada K, Masaki T, Takakura K (1991) Prevention of cerebral vasospasm by actinomycin D. J Neurosurg 74: 940–943
9. Shigeno T, Clozel M, Sakai S, Saito A, Goto K (1995) The effect of bosentan, a new potent endothelin receptor antagonist, on the pathogenesis of cerebral vasospasm. Neurosurgery 37: 87–91
10. Yanagisawa M, Kurihara H, Kimura S, Tomobe Y, Kobayashi M, Mitsui Y, Yazaki Y, Goto K, Masaki T (1988) A novel vasoconstrictor peptide produced by vascular endothelial cells. Nature 322: 411–415

Correspondence: Tatsuo Mima, M.D., Department of Neurosurgery, Kochi Medical School, Nankoku City, Kochi 783, Japan.

Acta Neurochir (1997) [Suppl] 70: 68–70
© Springer-Verlag 1997

Traumatic Brain Swelling in Head Injured Patients: Brain Edema or Vascular Engorgement?

A. Marmarou, P. Barzo, P. Fatouros, T. Yamamoto, R. Bullock, and **H. Young**

Division of Neurosurgery and Radiology, Medical College of Virginia, Virginia Commonwealth University, Richmond, VA, U.S.A.

Summary

Brain edema and vascular engorgement have been used interchangeably to describe brain swelling associated with severe brain trauma and their relative contribution of these compartments to the swelling process remains controversial. In this report, imaging techniques for measurement of brain water and blood volume have been used to study the relative contribution of blood volume and tissue water to the swelling process in severely brain injured patients. More specifically, magnetic resonance techniques for non-invasive tissue water measures founded on mathematical models and later substantiated in laboratory and clinical studies were used for measure of brain tissue water. These studies were combined with measures of cerebral blood volume utilizing indicator dilution methods. Studies indicated that brain water was increased while blood volume decreased. These studies provide compelling evidence that the major contributor to brain swelling is brain edema and not blood volume. Therapies should now be targeted toward preventing edema development and enhancing edema resolution.

Keywords: Brain swelling; brain edema; vascular engorgement; traumatic brain edema.

Introduction

The cause of brain swelling following traumatic brain injury is unresolved. Since the early work of Langfitt and others in the late sixties, the swelling process has been attributed to increased blood volume secondary to vasoparalysis. Others have provided more recent experimental and clinical evidence that edema plays a major role in the swelling process [2]. During the past several years, the precise resolution of this problem has been difficult as methodology for simultaneous measurement of brain water and blood volume in patient studies has been lacking. As a result, both blood volume and edema have been implicated but their relative contribution remains controversial. However, recent studies have confirmed the accuracy and reliability of brain water measurement by magnetic resonance techniques [2]. In addition, new methods for blood volume measurement have been developed that are applicable to the severely brain injured patient [1]. Taken in concert, these technological advances have enabled studies of the brain swelling process. In this report, we utilize these methods for determining the relative contribution of brain edema and blood volume to brain swelling in severely head injured patients.

Methods

Severely brain injured patients, (GCS < 8) following stabilization in the intensive care setting, were transported to the CT and MRI imaging suites using a specially designed cart. The cart provided for monitoring of blood pressure, heart rate, EKG, oxygen saturation, respiration and intracranial pressure. In addition, the cart contained spare oxygen, which was used in conjunction with a portable, MRI compatible, respirator for maintaining stable oxygenation and ventilation of the patient during transport. The transport team consisted of the neurosurgical resident, intensive care nurse, respiratory technician and additional clinical research staff. Only those considered sufficiently stable for the two hour imaging study were selected and all procedures were approved by an internal review board. Upon arrival in the imaging suite, all portable equipment was placed on standard power supply and oxygen connection. The order of studies was based on availability of CT for measurement of blood flow and blood volume and MRI suite for measurement of brain water was based on scheduling practice.

Both brain water and blood volume was measured during the first 7 days post admission. In total, 109 studies were performed in patients ranging from 16 to 77 years of age. The brain water measurements were based on accurate determinations of longitudinal relaxation time (T1) and subsequent conversion to water expressed in gm H_2O per gram tissue by means of a theoretical equation involving a fast exchange two state model. The equation was confirmed in both animal and human studies in comparison with standard gravimetric technique.

The measurement of cerebral blood volume was based on indicator dilution techniques. Specifically, the mean transit time was computed by dynamic CT following a rapid intravenous administration of a 50 cc iodine bolus. CBV was then calculated on a pixel by pixel basis by multiplication of CBF and mean transit time images in accordance with the central volume principal.

Results

The studies were conducted without complication. On occasion, patients experienced brief episodes of elevated ICP and were managed with csf drainage to maintain ICP and CPP within thresholds.

Brain water content as assessed by magnetic resonance techniques was increased compared to those of control patients. Brain tissue water averaged $79.1 \pm 2.3\%$ gm H_2O/gm tissue. The average increase in brain water content equaled $1.6\% \pm 1.4\%$ S.D. gm H_2O/gm tissue. In contrast, blood volume in head injured patients decreased. Brain blood volume in head injured patients averaged 4.2 ± 1.3 ml/100 gm tissue.

The average reduction in blood volume equaled 1.1 ± 1.4 ml/100 gm tissue. The corresponding measures of brain water and blood volume are shown in Fig. 1.

Discussion

These studies are the first to demonstrate the relative contribution of brain edema and blood volume to the swelling process in severely brain injured patients. The findings, combining all patient studies, indicate that traumatic brain swelling is associated with increased brain water and decreased blood volume.

Brain swelling and intracranial pressure rise, particularly in cases of traumatic injury, remains a critical problem. With traumatic injury, three forms of brain edema are thought to contribute to the elevated tissue water; vasogenic edema, characterized by a breakdown of the blood brain barrier and exudation of intravascular fluids into the extracellular space; cytotoxic edema, identified by intracellular swelling and most pronounced with metabolic crisis and ischemia; and neurotoxic edema, increased cellular water mitigated by membrane failure secondary to excess neurotransmitter release. In these studies, barrier breakdown identified by injection of Gd-DTPA was not demonstrated with exception of a slight halo in those patients with contusion. (not shown) Thus, it is reasonable to assume that the blood brain barrier at time of measurement was not compromised. Moreover, most studies were conducted beyond 24 hours post injury when it was most likely that the barrier re-

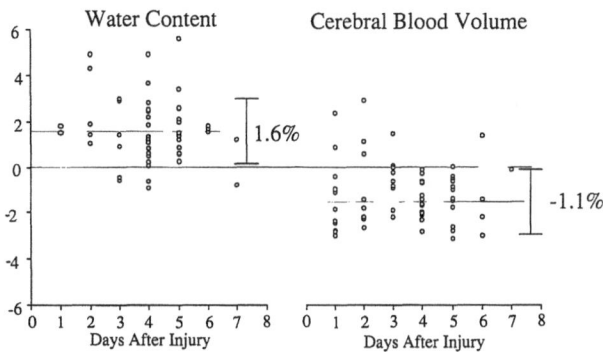

Fig. 1. The percentage change in brain water content as assessed by MRI technique and blood volume as measured by CT and indicator dilution technique. Brain water is increased and blood volume is reduced in severely head injured patients (n = 109)

mained intact. More detailed clinical studies of barrier opening are required to help resolve this issue. The findings of the present study clearly demonstrate the development of brain edema; however, the method does not identify if the edema is of vasogenic or cytotoxic origin. It may be possible in future studies to distinguish extracellular from intracellular using diffusion weighted imaging as has been done in experimental studies.

The underlying mechanisms leading to reduced blood volume remain elusive. Studies of vascular reactivity by Yoshihara *et al.* have shown that the resistance vessels appear to be in a persistent state of vasoconstriction and this is consistent with a reduction in blood volume [3]. One possibility is that the increased water contributing to the swelling process acts to compress the vessels. However, as the majority of patients were not at elevated pressure, this process of compression would have to occur in the absence of sustained pressure rise.

In summary, these studies indicate that the major contributor to traumatic brain swelling is brain edema and not vascular engorgement. Therapies should now be targeted toward preventing edema development and enhancing edema resolution.

Acknowledgement

This research was supported in part by Grant P01 NS12587 and R01 NS19235 from the National Institutes of Health.

References

1. Fatouros P, Schroeder ML, Muizelaar JP, Kuta AJ, Cothran SJ (1995) Dynamic computed tomography and cerebral blood volume. In: Tomanaga M, Tanaka A, Yonas H (eds)

Quantitative cerebral blood flow measurements using stable Xenon-CT: clinical applications. Futura, Armonk, NY, pp 95–110

2. Marmarou A, Fatouros P, Ward J, Appley A, Young H (1990) In-vivo measurement of brain water by MRI. In: Reulen JH, Baethman A, Fenstermacher J, Marmarou A, Spatz M (eds) Brain edema VIII. Acta Neurochiur (Wien) [Suppl] 51: 123–124

3. Yoshihara M, Bandoh K, Marmarou A (1995) Cerebrovascular carbon dioxide reactivity assessed by intracranial pressure dynamics in severely head injured patients. J Neurosurg 82: 386–393

Correspondence: Anthony Marmarou, Ph.D., Division of Neurosurgery, Medical College of Virginia, P.O.Box 980508, Richmond, VA 23298-0508, U.S.A.

Acta Neurochir (1997) [Suppl] 70: 71–74
© Springer-Verlag 1997

Evaluation of Homeostatic Changes in CSF Circulation: *In vivo* Analysis of the Effect of Neurotransmitter Accumulation in the Extracellular Space Following Transient Global Ischemia

T. Yamamoto, A. Marmarou, M. F. Stiefel, O. Tsuji, and **R. Bullock**

Division of Neurosurgery, Medical College of Virginia, Richmond, VA, U.S.A

Summary

Accumulation of potassium and excitatory amino acids (EAA) in the extracellular space (ECS) following ischemia has been well documented. Careful monitoring of these transients is crucial to gain a better understanding of CNS pathophysiology. This study was initiated to determine if CSF concentrations of EAAs reflect those measured in the ECS. Transient global ischemia, 20 minutes in duration, was produced by clamping the left subclavian and innominate arteries combined with hemorrhagic hypotension. The accumulation of glutamate and electrolytes were measured in CSF and the extracellular fluid (ECF) of cerebral cortex. Microdialysis (MD) was utilized to measure the extracellular concentrations while direct sampling of CSF was provided via cannulation of the cisterna magna. Hydrogen clearance and laser doppler methods were used to monitor regional cortical CBF.

Our results show that extracellular concentrations of potassium ($[K^+]_{ECF}$) and glutamate significantly increased following the initiation of ischemia ($p < 0.05$). The extracellular concentration of these substances decreased with the restoration of CBF. In CSF, a similar trend was observed following re-circulation ($p < 0.05$). However, CSF glutamate levels did not return to pre-ischemic values.

Keywords: Cerebral ischemia; extracellular glutamate; cerebrospinal fluid; homeostatic changes.

Introduction

The maintenance of extracellular and CSF composition is crucial for normal neuron function. There are numerous transport mechanisms and ion channels in cells such as astrocytes and at both the blood-brain barrier (BBB) and blood-CSF barriers [1, 3–5]. These transporters help to maintain and regulate the composition of the extracellular and CSF which bathe and protect the cells of the CNS.

With unrestricted movement between the CSF and ECF we hypothesize that alterations in ECF composition should be reflected in CSF. Any difference in composition should be due to the efficiency of homeo-static mechanisms which regulate EAAs and ionic levels in the compartments, respectively. The objective of this study was to compare ECS composition with that of CSF to determine to what degree CSF reflects global cerebral changes.

Materials and Methods

Male and female cats weighing 2.5 to 6.0 kg (n = 12) were initially anesthetized via a bolus injection of intravenous Brevital (10 mg/kg). After initial anesthesia was obtained the animal was intubated and mechanically ventilated through an endotracheal tube. Arterial blood gases (ABG) were maintained throughout the experiment with a PO_2 of 100 to 120 mmHg, and a pCO_2 of 30 to 35 mmHg.

Following stabilization of ABG, ABP and temperature a perpendicular incision on the left side of the animal was made between the second and third ribs. Snare ligatures were applied to the left subclavian and innominate artery approximately 5 to 10 mm distal to the heart. After closure of the incisions, the animal was placed into a stereotaxic frame and probes for ICP, CBF and MD were positioned in cortex.

Repetitive CSF sampling was obtained via a 25-gauge butterfly needle inserted into the cisterna magna. Insertion of MD probes was followed by a 90-minute stabilization period. ECF and CSF samples were collected every 10 or 15 minutes. Ionic concentration of CSF and the ECF dialysate were measured by flame photometer. Glutamate concentrations from the respective samples are measured via HPLC.

Cerebral ischemia was induced via arterial occlusion and hypotension and maintained for 20 minutes. Systemic hypotension was attained by withdrawing blood until mABP decreases to 80 mmHg. The brain was re-perfused by first gradually infusing blood into the animal followed by removal of the arterial snares.

Results

General Physiological Parameters

CBF, mABP and ICP of both groups are shown in Table 1. Ischemia produced significant changes in

Table 1. *General Physiological Parameters and Regional CBF*

	Control group	Base line	During	Recirculation			
	(mean ± SE)	(mean ± SE)	ischemia	30 min	60 min	90 min	120 min
m-ABP	103.7 ± 5.78	114.8 ± 5.06	72.8 ± 4.96	99.2 ± 1.25	93.9 ± 3.16	94.1 ± 1.33	97.3 ± 2.03
ICP	3.94 ± 0.60	1.7 ± 0.45	−5.4 ± 2.09[a]	6.3 ± 1.12[a]	2.2 ± 0.58	1.00 ± 0.71	6.79 ± 0.34[a]
r-CBF$_{(H2)}$[b]	74.3 ± 6.20	77.1 ± 4.32	2.9 ± 2.19[a]	59.8 ± 14.19	70.4 ± 3.00	61.18 ± 4.71	78.7 ± 4.73
r-CBF$_{(LD)}$[b]	38.8 ± 6.26	40.0 ± 17.6	1.25 ± 1.27[a]	34.5 ± 18.40	48.5 ± 17.14	40.5 ± 13.33	38.5 ± 20.97

[a] $p < 0.05$, compared to baseline values.
[b] *H2* Hydrogen clearance; *LD* laser Doppler.

CBF and ICP ($p < 0.05$) with CBF decreasing to values less than 10 ml/100 g/min ($p < 0.05$). Reestablishment of CBF was followed by periods of hypotension and elevated ICP. CBF slowly returned towards baseline over a 60 minute period following the termination of ischemia.

Changes in Electrolytes

The adjusted ECF concentrations were calculated using *in vitro* recovery values of each MD probe for Na⁺ and K⁺, respectively. Baseline values which were obtained by averaging the first 4 samples, did not differ significantly (Control; Na⁺ = 161 ± 9.6 mEq/l, K⁺ = 2.29 ± 0.23 mEq/l, Ischemia; Na⁺ = 143 ± 20.3 mEq/l, K⁺ = 2.40 ± 1.68 mEq/l, Na⁺; $p = 0.54$, K⁺; $p = 0.75$).

The time course for the percent change of $[K^+]_{ECF}$ in both sham and experimental groups is shown in Fig. 1. The initiation of ischemia immediately produced significant changes in $[K^+]_{ECF}$. A 250% increase, the largest change in extracellular potassium, was observed approximately 20 minutes after ischemia. $[K^+]_{ECF}$ decreased towards baseline immediately following the termination of ischemia, reaching control values in approximately 30 minutes ($T_{1/2KECF} = 15.0$ min).

The baseline values of $[K^+]_{CSF}$ were 2.95 ± 0.19 mEq/l and 2.71 ± 0.28 mEq/l in sham and ischemia groups respectively. In the experimental group a significant elevation in $[K^+]_{CSF}$ was first observed at 20 minutes after the initiation of ischemia ($p < 0.05$). Following re-circulation $[K^+]_{CSF}$ rapidly increased 155% above baseline.

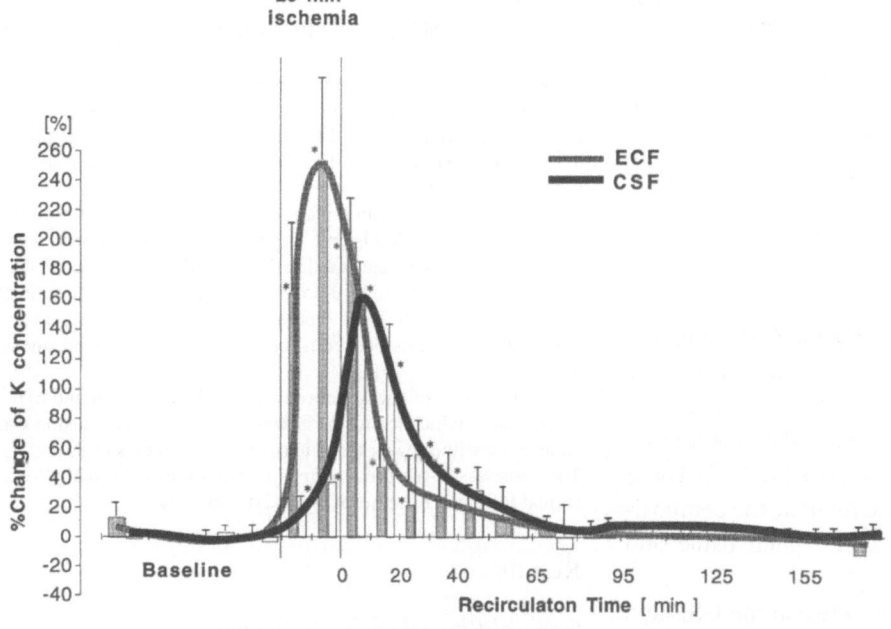

Fig. 1. The outline the time course of Potassium concentration percent changes in both ECF and CSF. The shaded bar (mean ± S.D.) is the percent change in ECF, and the open bar (mean ± S.D.) is the change in CSF. First four samples was averaged for base line values. * Indicates significant difference from baseline values ($p < 0.05$)

CSF values slowly returned towards baseline over a 40 minute interval ($T_{1/2 KCSF}$ = 13.3 min).

The sodium concentration ($[Na^+]_{ECF}$) in the sham group remained stable throughout the experiment. In the ischemic group, baseline $[Na^+]_{ECF}$ and $[Na^+]_{CSF}$ (160 ± 14.0 mEq/l) were not significantly different from control (167 ± 3.8 mEq/l, P = 0.13). During ischemia no significant changes in either $[Na^+]_{ECF}$ or $[Na^+]_{CSF}$ were observed ($[Na^+]_{ECF}$; p = 0.36, $[Na^+]_{CSF}$; p = 0.54).

Changes in EAAs

The measured base line glutamate levels in ECF and CSF were 9.39 ± 2.50 µmol/l and 1.02 ± 0.51 µmol/l, respectively. The induction of ischemia caused a rapid increase in extracellular glutamate. The greatest change was observed 20 minutes after ischemia was initiated. Following the restoration of CBF, one hour was required for extracellular glutamate to decrease to baseline. Although somewhat delayed, a similar trend to that observed in the ECF was seen in CSF. The maximum $[Glu]_{CSF}$ was observed approximately 30 minutes after the peak in ECF. Upon recirculation, glutamate slowly decreased towards baseline, however, it remained elevated for the duration of the experiment.

Discussion

It is widely accepted that ischemic insults in the CNS cause an accumulation of K^+ and EAAs in the ECF [1, 2, 13]. However, it is not well known how the pathophysiology of global ischemia effects CSF homeostasis and the degree to which CSF mirrors ECF changes. The present study shows that during the ischemic insult the accumulation of $[K^+]_{ECS}$ is closely reflected in CSF. Although a slight time delay is observed, the rise in $[K^+]$ in the respective compartments are not significantly different (p = 0.10).

Accumulation in ECF

The glutamate concentrations in ECF measured in this study are in good agreement with those reported previously [10–12]. Our results show that following a rise in $[Glu]_{ECF}$ a concomitant increase in $[Glu]_{CSF}$ is observed. The data reveals that the trends observed in CSF, rather than the measured concentration, are a reflection of the glutamate changes occurring in the ECS. The calculated concentrations of the respective fluids did not closely approximate each other, while the magnitude of change, 300% and 330%, in ECS and CSF respectively was similar.

The elevated levels of $[K^+]_{ECF}$ and $[Glu]_{ECF}$ are a result of cellular damage. As discussed by Shimada et al., a reduction of CBF to values less than 10 ml/100 g/min is below the threshold for ion pump failure and membrane breakdown [10, 13]. As a result, sodium and potassium move down their electrochemical gradients, potassium exiting the cell as sodium and chloride enter. The increase in $[Glu]_{ECF}$ is believed to result from excessive synaptic release compounded by impaired cellular uptake [4, 5]. Furthermore, damaged cell membranes may also allow for glutamate to leak into the ECF resulting in membrane depolarization and a larger potassium efflux.

The influx of sodium and chloride resulting from ion pump failure is accompanied by the isosmotic movement of water. This accumulation of water leads to cell swelling and a subsequent decrease in ECF volume. Hossmann et al. confirmed that extracellular sodium decreases significantly during ischemia [6]. In the present study, however, significant changes in extracellular sodium were not observed. One possibility is that the microdialysis technique employed may be not suitable for monitoring small sodium changes occurring in ECS.

Clearance of the ECF

Astrocyte uptake is believed to be the primary method for removing glutamate and potassium from the extracellular space [1, 5]. To maintain extracellular potassium, astrocytes utilize; (1) Na-K ATPase, (2) Na-K-2Cl co-transport, and (3) spatial buffering (inward rectifying K^+ channels) [3, 8, 13]. ATP levels are restored when, via recirculation, oxygen and glucose are delivered to cells. The presence of ATP allows the Na-K ATPase to remove potassium from the ECF and re-establish ion gradients.

Clearance of Potassium and Glutamate from ECF

Potassium and glutamate may also be cleared from the ECF by moving through ECS. Reduction of ECS volume and increased tortuosity of diffusion limits the diffusion of potassium and glutamate through the ECS. However, the direct communication between the ECF and CSF could be a mechanism for removing increased potassium and glutamate from ECS as well as accumulating in the CSF. Previous studies have shown that in the presence of a pressure gradient between the ECF and CSF, materials are capable of being transported via bulk flow into CSF [8].

An additional route of clearance from the ECF may be via the vasculature. Capillary endothelial cells posses numerous transport mechanisms and ion channels capable of removing potassium from the ECS. Moreover, astrocyte endfeet ensheathe cerebral blood vessels enabling potassium to be moved into the vasculature via special buffering.

Accumulation in CSF

The CSF showed its greatest accumulation of potassium following reperfusion. The most plausible explanations for the accumulation of potassium in CSF are: (1) spatial buffering by astrocytes, (2) movement through the extracellular space via diffusion or bulk flow. With the global ischemia model used in this study potassium accumulation in the ECF is widespread. As a result, spatial buffering of potassium to other regions of brain is limited. However, astrocyte endfeet which abut the pial membrane as well as the ependymal cells lining the ventricles provide a means for potassium to enter CSF.

Injury to the choroid plexus must also be considered as a potential reason for the accumulation of potassium and glutamate in the CSF. The choroid plexus is vital for maintaining CSF composition [9]. Failure of CSF homeostatic mechanisms at the blood-CSF barrier, may contribute to or inhibit the elimination of substances from the CSF. Disruption of CSF homeostatic mechanisms may explain why $[Glu]_{CSF}$ failed to return to control levels following the restoration of CBF.

Although the exact mechanisms for the change in glutamate and potassium concentrations have not been elucidated, this study clearly shows that potassium and glutamate transients in CSF are a reflection of processes occurring in the ECS during global pathophysiology.

Acknowledgment

This research was supported in part by Grants P01 NS12587 and R01 NS19235 from the National Institutes of Health. Additional facilities and support were provided by the Richard Roland Reynolds Neurosurgical Research Laboratories.

References

1. Choi DW (1988) Glutamate toxicity and diseases of the nervous system. Neuron 1: 623–634
2. Choi DW, Maulucci-Gedde M, Kriegstein AR (1987) Glutamate neurotoxicity in cortical cell culture. J Neurosci 7: 357–368
3. Clausen T (1992) Potassium and sodium transport and pH regulation. CAN J Physiol Pharmacol 70: S219–S222
4. Drejer J, Benveniste H, Diemer HN, Schousboe A (1985) Cellular origin of ischemia-induced glutamate release from brain tissue *in vivo* and *in vitro*. J Neurochem 45: 14–151
5. Hagberg H, Lehmann A, Sandberg M, Nyström B, Jacobson I, Hamberger A (1985) Ischemia-induced shift of inhibitory and excitatory amino acid from intra- to extracellular compartments. J Cereb Blood Flow Metab 5: 413–419
6. Hossman K, Sakaki S, Zimmermann V (1977) Cation activities in reversible ischemia of the cat brain. Stroke 8: 77–81
7. Marmarou A, Hochwald G, Nakamura T, Tanaka K, Weaver J, Dunbar J (1994) Brain edema resolution by CSF pathways and brain vasculature in cats. Am J Physiol 267: H514–H520
8. Newman EA (1986) High potassium conductance in astrocyte endfeet. Science 233: 453–454
9. Segal BM, Preston EJ, Collis SC, Zlokovic VB(1990) Kinetics and Na independence of amino acid uptake by blood side of perfused sheep choroid plexus. Am J Physiol 258: F1288–F1294
10. Shimada N, Graf R, Rosner G, Heiss W (1993) Ischemia-induced accumulation of extracellular amino acids in cerebral cortex, white matter, and cerebrospinal fluid. J Neurochem 60: 66–71
11. Shimada N, Graf R, Rosner G, Heiss W (1990) Differences in ischemia-induced accumulation of amino acids in the cat cortex. Stroke 21: 1445–1451
12. Roettger RV, Goldfinger DM (1991) HPLC-EC determination of free primary amino acid concentration in cat cisternal cerebrospinal fluid. J Neurosci Methods 39: 263–270
13. Walz W, Hertz L (1983) Intracellular ion changes of astrocytes in response to extracellular potassium. J Neurosci Res 10: 411–423

Correspondence: Anthony Mamarou, Ph.D., Division of Neurosurgery, Medical College of Virginia, P.O. Box 980508, Richmond, VA 23298-0508, U.S.A.

Acta Neurochir (1997) [Suppl] 70: 75–77
© Springer-Verlag 1997

Detection of Brain Atrophy Following Traumatic Brain Injury Using Gravimetric Techniques

K. Hayasaki[1], A. Marmarou[1], P. Barzó[1], P. Fatouros[2], and F. Corwin[2]

Division of [1] Neurosurgery and [2] Radiology, Medical College of Virginia, Richmond, VA, U.S.A.

Summary

We hypothesized, that with atrophy, the correlation between water content and specific gravity of brain solids would break down signifying the onset of the atrophic process. The correlation between tissue water content, specific gravity of solids and ventricular size was studied in an impact acceleration model of closed head injury of the rat. Adult Sprague Dawley rats weighing 350 to 375 grams (n = 63) were separated into two groups: Group I: Sham (n = 21), Group II: Trauma (n = 42). Water content was assessed using both gravimetric method and drying-weighing method at 1 hour, on days 1, 3, 7, 14, 28, and 42 in the trauma group as well as in the control group. Ventricular size was measured in cm² on the MRI computer console in the coronal section at the coronal suture at the same time points. In the trauma group we found a significant increase (p < 0.01) in water content during the first week except on day 3 and there was a good correlation between the results of water content using both methods (p < 0.001). However, this relationship was poorly correlated after day 14 (p = 0.25). Although the ventricular size was the smallest at 1 hour post trauma, it significantly increased over the next 3 days (p < 0.001). On day 7 and 14 ventricular size decreased to normal size, yet gradually increased and then reached a significantly larger size on 42 days post trauma again (p < 0.01). We may consider, that brain edema following CHI begins immediately following trauma and resolves within 2 weeks. After 14 days degenerative change occurs in the cortex, as detected by specific gravity measurements which signifies the onset of the atrophic process and subsequent post traumatic ventricular dilatation.

Keywords: Traumatic brain injury; brain atrophy; specific gravity; ventriculomegaly.

Introduction

Ventricular dilatation represents one of the most frequently observed sequelae of severe head injury. In clinical settings, distinction between hydrocephalus and brain atrophy, as the two possible causes of post-traumatic ventriculomegaly (PTV), has been difficult. Recently, we have developed a model of closed head injury (CHI) in rats that produces diffuse brain injury followed by ventriculomegaly at six weeks post injury

[4, 8]. The objective of this study was to study the relationships between tissue water, specific gravity of solids and ventricular size to help clarify the sequence of events leading to PTV.

Material and Methods

Impact Acceleration Injury

Adult Sprague Dawley rats weighing 350 to 375 grams (n = 63) were separated into two groups: Group I: Sham (n = 21), Group II: Trauma (n = 42). Rats were initially anesthetized with halothane, then intubated and artificially ventilated with a gas mixture of N_2O (70%), O_2 (30%), and halothane (0.5–1.5%). An impact acceleration model was used to induce traumatic brain injury. From a two-meter height, a 450 gram brass weight was allowed to drop freely through a plexiglass tube onto a stainless steel helmet firmly fixed to the skull vault of the rat.

Determination of the Ventricular Size

MRI imaging was performed using a 2.35T, 40 cm bore magnet (Biospec, Bruker Instruments, Billeriaca, MA) equipped with a 12 cm inner diameter. Radiofrequency excitation and reception were performed using a 7 cm inner-diameter "bird cage" design resonator. At 1 hour, on day 1, 3, 7, 14, 28, and 42 in the trauma group as well as in the control group, ventricular size was measured in cm² on the MRI computer console in a 3 mm coronal section at the level of the coronal suture.

Gravimetric Analysis

Nelson *et al.* [10] proposed the following equation:

$$\text{gm } H_2O \,/\, \text{gm tissue} = 1 - \{(\text{sp gr}_t - 1) \,/\, (1 - 1 \,/\, \text{sp gr}_s) \,\text{sp gr}_t\}, \quad (1)$$

where sp gr_t = specific gravity of the wet tissue, and sp gr_s = specific gravity of the tissue solids.

Marmarou [7] reported this equation can be restructured such that the brain-tissue water can be expressed in the form of a straight line (Fig. 1a). Tissue water is linearly related to the reciprocal of the specific gravity of the wet tissue sample and the general form of the straight line is given by Eq. 2:

$$\text{gm } H_2O \,/\, \text{gm tissue} = m \,/\, \text{sp gr}_t + b, \quad (2)$$

where the slope m equals (sp gr$_s$) / (sp gr$_s$ – 1), and the intercept b equals 1 / (sp gr$_s$ – 1).

The specific gravity of solids for rat cortex measured in our laboratory equals 1.2617. From this data the values of slope m and intercept b of Eq. 2 were computed to form the basic equation for measurement of water content using specific gravity of wet tissue only (m = 4.8212, b = 3.8212). Thus, for the rat cerebral cortex,

$$\text{gm } H_2O / \text{gm tissue} = (4.8212 / \text{sp gr}_t) - 3.8212. \quad (3)$$

Water Determination

The rats were deeply anesthetized and then sacrificed using 2 cc of saturated KCl administered transcardially, at the same time points as mentioned above. Brain was removed quickly and stored in an airtight container at –80 n. Within 20 minutes the frozen brains were sliced using standardized procedures in 5 slices from frontal to occipital pole. After defrosting the brains, microgravimetric analysis was performed at the cortex of the brain slice under the helmet. Specific gravity of wet tissue was determined sequentially in a gradient column of bromobenzene and kerosene. The water content was calculated using Eq. 3. Water content by conventional drying-weighing method [3] was measured on the remaining 4 brain slices.

Results

In the control group the ventricular size measured MRI technique remained the same (0.33 ± 0.04 cm^2) throughout the 6 week period and did not show any significant change. In the trauma group the ventricular size was reduced at 1 hour (0.24 ± 0.05 cm^2, p < 0.05)

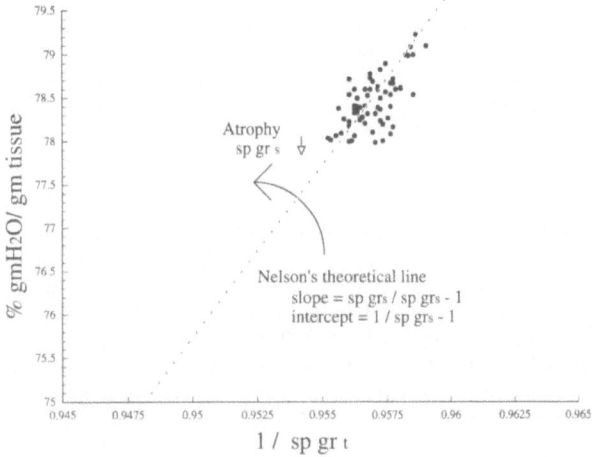

Fig. 1. Relationship between tissue water content and specific gravity. Graphic description of Nelson's equation relating tissue water content (am H$_2$O/gm tissue) to the specific gravity of solid (sp gr$_s$) and fresh tissue (sp gr$_t$). With a constant value of sp gr$_s$, water content is linearly related to the reciprocal of fresh tissue sp gr$_t$. A specific gravity of 1.0 corresponds to 100% H$_2$O. When tissue water is zero, sp gr$_s$ remains and the x axis intercept of the graph of 0% H$_2$O equals 1/sp gr$_s$. When the line rotates counterclockwise, the value of sp gr$_s$ becomes smaller as would occur with brain atrophy. Specific gravity values of cortex sample within 14 days are shown plotted with corresponding values of water content evaluated by drying-weighing method. The distribution of experimental data points closely follows the theoretical Equation 1 (broken line)

post trauma compared to baseline measurement (0.32 ± 0.06). Ventricular size significantly increased during the next 3 days (0.47 ± 0.12 cm^2, p < 0.001). On day 7 and 14 ventricular size decreased to normal size, but gradually increased and reached a significantly larger size at 42 days (0.36 ± 0.07, p < 0.01) post trauma (Table 1).

We found a significant increase (p < 0.01) in water content using the gravimetric method and wet/dry method during the first week except on day 3. There was a good correlation (p < 0.001) between the results of water content measured by both methods; however, this relationship showed a poor correlation after day 14 (p = 0.25). We plotted these data in a graphical format

Table 1. *Changes in Ventricular Size*

	Control	Trauma
Baseline	0.33 ± 0.04	0.32 ± 0.06
1 hour	0.30 ± 0.08	0.24 ± 0.05*
3 days	0.32 ± 0.06	0.47 ± 0.12***
7 days	0.31 ± 0.06	0.26 ± 0.11
14 days	0.31 ± 0.09	0.32 ± 0.15
28 days	0.31 ± 0.07	0.32 ± 0.09
42 days	0.34 ± 0.01	0.36 ± 0.07**

The ventricular size measured by MRI remained the same during the 6 weeks and did not show any significant change in control group. The ventricular size was changing during the 6 week period after head injury in trauma group. It was the smallest at 1 hour post trauma and the largest at 3 and 42 days post trauma.
*** p < 0.001, ** p < 0.01, * p < 0.05.

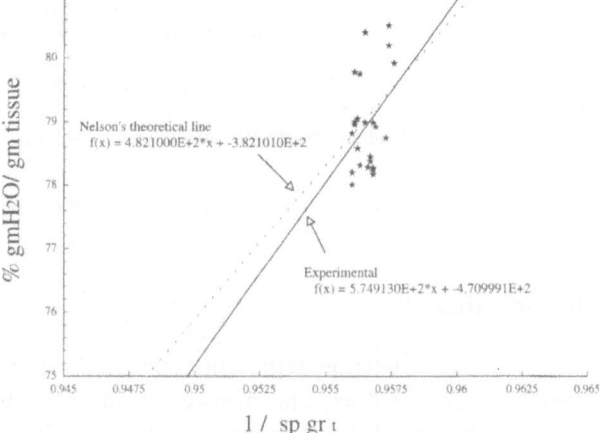

Fig. 2. Effect of atrophy on specific gravity. Specific gravity values of cortex sample on day 28 and 42 are shown plotted with corresponding values of water content evaluated by drying-weighing method. The linear regression of experimental data points (solid line) is compared to the theoretical Nelson's Equation 1 (broken line)

similar to Fig. 1a. The data within 14 days were distributed on the theoretical line (Fig. 1b); however, data recorded after 14 days did not follow this relationship (Fig. 1c). Slope m' of the experimental line equals 5.7491.

Discussion

It is well-known that ventriculomegaly often occurs after severe head injury. Some investigators posit that ventricular enlargement is due to the reduction in the volume of white and grey matter and thinning of the corpus callosum as the result of diffuse axonal injury [1, 2, 6]. Others have reported PTV occurs early and then stabilizes in diffuse axonal injured patients at 3 months [9, 11]. We observed changes in ventricular size throughout the 6 week period following traumatic brain injury (Table 1). Although the ventricular size was reduced at 1 hour post injury, it then increased during the next 3 days significantly ($p < 0.001$) above baseline measures. On day 7 and 14, ventricular size decreased to normal measures, a gradual increase was then observed and reached a significantly ($p < 0.01$) larger size on day 42 post trauma again. These data suggest that two types of PTV may have occurred. The early ventriculomegaly which peaked on day 3 may be due to an obstruction in CSF pathways by subarachnoid hemorrhage. As reported by Foda [5], the late ventriculomegaly in the chronic stage develops as a result of the reduction in brain bulk caused by the degeneration in white and grey matter after head injury and not as a result of an active hydrocephalic process.

In this study, we measured water content changes using gravimetric method and the conventional drying-weighing method (Fig. 2). In the trauma group there was a significant increase ($p < 0.01$) in water content during the first week except on day 3, and these results of water content measured by both methods had a good correlation ($p < 0.001$). Subsequently, water content increased, and was coupled with ventriculomegaly after day 14; however, the correlation was poor ($p = 0.25$). We consider the cause of this poor correlation to be attributed to the change of specific gravity of solids due to brain atrophy. The slope of experimental line derived by the data of day 28 and 42 is 5.7491. According to this value, the specific gravity of solids in the late phase equals 1.2106 which is smaller than the control

value (1.2617). This reduction of the solid specific gravity after day 14 signifies the onset of the atrophic process following traumatic brain injury and is synchronous with the development of port-traumatic ventriculomegaly.

Acknowledgement

This research was supported in part by Grant R01 NS19235 from the National Institutes of Health. Additional facilities and support were provided by the Richard Roland Reynolds Neurosurgical Research Laboratories.

References

1. Berryhill P, Lilly MA, Levin HS, Hillman GR, Mendelsohn D, Brunder DG, Fletcher JM, Kufera J, Kent TA, Yeakley J, Bruce D, Eisenberg HM (1995) Frontal lobe changes after severe diffuse closed head injury in children: a volumetric study of magnetic resonance imaging. Neurosurgery 37: 392–399
2. Beyerl B, Black PM (1984) Posttraumatic hydrocephalus. Neurosurgery 15: 257–261
3. Elliot KAC, Jasper H (1949) Measurement of experimentally induced brain swelling and shrinkage. Am J Physiol 157: 122–129
4. Foda M, Marmarou A (1994) A new model of diffuse brain injury in rats. Part II: Morphological characterization. J Neurosurg 80: 301–313
5. Foda M, Marmarou A (1994) Post-traumatic hydrocephalus following impact acceleration in the rat. In: Nagai H, Kamiya K, Ishii S (eds) Intracranial pressure IX. Springer, Tokyo, pp 305–307
6. Levin HS, Williams DH, Valastro M, Eisenberg HM, Crofford MJ, Handel SF (1990) Corpus callosal atrophy following closed head injury: detection with magnetic resonance imaging. J Neurosurg 73: 77–81
7. Marmarou A, Tanaka K, Shulman K (1982) An improved gravimetric measure of cerebral edema. J Neurosurg 56: 246–253
8. Marmarou A, Foda M, van den Brink W, Campbell J, Kita H, Demetriadou K (1994) A new model of diffuse brain injury in rats. Part I: Pathophysiology and biomechanics. J Neurosurg 80: 291–300
9. Masuzawa H, Kubo T, Nakamura N, Mayanagi Y, Ochiai C (1996) Diffuse ventricular enlargement outlines the late outcome of diffuse axonal injury. No Shinkei Geka 24: 227–233 (Jpn)
10. Nelson SR, Mantz M-L, Maxwell JA (1971) Use of specific gravity in the measurement of cerebral edema. J Appl Physiol 30: 268–271
11. Ochiai C, Ohno T, Nagai M (1993) Diffuse axonal injury caused by traffic accident: Long term serial CT findings and medicolegal problem. In: Nakamura N, Hashimoto T, Yasue M (eds) Recent advances in neurotraumatology. Springer, Berlin Heidelberg New York Tokyo, pp 180–183

Correspondence: Anthony Marmarou, Ph.D., Division of Neurosurgery, Medical College of Virginia, P.O. Box 980508, Richmond, VA 23298-0508, U.S.A.

Acta Neurochir (1997) [Suppl] 70: 78–79
© Springer-Verlag 1997

Altered Brain Oxygen Extraction with Hypoxia and Hypotension Following Deep Hypothermic Circulatory Arrest

M. M. O'Rourke, K. M. Nork, and C. D. Kurth

Department of Anesthesiology and Critical Care Medicine, The Children's Hospital of Philadelpia,
University of Pennsylvania, Philadelphia, PA, U.S.A.

Summary

The utilization of cardiopulmonary bypass in neonates, infants, and children often requires the use of deep hypothermia at 18°C with occasional periods of circulatory arrest. Thus, marked physiologic extremes of temperature and perfusion are induced. The safety of these techniques appears to be related to the reduction of metabolism, particularly cerebral metabolism. We studied the effect of deep hypothermic circulatory arrest and cardiopulmonary bypass on brain oxygenation using near-infrared spectroscopy. After hypothermic arrest, brain oxygen extraction during severe hypoxia and severe hypotension is diminished. However, these responses remain intact after cardiopulmonary bypass. Additionally, cardiopulmonary bypass, rather than deep hypothermic circulatory arrest, alters the cerebral oxygen response to hypercapnia. The primary goal of studying alteration of brain oxygenation during cardiopulmonary bypass and deep hypothermic circulatory arrest is to improve our understanding of the association between these methods and perturbations in hemodynamics and ventilation, so that effective brain protection strategies can be developed.

Keywords: Hypothermic circulatory arrest; cerebral oxygen extration; hypoxia; hypotension; cardiopulmonary bypass.

Introduction

Deep hypothermic circulatory arrest (DHCA) for repair of cardiac lesions in, neonates incurs a risk of neurologic sequelae. Brain injury may occur intraoperatively during cardiopulmonary bypass (CPB), DHCA, reperfusion, or postoperatively during hemodynamic or ventilatory perturbations. During the postoperative period, we studied the effects of hypocapnia, hypercapnia, hypoxia, and hypotension on cerebrovascular hemoglobin-O_2 saturation (ScO_2) as measured by near infrared spectroscopy hours after hypothermic CPB and DHCA.

Materials and Methods

We studied 3 groups of anesthetized newborn pigs (n = 28): Group 1: Control (no CPB, no DHCA); Group 2: CPB (deep hypothermic CPB; no arrest); Group 3: DHCA (deep hypothermic circulatory arrest-60 minute arrest period). Surgical preparation for all groups included: fentanyl/droperidol anesthesia, tracheostomy, femoral artery catheter, and right external jugular vein catheter. The CPB Method (CPB and DHCA Groups) included: right atrium and ascending aorta cannulation, cooling with CPB (150 cc/kg/min, alpha-stat method) over 15–20 minutes to 15–20°C (brain). The piglets were rewarmed with CPB over 25–30 minutes. CPB and DHCA Groups were studied 2 hours after discontinuing CPB. The Control Group was studied 4 hours after surgical preparation. In all groups, ventilation and inspired oxygen concentration were adjusted to achieve: hypocapnia ($paCO_2$ 25 torr), hypercapnia ($paCO_2$ 70 torr), moderate hypoxia (paO_2 40 torr), severe hypoxia (paO_2 25 torr), moderate hypotension (MAP 30 mmHg), and severe hypotension (MAP 20 mmHg).

Results

In the Control Group, ScO_2 decreased with hypocapnia and increased with hypercapnia reflecting increased oxygen extraction and decreased oxygen extraction by the brain, respectively. In the CPB Group, ScO_2 response to hypocapnia was similar to the Control Group. Unlike the Control Group, ScO_2 did not increase with hypercapnia ($p < 0.01$). In the DHCA group, SO_2 response to hypocapnia was similar to the Control and CPB Groups. The ScO_2 response to hypercapnia differed from Control ($p < 0.01$), as did the CPB Group (Control: $85.7 \pm 5.5\%$ vs. CPB: $65.1 \pm 6.3\%$ vs. DHCA: $55.6 \pm 9.3\%$; Fig. 1). In the Control Group, ScO_2 decreased with moderate hypoxia and severe hypoxia reflecting increased oxygen extraction by the brain. In the CPB Group, ScO_2 decreased with moderate and severe hypoxia, similar to the Control Group. In the DHCA Group, ScO_2 decreased similarly with moderate hypoxia as in the Control and CPB Groups. However, ScO_2 decreased less with severe hypoxia than the Control and CPB Groups ($p < 0.05$), reflecting

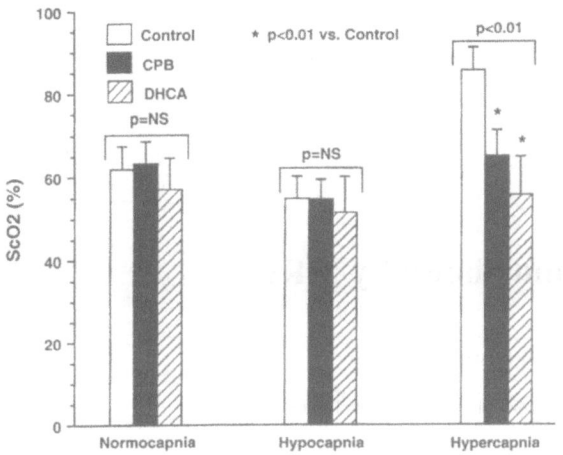

Fig 1. Brain oxygen response to hypocapnia/hypercapnia

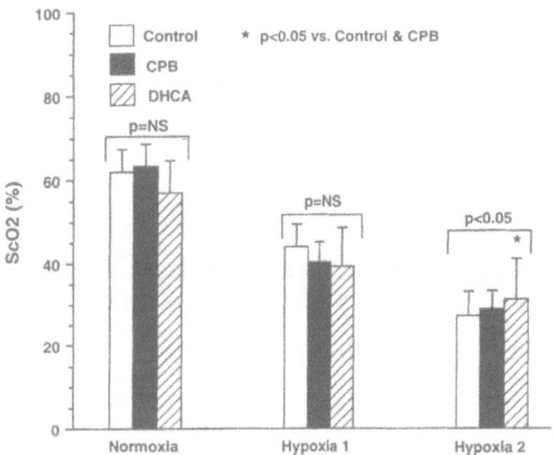

Fig. 3. Brain oxygen response to hypotension

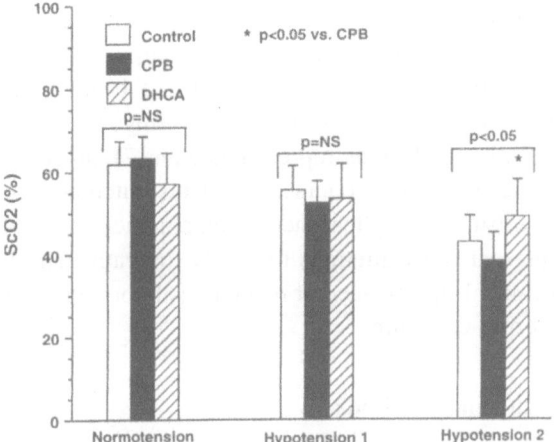

Fig. 2. Brain oxygen response to hypoxia

Discussion

These data suggest that after hypothermic arrest, the brain extraction of oxygen during severe hypoxia and severe hypotension is diminished. However, these responses remain intact after CPB. Cardiopulmonary bypass rather than DHCA alters the cerebral oxygen response to hypercapnia. Decreased ability to extract O_2 during ventilatory and hemodynamic perturbations may contribute to brain injury postoperatively.

Acknowledgment

The RunMan™ Unit is available from NIM, Inc., Philadelphia, Pennsylvania. This project was supported by the Nicholson Foundation, The Children's Hospital of Philadelphia, Philadelphia, PA.

References

1. Kurth CD, Steven JM, Swedlow D (1996) New frontiers in oximetry. Am J Anesthesiol 23: 169–175
2. Whitaker EA, Mault JR, Heinle JS, Lodge AJ, Greeley WJ, Jobsis-VanderVliet F, Ungerleider RM (1993) Near-infrared spectroscopy for noninvasive cerebral metabolic monitoring during congenital heart repair. Surgical Forum XLIV: 211–212

Correspondence: Maureen M. O'Rourke, Department of Anesthesiology and Critical Care Medicine, The Children's Hospital of Philadelphia, University of Pennsylvania, Philadelphia, PA 19104, U.S.A.

decreased extraction of oxygen (Control: $27.2 \pm 6.1\%$ vs. CPB: $29.0 \pm 4.4\%$ vs. DHCA: $31.4 \pm 9.8\%$; Fig. 2). In the Control Group, ScO_2 did not decrease with moderate hypotension, but decreased with severe hypotension reflecting increased oxygen extraction by the brain. In the CPB Group, ScO_2 response was similar to the Control Group during moderate and severe hypotension. In the DHCA Group, ScO_2 decreased less than the Control and CPB Groups during severe hypotension (Control: $43.0 \pm 6.4\%$ vs. CPB: $38.5 \pm 6.8\%$ vs. DHCA: $49.1 \pm 9.0\%$; $p < 0.05$). The response to moderate hypotension was similar (Fig. 3).

Acta Neurochir (1997) [Suppl] 70: 80–83

Posttraumatic Edema in the Corpus Callosum Shown by MRI

T. Tokutomi[1], **M. Hirohata**[1], **T. Miyagi**[1], **T. Abe**[2], and **M. Shigemori**[1]

Departments of [1] Neurosurgery and [2] Radiology, Kurume University School of Medicine, Kurume, Japan

Summary

MRI was performed on 120 patients who sustained closed head injury of varying severity. Patients ranged in age from 4 to 87 years (average, 32 years). All patients had an initial MRI within 28 days (median 12 days) of injury. MRI disclosed areas of abnormal signals in the corpus callosum of 21 (18%) of the 120 patients; 1 (2%) of the 44 patients who sustained mild injuries (GCS $\geq$ 13), 3 (10%) of the 31 moderate injuries (GCS 9~12), and 17 (38%) of the 45 severe injuries (GCS $\leq$ 8) (p < 0.0001). All but 2 of the 21 patients with corpus callosum lesions had other parenchymal lesions that were visualized by MRI. Of these 21 patients, MRI was repeated in 19. In 13 of the 19 patients, repeat MRI scans at 25 to 42 days after injury showed the disappearance of lesions that had on the first MRI shown a high signal on T2-weighted and FLAIR images and a normal signal on T1-weighted images. The MRI findings and time sourse of the disappearance of the corpus callosum lesions mirrored those of paracontusional edema in the subcortical white matter. Patients in whom the corpus callosum lesion disappeared had a better outcome than those in whom the lesion remained (good recovery/moderate disability; 92% vs 63%). The present MRI results suggest that some lesions in the corpus callosum following closed head injury are reversible, thus resembling edema that may be produced by a relatively mild shear strain force to the corpus callosum.

Keywords: Brain edema; corpus callosum; head injury; MRI.

Introduction

Recent neuropathological studies of head trauma have implicated lesions in the corpus callosum as a characteristic feature of diffuse axonal injury produced by shearing forces. Thus, these lesions are considered to be similar to lesions in the dorsolateral quadrant of the upper brainstem and diffuse Wallerian degeneration of the white matter [1–3]. Computed tomographic (CT) scanning, however, is not sufficiently reliable or sensitive to detect such lesions. In contrast, magnetic resonance imaging (MRI) has revealed such small parenchymal lesions because of its precise anatomical and pathological sensitivity [4, 6]. In a recent MRI study [5], corpus callosum lesions were present in 47% of patients with closed head injury. Follow-up MRI have shown that some lesions in the corpus callosum seen on the original MRI after closed head injury diminish or even disappear. These findings have suggested that the lesions represent edema [7], however, the frequency, time course, effect on outcome, and mechanism of this phenomenon remain unclear. Thus, the present study attempts to clarify the pathogenesis and clinical significance of reversible abnormalities in the corpus callosum.

Patients and Methods

MRI studies of 120 head-injured patients were reviewed. The patients consisted 86 males and 34 females, ranging in age between 4 and 87 years (average, 32 years). Noncontrast CT scans were obtained in all patients within 1 hour after admission. All patients had an initial MRI within 28 days (median 12 days) of injury. Of these, MRI analysis was repeated in 43 patients (36%). MRI was performed using either a 0.5-Tesla superconductive system (Shimadzu Magnex 50 Hp) or 1.5-Tesla superconductive system (Shimadzu Magnex 150 Hp). The imaging used T1-weighted, T2-weighted, and FLAIR sequences.

Parenchymal lesions detected by MRI were classified into cortical and central lesions. Central lesions were further subclassified according to location: (1) corpus callosum injury, (2) isolated deep white matter injury, (3) basal ganglia injury, and (4) brainstem injury.

The severity of injury was defined according to the Glasgow Coma Scale (GCS) [11] at 6 hours after injury or preoperative GCS as follows: no deterioration from a GCS score of 13 to 15 was classified as mild, a GCS score of 9 to 12 without subsequent deterioration as moderate, and a GCS score of 8 or less as severe. Thirty patients underwent surgery for intracranial hematomas and were clinically categorized as evacuated mass (EM). The remainder were categorized as diffuse injury (DI). Outcome was assessed by the Glasgow Outcome Scale (COS) [8] at 6 months after injury.

The Chi-squared test was used to detect differences in lesions shown by MRI among the groups as well as to determine differences in GOS and clinical classification (EM or DI) among the groups. Student's t-test was used for determine the variation of age with the groups. Statistical significance was established at the p < 0.05 level.

Results

Forty-five patients suffered severe injuries, 31 were judged as moderate, and 44 as mild. There were no significant differences in age distribution among the three groups (mean ± SD, 28 ± 23, 35 ± 22, 34 ± 22 years). MRI revealed areas of abnormal signals in the corpus callosum of 21 (18%) of the 120 patients. These 21 patients were composed 17 (38%) of the 45 patients who sustained severe injuries, 3 (10%) of the 31 moderate injury patients, and 1 (2%) of the 44 mild injury patients. The incidence of the corpus callosum lesions among the three groups was significantly different (p < 0.0001).

Fourteen (67%) of callosal lesions were found in the posterior portion of the corpus callosum (body to splenium). Four (19%) of callosal lesions were found in the genu of the corpus callosum. All but 2 of the 21 patients with corpus callosum lesions had other parenchymal lesions visualized by MRI. These included cortical contusions (11 cases), and small hemorrhages in the deep white matter (5 cases), basal ganglia (5 cases), and upper brainstem (5 cases). Thirteen (62%) of the 21 patients had other central lesions.

Of the 21 patients with callosal lesions, MRI analysis was repeated in 19. In 13 (68%) of the 19 patients, repeat MRI scans at 25 to 42 days after injury showed the disappearance of abnormal intensity in the corpus callosum which had previously appeared as a high signal on T2-weighted and FLAIR images and as a normal signal on T1-weighted images. All but one callosal lesion in the mild and moderate severity groups had disappeared. The MRI findings and time course of the disappearance of the corpus callosum lesions mirror those of paracontusional edema in the subcortical white matter (Fig. 1). In those patients who showed continuing abnormal intensity on T1-weighted, T2-weighted and FLAIR images, the lesions were considered to be hemorrhagic (Fig. 2).

The outcome of each group from the 120 patients is shown in Table 1. The correlation between the outcome and callosal lesions was analyzed only in the severe group, because of the small number of the patients with corpus callosum injuries in the another groups. Corpus callosum injury did not affect the outcome in the severe group (Table 2). However, patients in whom the corpus callosum lesions disappeared had a better outcome than those in whom the corpus callosum lesions remained (good recovery/moderate disability; 92% vs 63%).

The severe group included 16 patients with EM and 29 with DI. Six (37.5%) of the patients with EM and 11

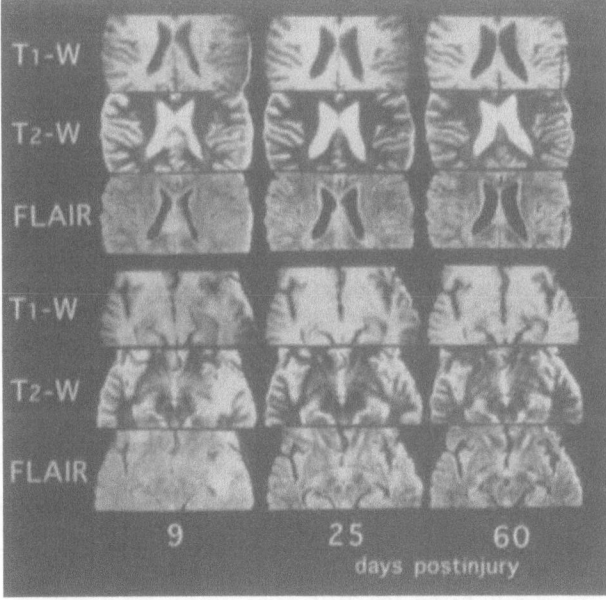

Fig. 1. 12-year-old boy with moderate injury. Repeat MR scans at 25 and 60 days after injury show the disappearance of abnormal intensity in the corpus callosum which previously appeared as a high signal on T2-weighted and FLAIR images and as a normal signal on T1-weighted images of initial MRI (9 days postinjury). The findings and time course of the disappearance of the corpus callosum lesion mirror those of the temporal subcortical lesion that represent paracontusional edema

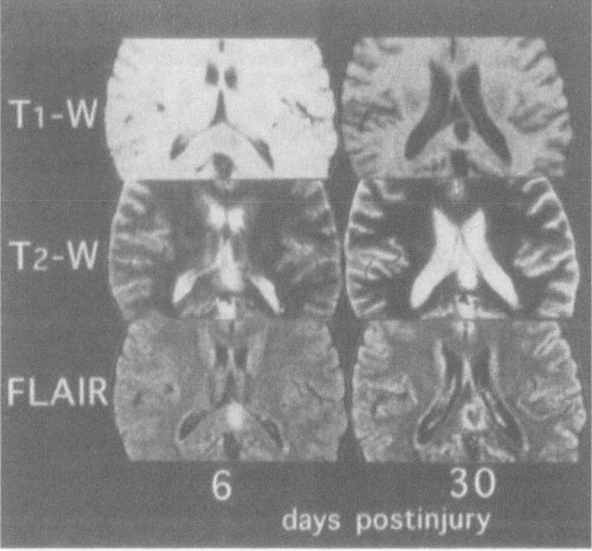

Fig. 2. 18-year-old womam with severe injury. Repeat MRI at 30 days after injury show continuing abnormal intensity in the corpus callosum on T1-weighted, T2-weighted and FLAIR images that previously appeared as a low signal on T1-weighted and a high signal on T2-weighted and FLAIR images of initial MRI (6 days after injury). The lesions are considered to be hemorrhagic

Table 1. *Glasgow Outcome Scale Score (GOS) Correlated with Severity Groups*

GOS	Mild		Moderate		Severe	
	No.	%	No.	%	No.	%
Good recovery	43	98	26	84	25	56
Moderate disability	1	2	5	16	7	16
Severe disability	–	–	–	–	5	11
Vegetative state	–	–	–	–	6	13
Dead	–	–	–	–	2	4
Totals	44	100	31	100	45	100

Table 2. *Glasgow Outcome Scale Score (GOS) Correlated with Corpus Callosum Injury (CCI) in the Severe Group*

GOS	With CCI		Without CCI	
	No.	%	No.	%
Good recovery	10	59	15	54
Moderate disability	3	18	4	14
Severe disability	2	12	3	11
Vegetative state	2	12	4	14
Dead	–	–	2	7
Totals	17	100	28	100

(38%) of those with DI had corpus callosum injuries. There was no significant difference between the groups.

Discussion

In the present report, traumatic lesions of the corpus callosum were detected in 17.5% of 120 patients and in 38% of the 45 patients with severe injuries. Other MRI studies have reported 47% frequency of callosal injuries (Gentry *et al.*) [5], and 24% frequency of callosal injuries (Mendelsohn *et al.*) [9]. This disparity may be explained by several factors such as patient age, severity and cause of injury. Genry *et al.* [5] reported that acute callosal lesions detected by MRI were most commonly (67.7%) nonhemorrhagic lesions. The frequency in the present study was similar. We believe that the nonhemorrhagic lesions that disappeared on follow-up MRI are edema, and therefore recovery should occur within 4 weeks of injury.

Corpus callosum injury occurred significantly more often in severely injured patients, although this did not adversely affect the outcome. Traumatic lesion of the corpus callosum is well known to be a prominent macroscopic feature of diffuse axonal injury [1, 2], and shear-strain deformation produced by coronal head acceleration [3] or linear translation of acceleration [12] at the time of impact is now widely accepted as the mechanism of the injury. Shear strains develop easily in the corpus callosum region. In the present study, disappearance of callosal lesions shown by follow-up MRI was more frequently observed in mild to moderate injured patients, and it was paralleled by improvement in outcome. These findings suggest that the disappearance of the callosal lesions that are believed to be edema may be produced by a relatively mild force of shear strain to the corpus callosum.

In our results, of the patients with callosal injuries, 62% had other associated central lesions. Although the diagnosis of diffuse axonal injury remains essentially pathological, traumatic callosal lesions detected by MRI could be a "marker" of diffuse axonal injury. Shigemori *et al.* [10] reported that postmortem examination revealed that 50% of focal brain injury including evacuated subdural hematoma, epidural hematoma, and traumatic intracerebral hematoma showed histological evidence of diffuse axonal injury. In the present study, the frequency of callosal injury in both DI and EM patients of the severe group were almost the same. Thus, present results indicate that diffuse axonal injury should be considered to be common subjacent damage in severe head injury, regardless of the clinical category.

References

1. Adams JH, Graham DI, Murray LS, Scott G (1982) Diffuse axonal injury due to non-missile head injury in humans. An analysis of 45 cases. Ann Neurol 12: 557–563
2. Adams JH, Doyle D, Ford I, Gennarelli TA, Graham DI, McLellan DR (1989) Diffuse axonal injury in head injury. Definition, diagnosis and grading. Histopathology 15: 49–59
3. Gennarelli TA, Thibault LE, Adams JH, Graham DI, Thompson CJ, Marcincin RP (1982) Diffuse axonal injury and traumatic coma in the primate. Ann Neurol 12: 564–574
4. Gentry LR, Godersky JC, Thompson B, Dunn VD (1988) Prospective comparative study of intermediate-field MR and CT in the evaluation of closed head trauma. AJNR 9: 91–100
5. Gentry LR, Thompson B, Godersky JC (1988) Trauma to the corpus callosum: MR features. AJNR 9: 1129–1138
6. Han JS, Kaufman B, Alfidi RJ (1984) Head trauma evaluated by magnetic resonance and computed tomography. A comparison. Radiology 150: 71–77
7. Hankins L, Taber KH, Yeakley J, Hayman LA (1996) Magnetic resonance imaging in head injury. In: Narayan RK, Wiberger JE, Povlishock JT (eds) Neurotrauma. McGraw-Hill, New York, pp 151–161
8. Jennet B, Bond M (1975) Assessment of outcome after severe brain damage. A practical scale. Lancet 1: 480–484
9. Mendelsohn DB, Levin HS, Harward H, Bruce D (1992) Corpus callosum lesions after closed head injury in children:

MRI, clinical features and outcome. Neuroradiology 34: 384–388

10. Shigemori M, Tokutomi T, Kuramto S, Moriyama T, Kikuchi N, Sasaguri Y (1991) Diffuse axonal injury and early intracranial sequelae in severe head injury. Neurol Med Chir (Tokyo) 31: 309–395

11. Teasdale G, Jennett B (1974) Assessment of coma and impaired consciousness. A practical scale. Lancet 2: 81–84

12. Zarkovic K, Jadro-Santel D, Grcevic N (1991) Distribution of traumatic lesions of corpus callosum in "inner cerebral trauma". Neurolog Croat 40: 129–155

Correspondence: Takashi Tokutomi, M.D., Department of Neurosurgery, Kurume University School of Medicine, 67 Asahi-machi, Kurume-shi, Fukuoka-ken 830, Japan.

Acta Neurochir (1997) [Suppl] 70: 84–86
© Springer-Verlag 1997

Detection of Lipid Peroxidation and Hydroxyl Radicals in Brain Contusion of Rats

S. Nishio, M. Yunoki, Y. Noguchi, M. Kawauchi, S. Asari, and **T. Ohmoto**

Department of Neurological Surgery, Okayama University Medical School, Okayama, Japan

Summary

To examine the relationship between the free radicals and brain tissue damage, we investigated the intensity of brain hydroxyl (OH) radical generation and lipid peroxidation in the rat contusion injury model. A unilateral contusion was induced by a weight-drop method. All rats were decapitated six hours after the injury, and brain samples were taken from three portions (core, peripheral, and distal) to examine the specific gravity as an indicator of brain edema, generation of OH using an electron paramagnetic resonance spectrometer (EPR), and malondialdehyde (MDA) and 4-hydroxyalkenals production. Analysis of the specific gravity revealed cerebral edema on the ipsilateral side in the injured group. The signal intensity of EPR in the core and peripheral portions in the contusion group was significantly higher than that in the distal portion of the contusion group and that of all portions in the control animals.

No significant difference was observed between the core and peripheral portions of the contusion group. The MDA and 4-hydroxyalkenals production was significantly higher in the core and peripheral portions than in the distal portion of the contusion group and that of all portions of the control group.

The degree of posttraumatic brain edema was closely correlated with the increase of DMPO-OH adduct, MDA, and 4-hydroxyalkenals. These results support the current concept that free radical production following traumatic brain injury may induce lipid peroxidation and may be the direct cause of edema formation.

Keywords: Hydroxyl radical; EPR; lipid peroxidation; brain contusion.

Introduction

Oxygen free radicals have been postulated to play a role in the pathophysiology of acute head injury. They attack the major classes of cellular components, such as lipids [6, 8], proteins [20], and nucleic acids [7]. To examine the relationship between the free radicals and lipid peroxidative brain tissue damage, we investigated the intensity of brain hydroxyl radical (OH) generation and lipid peroxidation in the rat contusion injury model.

Materials and Methods

Male Sprague-Dawley rats (250–320 g) were divided into two groups: contusion group (n = 12) and control group (n = 11). A burr hole 5 mm in diameter was made on the right parietal portion in each rat. The contusion was induced by a weight-drop method, in which a 20 g metallic cylinder 4.5 mm in diameter was dropped from a height of 30 cm through a guide tube onto the exposed dura. The control group carried out a sham operation. All rats were decapitated six hours after the injury. Brain samples were taken from three portions; the center of the injury (core), 2 mm posterior to the injury (peripheral), and the contralateral hemisphere (distal). To detect the generation of OH radicals, the tissue samples were homogenized in a buffer solution and 1 mM H_2O_2 was added. After addition of DMPO (5,5-dimethyl-1-pyrroline-N-oxide) to the homogenate samples, spin-adducts were detected using an electron paramagnetic resonance spectrometer (JES-FElXG: JEOL Ltd.,Tokyo, Japan). The conditions of spectrometry were as follows: magnetic field, 3356 ± 50 Gaus; microwave power, 8 mW; modulation amplitude, 0.8 Gaus; modulation frequency, 100 kHz; response, 0.1; sweep time, 1 min; room temperature. Lipid peroxidation in the samples was estimated from the amounts of malondialdehyde (MDA) and 4-hydroxyalkenals using the LPO-586 method [4] (Bioxytech S.A., France), and the specific gravity was measured by Marmarou's method [14] as an indicator of brain edema formation.

Results

EPR spectra of DMPO-OH adducts (four peaks) were detected at 3356 ± 50 Gaus in all samples. The signal intensity of the second peak was measured and corrected by the tissue protein of each sample. The signal intensity in the core (0.580 ± 0.164) and peripheral (0.508 ± 0.135) portions of the contusion group was higher than that in distal portion of the contusion group and all portions of the control animals ($p < 0.05$) (Table 1). No significant difference was observed between the core and the peripheral portions of the contusion group.

The MDA and 4-hydroxyalkenals production was significantly higher in the core (4.51 ± 1.84 mmol/g)

and peripheral (3.18 ± 1.52 mmol/g) portions of the contusion group than in the distal portion of the contusion group and all portions of the control group ($p < 0.05$) (Table 2).

Analysis of the specific gravity revealed significant cerebral edema on the ipsilateral side in the injured group (core 1.036 ± 0.001, peripheral 1.041 ± 0.002, $p < 0.01$) (Table 3). The degree of posttraumatic brain edema was closely correlated with the increase of DMPO-OH adduct, MDA, and 4-hydroxyalkenals.

Discussion

Previous investigators have measured the production of various free radicals using nitroblue tetrazollum reduction [2, 13], chemiluminescence [12], salicylate trapping [1, 3, 9–11], cytochrome c electrodes [5], and electron paramagnetic resonance spectroscopy [18, 19]. In the present study, we used an electron spin trapping method for measuring the levels of OH in tissue in attempt to detect the generation of this key radical in the rat contusion brain injury model. By this technique, we could directly detect free radicals in the rat brain. As a spin trap, DMPO has been used frequently because it forms relatively long-lived radical adducts and has no photoirradiation effects.

Due to the rapid metabolic degradation of DMPO and many radical scavengers in the brain, we chose a method to detect free radicals by homogenizing the cortex with a DMPO and H_2O_2 solution after decapitation. This method enabled us to measure the difference among the core, peripheral, and distal portions. If we inject DMPO into animals, the *in vivo* concentration change of DMPO may be too rapid to measure the difference in the free radical formation under the same conditions.

Kontos and Povlishock have demonstrated the appearance of superoxide radical in the cerebral extracellular space in the cat fluid percussion brain injury model using a cranial window technique [13]. They postulated that the superoxide underwent dismutation in the extracellular space to hydrogen peroxide. While iron in CSF catalyzed the interaction of hydrogen peroxide with superoxide, giving rise to OH radical (Haber-Weiss reaction). They thought that OH radical is the most likely cause of vascular injury after fluid percussion injury. In the present study, this reaction was probably the cause of production of the free radicals.

Puppo *et al.* [15] reported the ability of oxyhaemoglobin to generate a reactive oxidant [4] in the presence of low concentrations of H_2O_2, and the ease with which

Table 1. *Hydroxyl Radicals* (peak intensity / mg protein)

	Core	Peripheral	Distal
Control group	0.324 ± 0.099	0.349 ± 0.117	0.283 ± 0.108
Contusion group	0.580 ± 0.164[b]	0.508 ± 0.135[a]	0.313 ± 0.123

[a] $p < 0.05$ vs distal portion and all portions of control group.
[b] $p < 0.01$ vs distal portion and all portions of control group.

Table 2. *Lipid Peroxidation* (mmol/g)

	Core	Peripheral	Distal
Control group	1.473 ± 0.805	1.552 ± 0.678	1.345 ± 0.365
Contusion group	4.506 ± 1.837[b,c]	3.179 ± 1.522[a]	1.077 ± 0.538

[a] $p < 0.05$ vs distal portion and all portions of control group.
[b] $p < 0.001$ vs distal portion and all portions of control group.
[c] $p < 0.05$ vs peripheral portion of contusion group.

Table 3. *Specific Gravity*

	Core	Peripheral	Distal
Control group	1.045 ± 0.001	1.044 ± 0.001	1.044 ± 0.001
Contusion group	1.036 ± 0.001[b]	1.041 ± 0.002[a]	1.046 ± 0.002

[a] $p < 0.01$ vs distal portion and all portions of control group.
[b] $p < 0.001$ vs other portions of both group.

methaemoglobin): released iron in a form that can stimulate lipid peroxidation and OH radical formation. In our model, a small hematoma was sometimes seen on the brain surface or subdural space. To avoid the direct influence of the hematoma, we removed it as possible as it appeared. However, the recorded signals might have resulted from OH radical production by iron released from damaged tissues or blood cells in the brain. Another possibility is that NO generation in damaged tissues could lead to mobilization of iron from ferritin disrupting the intracellular iron homeostasis and increasing the level of free radicals [16]. Other origins of free radicals production after brain contusion may exist. The stimulation of xanthine-xanthine oxidase system in the cerebral vessels, activated neutrophils, cathecholamine oxidation, and arachidonic acid metabolism could all be the sources of oxygen free radicals.

In our study, we measured the values of MDA and 4-hydroxyalkenals six hours after brain contusion. The values increased, indicating lipid peroxidation. Sakamoto *et al.* [17] could detect the oxygen-derived radicals using the spin-trapping, and estimate the levels of lipid peroxidation by measuring thiobarbituric acid reactive substance (TBAR) in the rat model of forebrain ischemia-reperfusion injury. They demonstrated a burst of free radical formation and an increase of lipid peroxidation on reperfusion. They also demonstrated that the lipid peroxidation was proportionate to the free radical production during ischemia and reperfusion. We found a correlation among the increase in the peak intensity of spin-adduct formation, the increase in lipid peroxidation and the extent of brain edema formation six hours after brain contusion. These observations suggest that the free radicals may play an important role not only in the primary tissue damage but also in the secondary damage through the activation of lipid peroxidation following traumatic brain injury, and that this may be the cause of subsequent vasogenic edema.

Conclusions

The generation of OH radicals or the substances essential for OH radical production through Fenton reaction, such as metal ions, was monitored by spin trapping with DMPO in the rat model of contusion brain injury. The degree of posttraumatic brain edema was closely correlated with the increase of DMPO-OH adduct, MDA, and 4-hydroxyalkenals. These results support the current concept that free radical production following traumatic brain injury may induce lipid peroxidation and may be the direct cause of edema formation.

References

1. Althaus JS, Andrus PK, Williams CM, VonVoigtlander PF, Cazers AR, Hall ED (1993) The use of salicylate hydroxylation to detect hydroxyl radical generation in ischemic and traumatic brain injury. Reversal by tirilazad mesylate (U-74006F). Mol Chem Neuropathol 20: 147–162
2. Armstead WM, Mirro R, Busija DW, Leffler CW (1988) Postischemic generation of superoxide anion by newborn pig brain. Am J Physiol 255 (2 Pt 2): 4401–4403
3. Cao W, Carney JM, Duchon A, Floyd RA, Chevion M (1988) Oxygen free radical involvement in ischemia and reperfusion injury to brain. Neurosci Lett 88: 233–238
4. Esterbauer H, Cheeseman KH (1990) Determination of aldehydic lipid peroxidation products: malonaldehyde and 4-hydroxynonenal. Methods Enzymol 186: 407–421
5. Fabian RH, DeWitt DS, Kent TA (1995) *In vivo* detection of superoxide anion production by the brain using a cytochrome c electrode. J Cereb Blood Flow Metab 15: 242–247
6. Floyd RA (1990) Role of oxygen free radicals in carcinogenesis and brain ischemia. Faseb J 4: 2587–2597
7. Floyd RA, Schneider JE (1990) Hydroxyl free radical damage to DNA. In: Membrane lipid oxidation 1. Vigo-Pelfrey, Florida
8. Girotti AW (1985) Mechanisms of lipid peroxidation. J Free Radic Biol Med 1: 87–95
9. Globus MY, Alonso O, Dietrich WD, Busto R, Ginsberg MD (1995) Glutamate release and free radical production following brain injury: effects of posttraumatic hypothermia. J Neurochem 65: 1704–1011
10. Globus MY, Busto R, Lin B, Schnippering H, Ginsberg MD (1995) Detection of free radical activity during transient global ischemia and recirculation: effects of intraischemic brain temperature modulation. J Neurochem 65: 1250–1256
11. Hall ED, Andrus PK, Yonkers PA (1993) Brain hydroxyl radical generation in acute experimental head injury. J Neurochem 60: 588–594
12. Imaizumi S, Kayama T, Suzuki J (1984) Chemiluminescence in hypoxic brain – the first report. Correlation between energy metabolism and free radical reaction. Stroke 15: 1061–1065
13. Kontos HA, Povlishock JT (1986) Oxygen radicals in brain injury. Cent Nerv Syst Trauma 3: 257–263
14. Marmarou A, Tanaka K, Shulman K (1982) An improved gravimetric measure of cerebral edema. J Neurosurg 56: 246–253
15. Puppo A, Halliwell B (1988) Formation of hydroxyl radicals from hydrogen peroxide in the presence of iron. Is haemoglobin a biological Fenton reagent? Biochem J 249: 185–190
16. Reif DW, Simmons RD (1990) Nitric oxide mediates iron release from ferritin. Arch Biochem Biophys 283: 537–541
17. Sakamoto A, Ohnishi ST, Ohnishi T, Ogawa R (1991) Relationship between free radical production and lipid peroxidation during ischemia-reperfusion injury in the rat brain. Brain Res 554: 186–192
18. Sen S, Goldman H, Morehead M, Murphy S, Phillis JW (1994) alpha-Phenyl-tert-butyl-nitrone inhibits free radical release in brain concussion. Free Radic Biol Med 16: 685–691
19. Sen S, Phillis JW (1993) alpha-Phenyl-tert-butyl-nitrone (PBN) attenuates hydroxyl radical production during ischemia-reperfusion injury of rat brain: an EPR study. Free Radic Res Commun 19: 255–265
20. Wolff SP, Garner A, Dean RT (1986) Free radicals, lipids, and protein degradation. Trends Biol Sci 11: 27–31

Correspondence: Shinsaku Nishio, M.D., Department of Neurological Surgery, Okayama University Medical School, 2-5-1, Shikata-cho, Okayama 700, Japan.

Acta Neurochir (1997) [Suppl] 70: 87–90
© Springer-Verlag 1997

Time Course of Tissue Elasticity and Fluidity in Vasogenic Brain Edema

T. Kuroiwa[1], **M. Ueki**[1], **H. Ichiki**[1], **M. Kobayashi**[1], **H. Suemasu**[2], **I. Taniguchi**[3], and **R. Okeda**[1]

[1] Department of Neuropathology, [2] Department of Neurophysiology, Medical Research Institute, Tokyo Medical and Dental University, and [3] Faculty of Engineering, Sophia University, Tokyo, Japan

Summary

We examined chronological changes in regional tissue elasticity (stiffness) and fluidity (1/viscosity) of the white matter during the development and resolution of vasogenic brain edema. Cryogenic injury was created in the cortex of cat brain, and the brain was prepared for measurement of regional tissue elasticity and fluidity. The results were then compared with the histology and tissue water content. Vasogenic edema developed in the white matter under the lesioned cortex (4–24 h) and was resolved by day 10. Regional tissue elasticity decreased significantly during the initial 24 h (45.3 ± 32.5% of the control (mean ± S.D.), and then increased to 158.6 ± 32.3% of the control level at day 10. Regional tissue fluidity increased to 376.7 ± 240.4% of the control level during the initial 24 h and decreased to 77.7 ± 17.9% of the control level at day 10. Histological examination of the white matter revealed widening of the inter-fiber space at 4–24 h after lesioning and astrocytosis at day 10. Thus vasogenic edema causes an increase of tissue fluidity with a decrease of tissue elasticity. Reactive astrocytosis after the resolution of edema causes an increase of tissue elasticity with mild decrease in tissue fluidity.

Keywords: Tissue elasticity; tissue fluidity; Maxwell-Voigt model; vasogenic edema; astrocytes; sclerosis.

Introduction

Edema formation and its resolution constitute the healing process in many injured tissues/organs. However, in the brain, which is located inside the skull, the process occasionally results in fatal complications such as cerebral herniation, secondary hemorrhage and infarction, when the increase in volume and pressure exceeds the range of compensation. To analyze the mechanisms of these processes, a basic knowledge of the biomechanical properties of brain tissue under pathological as well as physiological conditions is important. Such data are also indispensable for computer simulation of intracranial processes in the fields of neurosurgery and neuropathology. In this study we examined chronological changes in regional tissue elasticity (stiffness) and fluidity (1/viscosity) of the white matter during the development and resolution of vasogenic edema. We observed an approximately four-fold increase of tissue fluidity with a reciprocal decrease of tissue elasticity in the edematous white matter. After resolution of edema, tissue elasticity increased with the development of astrocytosis.

Materials and Methods

Eighteen cats of both sexes weighing 3.0–4.5 kg were used in the experiment. For inducing cryogenic injury, the animal was anesthetized with ketamine (30 mg/kg) and the left femoral artery was cannulated for arterial blood sampling and blood pressure monitoring. The left femoral vein was cannulated for injection of drugs. Each animal was placed on a stereotaxic frame, and a cranial window (1 cm in diameter) was made over the left ectosylvian gyrus. A cold lesion was created by placing a metal plate cooled to –40°C with acetone-dry ice onto the dura mater over the ectosylvian gyrus for 60 seconds. To examine the extent of vasogenic edema, 2% Evans blue (EB) solution in saline (2 ml/kg) was injected shortly after lesioning. The animal was sacrificed at 4 h (n = 5), 24 h (n = 5) or 10 d (n = 5) after lesioning by an overdose injection of pentobarbital. The brain was removed and cut coronally at the center of the lesion. A coronal slice was immersion-fixed and prepared for histological examination by hematoxylin-eosin, Kluever-Barrera and glial fibrillary acid protein (GFAP) staining. Another coronal slice with the corresponding mirror surface was placed in a chamber filled with silicone oil, and several regions of interest were selected in the white matter of the lesioned cortex and the deeper white matter. The data needed for calculation of tissue elasticity and fluidity according to the Maxwell-Voigt model was measured by an indentation method [1, 5]. After measurement, tissue samples (each approximately 10 mg) from the above regions of interest were dissected out and transferred to a kerosene-monobrombenzene gradient column for measurement of the specific gravity (SG). Tissue water content was calculated from the SG values according to a formula proposed by Marmarou [4]. Three control animals were treated similarly except for cold lesioning.

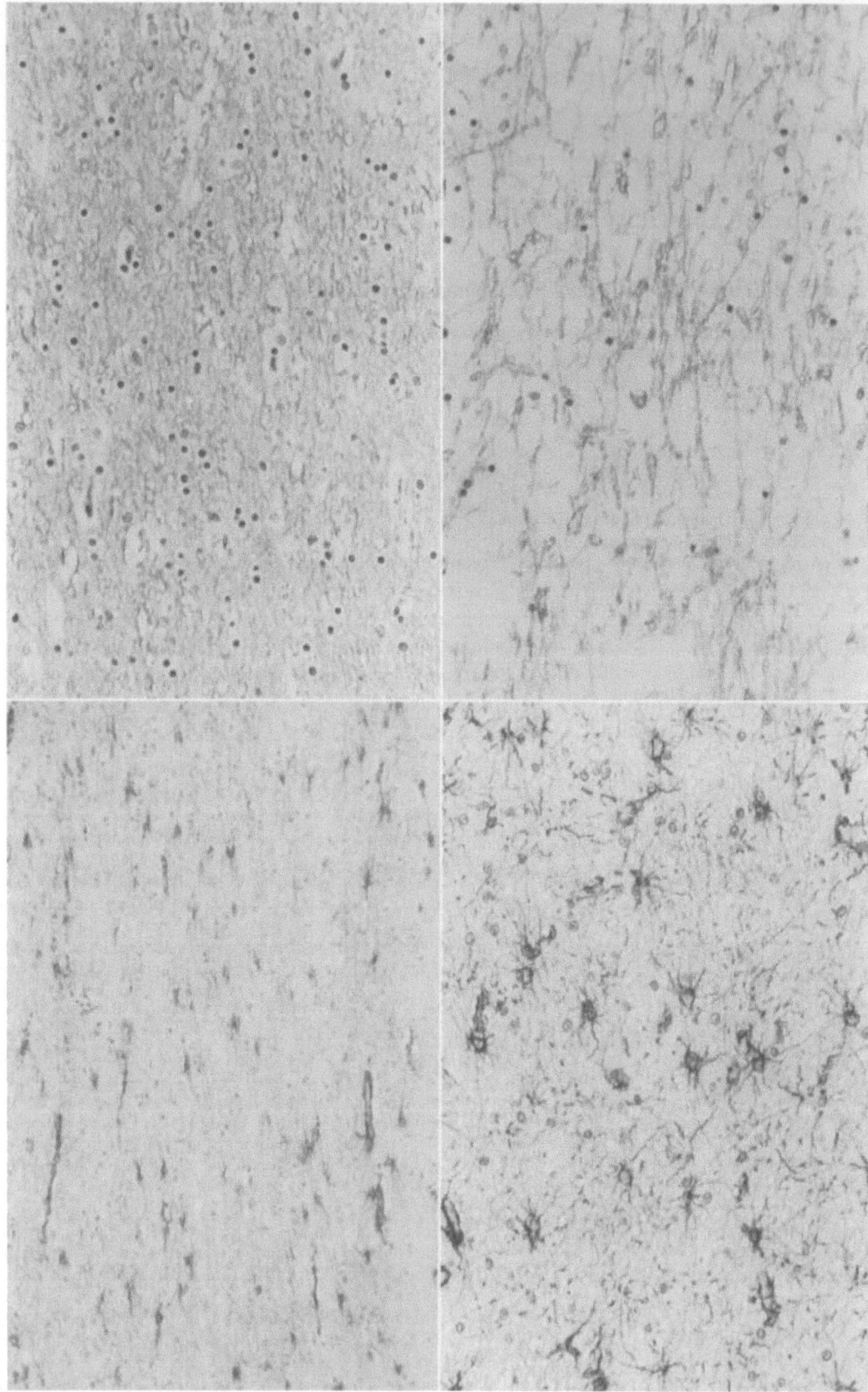

Fig. 1. White matter of the normal brain, KB staining (upper left), 4 h after cold lesion, KB staining (upper right). Note the widening of the inter-fiber space at 4 h after lesioning. White matter of the normal brain, GFAP staining (lower left) and 10 d after lesion (lower right). After resolution of edema, astrocytosis was evident in the white matter

Results

Physiological parameters were kept within the normal ranges during lesioning. The EB-stained area, corresponding to the distribution of extravasated serum protein, was observed in the white matter under the lesioned cortex at 4 h. The area extended to the adjacent deeper white matter at 24 h and 10 d. The specific gravity measurement showed brain edema in the area with EB staining at 4 h and 24 h. No edema was observed in any area with EB staining in the 10 d group. Histological examination revealed widening of the inter-fiber space in the edematous white matter at 4 h and 24 h. At 10 days after lesioning, GFAP staining showed reactive astrocytsis in the area showing EB staining (Fig. 1).

Biomechanical analysis showed decrease of tissue elasticity to 52.5 ± 29.5% and 45.3 ± 32.5% of the control level at 4 h and 24 h after lesioning, respectively. The value increased to 158.6 ± 32.3% of the control level at 10 d. Tissue fluidity increased to 230.1 ± 150.6% and 376.7 ± 240.4% of the control level at 4 h and 24 h, respectively. The value decreased to 77.7 ± 17.9% of the control level at 10 d after lesioning (Fig. 2).

Discussion

Tissue elasticity and fluidity were calculated according to the Maxwell-Voigt three-element model from data obtained by an indentation method [1]. The threeelement model has been widely used to simulate the biomechanical properties of various materials to a combination of three elements i.e., one dash-pot (fluidity) connected in parallel to one spring (elasticity) and in series with another spring (elasticity). The result shows only the biomechanical properties of brain tissue slices *ex vivo*. Many *in vivo* factors such as changes in CSF and blood pressure cannot be taken into account in this method. However, data from individual analysis of each factor are indispensable for mathematical analysis of the injury process caused by mechanical stresses in the living brain. We have previously reported that tissue elasticity decreases in parallel with the increase of tissue water content in vasogenic edema [2, 3]. Since the speed of displacement of brain tissue is a very important factor determining the outcome of brain edema and swelling, fluidity should also be an important factor in the mechanism of edema-mediated brain injury. We attempted in this study to measure the fluidity of edematous brain tis-

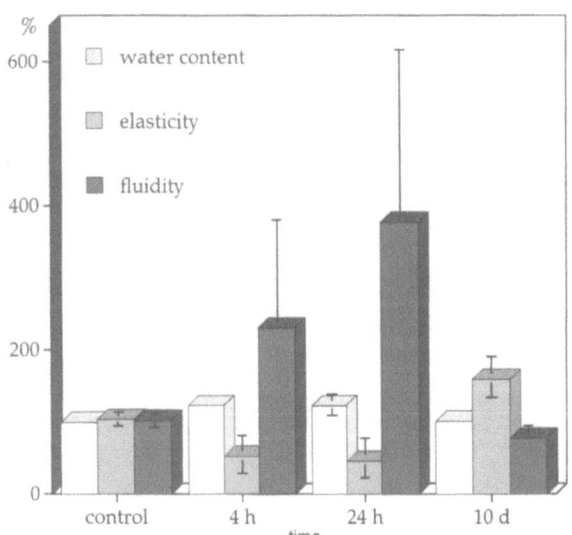

Fig. 2. Chronological change of the tissue water content, tissue elasticity (stiffness) and tissue fluidity. Note that vasogenic edema causes an increase of tissue fluidity with a decrease of tissue elasticity. Reactive astrocytosis after the resolution of edema causes an increase of tissue elasticity with mild decrease in tissue fluidity

sue. The increase of tissue water content from 63.6% to 78.2% (Δ = 14.6) corresponded to the decrease of tissue elasticity to 45.3% of the control level and the increase of tissue fluidity to 376.7% of the control level. Thus we found that tissue fluidity of the white matter is very sensitive to vasogenic-type brain edema. The term "sclerosis" is often used in various pathological changes, e.g., atherosclerosis and nephrosclerosis. Several pathological changes such as calcification and fibrosis are responsible for the sclerosing or hardening of the tissue. The term "sclerosis" is also commonly used in neuropathology. Sclerosing panencephalitis, hippocampal sclerosis and multiple sclerosis are examples. Although various pathological changes such as neuronal loss and demyelination are found in these disorders, the corresponding pathological change common to all of them is astrocytosis. To date, no quantitative analysis has confirmed the increase of brain tissue elasticity in astrocytosis. The present study clearly showed that tissue elasticity is indeed increased during the development of astrocytosis. The data also showed that approximately a 1.5-fold increase of tissue elasticity due to astrocytosis causes a mild decrease in tissue fluidity.

References

1. Aoyagi N, Masuzawa H, Sano K, Norihira M, Kobayashi H (1980) Compliance of the brain. Brain Nerve (No to Shinkei) 32: 47–56

2. Kuroiwa T, Taniguchi I, Okeda R (1991) Regional tissue compliance of edematous brain after cryogenic injury in cats. Intracranial pressure VIII. Springer, Berlin Heidelberg New York Tokyo, pp 127–129

3. Kuroiwa T, Ueki M, Suemasu H, Taniguchi I, Okeda R (1994) Biomechanical characteristics of brain edema. Acta Neurochir (Wien) [Suppl] 60: 158–161

4. Marmarou A, Tanaka K, Schulman K (1982) An improved gravimetric measure of cerebral edema. J Neurosurg 56: 246–253

5. Walsh EK, Schettini A (1976) Elastic behavior of brain tissue *in vivo*. Am J Physiol 230: 1058–1062

Correspondence: Toshihiko Kuroiwa, M.D., Yushima 1-5-45, Bunkyo-ku, Tokyo 113, Japan.

Acta Neurochir (1997) [Suppl] 70: 91–93
© Springer-Verlag 1997

The Penumbra Zone of a Traumatic Cortical Lesion: a Microdialysis Study of Excitatory Amino Acid Release

M. Stoffel, J. Eriskat, M. Plesnila, N. Aggarwal, and **A. Baethmann**

Institute of Surgical Research, Klinikum Grosshadern, Ludwig-Maximilians-University, Munich, Federal Republic of Germany

Summary

A cortical tissue necrosis from focal trauma expands to 150% of its initial volume within 24 hrs. It is currently unknown, whether this phenomenon is part of the primary traumatic lesion or if it involves secondary mechanisms such as the release of excitatory amino acids into the traumatic penumbra zone. A microdialysis probe was inserted for that purpose in an oblique angle into the cortex of Sprague-Dawley rats, approximately 2 mm below the brain surface. One day later a highly standardized cortical freezing lesion was induced at the brain cortex above the microdialysis probe. Dialysate was collected prior to, during, and after trauma in 10 min intervals. In each animal, it was confirmed histologically, that the tip of the microdialysis probe was localized in the grey matter in close vicinity to the primary lesion. Following induction of the trauma a statistically significant increase of the dialysate level of aspartate, glutamate, glycine, and serine was observed, whereas that of alanine was not altered throughout the experiment. The posttraumatic increase of the excitatory neurotransmitters aspartate and glutamate indicates that these amino acids are involved in the secondary lesion growth after trauma. Confirmation of this hypothesis would require that specific antagonization of these excitotoxic amino acids is inhibiting growth of the lesion.

Keywords: Brain injury; penumbra; excitatory amino acids; microdialysis.

Introduction

Brain damage from a traumatic insult is not restricted to the primary necrotic lesion of the impact, but in addition the result of secondary mechanisms enhancing the initial pathology. The secondary growth of a focal cortical contusion deserves special attention in this context. Experiments of our laboratory have confirmed that a tissue necrosis induced by a focal trauma of brain cortex is expanding during the subsequent 24 hrs [3]. Predominent direction of this expansion is towards the corpus callosum. As it is unclear yet, whether the phenomenon is part of the primary traumatic brain injury – albeit evolving with delay – or a manifestation of secondary brain damage, experiments are required to analyse the pathophysiology of this intriguing process. Excitotoxic amino acids are important mediator compounds of neuronal damage in various pathological conditions such as cerebral ischemia and trauma [1, 2, 7–9]. Objective of the subsequent study was, therefore, to assess the release of glutamate and aspartate in the grey matter underneath a focal traumatic lesion, i.e. in the area of secondary expansion of the necrosis.

Material and Methods

Male Sprague-Dawley rats (n = 5) of 230 to 390 g body weight (b.w.) were anaesthetized with chloralhydrate (360 mg/100 g b.w.) and mounted on a stereotaxic frame. Two burr holes were drilled in the right parietal bone using stereotactic coordinates. The first trephination (3 mm lateral and caudal to bregma) was to expose the intact dura for induction of the trauma. Through the second burr hole (2.5 mm caudal from the centre of the first) a microdialysis probe (CMA 11, o.d. 0.25 mm, membran length 4 mm, Carnegie Medicine, Sweden) was inserted into the right parietal cortex in an angle of 50°, and fixed to the skull with dental cement. Thereafter, the scalp was sutured and the animals were allowed to regain consciousness. 24 hrs later the animals were intubated and mechanically ventilated using 0.8% halothane and an O_2/N_2O mixture. The body temperature was kept constant at 37.5°C by means of a feedback controlled heating pad. Systemic blood pressure, blood gases, and body temperature were monitored. The microdialysis probe was connected to a microinjection pump (Carnegie Medicine, Sweden) and perfused with Krebs buffer (NaCl: 122 mM, KCl: 3.0 mM, $CaCl_2$: 1.8 mM, $NaHCO_3$: 25 mM, KH_2PO_4: 0.4 mM, $MgSO_4$: 1.2 mM) adjusted to pH 7.4 at a flow rate of 2 μl/min. After a 30-min-equilibration period samples were collected in 10-min-intervals for 1 h to acquire baseline values under control conditions prior to trauma. Subsequently, a highly standardized cortical lesion was induced by focal freezing of the brain surface by attachment of a copper cylinder (–68°C) 2.5 mm rostral to the insertion coordinates of the microdialysis probe. Thereby, the tip of the microdialysis probe localized in the depth of parietal cortex was in close vicinity to the cold-induced primary lesion. Dialysis was continued until termination of the experiment with sacrifice of the animals and removal of the brain. The predetermined position of the dialysis probe adjacent to the primary lesion was confirmed by histological control. Quantitative analysis of the level of amino acids in dialysate samples was carried out by employment of HPLC with fluorescence detection using a modified method by Lindroth and Mopper [5].

Results

The concentration of the excitatory neurotransmitters aspartate and glutamate in the dialysate, obtained from the interstitial space of parietal cortex, was 0.48 ± 0.21 and 1.38 ± 0.64 μM, respectively, under baseline conditions (Table 1). The focal trauma led to a 5.4-fold increase of the aspartate concentration, i.e. to 2.57 ± 1.15 μM, and a 4.6-fold increase of the glutamate concentration, i.e. to 6.31 ± 2.82 μM. The increase versus control is statistically significant ($p < 0.05$). Following the initial sharp elevation of glutamate and aspartate in the dialysis fluid immediately after trauma the concentrations of these transmitters returned back to baseline. The time course of the changes of the glycine and serine concentration in this fluid was quite similar. The concentrations of both amino acids were found to increase by 3.5 times in the first fraction sampled after induction of the cold lesion. On the other side, the alanine concentration of alanine was not markedly affected throughout the experimental observation period.

Discussion

As seen, a focal trauma of brain cortex induces marked and prompt release of excitatory amino acids in the adjacent viable tissue. In addition, glycine which is known to enhance the excitatory effect of glutamate at the NMDA-receptor, and serine, a precursor of the glutamateand glycine-biosynthesis, were also significantly increased, although not as pronounced as glutamate. On the other side, the level of alanine was not affected throughout the total experimental observation period, indicating that the traumatic release of the excitatory amino acids might be viewed as a specific response.

Due to the high level of standardization and reproducibility of the cold lesion model in producing a circumscribed area of necrosis, it was possible to measure changes of the extracellular amino acid composition in the penumbra directly underneath the primary lesion, i.e. in tissue, which may secondarily perish [3]. In contrast to mechanical brain trauma models [4, 6, 7] it is not necessary to remove the microdialysis probe prior to trauma followed by reinsertion thereafter. Accordingly, the present experiment is advantagous as additional tissue trauma caused by reinsertion of the probe e.g. off the original track is avoided, as for example reported by Palmer *et al.* using a standardized controlled cortical impact model [7]. Moreover, to the best of our knowledge, cold injury of the brain is the

Table 1. *Effect of Focal Cortical Lesion on the Amino Acid Concentration in the Tissue Underneath the Primary Necrosis (Given as Dialysate Concentration)*

Sampling start [min]	Asp [μM]	Glu [μM]	Gly [μM]	Ser [μM]	Ala [μM]
Baseline	0.48 ± 0.21	1.38 ± 0.64	1.21 ± 0.56	1.76 ± 0.82	1.64 ± 0.77
0	2.57 ± 1.15[a]	6.31 ± 2.82[a]	4.19 ± 1.88[a]	6.10 ± 2.73[a]	2.36 ± 1.05
10	0.62 ± 0.28	2.78 ± 1.24	1.62 ± 0.73	2.68 ± 1.20	1.46 ± 0.65
20	0.46 ± 0.23	3.48 ± 1.56	1.79 ± 0.80	3.91 ± 1.75	1.62 ± 0.73
30	0.73 ± 0.33	2.73 ± 1.22	2.71 ± 1.21	2.26 ± 1.01	2.15 ± 0.96
40	0.81 ± 0.36	2.68 ± 1.20	2.04 ± 0.91	2.53 ± 1.13	2.17 ± 0.97
50	0.98 ± 0.44	2.73 ± 1.22	2.42 ± 1.08	3.68 ± 1.84	1.77 ± 0.79
60	0.62 ± 0.28	2.64 ± 1.18	3.64 ± 1.82	4.35 ± 2.17	2.00 ± 0.89
70	0.58 ± 0.29	2.21 ± 1.10	1.78 ± 0.89	1.85 ± 0.93	2.04 ± 1.02
80	0.53 ± 0.24	2.34 ± 1.05	2.42 ± 1.08	2.86 ± 1.28	1.57 ± 0.70
90	0.40 ± 0.20	2.24 ± 0.10	2.67 ± 1.20	2.89 ± 1.29	2.04 ± 0.91
100	0.49 ± 0.22	2.15 ± 0.96	2.66 ± 1.33	2.71 ± 1.21	2.00 ± 1.00
110	0.33 ± 0.15	1.96 ± 0.88	1.63 ± 0.73	2.56 ± 1.15	2.23 ± 1.00
120	0.55 ± 0.39	0.78 ± 0.55	0.89 ± 0.63	0.84 ± 0.59	2.94 ± 2.08

[a] Statistically significant difference compared to basal values according to Wilcoxon paired rank sum test at $p < 0.05$.

only currently available model, which is inducing a lesion reproducible enough to measure the time course of the expansion of the tissue necrosis.

In summary, the increase of the release of excitatory amino acids into the interstitial space of perifocal brain tissue in response to trauma indicates a possible role of these substances in the secondary growth of the resulting brain tissue necrosis. Currently conducted administration of specific antagonists can be expected to provide further evidence on whether the posttraumatic extracellular accumulation of excitotoxic amino acids plays a role in the secondary brain lesion expansion. Moreover, respective findings would have clinical significance for the improvement of the therapeutical specificity and effectivity of rescuing brain tissue from secondary extinction.

Acknowledgment

Supported by BMBF-Verbund "Neurotrauma" München, FKZ: 01 KO 94026.

References

1. Benveniste H, Drejer J, Schousboe A (1984) Elevation of the extracellular concentrations of glutamate and aspartate in rat hippocampus during transient cerebral ischemia monitored by intracerebral microdialysis. J Neurochem 43: 1369–1374
2. Choi DW (1990) Methods for antagonizing glutamate neurotoxicity. Cerebrovasc Brain Metab Rev 2: 105–147
3. Eriskat J, Schurer L, Kempski O, Baethmann A (1994) Growth kinetics of a primary brain tissue necrosis from a focal lesion. Acta Neurochir (Wien) [Suppl] 60: 425–427
4. Katayama Y, Becker DP, Tamura T, Hovda DA (1990) Massive increases in extracellular potassium and the indiscriminate release of glutamate following concussive brain injury. J Neurosurg 73: 889–900
5. Lindroth P, Mopper K (1979) High performance liquid chromatographic determination of subpicomole amounts of amino acids by precolumn fluorescence derivatization with ophthaldialdehyde. Anal Chem 51 (11): 1667–1674 (Abstract)
6. Nilsson P, Hillered L, Ponten U, Ungerstedt U (1990) Changes in cortical extracellular levels of energy-related metabolites and amino acids following concussive brain injury in rats. J Cereb Blood Flow Metab 10: 631–637
7. Palmer AM, Marion DW, Botscheller ML, Swedlow PE, Styren SD, DeKosky ST (1993) Traumatic brain injury-induced excitotoxicity assessed in a controlled cortical impact model. J Neurochem 61: 2015–2024
8. Smith SE, Meldrum BS (1995) Cerebroprotective effect of lamotrigine after focal ischemia in rats. Stroke 26:117–122
9. Xue D, Huang ZG, Barnes K, Lesiuk HJ, Smith KE, Buchan AM (1994) Delayed treatment with AMPA, but not NMDA, antagonists reduces neocortical infarction. J Cereb Blood Flow Metab 14: 251–261

Correspondence: Alexander Baethmann, M.D., Ph.D., Institute for Surgical Research, Klinikum Grosshadern, Marchioninistrasse 15, D-81366 München, Federal Republic of Germany.

Acta Neurochir (1997) [Suppl] 70: 94–95
© Springer-Verlag 1997

Assessment of Regional Cortical Blood Flow Following Traumatic Lesion of the Brain

J. Eriskat, N. Plesnila, M. Stoffel, and **A. Baethmann**

Institute for Surgical Research, Klinikum Grosshadern, Ludwig-Maximilians-University, Munich, Federal Republic of Germany

Summary

A brain tissue necrosis from trauma gradually expands during the subsequent 24 h. Among others, deterioration of perifocal blood flow could be involved in the secondary extinction of initially viable brain tissue. A highly standardized freezing lesion was made in cerebral cortex of rats for frequent measurements of regional cortical blood flow with high spatial resolution by laser Doppler scanning flowmetry. Following trauma a profound decrease in cerebral blood flow was found, not only in the lesion proper but also in the perifocal and distant brain areas, which would support a role of ischemia in the secondary lesion growth. Further studies, however, are required, particularly on whether therapeutic improvement of perifocal flow is affecting expansion of the traumatic tissue necrosis.

Keywords: Brain injury; cortical blood flow; laser Doppler method; experimental model.

Introduction

A brain tissue necrosis from focal trauma gradually expands during the subsequent 24 h [2]. Depending on the model and species utilized, increases of the resulting cerebral necrosis within 24 h were amounting to 150% in rats [6, 10] or even 300% in rabbits [11]. A deterioration of perifocal blood flow leading to ischemia could be involved in the secondary extinction of initially viable brain tissue. For testing this hypothesis, a highly standardized freezing lesion was induced in cerebral cortex of rats resulting in histopathologically distinct areas: (a) primary lesion of irreversibly injured parenchyma, (b) perifocal tissue with progressive necrosis (penumbra), and (c) distant tissue without morphological alterations. The model was utilized for frequent measurements of regional aortical blood flow (rCBF) with high spatial resolution by employment of laser Doppler flowmetry [8]. Accordingly, the exposed brain surface was subjected to scanning by the laser Doppler flow probe utilizing a computerized guidance system.

Materials and Methods

Male Sprague-Dawley rats (250–300 g b.w.) were anesthetized with a mixture of 0.8% Halothane, 30% O_2 and 70% N_2O, intubated and mechanically ventilated. After fixation of the skull in a stereotactic frame a 4 mm × 9 mm rectangular trephination over the right parietal cortex was made with a dental drill under continuous cooling without damaging the underlying dura or brain. A catheter was inserted into the tail artery for continuous monitoring of blood pressure and drawing of blood samples for measurement of arterial blood gases. Body temperature was monitored and maintained between 37.0°C and 37.5°C by a servo controlled heating pad. rCBF was assessed by laser Doppler scanning flowmetry according to KEMPSKI over the right parietal cortex at 60 different points. The points were arranged as a 6 × 10 matrix forming a rectangular area of 2.5 × 4.5 mm² above, adjacent to, and distant from the lesion. The needle probe of the laser Doppler monitor (Perimed 4001 Master) was attached to a computer controlled micromanipulator (Wagner Instrumentenbau KG, Schöffenbach Germany), allowing to move its tip in all three dimensions at an accoracy of only few micrometers. The distance between the dura mater and the LD probe was minimized under the operating microscope without touching the underlying dura. A measuring period for each point was 4 seconds. To avoid movement artifacts of the LD probe, a delay of one second was allowed before each measurement. A fast analog-to-digital conversion board permitted sampling of flow data with a ruuning average of 4 s, i.e. over approximately 6 breathing cycles. Therefore, duration of one complete sweep over the matrix was 5 minutes. Three different regions of interest were distinguished, namely the area of necrosis and the perifocal and remote brain surface according to their distance from the center of the lesion. A computer program was developed for continuous data acquisition, positioning of the LD probe by the micromanipulator, and display of physiologic variables. In addition, algorithms were established for drawing of color coded maps of the LD data, calculation of frequency histograms and of the median values.

Results

Prior to injury the flow data obtained from 60 measuring sites at the brain surface had a bimodal histogram distribution. A large peak representing the majority of flow valnes had a range from 350 to 750 LD-units on a scale from 0 to 999, while a smaller peak was approaching the upper limit of the LDF scale. The latter was reflecting large blood vessels which were dominating the LD signal. After induction of the lesion widespread flow depression could be observed. LDF decreased immediately after trauma reaching a minimum of about 50% of the baseline at 20 and 35 min. More than 40% of the LDF values were falling below the lower limit of the LD values observed during the control period, demonstrating the marked increase of "low-flow" areas. The considerable impairment of rCBF after trauma appeared to indiscriminately affect all scanning areas, the focal, perifocal, and remote brain, however, with some recovery of flow in the perifocal and distant brain.

Discussion

The current findings demonstrate that a traumatic focal lesion of the brain is associated with a marked decrease of blood flow in the adjacent brain, however, not only there but also in the remote areas which were studied for up to 60 minutes. It could be shown that systematic scanning of the brain surface by laser Doppler flowmetry is a valuable tool for investigating blood flow disturbances from a focal lesion at a high spatial and temporal resolution. Compared to laser Doppler measurements using a stationary probe, this method provides for a better spatial resolution together with the possibility to establish frequency histograms of the many single flow values. Kempski *et al.* [5] have shown that a minimum of 25 laser Doppler measurements is required to obtain reliable information on the regional cerebral blood flow.

These present experimental observations are in good agreement with findings on CBF alterations studied by different methods in a variety of models of focal brain injury [1, 3, 6, 9, 12, 13]. Yet the mechanisms underlying the widespread depression of rCBF are not fully understood. It is conceivable, however, that vasoactive factors acting at the microvasculature, such as PAF [4], platelet aggregation [1], or release of endothelin [7] are involved. It is concluded that the currently observed blood flow response together with the release of toxic mediator compounds and the development of acidosis are involved in the secondary expansion of a traumatic tissue necrosis into the perifocal brain. Nevertheless, longer observation periods as well as experimental approaches of therapeutically influencing posttraumatic depression of blood flow are necessary to confirm or reject, respectively, whether the development of cerebral ischemia is a major mechanism of secondary lesion growth.

Acknowledgement

Supported by BMBF-Verbund "Neurotrauma" München, FKZ 01 KO 94026.

References

1. Dietrich WD, Alonso O, Busto R, Prado R, Dewanjee S, Dewanjee MK, Ginsberg MD (1996) Widespread hemodynamic depression and focal platelet accumulation after fluid percussion injury: a double-label autoradiographic study in rats. J Cereb Blood Flow Metab 16 (3): 481–489
2. Eriskat J, Schürer L, Kempski O, Baethmann A (1994) Growth kinetics of a primary brain tissue necrosis from a focal lesion. Acta Neurochir (Wien) [Suppl] 60: 425–427
3. Frei HJ, Wallenfang T, Pöll W, Reulen HJ, Schubert R, Brock M (1973) Regional cerebral blood flow and regional metabolism in cold induced oedema. Acta Neurochir (Wien) 29 (1): 15–28
4. Frerichs KU, Lindsberg PJ, Hallenbeck JM, Feuerstein GZ (1990) Platelet-activating factor and progressive brain damage following focal brain injury. J Neurosurg 73: 223–233
5. Kempski O, Heimann A, Strecker U (1995) On the number of measurements necessary to assess regional cerebral blood flow by local laser Doppler recordings: a simulation study with data from 45 rabbits. Int J Microcirc Clin Exp 15 (1): 37–42
6. Lindsberg PJ, Frerichs KU, Burris JA, Hallenbeck JM, Feuerstein G (1991) Cortical microcirculation in a new model of focal laser-induced secondary brain damage. J Cereb Blood Flow Metab 11 (1): 88–98
7. Spatz M, Yasuma Y, Strasser A, McCarron RM (1996) Cerebral postischemic hypoperfusion is mediated by ET-A receptors. Brain Res 726 (1–2): 242–246
8. Ungersböck K, Heimann A, Strecker U, Kempski O (1993) Mapping of cerebral blood flow by laser-Doppler flowmetry. In: Tomita M, Mchedlishvili G, Rosenblum WI, Heiss WO, Fukuuchi Y (eds) Microcirculatory stasis in the brain. Elsevier, Amsterdam, pp 405–413
9. Vinas FC, Dujovny M, Hodgkinson D (1995) Early hemodynamic changes at the microcirculatory level and effects of mannitol following focal cryogenic injury. Neurol Res 17 (6): 465–468
10. Vonhof S (1995) Die zerebrale Proteinbiosynthese nach Schädel-Hirn-Trauma: eine experimentelle Untersuchung zur Quantifizierung der sekundären Hirngewebsnekrose. Inauguraldissertation. Ludwig-Maximilians-Universität, München
11. Wyrwich W (1994) Die Entwicklung einer sekundären Hirngewebsnekrose nach primärem Trauma. Methodische Ansätze ihrer Quantifizierung. Inauguraldissertation. Ludwig-Maximilians-Universität, München
12. Yamakami I, McIntosh TK (1991) Alterations in regional cerebral blood flow following brain injury in the rat. J Cereb Blood Flow Metab 11 (4): 655–660
13. Yamamoto L, Soejima T, Meyer E, Feindel W (1976) Early hemodynamic changes at the microcirculatory level following focal cryogenic injury over the cortex. In: Pappius HM, Feindel W (eds) Dynamics of brain edema. Springer, Berlin Heidelberg New York, pp 59–62

Correspondence: Alexander Baethmann, M.D., Ph.D., Institute for Surgical Research, Klinikum Grosshadern, Marchioninistrasse 15, D-81366 München, Federal Republic of Germany.

Acta Neurochir (1997) [Suppl] 70: 96–97
© Springer-Verlag 1997

Comparison of the Interleukin-6 and Interleukin-10 Response in Children After Severe Traumatic Brain Injury or Septic Shock

M. J. Bell, P. M. Kochanek, L. A. Doughty, J. A. Carcillo, P. D. Adelson, R. S. B. Clark, M. J. Whalen, and S. T. DeKosky

Safar Center for Resuscitation Research, and the Departments of Anesthesiology and Critical Care Medicine, Neurological Surgery, Pediatrics, and Psychiatry, The University of Pittsburgh, and Children's Hospital of Pittsburgh, Pittsburgh, PA, U.S.A.

Summary

Inflammation may play an important role in the evolution of damage after traumatic brain injury (TBI). IL-6 and IL-10 are markers of inflammation that are pro- and anti-inflammatory in nature, respectively. They have been used as an index of the degree of inflammation in diseases including sepsis and meningitis. We hypothesized that both IL-6 and IL-10 would be increased in the cerebrospinal fluid (CSF) of children after TBI. We measured ventricular CSF concentrations of these metabolites (ELISA) each of the first 3 days after TBI in 15 children. CSF IL-6 was increased on day 1 ($p < 0.05$ vs days 2 or 3). CSF IL-10 was similarly increased on day 1 ($p < 0.05$). CSF IL-6 after TBI is similar to serum IL-6 levels previously reported in children with septic shock. In contrast, the CSF IL-10 response was markedly attenuated following TBI compared to sepsis. These data suggest a unique balance between pro- and anti-inflammatory cytokines in brain after TBI.

Keywords: Traumatic brain injury; interleukin response; pediatric; cerebrospinal fluid.

Introduction

Secondary injury after TBI in children is mediated by many mechanisms. Cytokines are inflammatory mediators involved in the injury response. However, cytokines may also upregulate antioxidant defense mechanisms and repair. The balance between pro- and anti-inflammatory cytokines plays an important role in determining outcome in children during inflammatory processes such as septic shock. The nature of the participants in injured brain during the inflammatory response to TBI in children remains to be defined.

IL-6 is a cytokine that has predominantly pro-inflammatory effects outside of the CNS. Plasma levels of IL-6 are strongly correlated with mortality and morbidity in sepsis. Also, CSF levels have been directly correlated with poor outcome in stroke. IL-6, in CNS may also have some neurotrophic properties.

IL-10 is a potent anti-inflammatory cytokine which inhibits macrophage cytokine, oxygen radical, and nitric oxide production. The role of this potent anti-inflammatory cytokine in the CNS, and the relationship between TBI and IL-10 production has not been investigated in children or adults.

We hypothesized that severe TBI in children produces an inflammatory response in brain that includes both pro- and anti-inflammatory cytokines and is detectable in ventricular cerebrospinal fluid (CSF).

Methods

Children (n = 15) with severe TBI (GCS < 8) were studied. All received standard neurointensive care including mild hyperventilation ($PaCO_2$ = 30–35 mmHg), mannitol, and a ventricular catheter. Barbiturates were used as indicated. CSF was drained continuously at 3 cm above the level of the midbrain. Therapy was directed to maintain CPP = 70 mmHg in children and 50 mmHg in infants.

CSF was collected every 24 h for 3 days and immediately centrifuged. IL-6 and IL-10 concentrations were determined in the supernatant by commercially available ELISA (Pharmigen). Repeated-measures ANOVA and Neuman-Keuls test were used to compare CSF cytokine levels over time.

Results

Age ranged from 1 month to 13 years. Seven of the 15 children survived. Mechanism of injury included abuse, bicycle vs motor vehicle, and motor vehicle accident. CSF IL-6 was increased on day 1 ($p < 0.05$ vs days 2 or 3). CSF IL-10 was similarly increased on day 1 ($p < 0.05$).

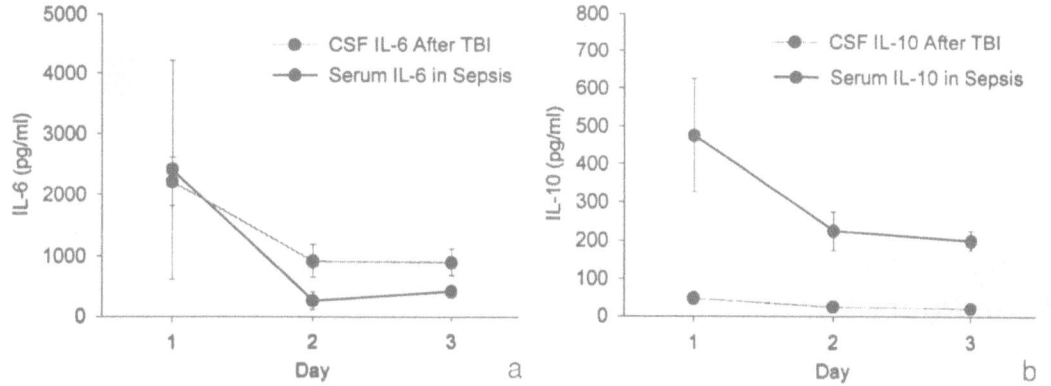

Fig. 1. (a) Comparison of IL-6 levels in ventricular CSF from children with severe TBI with serum from children with septic shock. (b) IL-10 levels in ventricular CSF from children with severe TBI and serum from children with septic shock. The magnitude and time course of the increase in IL-6 in head injury and sepsis are remarkably similar, despite the fact that a non-infectious process (head trauma) is being compared to an infectious process (sepsis) occurring outside of the CNS. In contrast, systemic IL-10 levels during sepsis in children are markedly greater (about 10-fold) than thoso observed in CSF of head injured children

Based on a prior publication by investigators in our group [1], CSF IL-6 in children after TBI was similar both in magnitude and in time course to serum IL-6 in children (n = 53) during septic shock. In contrast, the increase in CSF IL-10 in children after TBI was minimal compared to the increase in serum IL-10 in children during septic shock (Fig. 1).

Discussion

This is a preliminary report representing the first data showing that IL-6 is increased after TBI in children. The increase is marked, peaks on the first day after injury, and similar in magnitude to that observed in adults after TBI [2–4] and similar in magnitude and time course to the increase in serum during septic shock in children. This is also the first report of increased levels of IL-10 in either children or adults after TBI. Although an increase in IL-10 is seen on the first day after TBI in children, the magnitude of this increase is small compared to the large increase seen in serum of children during septic shock [1]. These results suggest the production of a unique cytokine profile in the CNS after TBI, and possibly an imbalance between pro- and anti-inflammatory cytokines.

Whether these results reflect differences in response to divergent inflammatory stimuli (trauma vs infection), an age-related difference in the inflammatory response to TBI, or differences between the inflammatory response inside vs outside of the CNS remains to be determined [5].

References

1. Doughty LA, Kaplan SS, Carcillo JA (1996) Inflammatory cytokine and nitric oxide responses in pediatric sepsis and organ failure. Crit Care Med 24: 1137–1143
2. Kossmann T, Hans VHJ, Imhof H-G, et al (1995) Intrathecal and serum interleukin-6 and the acute-phase response in patients with severe traumatic brain injuries. Shock 4: 311–317
3. Kossman T, Hans VHJ, Lenzlinger PM, et al (1995) Analysis of immune mediator production following traumatic brain injury. Proceedings of the 5th Wiggers Bernard Conference. Vienna, Austria
4. McClain C, Cohen D, Phillips R, et al (1991) Increased plasma and ventricular fluid interleukin-6 levels in patients with head injury. J Clin Lab Med 118: 226–231
5. Rothwell NJ, Luheshi G, Toulmond S (1996) Cytokines and their receptors in the central nervous system: physiology, pharmacology, and pathology. Pharmacol Ther 69: 85–95

Correspondence: Patrick M. Kochanek, M.D., Safar Center for Resuscitation Research, University of Pittsburgh, 3434 Fifth Ave., Pittsburg, PA 15260, U.S.A.

Acta Neurochir (1997) [Suppl] 70: 98–101
© Springer-Verlag 1997

Changes of MPO Activity and Brain Water Accumulation in Traumatic Brain Injury Experiments

B. J. Darakchiev, M. Itkis, T. Agajanova, A. Itkis, and **R. J. Hariri**

Center for Trauma Research, Division of Neurosurgery, Department of Surgery, The New York Hospital and Cornell University Medical College, New York, NY, U.S.A.

Summary

Comparison of brain tissue water content (BWC) data with myeloperoxidase activity assay (MPO) allows for analysis of the complex pathophysiological mechanisms of cerebral edema following catastrophic brain injuries. The neuroprotective effect of an experimental anti inflammatory drug (FL1003, butyrolactone) was tested in a traumatic brain injury (TBI) model using BWC and MPO analysis.

We conducted these studies on a mini-pig model of severe TBI that is well characterized in our laboratory. The animals were divided into three animal groups: no injury, no treatment (control), injured and treated with FL1003, and injured, untreated with FL1003. They were maintained with fluids for 24 hours under general anesthesia. We employed the MPO assay to identify the degree of inflammatory cellular response (polymorphonuclear leukocytes, PMNLs) 24 hours following TBI and calculated brain density from the data of the gravimetric (Percoll) column method for BWC on brain samples. Our results demonstrated increased infiltration of PMNLs and a shift of water into the extravascular space in the injured animals. These changes were significantly ($P < 0.05$) attenuated in the animal group treated with FL1003.

Keywords: Traumatic brain injury; myeloperoxidase; brain water accumulation; mini-pig model.

Introduction

Cerebrovascular dysfunction has been observed following almost any kind of injury to the brain, whether ischemic, traumatic, or otherwise. One of its main hallmarks is the loss of endothelial cell integrity resulting in extravasation of fluid and solute into the interstitium [21]. Although the precise mechanism responsible for the increased permeability remains unclear, there is an increasing accumulation of data implicating inflammatory events mediating the opening of endothelial tight junctional complexes.

The role of polymorphonuclear leukocytes (PMNLs) in this cascade of events has been an issue of long standing contradiction and controversy [4, 14]. The contemporary interpretation of the leukocytic contribution to the endothelial dysfunction in brain trauma and ischemia has changed considerably with the understanding of the mechanisms of their adhesion and migration [25, 26]. Previous work demonstrated perivascular accumulation of inflammatory cells, specifically PMNLs and monocytes, following cerebral ischemia and stroke [10, 14].

Myeloperoxidase is a reliable marker enzyme for polymorphonuclear leukocytes and is found within their azurophilic granules. The MPO assay has been demonstrated to be a reproducible and objective method for quantifying PMNL accumulation in myocardial infarction [1, 23, 24], skin inflammation [5, 6], lung infection [9], and intestinal inflammation [15]. Barone *et al.* [2] modified the MPO assay for use in brain tissue. Since then, this technique has been employed to quantify neutrophil accumulation in the brain in the setting of ischemic and traumatic brain injuries and the dynamics of these injuries [3, 4, 7, 20].

We have recently shown that following mechanical brain injury, up-regulation of leukocyte-endothelial cell adhesion occurs, which promotes margination and ultimately diapedesis of neutrophils in the extravascular space [11–13]. We hypothesize that, following TBI, production of eicosanoid and cytokine pro-inflammatory mediators by astrocytes and PMNLs mediates the dysregulation of the endothelial cell-maintained semiselective permeability of the cerebral microvasculature by purely inflammatory mechanisms. Therefore, anti inflammatory pharmacotherapy may beneficial in the treatment of post-traumatic cerebrovascular dysfunction. Recently a butyrolactone derivative of ascorbic acid (FL1003, provided by Forest Laboratories, New

York, NY) has been synthesized and shown to inhibit the production of various inflammatory mediators *in vitro*.

We performed this study using the TBI model on mini pigs to show the increased accumulation of PMNLs in the cerebral parenchyma 24 hours following traumatic brain injury, demonstrate any correlation between increased leukocyte infiltration and brain water content in the injured brain, and test the beneficial neuroprotective action of the novel anti inflammatory drug (FL1003) on leukocyte extravasation and eventually on endothelial cell permeability. We used a modified MPO assay for brain tissue by Barone *et al.* [2] as a tool for quantifying the degree ot leukocyte infiltration, and gravimetric (Percoll) column for brain water accumulation as an index of developing brain edema.

Materials and Methods

Our studies were performed on eighteen female miniature, sexually mature Yucatan swine (Charles River Laboratories, Wilmington, Mass). Experiments were conducted in accordance with the Animal Welfare Act and approved by the Institutional Animal Care and Use Committee of Cornell University Medical College. Animals were premedicated with ketamine and xylazine, weighted, anesthetized with isoflurane by mask and intubated. They were ventilated to maintain normal arterial blood gas (ABG) levels. The left femoral artery and vein, and central vein (int. jugular v.) were cannulated for the monitoring of various physiologic pressures and access for ABG sampling. Biventricular cannulation was then performed for intracranial pressure (ICP) monitoring and cerebrospinal fluid (CSF) access. Animals were kept normothermic with a heating lamp and euvolemic with intravenous (i.v.) Lactated Ringer's solution to maintain central venous pressure (CVP) between 2 and 5 mmHg. A cystotomy was performed for urine output monitoring, and urine output was maintained at ≥ 0.5 ml/kg/hour. Animals were allowed to equilibrate for a 30-minute period before experimental injury. In fifteen animals TBI was produced by 2.5 atm barotrauma via right frontal injury screw using the fluid wave percussion method described by Sullivan *et al.* [27]. These animals were followed for a 24-hour period post-injury and sacrificed by anesthetic overdose. Brains were removed immediately at the end of the experiment; samples were taken from each lobe and placed in hermetic containers to prevent evaporation, frozen in liquid nitrogen, and stored at –80°C for further analysis.

Experimental Groups

Group I (n = 10): sham cootrol;
Group II (n = 8): TBI and FL1003, 100 mg/kg i.v. bolus 1 hour following injury;
Group III (n = 7): TBI alone.

Myeloperoxidase Activity Assay (MPO)

We utilized the modified myeloperoxidase activity assay [2] to identify the infiltration of polymorphonuclear leukocytes (PMNLs) into brain parenchyma following traumatic injury.

First, we obtained 6 mm, 0.5–1.0 g coronal sections from each cerebral lobe sample. Each specimen was homogenized in 8 ml of 50 mM potassium phosphate buffer (pH 6.0) and centrifuged at 2500 g for 10 min, then similarly recentrifuged. The supernatant was discarded and brain tissue pellets were resuspended in 2.5 ml hexadecyltrimethylammonium bromide (HTAB, 0.5% HTAB in 50 mM potassium phosphate buffer). Three rapid freeze-thaw cycles were performed before final centrifugation at 2500 g for 10 min. Finally, 100 ml of the supernatant was added to 2.5 ml of 50 mM potassium-phosphate buffer with 0-diasinidine hydrochloride (0.167 mg/ml) and H_2O_2 (0.0005%). Changes in absorbance were spectrophotometrically determined as a mean of three readings (every 2 min) at 460 nm (Spectronic, Milton Roy Cornpany). One unit of MPO activity is equal to the amount that degrades 1 mmol of H_2O_2/min at 25°C.

Brain Water Content Determination

Brain water content was studied on brain samples taken from the same regions as those used in the MPO measurements. We used brain density as an indicator for brain water accumulation. Brain density was determined using a specific gravity bromobensine-kerosine column [17, 18]. The calibration of these columns was done by means of specifically precalibrated glass beads with the following densitiy: 1.0202, 1.0302, 1.0400, 1.0425, 1.0450, 1.0475 and 1.0497 g/cm³, respectively. Each column was used only if the linearity was sufficient (i.e., the minimal correlation coefficient was not less than r = 0.97, and resolution of the column was not less than 2.5e–04. g/cm³). The brain density data was measured by the depth of brain samples after 1 min in the column.

Statistical Analysis

All the registered data was stored in worksheets and processed statistically using Microsoft Excel software. Regression analysis and ANOVA tests were processed by means of SPSS 6.0. All data are expressed as a mean ± SD. Differences were considered statistically significant if $P < 0.05$.

Results

Figures 1 and 2 depict the MPO and brain density data. Letters A, B and C represent the three groups of animals: Group I: sham control (no injury, no drug), Group II: TBI and FL1003 (injury, drug treated animals), and Group III: TBI alone (injury, no drug) in both figures respectively. Figure 2 was obtained by means of an imaging program developed by our research group using Visual Basic for Microsoft Excel 5.0. This program allowed for the interactive development of 56 color gradations and minimal and maximal values of analyzing parameters, while maintaining separate brain images for cortex and white matter. The bar graph below the image demonstrates average BWC values of the different brain regions with their standard deviations.

Twenty-four hours after the injury, MPO activity was most increased in the injured, non-treated Group III (0.12 U/g) with minimal change in the controls (Group I, 0.0035 U/g). The MPO values in Group II

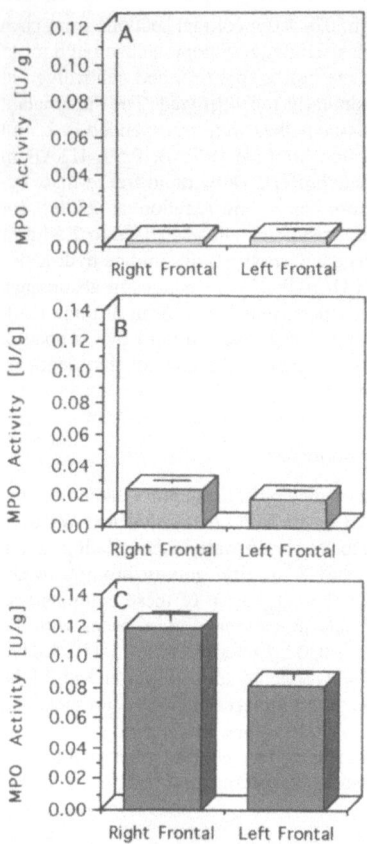

Fig. 1. MPO activity assay – MPO changes 24 hours post-TBI in the three groups of animals (see explanation in text)

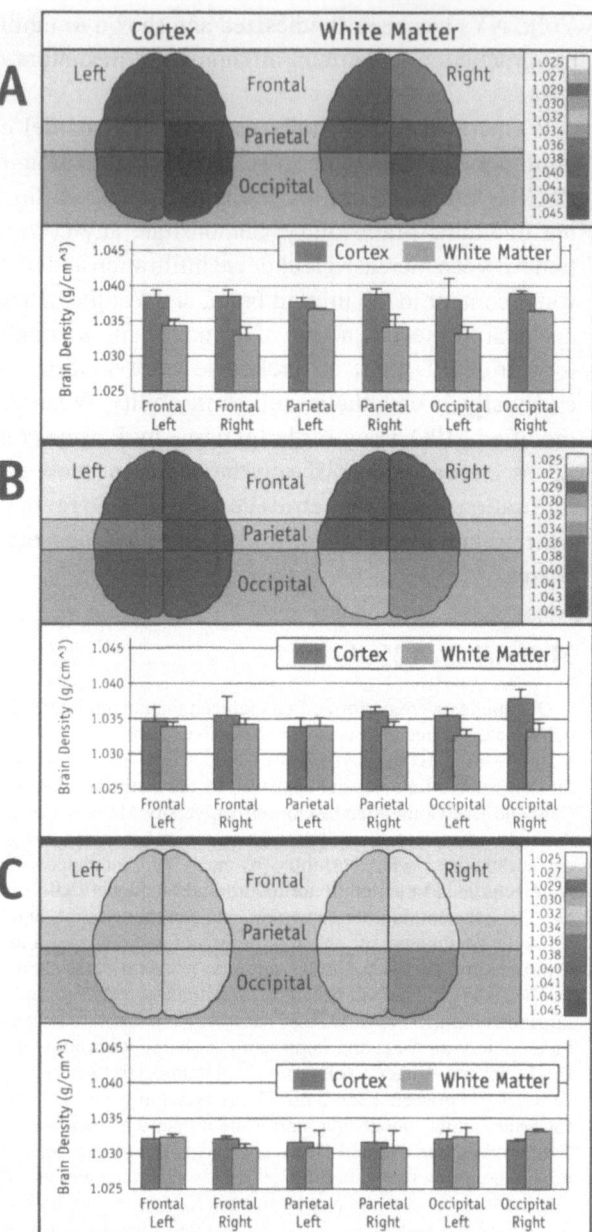

Fig. 2. Brain density changes depicted as gray gradations where cortex and white matter are presented separately in the different brain regions (see the text)

(injured and treated with FL1003) also increased (0.024 U/g), but less than in Group III (the injured, non-treated group). These values represent the MPO activity in the right frontal lobe where the injury was delivered. The MPO assay on samples from the other brain regions closely followed the results of the right frontal lobe, with slightly decreased values (see Fig. 1).

Brain density results demonstrated a good correlation with MPO activity: brain water accumulation was highest in the injured, untreated group, lower in the injured, treated group, and minimal in the controls (see Fig. 2). Our data showed that brain density was more increased in the cortex than in the white matter; we found this to be consistent with the majority of TBI experiments. The average difference between densities of gray and white matter in the same region was 0.00394053 ± 0.00129 ($P = 0.0006$). Unlike the MPO data however, brain density did not correlate well with the site of the impact (right frontal lobe). In the controls BWC was almost evenly distributed, whereas in the injured, treated group and injured, non-treated group the values were lowest for the left parietal lobe and right frontal lobe, respectively.

Discussion

The focus of this study was not on the mechanisms and location of PMNLs but to demonstrate their accumulation and correlation with brain edema development following traumatic brain injury. Our results are in accord with the previously performed studies by Biagas *et al.* [4], Barone *et al.* [2, 3], and Clark [7]. We observed a five-fold increase in MPO activity and 0.9 fold decrease in brain density 24 hours after TBI. This suggests that the defect in the endothelial permeability is related, if not entirely dependent on, the sequestration and accumulation of PMNLs in the brain parenchyma post-traumatically. The changes in the parameters of interest were expressed most at the site of the injury. Our data showed cellular response was more localized, whereas water accumulation was more evenly distributed, in the different brain regions.

Another goal of the study was to test new therapeutic modalities in the treatment of catastrophic brain injuries. The novel anti-inflammatory drug FL1003 (γ-butyrolactone) showed a beneficial effect on the trauma-induced cellular infiltration and the shift of water from the vascular space. In the treated group it caused a significant decrease ($P < 0.05$) of the MPO level (0.02 U/g) and moderately affected the brain density (1.035 g/cm^3). However, as is evident from Fig. 2, the increase in brain density in the treated group was not as pronounced as the attenuation of MPO. This could be explained by a more complex mechanism participating in the "vascular leak" than merely inflammatory cell and cell products' enhanced process. We have shown previously [16] that γ-butyrolactone can positively influence the clinical consequences of TBI (cerebrovascular permeability, vasomotor dysfunction). This neuroprotective effect has been confirmed in our recent studies [8], including this one. Thus, based on the current understanding of the pathophysiology of TBI, the anti inflammatory action of FL1003 may prove to be therapeutically beneficial in the treatment of severe head injury.

References

1. Allan G, Bhattacherjee P, Brook CD, et al (1985) Myeloperoxidase activity as a quantitative marker of polymorphonuclear leukocyte accumulation into an experimental myocardial infarct – the effect of ibuprofen on infarct size and polymorphonuclear leukocyte accumulation. J Cardiovasc Pharmacol 7: 1151–1160

2. Barone FC, Hillegass LM, Price WJ, et al (1991) Polymorphonuclear leukocyte infiltration into cerebral focal ischemic tissue: myoloperoxidase activity assay and histologic verification. J Neurosci Res 29: 336–345

3. Barone FC, Hillegass LM, Tzimas MN, et al (1995) Time-related changes in myeloperoxidase activity and leukotriene B$_4$ receptor binding reflect leukocyte influx in cerebral focal stroke. Mol Chem Neuropathol 24: 13–30

4. Biagas KV, Uhl MW, Schiding JK, et al (1992) Assessment of posttraumatic polymorphonuclear leukocyte accumulation in rat brain using tissue myeloperoxidase assay and vinblastine treatment. J Neurotrauma 9: 363–371

5. Bradley PP, Priebat DA, Christensen RD, et al (1982) Measurement of cutaneous inflammation: estimation of neutrophil content with an enzyme marker. J Invest Dermatol 78: 206–209

6. Change J, Carlson RP, O'Neil-Davis L, et al (1986) Correlation between mouse skin inflammation induced by arachidonic acid and eicosanoid synthesis. Inflammation 10: 205–214

7. Clark RSB, Schiding JK, Kaczarowski SL, et al (1994) Neutrophil accumulation after traumatic brain injury in rats: comparison of weight drop and controlled cortical impact models. J Neurotrauma 11: 499–506

8. Cohen SM, Hariri RJ, Darakchiev BJ, Barie P (1996) Changes in systemic vascular permeability and intravascular volume requirements following traumatic brain injury (TBI). Surgical Forum Proceedings

9. Goldblum SE, Kuli-Meng W, Jay M (1985) Lung myeloperoxidase as a measure of pulmonary leukostasis in rabbits. J Appl Physiol 59: 1978–1985

10. Hallenbeck JM, Dutka AJ, Tanishima T, et al (1986) Polymorphonuclear leukocyte accumulation in brain regions with low blood flow during the early postischemic period. Stroke 17: 246–253

11. Hariri RJ, Ghajar JBG, Pomerantz K, et al (1989) Human glial cell production of lipoxigenase-generated eicosanoids: a potential role in the pathophysiology of vascular changes following traumatic brain injury. Trauma 29: 1203–1210

12. Hariri RJ, Chang VA, Barie PS, et al (1994) Traumatic injury induces interleukin-6 production by human astrocytes. Brain Res 636: 139–141

13. Hariri RJ (1994) Cerebral edema. Neurosurg Intensive Care 5: 687–706

14. Kochanek PM, Hallenbeck JM (1992) Polymorphonuclear leukocytes and monocytes/macrophages in the pathogenesis of cerebral ischemia and stroke. Stroke 23: 1367–1379

15. Krawisz JE, Sharon P, Stenson WF (1984) Quantitative assay for acute intestinal inflammation based on myeloperoxidase activity. Gastroenterology 87: 1344–1350

16. Lavyne MH, Hariri RJ, Tankosic T, et al (1983) Effect of low dose γ-butyrolactone therapy on forebrain neuronal ischemia in the unrestrained, awake rat. Neurosurgery 12: 430–434

17. Marmarou A, Poll W, Shulman K, et al (1978) A simple gravimetric technique for measurement of cerebral edema. J Neurosurg 49: 530–537

18. Marmarou A, Tanaka K, Shulman K (1982) An improved gravimetric measure of cerebral edema. J Neurosurg 56: 246–253

19. Maruo N, Morita I, Shirao M, et al (1992) IL-6 increases endothelial permeability in vitro. Endocrinology 131: 710–714

20. Matsuo Y, Onodera H, Shiga Y, et al (1994) Correlation between myeloperoxidase-quantified neutrophil accumulation and ischemic brain injury in the rat. Effects of neutrophil depletion. Stroke 25: 1469–1475

21. Miller JD (1993) Traumatic brain swelling and edema. In: Copper PR (ed) Head injury. Williams and Wilkins, Baltimore, pp 331–353

22. Montesano R, Orci L, Vassalli P (1985) Human endothelial cell cultures: phenotypic modulation by leukocyte interleukins. J Cell Physiol 122: 424–434

23. Mullane KM, Kraemer R, Smith B (1985) Myeloperoxidase as a quantitative assessment of neutrophil infiltration into ischemic myocardium. J Pharmacol Methods 14: 157–167

24. Smith EF III, Egan JW, Bugelski PJ, et al (1988) Temporal relation between neutrophil accumulation and myocardial reperfusion injury. Am J Physiol 255: H1060–H1068

25. Springer TA (1990) Adhesion receptors of the immune system. Nature 346: 425–434

26. Springer TA, Lasky LA (1991) Sticky sugars for selectins. Nature 349: 196–197

27. Sullivan HG, Martinez J, Becker DP, et al (1976) Fluid percussion model of mechanical brain injury in the cat. J Neurosurg 45: 520

Correspondence: Borimir J. Darakchiev, M.D., 436 East 69th Street, Apt. 2-K, New York, NY 10021, U.S.A.

Acta Neurochir (1997) [Suppl] 70: 102–105
© Springer-Verlag 1997

Hemodynamic Depression and Microthrombosis in the Peripheral Areas of Cortical Contusion in the Rat: Role of Platelet Activating Factor

T. Maeda, Y. Katayama, T. Kawamata, N. Aoyama, and **T. Mori**

Department of Neurological Surgery, Nihon University School of Medicine, Tokyo, Japan

Summary

Cerebrovascular damages leading to subsequent reductions in regional cerebral blood flow (rCBF) may play an important role in secondary cell damages following traumatic brain injury (TBI). Recent studies have demonstrated that rCBF markedly decrease in experimental model of TBI (e.g. fluid percussion injury, acute subdural hematoma, contusion). However, precise mechanisms underlying post-traumatic CBF reduction remain unclear. In the present study, the rCBF changes and microthrombosis formation were investigated in a cortical contusional model in rats, and the effects of etizolam (platelet activating factor antagonist) on microthrombosis were tested. The rCBF in the peripheral areas increased transiently, and decreased to ischemic level 3 hours post- injury. The histological examinations revealed microthrombosis formation in the contused area, extending from the center to the peripheral areas within 6 hours post-injury. The rCBF decrease and the contusion necrosis volume were significantly attenuated by etizolam administration. These results indicate that platelet activating factor is involved in microtorombosis formation and hemodynamic depression, and resultant ischemic damages within areas surrounding the contusion.

Keywords: Platelet activating factor; cerebral contusion; cerebral blood flow.

Introduction

In cerebral contusion, various kinds of secondary neural tissue damage are progressively produced in the peripheral areas surrounding the primary site of contusion [7, 10–12, 14]. Previous studies have indicated that cerebral blood flow (CBF) is impaired within a wide area surrounding the contusion, and such CBF impairment may play a vital role in the development of secondary tissue damage following the injury [1, 3–5, 9]. The precise mechanisms underlying the contusion-induced CBF impairment, however, remain unclear.

Platelet activating factor (PAF) is involved in the pathophysiology of central nervous system disorders.

Brain injury induces endothelial damage and release of PAF from the injured tissues as well as towards the endothelial cells, which in turn induces further endothelial damage. PAF has a variety of cytotoxic properties, causing vasoconstriction, blood-brain barrier (BBB) disruption, neutrophils adhesion and thrombosis formation [8, 9, 13]. Release of PAF, following the trauma may thus be involved in the reduction of CBF, so that and secondary cell damage becomes more exaggerated following cortical contusion. In the present study, we investigated the rCBF changes and consequent secondary tissue damage employing a cortical contusion model in rats, and the effects of the PAF antagonist, etizolam, were tested.

Material and Methods

Male Wistar rats were anesthetized by 1% halothane inhalation. Cerebral contusion was produced in the parietal cortex using a controlled cortical impact device (diameter of injury tip = 5 mm, velocity = 6 m/sec, penetration depth = 3 mm) [6]. Before and after the injury induction, the rCBF levels in the central area and peripheral area (3 mm distant from the center) of the contusion were monitored continuously using laser-Doppler flowmetry. Following injury induction, the animals were kept alive for 1, 6, and 24 hours, and were then killed by *in vivo* perfusion fixation under deep anesthesia. Coronal sections were cut at a thickness of 10 μm and stained with hematoxylin and eosin (HE). The histology was evaluated under a light microscope.

In another group of animals, the PAF antagonist, etizolam (4 mg/kg), was administered trans-orally immediately following the injury induction [15]. Twenty-four hours later, the size of the contusional necrosis was estimated on coronal sections by 2,3,5-triphenyl tetrazolium chloride (TTC) staining.

Results

At 1 hour after the injury induction, a number of sites with microthrombosis formation were already evident

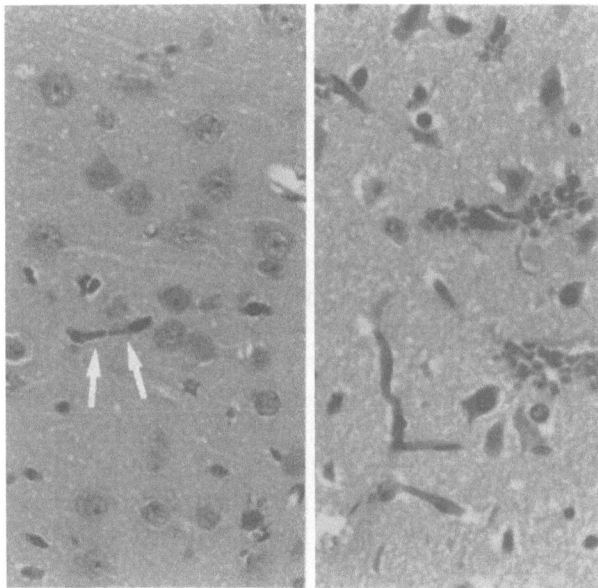

Fig. 1. Photomicrograph of the peri-contusion area 3 mm distant from the contusion, at 6 hours post-trauma (left). A number of sites with microthrombosis (arrow) have began to appear. At 24 hours post-trauma (right), edema formation was also noted in the peri-contusion areas (HE stain, × 250)

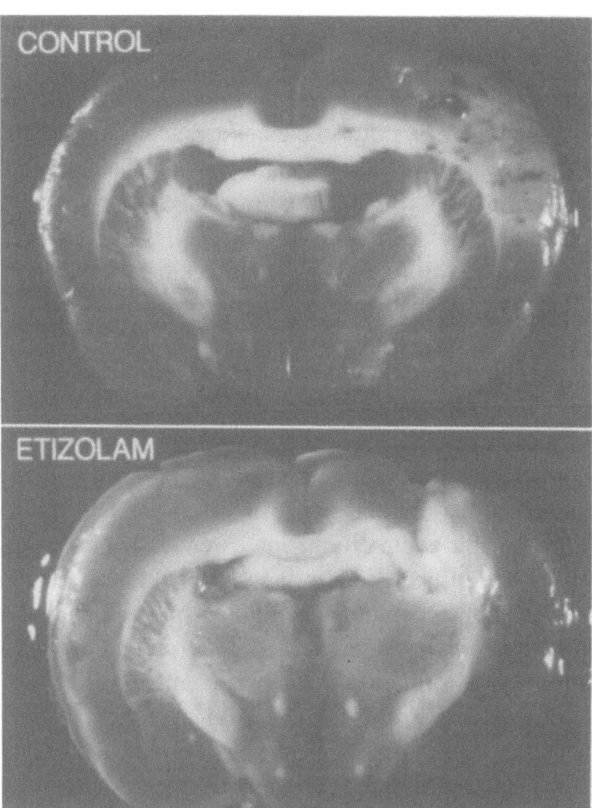

Fig. 2. Representative sections of TTC-stained materials from a non-treated control (upper) and an etizolam-treated animal (lower). Contusional necrosis is evident as light-staining areas

in the center of the contusional tissue. There were various vascular and perivascular alterations, such as petechial hemorrhage and neural tissue damage caused by the direct impact.

At 6 hours after the injury, in the peri-contusion areas 2–3 mm distant from the contusion, a number of sites with microthrombosis began to appear but no obvious damage to the neural tissue was observed (Fig. 1, left). At 24 hours post-trauma, edema formation was also noted in the peri-contusion areas (Fig. 1, right). The microthrombosis and edema formation were generally exacerbated as compared to those in the 6-hour animals. These findings indicated that microthrombosis and edema formation had progressively extended from the center to the peripheral areas of the contusion.

The rCBF in the central area of the contusion declined to an ischemic level immediately post-injury. In the peripheral area, the rCBF increased transiently, and then decreased to an ischemic level within 3 hours post-injury. Etizolam administration significantly attenuated the rCBF decrease in the pen-contusion areas, but not that in the center of the contusion.

Administration of etizolam immediately after the injury significantly reduced the size of the contusional necrosis as compared to that in the control ($p < 0.05$) (Figs. 2, 3).

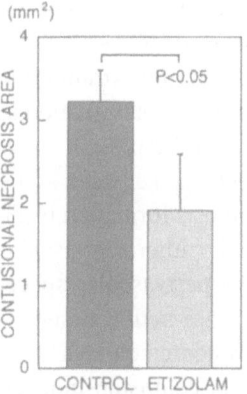

Fig. 3. Quantitative analysis revealed that etizolam administration significantly reduced the size of the contusional necrosis ($p < 0.05$), indicating that PAF antagonist can attenuate secondary tissue damage following contusion

Discussion

The present study demonstrated that, in addition to neural tissue damage, microthrombosis formation occurs as a major pathological alteration following cerebral contusion. This microvascular alteration extended progressively to the peri-contusion areas far beyond the evidently contused tissue. Such microthrombosis is the first pathological change to be seen in the peri-contusion areas, prior to the appearance of neural tissue alterations such as edema formation. These pathological alterations were accompanied by a progressive reduction of rCBF.

Previous histopathological studies have repeatedly demonstrated that ischemic brain damage is associated with cerebral contusion [1, 3, 7, 19 11, 14]. Such ischemic changes have been attributed to vascular injury within the contused brain tissue and/or a decreased cerebral perfusion pressure caused by an increase in intracranial pressure. The results of the present study indicated that microthrombosis formation and resultant ischemic edema formation extended from the primary site of contusion to the peri-contusion areas in which no histopathological findings of cerebral contusion were observed primarily. Furthermore, the microthrombosis formation in the peri-contusion areas was more extensive at 24 hours than at 1 hour. These changes suggest that secondary ischemic neural damage is produced in the peri-contusion areas, and that a possible opportunity to prevent the ischemic brain damage associated with cerebral contusion may exist. Effective treatments are clearly needed at an early stage following the contusion.

Hekmatpanah *et al.* reported that microvascular obstruction after contusion appeared to be caused by extravascular pressure from destroyed and swollen tissue, petechial hemorrhage, and dissecting extraluminal clots [11]. However, the microthrombosis formation in the pericontusion areas observed in the present study cannot be explained by such mechanisms, since at the early stage after injury the thrombosis formation is the sole histological abnormality, and neither perivascular alterations (e.g. dilatation of the perivascular space, perivascular clot formation, etc.) nor neural tissue alterations were evident in the peri-contusion areas.

Another possible mechanism for contusion-induced microthrombosis formation could involve alterations of the intravascular aggregatory activity caused by endothelial dysfunction in traumatized vessels [12]. The results of the present study demonstrated that administration of a PAF antagonist significantly reduced the size of the contusional necrosis, indicating that activation of PAF may have participated in the secondary tissue damage following cerebral contusion. PAF (1-O-alkyl-2-acetyl-sn-glycoryl-3-phosphoryl-choline) is an endogenous lipid that potently constricts blood vessels, increases the microvascular permeability, activates granulocytes, and stimulates platelet aggregation [8]. Furthermore, it has been reported that PFA exerts direct cytotoxic effects on neurons resulting in edema formation, and can modify the blood flow and brain metabolism [2, 8, 9]. The effects of etizolam administration suggest that activation of PAF is indeed involved in the pathogenesis of post-traumatic microthrombosis and edema formation in the peri-contusion areas. Further studies are needed to confirm the specificity of PAF antagonist actions on traumatic brain damage.

We conclude that in cerebral contusion, hemodynamic depression resulting in the secondary tissue damage seen in the peri-conlusion areas is closely related to the extension of microthrombosis formation, and PAF plays an important role in these events.

Acknowledgement

This work was supported by a Grant-in-Aid for Scientific Research from the Ministry of Education, Science and Culture of Japan (No. 07671547).

References

1. Arvigo F, Cossu M, Fazio B, Gris A, Pau A, Rodriguez G, Rosadini G, Sehrbundt Viale E, Siccardi D, Turtas S, Valsania V, Viale GL (1985) Cerebral blood flow in minor cerebral contusion. Surg Neurol 24: 211–217
2. Buchanan DC, Kochanek PM, Nemoto EM, Melick JA, Schoettle RJ (1989) Platelet-activating factor receptor blockade decreases early posttraumatic cerebral edema. Ann NY Acad Sci 559: 427–428
3. Dickman CA, Carter LP, Baldwin HZ, Harrington T, Tallman D (1991) Continuous regional cerebral blood flow monitoring in acute craniocerebral trauma. Neurosurgery 28: 467–472
4. Dietrich WD, Alonso O, Halley M (1994) Early microvascular and neuronal consequences of traumatic brain injury: a light and electron microscopic study in rats. J Neurotrauma 11: 289–301
5. Dietrich WD, Alonso O, Busto R, Prado R, Dewanjee S, Dewanjee MK, Ginsberg MD (1996) Widespread hemodynamic depression and focal platelet accumulation after fluid percussion brain injury: a double-label autoradiographic study in rats. J Cereb Blood Flow Metab 16: 481–489
6. Dixon CE, Clifton GL, Lighthall JW, Yaghmai AA, Hayes RL (1991) A controlled cortical impact model of traumatic brain injury in the rat. J Neurosci Meth 39: 253–262
7. Evans JP, Scheinker IM (1945) Histologic studies of the brain following head trauma. I. Post-traumatic cerebral swelling and edema. J Neurosurg 2: 306–314
8. Feuerstein G, Tian-Li Y, Lysko PG (1990) Platelet-activating factor: a putative mediator in central nervous system injury? Stroke 21 [Suppl III]: III90–III94
9. Frerichs KU, Lindsberg PJ, Hallenbeck JM, Feuerstein GZ (1990) Platelet-activating factor and progressive brain damage following forcal brain injury. J Neurosurg 72: 223–233
10. Graham DI, Adams JH, Doyle D (1978) Ischemic brain damage in fatal non-missile head injuries. J Neurol Sci 39:213–234

11. Hekmatpanah J, Hekmatpanah CR (1985) Microvascular alterations following cerebral contusion in rats. J Neurosurg 62: 888–897
12. Huber A, Dorn A, Witzmann A, Cervós-Navarro J (1993) Microthrombi formation after severe head trauma. Int J Legal Med 106: 152–155
13. Kochanek PM, Nemoto EM, Melick JA, Evans RW, Bruke DF (1988) Cerebrovascular and cerebrometabolic effects of intracarotid infused platelet-activating factor in rats. J Cereb Blood Metab 8: 546–551
14. Lindenberg R, Freytag E (1957) Morphology of cortical contusions. AMA Arch Pathol 63: 23–42
15. Tahara T, Mikashima H, Terasawa M, Maruyama Y (1987) PAF antagonist activity of some thieno [3,2-f] [1,2,4] triazolo [4,3-a] [1,4] diazepines. Chem Pharm Bull 35: 2119–2121

Correspondence: Takeshi Maeda, M.D., Department of Neurological Surgery, Nihon University School of Medicine, 30-1 Oyaguchi Kamimachi, Itabashi-ku, Tokyo 173, Japan.

Acta Neurochir (1997) [Suppl] 70: 106–108
© Springer-Verlag 1997

Characterisation of Brain Edema Following "Controlled Cortical Impact Injury" in Rats

A. W. Unterberg, R. Stroop, U.-W. Thomale, K. L. Kiening, S. Päuser, and **W. Vollmann**

Department of Neurosurgery, Virchow Medical Center, Humboldt University Berlin, Federal Republic of Germany

Summary

Significance, origin and nature of posttraumatic brain edema are still being debated. Recently, a "controlled cortical impact injury" (CCII) was introduced to model traumatic brain injury. Purpose of this study was to investigate the development and nature of brain edema following CCII. Traumatic brain injury was applied to the intact dura of the left hemisphere in Sprague-Dawley rats (n = 52, 250–350 g b.w.). Ketamine/xylazine-anesthesia or inhalation-anesthesia were used. A pneumatic impactor with a diameter of 5 mm contused the temporo-parietal cortex with a velocity of 7 m/s and an impact depth of 2 mm. 24 hours post injury the brains were removed. Posttraumatic hemispheric swelling and water content were determined gravimetrically, Evans blue extravasation spectrophotometrically, area and volume of ischemia by staining with TTC. MRI studies were performed with T1-, T2- and diffusion-weighted sequences.

Posttraumatic swelling following CCII was 14.3 ± 3.1%. Brain water content increased to 82.5 ± 0.5% in lesioned hemisphere compared to 79.9 ± 0.2% in control hemisphere. Following TTC staining, the average ischemic tissue volume was 56.7 ± 19.2 mm³. There was a moderate uptake of Evans blue into the lesioned hemisphere. MRI studies demonstrated edema in 35.4 ± 9.5 mm³ of the lesioned hemisphere. Gd-DTPA was taken up early after trauma only. A significantly decreased ADC (apparent diffusion coefficient) indicates the cytotoxic (ischemic) component of edema in this model.

In conclusion, CCII produces significant posttraumatic brain swelling and edema which is both, of vasogenic and cytotoxic nature. Thus, the CCII models the human cortical contusion more appropriately and opens new avenues for therapeutical studies focussing on cortical contusions.

Keywords: Controlled cortical impact injury; cerebral ischemia; vasogenic edema; cytotoxic edema; apparent diffusion coefficient (ADC); MRI; rats.

Introduction

Traumatic brain edema has been discussed for many years. Its significance has been questioned, but is meanwhile widely accepted [9, 10]. Nevertheless, the origin and nature of posttraumatic brain edema are still under debate [2, 8, 11]. For many years, the vasogenic type of edema has been stressed. Thus, the cortical freezing lesion according to Klatzo has served as an experimental model for a long time [7]. Since the cytotoxic and ischemic component have become of increasing interest, however, the freezing lesion has been used less frequent [9]. Recently, a controlled cortical impact injury has been developed as an experimental model for traumatic brain injury dominated by cortical contusions [3]. The objective of this study was therefore to investigate the development of brain edema following controlled cortical impact injury to characterize the amount and extent of brain edema, the state of the blood-brain-barrier and the subtype of edema dominating this experimental model. For this purpose, additional MRI-studies were performed, in particular, diffusion-weighted magnetic resonance imaging (DWI) was used to detect the type of edema that develops in this experimental traumatic brain injury.

Methods

For the study, Sprague-Dawley rats weighing 200–300 g were used. They were anesthetized either with ketamine/xylazine, or with N₂O and isoflurane. Altogether, 75 animals were used. In all animals, a medial skin incision was performed over the skull and the temporal muscle was incised and partially resected to enable an exposure of the temporal and parietal region of the skull. Thereafter, a left temporo-parietal trephination was performed with a diameter of approximately 7 mm to apply the impact to the exposed dura. The pneumatic impactor has a convexed tip surface and a diameter of 5 mm. The impact depth was set to 2 mm and the impactor velocity was 7 m/s. In the pre- and posttraumatic period, blood pressure was monitored via the tail artery and the animals were followed for up to 24 hours, in some instances up to 48 hours. If the brains were used for analysis, they were removed 24 hours post trauma.

Posttraumatic hemispheric swelling and water content in left and right hemisphere were then determined gravimetrically, Evans blue extravasation spectrophotometrically [12]. The area of ischemia under the contusion was determined by staining serial brain cuts of 2 mm by a 2% solution of 2,3,5 triphenyltetrazolium chloride (TTC). The areas were planimetrically measured and the volume of ischemia and tissue infarction was calculated.

In addition, magnetic resonance imaging (MRI) studies were performed using T1-weighted sequences (ST = 3.0 mm; TR = 500 ms; TE = 15 ms) with and without contrast enhancement, as well as T2 (ST = 1.5 mm; TR = 3330 ms; TE = 30 ms effectively 120 ms) and diffusion-weighted imaging (ST = 3.0 mm; δ =10 ms, Δ = 135 ms; b-Factor: 0, 500, 1000, 1500 s/mm^2). The MRI experiments were performed using a 2.35-Tesla, 40 cm bore magnet (Bruker Instruments).

Results

The impactor induced a unilateral hemorrhagic contusion leading to a posttraumatic swelling of $14.3 \pm 3.8\%$ (Fig. 1). All animals survived this degree of trauma. Brain water content rose significantly to $82.5 \pm 0.5\%$ in the left, lesioned hemisphere, compared to $79.9 \pm 0.2\%$ in the right, non-lesioned hemisphere (Fig. 1).

When Evans blue (1 ml/kg b.w. of a 2% solution) was given 1 hour before sacrifice at 24 hrs post trauma, 48.9 ± 8.0 ng/mg dry weight were detected in the

lesioned, left hemisphere (Fig. 2). TTC-staining of serial brain slices demontrated an area of tissue ischemia of 3.4 ± 0.7 to 10.8 ± 1.5 mm^3 of the lesioned hemisphere. Calculating the average ischemic tissue volumeyielded 56.7 ± 19.2 mm^3 in the left hemisphere.

MRI-Studies

T1-weighted ages with and without i.v.-application of gadolinium-DTPA were taken to analyze whether there was blood-brain barrier damage. At 90 minutes post trauma there was marked uptake of gadolinium in and around the contusion, while 24 hours after trauma the uptake of gadolinium was considerably less.

T2-weigthed images were used to determine the total edema volume of the hemisphere as well as the intensity of edema. They were taken 90 minutes, 24 and 72 hours after trauma. In T2-weighted images, 35.4 ± 9.9 mm^3 of the lesioned hemisphere revealed a

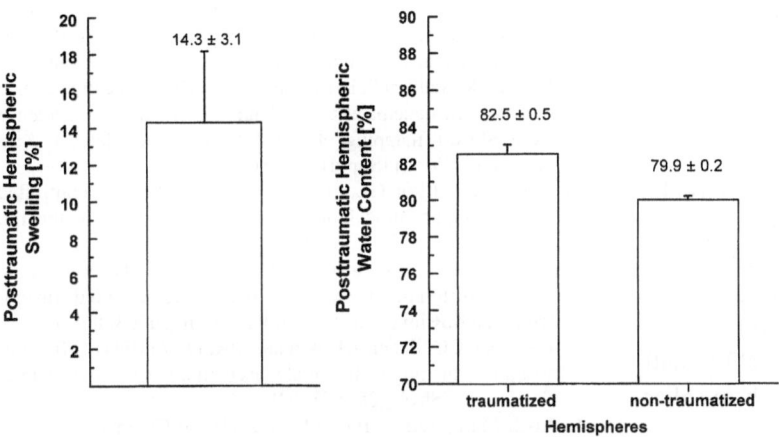

Fig. 1. Posttraumatic hemispheric swelling and hemispheric water content 24 hours after controlled cortical impact injury in rats (n = 9)

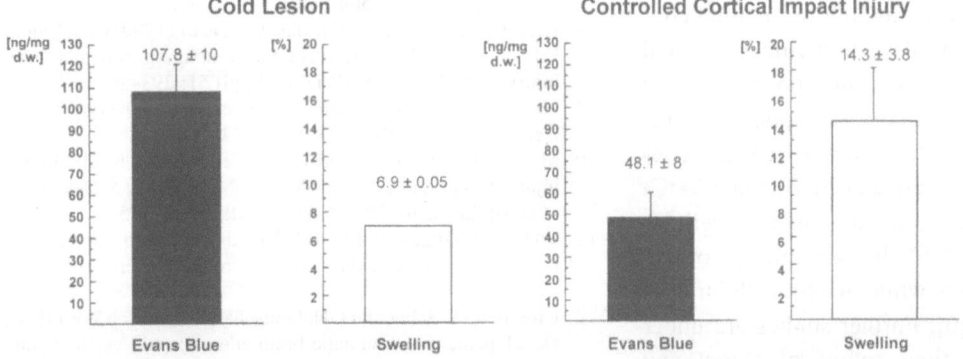

Fig. 2. Extravasation of Evans blue as marker of blood-brain barrier damage and posttraumatic swelling following cortical cold lesion according to Klatzo (n = 9) and controlled cortical impact injury (n = 9) in Sprague-Dawley rats. While a moderate cold lesion causes marked uptake of Evans Blue indicating massive blood-brain barrier leakage, a cortical impact injury leading to a markedly more pronounced posttraumatic swelling is associated with a less uptake of Evans blue. This indicates that the vasogenic edema component is significantly less following CCII

hyperintense signal indicating cerebral edema at 90 minutes post trauma. 24 hours after trauma, the extent as well as the intensity of edema had considerably increased, i.e. up to 57 ± 3 mm³ of the lesioned hemisphere.

Diffusion-weighted images were taken to characterize the subtype of edema. The apparent diffusion coefficient (ADC) dropped significantly at 90 minutes post trauma (cortex: 0.63 ± 0.07 10^{-3} mm² s⁻¹; basal ganglia: 0.54 ± 0.03 10^{-3} mm² s⁻¹; trauma: 0.32 ± 0.03 10^{-3} mm² s⁻¹) as well as 24 hours after trauma beneath the contusion indicating cytotoxic or ischemic edema.

Discussion

The controlled cortical impact injury produces significant posttraumatic brain swelling and edema which is both, of vasogenic and cytotoxic nature.

Comparing Evans blue extravasation and volume of infarction following controlled cortical impact injury and cortical freezing, there are considerable differences: In rats subjected to a cortical freezing lesion resulting in hemispheric swelling of $6.0 \pm 0.5\%$, there is marked uptake of Evans blue into the tissue, i.e. 107.8 ng/mg d.w. While the cortical impact injury resulted in a nearly two fold higher swelling, Evans blue extravasation was only half of that seen following cold lesion (Fig. 2). Thus, the vasogenic edema component is markedly less pronounced following cortical impact injury. On the other hand, the area of necrosis/infarction following a freezing lesion is considerably smaller, even if the same degree of posttraumatic hemispheric swelling is reached (data not shown).

The MRI-studies are in the same line. T2-weighted images indicate marked cerebral edema. As in the cold lesion model, it appears to be maximal 24–48 hours after trauma. Interestingly about 50% of the final edematous tissue volume reveals a hyperintense signal 90 minutes post trauma. At this time point, the area beneath the contusion has a decreased apparent diffusion coefficient indicating cytotoxic or ischemic edema [1, 4–6]. The apparent diffusion coefficient (ADC) is used to differenciate between intra- and extracellular water accumulation [1, 4–6]. In ischemic, cytotoxic edema, the ADC decreases while in extracellular edema the ADC increases [6]. Further studies are under way to investigate the time course of extent and amount of cytotoxic edema in this model.

A vasogenic component of edema is also adherent to the model. T1-weighted images indicate that there is significant gadolinium-DPTA uptake 90 minutes post trauma. Although gadolinium uptake is less pronounced 24 hours after trauma, there is still Evans blue extravasation indicative of blood-brain barrier dysfunction at this time point. It has to be mentioned, however, that the Evans blue uptake 24 hours post trauma is only about 20–25% of that seen in comparable freezing lesions. Thus, the vasogenic edema component is existent, but less important.

Taken together, the controlled cortical impact injury models human cortical contusions better than the freezing lesion, since it has been suggested that in humans contusions are surrounded by perifocal cytotoxic, rather than vasogenic edema [2, 8, 11]. This model opens new avenues for therapeutic studies, focussed not only on total cerebral edema, but also on posttraumatic ischemia and the different components of edema seen after trauma.

References

1. Benveniste HD, Hedlund LW, Johnson GA (1992) Mechanism of detection of acute cerebral ischemia in rats by diffusion-weighted magnetic resonance microscopy. Stroke 23: 746–754
2. Bullock R, Satharn P, Patterson J, *et al* (1990) The time course of vasogenic oedema after focal human head injury – evidence from SPECT mapping of blood brain barrier defects. Acta Neurochir (Wien) [Suppl] 51: 286–288
3. Dixon CE, Clifton GL, Lighthall JW, *et al* (1991) A controlled cortical impact model of traumatic brain injury in the rat. J Neurosci Meth 39: 253–262
4. Ebisu T, Naruse S, Horikawa Y, *et al* (1993) Discrimination between different types of white matter edema with diffusion-weighted MR imaging. J Magn Reson Imaging 3: 863–868
5. Hanstock CC, Faden AI, Bendall MR, *et al* (1994) Diffusion-weighted imaging differentiales ischemic tissue from traumatized tissue. Stroke 25: 843–848
6. Ito J, Marmarou A, Barzo P, *et al* (1996) Characterization of edema by diffusion-weighted imaging in experimental traumatic brain injury. J Neurosurg 84: 97–103
7. Klatzo I (1958) The relationship between edema, blood-brain barrier and tissue elements in local brain injury. J Neuropathol Exp Neurol 17: 548–564
8. Lang DA, Hedley DM, Teasdale GM, *et al* (1990) Gadolinium DTPA enhanced magnetic resonance imaging in human head injury. Acta Neurochir (Wien) [Suppl] 51: 293–295
9. Marmarou A (1994) Traumatic brain edema: an overview. Acta Neurochir (Wien) [Suppl] 60: 421–424
10. Miller JD, Corales RL (1981) Brain edema as a result of head injury: fact or fallacy? In: de Vlieger M, de Lange S, Beks JWK (eds) Brain edema. Wiley, New York, pp 99–115
11. Todd NV, Graham DI (1990) Blood-brain barrier damage in traumatic brain contusions. Acta Neurochir (Wien) [Suppl] 51: 296–299
12. Unterberg A, Schneider GH, Gottschalk J, Lanksch WR (1994) Developement of traumatic brain edema in old versus young rats. Acta Neurochir (Wien) [Suppl] 60: 431–433

Correspondence: A. W. Unterberg, M.D., Ph.D., Department of Neurosurgery, Virchow Medical Center, Humboldt University Berlin, Augustenburger Platz 1, D-13353 Berlin, Federal Republic of Germany.

Acta Neurochir (1997) [Suppl] 70: 109–111
© Springer-Verlag 1997

The Role of Adenosine During the Period of Delayed Cerebral Swelling After Severe Traumatic Brain Injury in Humans

P. M. Kochanek, R. S. B. Clark, W. D. Obrist, J. A. Carcillo, E. K. Jackson, Z. Mi, S. R. Wisniewski, M. J. Bell, and D. W. Marion

Safar Center für Resuscitation Research and the University of Pittsburgh Brain Trauma Research Center, Pittsburgh, PA, U.S.A.

Summary

Cerebrovascular failure with an increase in cerebral blood volume or hyperemia contributes delayed cerebral swelling after severe traumatic brain injury (TBI) in humans. One mediator that could be involved in this process is adenosine, which stimulates a concurrent reduction in cerebral metabolic rate and an increase in cerebral blood flow (CBF). We hypothesized that during the delayed phase after TBI in humans; 1) CSF adenosine concentration is associated with uncoupling of CBF and $CMRO_2$, and 2) adenosine formation is driven by mediator-stimulated cAMP production in injured brain. We serially measured CBF and $AVDO_2$, and CSF adenosine, lactate and cAMP after severe TBI in 13 humans. After 6–18 h, global CBF was increased and $AVDO_2$ was reduced vs all other time periods, defining the uncoupling phase as the period between 18 h and 5 days. CSF adenosine concentration was negatively associated with $AVDO_2$ and strongly associated with death (both $p < 0.05$), CSF lactate peaked during the initial 18 h, but remained increased for 5 days. CSF cAMP concentration was not increased (vs normal). The association between CSF adenosine concentration and death, and the correlation between uncoupling of CBF and oxidative metabolism and CSF adenosine concentration support our first hypothesis. In contrast, the low levels of cAMP in CSF observed in these patients, but persistently increased CSF lactate, refute our second hypothesis. We speculate that hyperglycolysis or occult ischemic foci are possible sources of ATP breakdown and adenosine formation, and that adenosine is playing a neuroprotective role.

Keywords: Traumatic brain injury; cerebral swelling; adenosine; hyperemia.

Introduction

Cerebrovascular failure with an increase in cerebral blood volume and/or hyperemia has been postulated to contribute importantly to the development of delayed cerebral swelling after severe traumatic brain injury (TBI) in humans [6, 8]. During this period, uncoupling of cerebral blood flow (CBF) and oxidative metabolism has been shown to occur, specifically, $CMRO_2$ is depressed while CBF is normal or increased [5, 8, 9]. One mediator that could be involved in this process is CBF is normal or increased [5, 8, 9]. One mediator that could be involved in this process is adenosine, which is a unique molecule that stimulates a concurrent reduction in cerebral metabolic rate and an increase in CBF [7, 11, 12]. At least two distinct pathways of adenosine production could be involved, including the production of adenosine from the breakdown of ATP (during hyperglycolysis or in occult ischemic foci) or the metabolism of cyclic-AMP (cAMP) produced by a host of mediators such as prostanoids and catechols.

Hypothesis: During the delayed phase of cerebral swelling, 1) CSF adenosine concentration is associated with uncoupling of CBF and $CMRO_2$, and 2) adenosine production is driven by mediator-stimulated cAMP production in the injured brain.

Methods

To define the association between adenosine and uncoupling of CBF and $CMRO_2$ during delayed cerebral swelling, we serially measured concentrations of adenosine (HPLC) in CSF (ventricular catheter) in 13 adults during the initial 5 days after severe TBI (GCS $\leq$ 7) and examined its association with CBF (^{133}Xe method), $CMRO_2$, and $AVDO_2$ measured simultaneously in these patients. Patients received contemporary neurointensive care management (The study was undertaken during the prospective randomized evaluation of moderate hypothermia on neurologic outcome after closed head injury).

Uncoupling was defined as $AVDO_2 \leq 4$ vol% [8]. In addition, to obtain clues as to both the possible source of adenosine and the underlying mechanisms behind the role of adenosine in delayed cerebral swelling, we measured CSF lactate and cAMP concentrations in these same samples.

Results

After 6–18 h posttrauma, global CBF was increased and $AVDO_2$ was reduced at all other time periods (both $p < 0.05$ by repeated measures ANOVA), defining the uncoupling phase as the period between 18 h and 5 days after TBI.

A total of 67 CSF samples were assayed for adenosine with an average of 5 per patient. CSF adenosine concentration was negatively associated with $AVDO_2$ ($p < 0.05$, generalized multivariate linear regression model). In addition, CSF adenosine concentration was strongly associated with death ($p < 0.001$). CSF adenosine was increased when $AVDO_2$ was ≤ 4 vs > 4 vol%, and in patients that died vs survivors (both $p < 0.05$). Furthermore CSF lactate concentration peaked during the initial 18 h after TBI, but remained increased (vs normal) until 5 days after TBI. CSF cAMP concentration was not increased (vs normal) at any time after TBI, and was actually depressed until 3 days after TBI.

Discussion

In this preliminary report, the highly significant association between CSF adenosine concentration and death, and the correlation between uncoupling of oxidative metabolism and CSF adenosine concentration strongly support our first hypothesis, and suggests an important biological role for adenosine in the brain during delayed cerebral swelling after severe TBI in humane. In contrast, the low levels of cAMP in CSF observed in these patients, but persistently increased CSF lactate refute our second hypothesis, and suggest that adenosine is produced from ATP breakdown during this phase (most likely from either hyperglycolysis or occult ischemic foci).

Adenosine has been shown to be important in coupling CBF to metabolic demands during functional activation [4]. Similarly, adenosine is an important endogenous neuroprotectant when it is formed during the breakdown of ATP during ischemia [2].

Based on the recent work of Pellerin and Magistretti [10] and Begsneider *et al.* [1], one possible explanation for the concurrent increase in CBF, reduction in $CMRO_2$ and increase in adenosine during the secondary cerebral swelling phase is that adenosine is participating in a coupled increase in CBF relative to glucose utilization (hyperglycolysis). This hyperglycolysis could be stimulated by glutamate, potassium, cytokines, or arachidonic acid (Fig. 1). Thus, adenosine could be facilitating the coupling of this response and

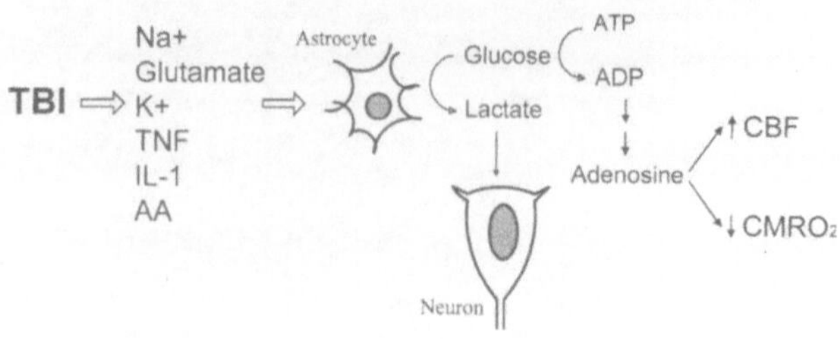

Fig. 1

inhibiting $CMRO_2$ during this phase. Increased CSF adenosine was associated with mortality in our study. If the mechanism proposed in the Fig. 1 is operating, it would suggest that adenosine is attempting to perform an endogenous neuroprotective role in the most severely injured patients. Finally, additional mediators capable of increasing CBF and reducing CMR, such as nitric oxide produced by inducible nitric oxide synmase, could also be involved in this complex process [3].

Although further studies are needed, these data are most consistent with and endogenous neuroprotectant role for adenosine during delayed cerebral swelling after severe TBI in humans.

Acknowledgment

We thank the Society of Critical Care Medicine, NINDS, 2P50 NS30318-04A1, and Children's Hospital of Pittsburgh (GCRC Grant 5MO1 RR00084) for support.

References

1. Bergsneider M, Kelly DF, Shalmon MJ, *et al* (1995) Early hyperglycolysis following severe human traumatic brain injury: a positron emission tomography study. J Neurotrauma 12: 371
2. Berne RM, Rubio R, Curnish RR (1974) Release of adenosine from ischemic brain. Effect on cerebral vascular resistance and incorporation into cerebral adenine nucleotides. Circ Res 35: 262–271
3. Clark RSB, Kochanek PK, Obrist WD, Wong HR, Billiar TR, Wisniewski SR, Marion DW (1996) Cerebrospinal fluid and plasma nitrite and nitrate concentrations after head injury in humane. Crit Care Med 24: 1243–1251
4. Dirnagl U, Niwa K, Lindauer U, Villringer A (1994) Coupling of cerebral blood flow to neuronal activation: role of adenosine and nitric oxide. Am J Physiol 267: H296–301
5. Lassen NA (1966) The luxury-perfusion syndrome and its possible relation to acute metabolic acidosis localised within the brain. Lancet 2: 1113–1115
6. Marmarou A (1992) Increased intracranial pressure in head injury and influence of blood volume. J Neurotrauma 9 [Suppl 1]: S327–332
7. Miller LP, Hsu C (1992) Therapeutic potential for adenosine receptor activation in ischemic brain injury. J Neurotrauma 9 [Suppl 2]: S563–577
8. Obrist WD, Langfitt TW, Jaggi JL, Cruz J, Gennarelli TA (1984) Cerebral blood flow and metabolism in comatose pa-

tients with acute head injury. Relationship to intracranial hypertension. J Neurosurg 61: 241–253

9. Obrist WD, Marion DW, Aggarwal S, Darby JM (1993) Time course of cerebral blood flow and metabolism in comatose patients with acute head injury. J Cereb Blood Flow Metab 13 [Suppl 1]: S571

10. Pellerin L, Magistretti PJ (1994) Glutamate uptake into astrocytes stimulates aerobic glycolysis: a mechanism coupling neuronal activity to glucose utilization. Proc Natl Acad Sci USA 91: 1062–10629

11. Phillis JW, Kostopoulos GK, Limacher JJ (1975) A potent depressent action of adenosine derivatives an cerebral cortical neurones. Eur J Pharmacol 30: 125–129

12. Winn HR, Rubio R, Berne RM (1981) The rote of adenosine in the regulation of cerebral blood flow. J Cereb Blood Flow Metab 1: 239–244

Correspondence: Patrick M. Kochanek, M.D., Safar Center for Resuscitation Research, University of Pittsburgh, 3434 Fifth Ave., Pittsburgh, PA15260, U.S.A.

Acta Neurochir (1997) [Suppl] 70: 112–114
© Springer-Verlag 1997

Near Infrared Spectroscopy (NIRS) in Patients with Severe Brain Injury and Elevated Intracranial Pressure

A Pilot Study

A. Kampfl, B. Pfausler, D. Denchev, H. P. Jaring, and **E. Schmutzhard**

Department of Neurology, Intensive Care Unit, University Hospital Innsbruck, Austria

Summary

Near infrared spectroscopy (NIRS) was used to asses changes in regional cerebral oxygen saturation (rSO_2) in 8 head injured patients with an intracranial pressure (ICP) higher or lower than 25 mmHg (n = 4 for each group). NIRS values in the high ICP group (> 25 mmHg) were significantly lower than in the low ICP group (< 25 mmHg). In contrast, arterial pO_2, pCO_2, peripheral oxygen saturation and transcranial Doppler sonography (TCD) values were similar in both groups. To further investigate changes in rSO_2 to changes in peripheral oxygen saturation and arterial pO_2, patients of both groups underwent an artificial hyperoxygenation (50% O_2) period of 3 minutes. Both groups revealed similar values in peripheral oxygen saturation, arterial pO_2, and TCD velocities at the end of the hyperoxygenation period. However, rSO_2 values in patients with an ICP > 25 mmHg were significant lower than in patients with an ICP < 25 mmHg after the hyperoxygenation period. In addition, patients with an ICP < 25 mmHg revealed a significant increase in rSO_2 values at the end of the hyperoxygenation period, not detectable in patients with an ICP > 25 mmHg. Our results suggest that NIRS may be an additional diagnostic tool in the non-invasive evaluation of impaired cerebral microcirculation in patients with increased intracranial pressure.

Keywords: Severe brain injury; elevated intracranial pressure; near infrared spectroscopy; cerebral oxygen saturation.

Introduction

Near infrared spectroscopy (NIRS) is a new method of noninvasively monitoring regional intracerebral oxygen saturation (rSO_2). Transcranial NIRS has been used to detect cerebral hypoxia [12], changes in cerebral blood volume [1] and to identify the presence of hypoxia after circulatory arrest [11]. In addition, NIRS has been used to detect metabolic brain injury in infants [4] and to measure cerebral blood flow in preterm infants [5, 9]. However, there is only limited experience using NIRS to detect changes in rSO_2 in head injured patients [6, 7]. To illustrate the effectiveness of NIRS to monitor intracerebral oxygen saturation in patients with severe head injury and increased intracerebral pressure (ICP) we simultaneously recorded signals of rSO_2, arterial pO_2, arterial oxygen saturation, cerebral perfusion pressure, and TCD velocities in 8 patients with ICP higher or lower than 25 mmHg. In addition, periods of artificial hyperoxygenation were used to compare changes in rSO_2 changes in arterial pO_2 and peripheral oxygen saturation.

Material and Methods

Patients

Over a 6 month period, 5 male and 3 female patients, ranging in age from 20 to 67 years and suffering from severe brain injury (Glasgow Coma Scale score < 6) were deemed suitable for our study. Patients were selected because they had no intracranial mass lesions, extracranial trauma, or scalp lacerations that would preclude safe application of surface probes. All selected patients had probes positioned within 12 hours of the injury.

Monitoring Procedures

a) Intracranial pressure (ICP): An epidural ICP probe (Spiegelberg probes) was placed 2 cm apart in the frontal region according to the side of maximum trauma seen on the admission computerized tomography (CT) scan. If similar bilateral CT changes were seen, the probe was placed in the right frontoparietal epidural space. b) Cerebral perfusion pressure (CPP): Arterial blood pressure was monitored continuously using radial artery catheters, transducers, and monitors. Cerebral perfusion pressure was calculated from digitized signals of mean arterial blood pressure (MAP) and ICP. c) Middle cerebral artery flow velocity: Monitoring of the middle cerebral artery flow velocities was undertaken using a mobile transcranial Doppler (TCD) device. d) Peripheral oxygen saturation: Peripheral saturation was monitored continuously with a pulse oximeter (Datex AS/3). e) Near infrared spectroscopy: Transcranial cerebral oximetry, a technique that evaluates regional saturation of oxygen (rSO_2) in the brain by the noninvasive method of near infrared spectroscopy (NIRS), was performed using an INVOS

3100A cerebral oximeter. The probe was situated on the patients forehead at the side of the maximum trauma seen on CT. If similar bilateral diffuse CT changes were seen, the probe was placed on the righ frontal region. f) Patient management: The patients were analgetized, sedated, and ventilated using a standard regime of midazolam, fentanyl and if necessary, atracrium. Moderate hyperventilation was initiated to achieve a $PaCO_2$ of 30–35 mmHg. Attempts were made to maintain a CPP of 60 mm Hg or more with inotropes, if Patients were divided into 2 groups: Patients with an ICP higher than 25mm Hg (= high ICP group), and patients with an ICP lower than 25mm Hg (= low ICP group; n = 4 for each group). Our protocol consisted of (1) a continuous arterial blood gas-, CPP, TCD, and NIRS check at the actual respirator setting (= 21% O_2) for approximately 30 minutes (= baseline). (2) The same parameters were checked after 3 minutes of hyperoxygenation with 50% O_2. Data were evaluated by Students t test. Values are given are mean ± SEM. Differences were considered significant when p < 0.05.

Results

Mean ICP values in the low ICP group were 19.9 ± 3.9 mmHg, in the high ICP group 31.2 ± 2.9 mmHg (p < 0.05). No statistical differences in flow velocities of the middle cerebral arteries and CPP levels were observed between both groups during the evaluation of thebaseline values, and at the end of the hyperoxygenation period. In contrast, rSO_2 values of the high ICP group were significantly lower than rSO_2 values of the low ICP group during the baseline evaluation (ICP > 25 mmHg: 67 ± 1%; ICP < 25 mmHg: 71 ± 2%; ** p < 0.01), and at the end of hyperoxygenation period (ICP > 25 mmHg: 70 ± 2%; ICP < 25 mmHg: 78 ± 0.75%; *** p < 0.001; Fig. 1A). rSO_2 values for the high ICP group were similar at all time points investigated (Fig. 1A). In contrast, patients with low ICP revealed a significant increase in rSO_2 at the end of the hyperoxygenation period (+ p < 0.05, in comparison to the baseline values; Fig. 1A). Interestingly, no signifi-

cant difference between the peripheral oxygen saturation and arterial pO_2 were observed in the low and high ICP groups during the evaluation of the baseline values, and the end of the hyperoxygenation period (Fig. 1B).

Discussion

Reduced cerebral blood flow and cerebral oxygen saturation following traumatic brain injury may be associated with poor clinical outcome. Therefore, reliable methods for the detection of reduced cerebral oxygen saturation are required. Many techniques for continuously monitoring cerebral circulation in head injured patients are available. For example, transcranial Doppler (TCD) sonography enables continuous monitoring of cerebral blood flow velocity in the intracerebral vasculature and has gained wide acceptance in the monitoring of cerebral perfusion in head injured patients [3]. However, this method gives no information concerning peripheral cortical perfusion. Jugular venous catheterization and venous saturation monitoring seemed to be a promising method for detection of cerebral oxygen desaturation periods [10]. However, this invasive technique remains prone to artifacts due to catheter movement, clot formation, and intimal impaction. In contrast, near infrared spectroscopy (NIRS) is a noninvasive technique for assessing cerebral regional oxygen saturation (rSO_2). Moreover, a recent report has provided evidence that NIRS is twice as sensitive for the detection of cerebral oxygen desaturation periods than invasive jugular venous saturation monitoring [7]. Our preliminary study demonstrated that in head injured patients with increased

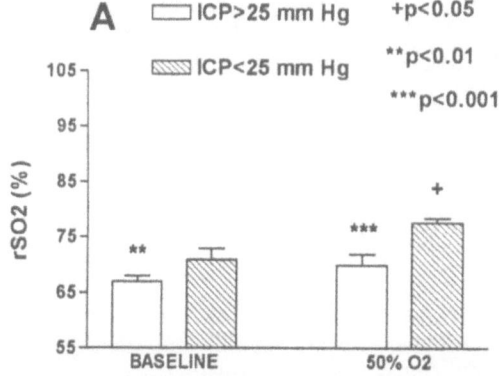 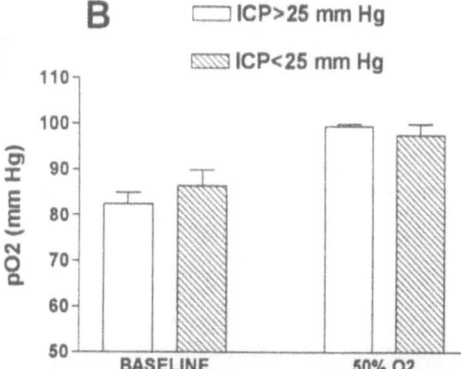

Fig. 1. (A) Regional cerebral oxygen saturation in head injured patients with an ICP higher (open bars) or lower (hatched bars) than 25 mmHg. rSO_2 values were significant lower in patients with an ICP > 25 mmHg than in patients with an ICP < 25 mmHg during the evaluation of the baseline values and at the end of the hyperoxygenation period. In addition, patients with an ICP < 25 mmHg revealed a significant increase in rSO_2 values at the end of the hyperoxygenation period. (B) Similar values in arterial pCO_2 were observed in both groups during the evaluation of the baseline values and the end of the hyperoxygenation period

intracerebral pressure (ICP) higher than 25 mmHg rSO$_2$ values were significant lower than in patients with an ICP lower than 25 mmHg. Interestingly, CPP, blood gas values and TCD velocities were similar in both groups. In addition, patients with an ICP < 25 mmHg revealed a significant increase in rSO$_2$ after the hyperoxygenation periods not seen in patients with an ICP > 25 mmHg. Although recent doubts have been expressed concerning the accuracy of the measurements made by the cerebral oximeter [2, 8], our results suggest that NIRS may be a valuable tool in the detection of impaired microcirculation and/or local brain tissue oxygenation in patients with increased intracerebral pressure, which may not be detectable by means of monitoring CPP, blood gas analysis, and monitoring TCD velocities. However, the clinical relevance of these findings awaits improved reliability and a much broader experience with this new technique.

References

1. Brazy JE (1991) Cerebral oxygen monitoring with near infrared spectroscopy: clinical application to neonates. J Clin Monit 7: 325–334
2. Brown R, Wright J, Royston R (1993) A comparison of two systems for assessing cerebral venous oxyhaemoglobin saturation during cardiopulmonary bypass in humans. Anesthesia 48: 697–709
3. Chan KH, Dearden NM, Miller JD (1993) Transcranial Doppler sonography in severe head injury. Acta Neurochir (Wien) 59: 81–85
4. Chance B, Smith DS, Delivoria-Papadoupoulos M, Younkin DP (1989) New techniques for evaluating metabolic brain injury in newborn infants. Crit Care Med 17: 465–471
5. Edwards AD, Wyatt JS, Richardson C, Delpy DT, Cope M, Reynolds ED (1988) Cotside measurement of cerebral blood flow in ill newborn infants by near infrared spectroscopy. Lancet 2: 770–771
6. Gopinath SP, Robertson CS, Grossman RG, Chance B (1993) Near-infrared spectroscopic localization of intracranial hematomas. J Neurosurg 79: 43–47
7. Kirkpatrick PJ, Smielewski P, Czosnyka M, Menon DK, Pickard JD (1995) Near-infrared spectroscopy use in patients with head injury. J Neurosurg 83: 963–970
8. Harris DNF, Bailey SM (1993) Near infrared spectroscopy in adults. Anesthesia 48: 694–696
9. Lou HC, Lassen NA, Friis-Hansen B (1979) Impaired autoregulation of cerebral blood flow in the distressed newborn infant. J Pediatr 94: 118–121
10. Robertson CS, Contant CF, Goksalan ZL, Narayan RK, Grossman RG (1992) Cerebral blood flow, arteriovenous oxygen difference, and outcome in head injured patients. J Neurol Neurosurg Psychiatry 36: 559–566
11. Smith DS, Levy W, Maris M, Chance B (1990) Reperfusion hyperoxia in brain after circulatory arrest in humane. Anesthesiology 73: 12–19
12. Williams IM, Picton AJ, Hardy SC, Mortimer AJ, McCollum CN (1994) Cerebral hypoxia detected by near infrared spectroscopy. Anesthesia 49: 762–768

Correspondence: A. Kampfl, M.D., Department of Neurology, Anichstrasse 35, A-6020 Innsbruck, Austria.

Acta Neurochir (1997) [Suppl] 70: 115–118
© Springer-Verlag 1997

MRI Diffusion-Weighted Spectroscopy of Reversible and Irreversible Ischemic Injury Following Closed Head Injury

P. Barzó[1], A. Marmarou[1], P. Fatouros[2], J. Ito[1], and F. Corwin[2]

[1] Division of Neurosurgery and [2] Department of Radiology, Medical College of Virginia, Richmond, VA, U.S.A.

Summary

The objective of this study was to detect the threshold between reversible and irreversible secondary insult of hypoxia and hypotension following closed head injury as measured by MRI.

Adult Sprague rats were separated into 3 groups: I: Sham (n = 6), II: Trauma and hypoxia coupled with mild hypotension of 40–50 mmHg (n = 6), III: Trauma and hypoxia coupled with severe hypotension of 30–40 mmHg (n = 6). The measurement of brain water content (BWC) was based on T1, whereas the differentiation between reversible and irreversible secondary insult on the measurement apparent diffusion coefficient (ADC).

The ADCs in both trauma and secondary insult groups decreased rapidly from a control level of $0.68 \pm 0.5 \times 10^{-3}$ to significantly different minimum levels of $0.52 \pm 0.5 \times 10^{-3}$ in Group II and $0.42 \pm 0.5 \times 10^{-3}$ mm^2/second in Group III at 30 minutes. In Group II rats there was a complete recovery in ADC as well as in their clinical conditions, whereas ADC in Group III rats remained at the minimum level and the animals were brain dead. The BWC was also significantly different at four hours post injury (Group II: $80.3 \pm 0.7\%$, Group III: $81.8 \pm 0.8\%$).

The data lead the authors to suggest that the threshold between reversible and irreversible posttraumatic secondary insult is very narrow, and the measurement of ADC can provide information that will enable the clinician to identify critical threshold beyond which recovey is not possible.

Keywords: Traumatic brain injury; magnetic resonance imaging; diffusion-weighted spectroscopy; reversible and irreversible ischemic injury.

Introduction

Second insults of hypoxia and hypotension occur in over 50% of head injured patients and the contribution of secondary insults to poor outcome from severe head injury has been well documented [1, 2]. Studies from the traumatic coma data bank have also related to diffuse swelling and high intracranial pressure.

Recently a new model producing diffuse brain injury with secondary insult has been developed in rats in our laboratory [3, 4]. In this model cerebral blood flow decreases as the systemic blood pressure falls, due to 30 minute secondary insult, and ischemia causes additional damage to the injured brain.

Diffusion-weighted MRI, which is based on the translational movement or diffusion of water, can rapidly detect and localize focal brain injury as a hyperintense region within a few minutes after the onset of ischemia [5]. Such hyperintense changes observed in the acute stage of ischemia reflect a decline of the ADC of water in ischemic brain tissue. This decline of ADC soon after an ischemic insult is presumed to be related to intracellular water accumulation (cytotoxic edema) or changes in membrane permeability caused by rapid failure of energy metabolism. Reversal of ADC reduction (increase in ADC to normal level) might be expected to occur following resuscitation dependent upon the severity of insult.

The objective of this study was to use single voxel diffusion-weighted spectroscopy (VOSY) and longitudinal relaxation time (T_1) by MRI to help detect the threshold between reversible and irreversible secondary insult of hypoxia and hypotension following closed head injury (CHI) as the evidence by the apparent diffusion coefficient (ADC).

Materials and Methods

Eighteen adult male Sprague-Dawley rats weighing 340 to 375 grams were divided into 3 groups: I. Sham (n = 6), II. Trauma and hypoxia coupled with mild hypotension of 40–50 mmHg (n = 6), III. Trauma and hypoxia coupled with severe hypotension of 30–40 mmHg (n = 6). Rats were initially anesthetized with halothane, then intubated and artificially ventilated with a gas mixture of N_2O (70%), O_2 (30%), and halothane (0.5–1.5%). Body temperature was maintained at 37°C $\pm$ 0.5°C. A new impact acceleration head injury model was used to produce trauma [6].

Experiments were performed using a 2.35 T, 40 cm bore magnet (Biospec, Bruker Instruments, Billerica, MA) equipped with a 12 cm inner diameter actively shielded gradient insert, with a G_{max} of 25 G/cm.

Two dimensional diffusion-weighted imaging employed a spin echo (SE) sequence.

For fast ADC measurements single voxel diffusion-weighted spectroscopy (VOSY) was used. Voxel dimensions (typically 5 mm × 5 mm × 5 mm) were selected to fit entirely within the brain. The VOSY employed a stimulated echo sequence.

Our experience in utilizing MRI for measurement of brain water is based upon laboratory and clinical studies directed toward non-invasive monitoring of brain edema formation and resolution (Marmarou).

Schedule of the measurements: Baseline diffusion weighted (both type) and T_1-weighted images (water map) were obtained. The rat was then removed from the magnet, subjected to head injury, and was returned to the magnet immediately after the trauma. VOSY was carried out in every minute and T_1-water determination at four 1-hour intervals post injury.

Results

ADC Changes

Control group: The ADCs measured by VOSY at baseline ($0.68 \pm 0.5 \times 10^{-3}$ mm²/second) did not show any significant changes during the four hour interval of the study. Group II (trauma coupled with mild hypotension): The baseline values were not different from those of the control group. During the first 10–30 minutes of secondary insult the ADC showed a significant decrease ($p < 0.001$), with a minimum value of $0.52 \pm 0.05 \times 10^{-3}$ mm²/sec at 30 minutes. After the resuscitation the MRI showed gradually increased ADC and, return to normal value was observed at four hours after the trauma (Fig. 1). Group III (trauma coupled with severe hypotension): During the secondary insult the decrease in ADC was more severe than in Group II with a significantly different minimum level of $0.42 \pm 0.05 \times 10^{-3}$ mm²/sec ($p < 0.001$). In contrast with the Group II animals where we observed complete recovery of ADC as well as their clinical conditions, the ADC in the Group III rats remained at the minimum level and the animals were brain dead at the end of the experiment (Fig. 1).

Water Content Changes

Control group: Water content of the whole brain was $77.8 \pm 0.4\%$ and did not change during the 4 hour period of the experiment (Fig. 2). Group II (Trauma coupled with mild hypotension): A significant water content increase was observed during the second half of the experiment ($80.3 \pm 0.7\%$, $p < 0.001$); however, it

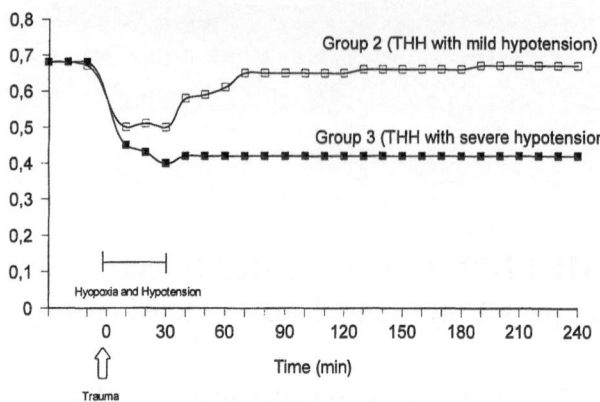

Fig. 1. Time course of apparent diffusion coefficients (ADC): ADC in both trauma with secondary insult group (Group II and III) decreased rapidly from the control value to significantly different levels. In Group II (trauma followed by hypoxia and mild hypotension) there was complete recovery in ADC, whereas ADC in Group III (trauma followed by hypoxia and severe hypotension) remained at the minimum level

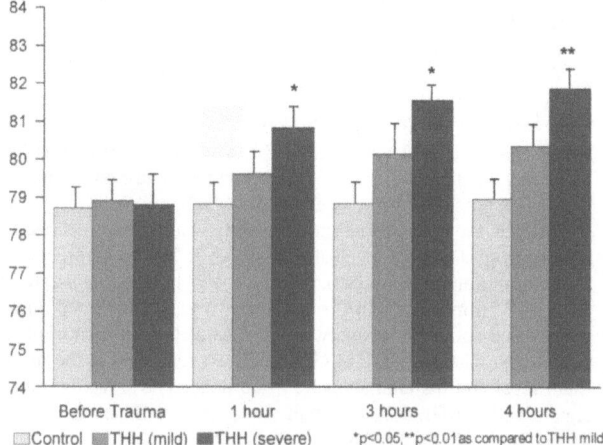

Fig. 2. Time course of brain water content: In the Control Group, water content did not change during the 4 hour period in the brain. In Group II and III water content of the brain increased significantly and reached its highest value at four hours post injury. After one hour following the insult, the difference between the two groups was statistically significant. Values showed mean standard deviation

was less pronounced as compared to the Group III animals (Fig. 2). Group III (trauma coupled with severe hypotension): Water content of the whole brain was significantly elevated as soon as at the end of the first hour post injury ($80.7 \pm 0.7\%$). This increase continued during the next few hours and reached its highest value of $81.8 \pm 0.8\%$ at the end of the experiment (Fig. 2). The brain swelling was diffuse, that is, the water map did not show any regional difference in water content.

Discussion

This study has, for the first time, systematically characterized the threshold between reversible and irreversible ischemic injury in posttraumatic secondary insult of hypoxia and hypotension as the evidence by the apparent diffusion coefficient. In general, 30 minutes of hypoxia ($pCO_2 \pm$ 40–50 mmHg) and severe hypotension of 30–40 mmHg after CHI was followed by irreversible derangements and brain death in all rats of this group where as rats with mild hypotension of 40–50 mmHg and hypoxia after CHI fully recovered. The present data shows that the threshold between reversible and irreversible secondary insult is very narrow and 10–20 mmHg increase in MABP as well as in perfusion pressure during hypoxia and hypotension can result in completely different outcome. This is of clinical importance and is in agreement with the clinical study of Chesnut et al. who observed 150% increase in mortality rate in those patients in which head injury was associated with severe secondary insult of hypotension and hypoxia [2].

Changes in cerebral circulation and metabolism after head injury have been studied both experimentally and clinically. Studies carried out to investigate metabolic derangement by MRI following head injury have reported, that trauma disturbs the normally close correlation between CBF and cerebral oxygen demand, rendering the brain unable to adequately increase CBF in response to increased metabolic demands. Hypoxia raises the cerebral metabolic rate and oxygen demand, and consequently requires an increase in CBF to maintain normal energy levels through oxidative metabolism. Combining hypotension with trauma prevents CBF from increasing as required to maintain normal oxidative energy metabolism, and forces an increase in anaerobic energy metabolism. This situation was defined by Siesj as hypoxic hypoxia [7]. The result is a cascade process of free radical release which can cause additional damage to the injured brain.

Diffusion-weighted imaging (DWI) is a relatively new MR modality that is sensitive to the microscopic motion of water molecules and permits quantification of this phenomenon through the calculation of apparent diffusion coefficient (ADC) images. The potential role of ADC measurement in cerebral ischemia is based on the observation that the apparent diffusion rate of water protons in ischemic brain is much lower than in normal brain. DWI has been used to demarcate very early (within 14 and 30 minutes) changes in the

evolution of cerebral ischemia in animals and in humans. Recently several authors demonstrated that the hyperintensity (low ADC) seen on early DWI in part may represent reversible ischemic injury and that varying degrees of decline in ADC values may reflect the severity of the ischemic tissue damage at each imaging timepoint [8, 9]. In this study we measured changes in absolute ADC values in a particular voxel of the brain during and after secondary insult following CHI. ADC values progressively increased after resuscitation and reached the normal level in animals with complete recovery, in contrast with the brain death animals in which the ADC remained low indicating irreversible injury. These findings were also supported by the significantly higher brain water content in Group in animals. Our result suggest that measurement of changes in ADC could serve as a mechanism to identify brain lesions sooner than was possible with standard MRI and potentially to target therapeutic intervention more effectively.

Taking all these results in concert we have to conclude that threshold between reversible and irreversible posttraumatic secondary insult is very narrow, and the measurement of ADC can provide information that will enable the clinician to differentiate between irreversible and potentially reversible injury before the initiation of specific therapy.

Acknowledgement

This research was supported in part by Grant P01 NS12587 and R01 NS19235 from the National Institutes of Health.

References

1. Miller JD (1985) Head injury and brain ischemia: implication for therapy. Br J Anaesth 57: 120–129
2. Chesnut RM, Marshall LF, Klauber MR, Blunt BA, Baldwin N, Eisenberg HM, Jane JA, Marmarou A, Foulkes MA (1993) The role of secondary brain injury in determining outcome from severe head injury. J Trauma 34: 216–222
3. Barzo P, Marmarou A, Fatouros P, Corwin F, Dunbar J (1996) MRI-monitored acute blood-brain barrier changes in experimental traumatic brain injury. J Neurosurg 85: 1113–1121
4. Ito J, Marmarou A, Barzo P, Fatouros P, Corwin F (1996) Characterization of edema by diffusion-weighted imaging in experimental traumatic brain injury. J Neurosurg 84: 97–103
5. Le Bihan D, Breton E, Lallemand D, Aubin ML, Vignaud J, Laval-Jeantet M (1988) Separation of diffusion and perfusion in intravoxel incoherent motion (IVIM) MR imaging. Radiology 168: 497–505
6. Marmarou A, Foda AE, van den Brink W, Campbell J, Kita H, Demetriadou K (1994) A new model of diffuse brain injury in rats. Part I: Pathophysiology and biomechanics. J Neurosurg 80: 291–300

7. Siesj BK, Zwetnow NN (1970) The effect of hypovolemic hypotension on extra- and intracellular acid-base parameters and energy metabolites in the rat brain. Acta Physiol Scand 79: 114–122

8. Hasegawa Y, Fischer M, Latour LL, Dardzinski BJ, Sotak CH (1990) MRI diffusion mapping of reversible and irreversible ischemic injury in focal brain ischemia. Neurology 44: 1484–1490

9. Rother J, de Crespigny AJ, D'Arceuil H, Iwai K, Moseley ME (1996) Recovery of apparent diffusion coefficient after ischemia-induced spreading depression relates to cerebral perfusion gradient. Stroke 27: 980–986

Correspondence: Anthony Marmarou, M.D., Division of Neurosurgery, P.O. Box 508, MCV Station, Sanger Hall, Room 8004, 1101 E Marshal St., Richmond, Virginia 23298, U.S.A.

Acta Neurochir (1997) [Suppl] 70: 119–122

Biphasic Pathophysiological Response of Vasogenic and Cellular Edema in Traumatic Brain Swelling

P. Barzó[1], A. Marmarou[1], P. Fatouros[2], K. Hayasaki[1], and F. Corwin[2]

[1] Division of Neurosurgery and [2] Department of Radiology, Medical College of Virginia, Richmond, VA, U.S.A.

Summary

The objective of this study was to quantify the temporal water content changes and document the type of edema (cellular versus vasogenic) that is occurring during both the acute and the late stages of edema development following closed head injury.

Adult Sprague rats (n = 50) were separated into two groups: *Group I:* Sham (n = 8), *Group II:* Trauma (n = 42). The measurement of brain water content (BWC) was based on T1, whereas the differentiation of edema on the measurement of the random, translational motion of water protons (apparent diffusion coefficients – ADC) by MRI.

In trauma animals, we found a significant increase in ADC (105%) as well as in BWC (0.7 ± 0.3%) during the first 60 minutes post injury indicating vasogenic edema formation. This transient increase; however, was followed by a continuing decrease in ADC beginning at 45 minutes post injury and reaching a minimum at days 7–14 (–103%). Since the BWC continued to increase during the next day (10.3%), it is suggested cellular edema formation started to develop soon after injury and became dominant between 1–2 weeks post injury.

In conclusion we may consider, that there is a predominantly vasogenic edema formation immediately after injury and later a more widespread and slower edema formation due to a predominantly cellular swelling.

Keywords: Traumatic brain injury; brain edema; magnetic resonance imaging; diffusion-weighted imaging brain water determination; posttraumatic ventriculomegaly.

Introduction

Vasogenic edema, secondary to blood-brain barrier compromise following traumatic brain injury, has long been thought to be the major contributor to the swelling process and subsequent rise in intracranial pressure [1, 2]. However, morphologic and magnetic resonance studies of edema following traumatic brain injury cast new light on the swelling process and it is our hypothesis that the role of vasogenic edema, in contrast to a cellular swelling, may have been overemphasized [3–5].

Two recently developed magnetic resonance imaging (MRI) techniques offer the opportunity of early detection and differentiation of the edema formation. The diffusion-weighted imaging (DWI), is sensitized to the random, microscopic translational motion of water protons and provides an image of the apparent diffusion coefficients (ADC) [19]. In a previous study it has been demonstrated that ADC is increased with vasogenic and decreased with cytotoxic forms of edema [4]. The second imaging technique based on precise estimates of tissue longitudinal relaxation time (T1) allows noninvasive measurements of brain water expressed in grams of water per gram of tissue [6, 7].

In the present study, a combination of these two techniques was used to quantify the temporal water content changes and document the type of edema that is occurring during both the acute and the late stages of posttraumatic edema development.

Materials and Methods

Fifty adult male Sprague-Dawley rats weighing 340 to 375 grams were divided into two groups: I. Control (n = 8) and II. Trauma (n = 42). Rats were initially anesthetized with halothane, then intubated and artificially ventilated with a gas mixture of N_2O (70%), O_2 (30%), and halothane (0.5–1.5%). Body temperature was maintained at 37°C ± 0.5°C. A new impact acceleration head injury model was used to produce trauma [8].

Experiments were performed using a 2.35 T, 40 cm bore magnet (Biospec, Bruker Instruments, Billerica, MA) equipped with a 12 cm inner diameter actively shielded gradient insert, with a G_{max} of 25 G/cm.

Two dimensional diffusion-weighted imaging employed a spin echo (SE) sequence. Each data set consisted of two parallel, coronal slices, (3 mm thick, 4 mm center separation), 128 × 128 matrix, TR/TE of 1500/33 ms and 40 mm^2 field of view. The ADC maps determined in the cortex, caudate nucleus and the thalamus were generated for each slice.

For fast ADC measurements *single voxel diffusion-weighted spectroscopy* (VOSY) was used. Voxel dimensions, (typically 5 mm × 5 mm × 5 mm) were selected to fit entirely within the brain in the same region where the coronal sections of the two dimensional diffusion-weighted imaging were chosen. The VOSY employed a stimulated echo sequence.

Our experience in utilizing *MRI for measurement of brain* water is based upon laboratory and clinical studies directed toward non-invasive monitoring of brain edema formation and resolution [6].

Schedule of the measurements: Baseline diffusion weighted (both types) and T1-weighted images (water map) were obtained. The rat was then removed from the magnet, subjected to head injury, and was returned to the magnet immediately after the trauma. VOSY were obtained sequentially (every minute) for one hour post injury. Conventional diffusion-weighted images and T1 images for water content determination were performed at the end of the first hour post injury, at 4 hours, on day 1, 3, 7, 14, 28, and 42.

Results

Water Content Changes

In the control group, water content of the whole brain, cortex and caudate nucleus were $77.8 \pm 0.4\%$, $78.2 \pm 0.2\%$ and $77.5 \pm 0.3\%$. The water content of the cortex was significantly higher than that of the caudate nucleus ($p < 0.001$). The water content did not change during the 6 week period in any of the regions or in the whole brain Fig. 1a. In the *trauma group* the water content immediately increased after trauma in each region as well as in the whole brain. This increase continued during the next 24 hours and reached its maximum value at the end of the first day. During the next two weeks the water content was significantly higher then the control values except on day 3 when a transient decrease was observed. Although, at the end of the week 6 we measured higher values in most of the animals, the difference was not significant in the whole brain. The brain swelling was diffuse, that is, the water map did not show any regional difference in water content.

ADC Changes

Control group: The ADCs measured by VOSY and DWI at baseline (0.70 ± 0.02 and $0.57 \pm 0.04 \times 10^{-3}$ mm²/sec) did not show any significant changes during the 6 week interval of the study (Fig. 1a). *Trauma group:* The baseline values were not different from those of the control group (VOSY ADC: $0.70 \pm 0.02 \times 10^{-3}$ mm²/sec; DWI ADC: $0.57 \pm 0.04 \times 10^{-3}$ mm²/sec). During the first 45 minutes post trauma the ADC measured by VOSY technique showed a significant increase ($p < 0.001$), with a maximum value of $0.77 \pm 0.04 \times 10^{-3}$ mm²/sec at 45 minutes. This transient elevation of the ADC was followed by a gradual decrease beginning at 40–60 minutes post injury, and the ADC crossed the baseline value at 24 hours. Beyond this time the ADC reduction continued

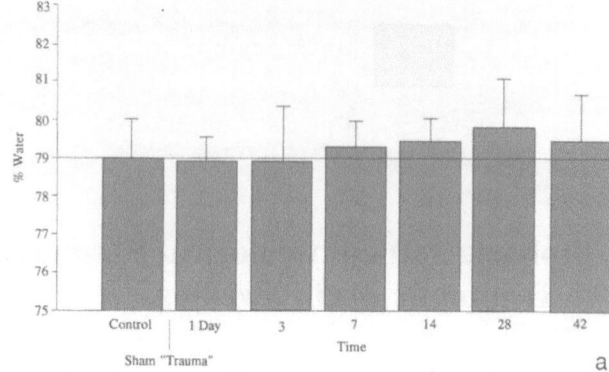

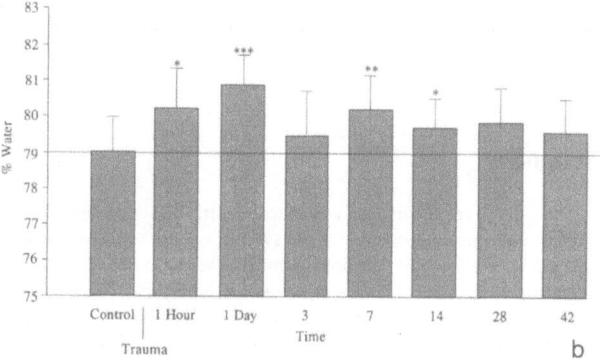

Fig. 1. Time course of brain water content. (a) Control group, the water content did not change during the 6 week period in any of the regions or in the whole brain. (b) Trauma group, the water content immediately increased after trauma and reached its maximum value at the end of the first day. During the next two weeks the water content was significantly higher then the control values except on day 3 when a transient decrease was observed. Values showed mean standard deviation

and a minimum value of $0.52 \pm 0.04 \times 10^{-3}$/mm²/sec (whole brain) was observed at 7–14 days post injury (by 2 dimensional DWI). Interestingly, return of ADC to normal value was observed only at 4 weeks after the trauma (Fig. 1b). The cerebral cortex and caudate nuclens showed the most pronounced decrease (cortex from 0.58 ± 0.02 to $0.53 \pm 0.03 \times 10^{-3}$ mm²/sec and the caudate nucleus, from 0.53 ± 0.02 to $0.49 \pm 0.03 \times 10^{-3}$ mm²/sec), and the mean value of maximal percentage change was 103%. The ADC change in the thalamus was not significant.

Discussion

Traumatic brain edema has usually been distinguished from other forms of edema by its origin, namely the leakage of plasma borne substances from the vasculature as a result of a breakdown of the BBB [9]. However, in light of more recent studies, it may be incorrect to strictly assign the term vasogenic to trau-

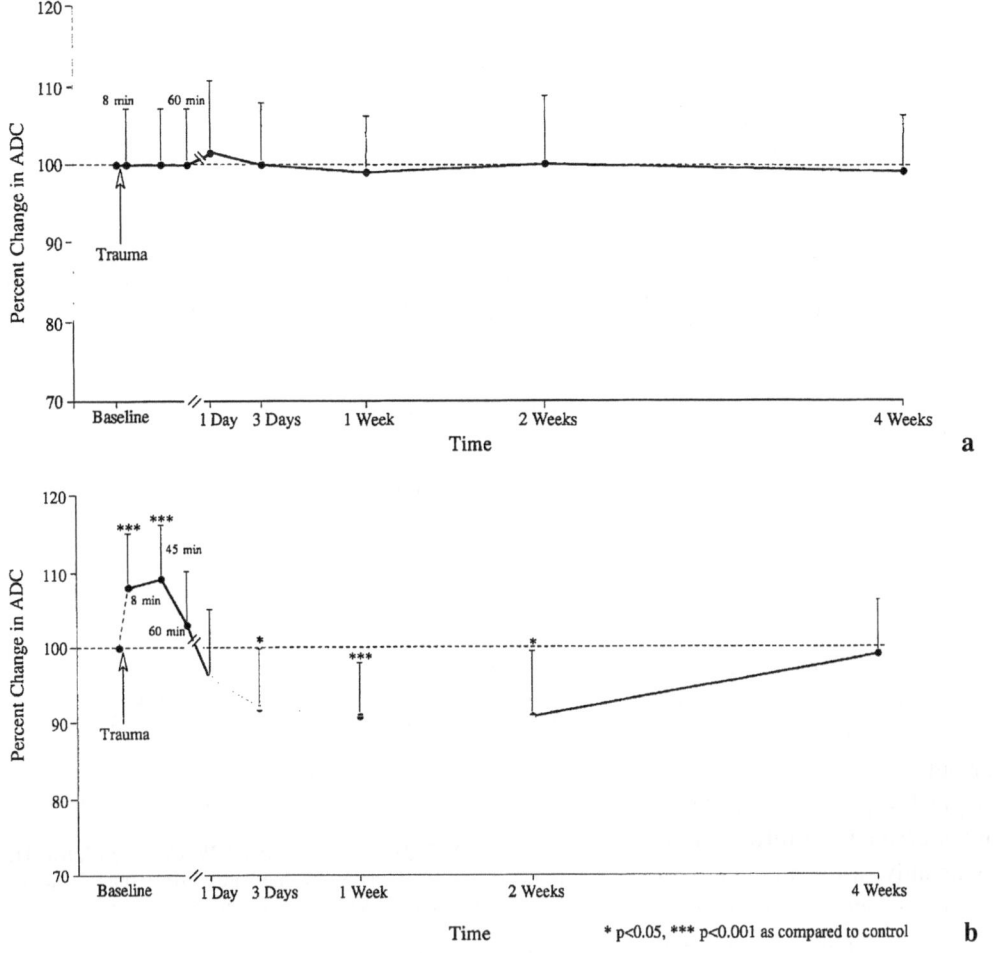

Fig. 2. Time course of apparent diffusion coefficients (ADC). (a) Control group, the ADC did not change during the 6 week period in any of the regions or in the whole brain. (b) Trauma group, during the first 45 minutes post trauma the ADC showed a significant increase. This transient elevation was followed by a gradual decrease beginning 40–60 minutes post injury, and the ADC crossed the baseline value at 24 hours. Beyond this time the ADC reduction continued and its minimum was observed at 7–14 days post injury

matic edema, as other forms of edema are now considered to play an important role in the swelling process. Cellular edema associated with ischemia has been designated cytotoxic according to the original classification by Klatzo [9]. Cellular swelling that occurs in the absence of ischemia is considered neurotoxic and may result as a consequence of ionic disruption associated with traumatic injury [10]. Thus at least three forms of edema, vasogenic (extracellular), ischemic and neurotoxic (both intracellular) may be contributing to the increased tissue water following trauma. In the present study, the changes in ADC after severe closed head injury suggest that the type of edema, cellular or vasogenic, is changing with time after the traumatic insult. We found a significant increase in ADC as well as in brain water content during the first 60 minutes post injury. In our previous study, in which the BBB was

tested with contrast agent (Gd-DTPA) in MRI, we demonstrated that the BBB opens at the time of the trauma and approaches closure at about 30 minutes post injury [3]. If we take all of these observations in concert we may conclude, that these results are consistent with an increase in the volume of the extracellular fluid and vasogenic edema formation.

Analysis of the ADC changes demonstrated that the transient increase was followed by a gradual decrease in ADC beginning at 40–60 minutes post injury and reaching a minimum at the day 7. Thereafter, the ADC remained negative until day 14 and by day 28 returned to baseline. Since the water content of the brain continued to increase during the next 24 hours after injury, we posit, that the fluid taken up by the cells must have been originated either from the blood circulation, or from the extracellular space. Based on these observations we conclude that cellular edema begins to develop at 40–60 minutes post injury and remains predominantly cytotoxic for up to 14 days. We use the term predominant as the ADC measures the net difference between cellular and extracellular forms of edema, and it is entirely possible that a vasogenic component may contribute a small portion to the total tissue water.

Although energy failure after trauma is less evident, the end result of ischemia and brain trauma is the same, that is cell dysfunction and cell death. Therefore, it can be assumed a sequence of events is occurring, in which several different precipitating factors lead to the same final common pathway of injury progression. Although information about the process of cytotoxic damage in traumatic brain injury is limited, considerable evidence exists, that loss of calcium homeostasis, release of excitotoxic amino acids and free radicals as well as acidosis give rise to parenchymal damage [10]. Therefore, in the absence of ischemia or barrier compromise (later than 30 minutes), and the presence of a decreased water diffusion distance it is reasonable to suspect neurotoxic edema playing a major role in the swelling process.

On the basis of these results we suggest, that there is a biphasic pathophysiological response to closed head injury. First, there is an increased water diffusion distance signifying a predominantly vasogenic edema formation immediately after injury. Second, a more widespread and slower edema formation due to a predominant cellular swelling which begins within one hour post injury and becomes dominant at 1–2 weeks post injury. These results provide compelling evidence that cellular edema plays a major role in the swelling process and that the contribution of vasogenic edema may be overemphasized in diffuse traumatic injury.

Acknowledgment

This research was supported in part by Grant P01 NS12587 and R01 NS19235 from the National Institutes of Health.

References

1. Klatzo I, Chui E, Fujiwara K (1980) Resolution of vasogenic brain edema. In: Cervós-Navaro J, Ferszt R (eds) Advances in neurology, vol 28. Brain edema. Raven, New York, pp 359–373
2. Reulen HJ, Graham R, Spatz M, Klatzo I (1977) Role of pressure gradients and bulk flow in dynamics of vasogenic brain edema. J Neurosurg 46: 24–36
3. Barzo P, Marmarou A, Fatouros P, Corwin F, Dunbar J (1996) MRI-monitored acute blood-brain barrier changes in experimental traumatic brain injury. J Neurosurg 85: 1113–1121
4. Ito J, Marmarou A, Barzo P, Fatouros P, Corwin F (1996) Characterization of edema by diffusion-weighted imaging in experimental traumatic brain injury. J Neurosurg 84: 97–103
5. Marmarou A (1994) Traumatic brain edema: an overview. In: Ito U, Baethmann A, Hossmann KA, Kuroiwa T, Marmarou A, Reulen HJ, Takakura K (eds) Brain edema IX. Acta Neurochir (Wien) [Suppl] 60: 421–424
6. Le Bihan D, Breton E, Lallemand D, Greiner P, Cabanis E, Laval-Jeantet M (1986) Magnetic resonance imaging of intravoxel incoherent motions: application to diffusion and perfusion in neurologic disorders. Radiology 161: 401–407
7. Fatouros PP, Marmarou A, Kraft KA (1991) *In vivo* determination by T1 measurements: effect of total water content, hydration fraction 1 and field strength. Magn Reson Med 17: 402–413
8. Marmarou A, Foda AE, van den Brink W, Campbell J, Kita H, Demetriadou K (1994) A new model of diffuse brain injury in rats. Part I: Pathophysiology and biomechanics. J Neurosurg 80: 291–300
9. Klatzo I (1967) Neuropathological aspects of brain edema. J Neuropathol Exp Neurol 26: 1–14
10. Siesj BK (1993) Basic mechanisms of traumatic brain damage. Ann Emerg Med 22: 959–969

Correspondence: Anthony Marmarou, Division of Neurosurgery, P.O. Box 980508, Sanger Hall, Room 8004, 1101 E Marshal St., Richmond, VA 23298, U.S.A.

Acta Neurochir (1997) [Suppl] 70: 123–125
© Springer-Verlag 1997

Intracranial Pressure in a Modified Experimental Model of Closed Head Injury

K. Engelborghs[1], **J. Verlooy**[1], **B. Van Deuren**[2], **J. Van Reempts**[2], and **M. Borgers**[1]

[1] Department of Neurosurgery, University of Antwerp, and [2] Department of Life Sciences, Janssen Research Foundation, Beerse, Belgium

Summary

Intracranial pressure (ICP) was studied in a modified experimental model of closed head injury, in which the dynamic process of impact versus impulse loading was separately controlled. In this model, mortality of Wistar rats was considerably higher as compared to Sprague-Dawley rats subjected to similar traumatic conditions. Therefore Sprague-Dawley rats were used for all further experiments. Twenty-four rats, divided into 4 groups, underwent either sham or gradually increasing impact-acceleration trauma. Four hours after closed head injury, ICP measurements showed a significant correlation between the severity of the traumatic challenge and the resultant pressure rise ($r^2 = 0.731$; $p < 0.001$). At the moment of impact there was a momentary blood pressure peak immediately followed by a transient period of hypotension. ICP measurements following directly to an impact-acceleration trauma, revealed an abrupt rise in ICP reaching pathological levels within 5 minutes. In conclusion, this modified model of closed head injury produces a predictable and reproducible pathologic ICP in Sprague-Dawley rats.

Keywords: Experimental head injury; intracranial pressure; impulse loading; animal model.

Introduction

This paper describes a modified experimental model of closed head injury in the rat which may be used as a tool to better understand the pathophysiological cascade after neurotrauma. In blunt head trauma, primary brain injury may result in focal or diffuse damage. Secondary events, occurring soon after the impact, are probably more detrimental to brain function than the initial mechanical insult. Several models of traumatic brain injury have been previously described in the literature [1, 2]. Amongst them, closed head injury and fluid-percussion models are regarded as the most commonly used. The latter preferentially produce a focal brain contusion and are complicated by artifacts resulting from the experimental methodology. There-fore a closed head injury model of impact-acceleration [3, 4] was chosen and modified to allow adjustment of the dynamic process of impact-acceleration, i.e. variable impact loading (contusion) and impulsive loading (concussion). Furthermore, besides a rise in intracranial pressure (ICP), an absolute prerequisite in this model, is the presence of morphological aberrations comparable to those encountered in clinical neuropathology.

Materials and Methods

Animal housing and treatment conditions complied with EU directive for Animal Wellfare #86/609.

Trauma Device

The trauma device is composed of two components. A first part is a hollow Plexiglas column with inner diameter of 20 mm and a length of 1.5 m. It contains a segmented steel cylinder with outer diameter of 19 mm, constructed to allow use of weights ranging from 50 g to 500 g. The steel cylinder falls freely from designated heights through the column by gravity. The impact-site of the cylinder, is a slightly deformable silicon disc of 9 mm diameter and 2 mm thickness. The entire set-up is firmly fixed to a horizontal platform and precisely leveled. The second part is a horizontal platform mounted on replaceable springs of variable elasticity. Onto the horizontal platform a stereotaxic head frame is fixed to allow accurate positioning of the rat. Six springs are asymmetrically positioned to allow a vertical downward displacement of the entire horizontal platform after impact, thereby avoiding critical hyperextension of the neck.

Induction of Head Trauma

Blunt trauma is induced on the unprotected skull of intubated halothane (1%) anesthetized Sprague-Dawley rats weighing between 360 g and 380 g. The inter-aural line was used as reference coordinate. The impact was leveled at the bregma of the rat skull. ICP was recorded using a Codman micro-sensor probe, inserted in the right parietal cortex. Blood pressure and rectal temperature were monitored. Histology was performed on brain tissue, perfusion-fixed in formaldehyde and routinely prepared for light- and electronmicroscopy.

Experimental Set-up

In a preliminary experimental series the consequences of traumatic impact (60 cm/400 g) were compared between Wistar and Sprague-Dawley rats (n = 10) 4 hours after the impact. In a second series, ICP levels were determined at 4 hours after 400 g impacts from 25, 40 and 55 cm in comparison with a sham condition (n = 6/group). In a third series, an impact force was chosen from which a predictable injury could be expected (47 cm, 400 g; n = 6). Its influence on ICP was continuously recorded during 4 hours in comparison to shams (n = 3). Throughout the whole procedure, rats were anesthetized with 1% halothane.

Results

Wistar rats showed a considerably higher mortality rate (50%) as compared to Sprague-Dawley rats (no mortality) undergoing the same impact-acceleration trauma. Preliminary experiments demonstrated that mortality was caused mainly by respiratory failure secondary to the development of severe pulmonary edema or by direct biomechanical brainstem trauma leading to persistent apnea. Direct brainstem trauma was usually accompanied by convulsions. The skull fracture incidence in both groups was 50%. In a second experiment, gradually increasing impact-acceleration conditions resulted in a significant correlation between ICP rise and severity of traumatic challenge at 4 hours. This is shown in figure one together with the line of

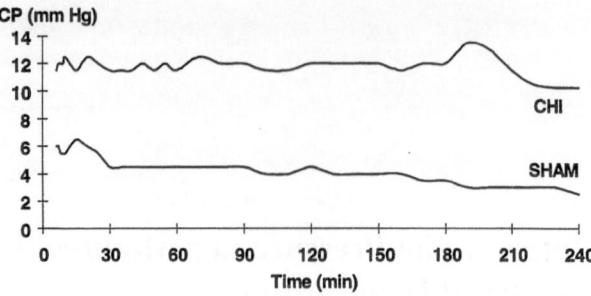

Fig. 2. Continuous intracranial pressure recordings in rats subjected to closed head injury of 47 cm and 400 g (n = 6) and sham-operated rats (n = 3)

best fit as determined by linear regression (Fig. 1, ICP = 4.9 ($\pm$ 0.74) + ($\pm$ 0.02) $\times$ Height, p < 0.001). In the 40 cm group 1 rat was accidentally lost at 4 h. In the 55 cm group 4 out of 6 rats had a closed linear skull fracture and 2 rats died within the first 1 hour following trauma. At the moment of impact there was a brief blood pressure surge immediately followed by a transient period of hypotension. Histological examination of the brains of the 55 cm group after 4 hours, did not show glial swelling, irreversible neuronal damage or axonal injury. In a third series, continuous ICP measurement after impact-acceleration trauma of 47 cm and 400 g revealed an abrupt pressure rise reaching pathological levels within 5 minutes (Fig. 2).

Discussion

This modified experimental model of closed head injury has shown that it is possible to produce a reliable, predictable and pathologic ICP with a limited amount of skull fractures and low mortality. The higher mortality within the Wistar strain as compared to the Sprague-Dawley strain, can be explained by a difference in skull anatomy, resulting in a different biomechanical response to the impact-acceleration trauma. We demonstrated a logical correlation between the severity of the head trauma and the rise in ICP after 4 hours. ICP measurements recorded immediately after closed head injury revealed a rapid rise in ICP. Further studies are needed to determine which pathological process may cause the sudden increase in ICP. The present traumatic conditions resulted in a pathological ICP, but did not lead to detectable histological changes such as cellular edema, irreversible neurodegeneration or diffuse axonal damage. However, recent studies indicate that increased impact-acceleration challenges result in higher ICP values and concomitant morpho-

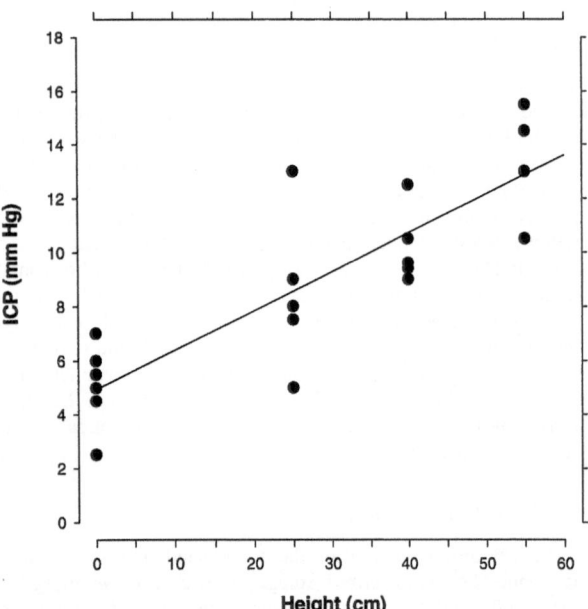

Fig. 1. Individual intracranial pressure measurements at 4 hours after gradually increasing traumatic challenge (height) with line of best fit

logical damage (manuscript in preparation). Since this model allows variations in the balance between impact and acceleration components, it can be regarded as a valuable tool to analyze the complex pathophysiological cascade of traumatic brain injury caused by different impact-acceleration settings.

References

1. Lighthall JW, Anderson TE (1994) *In vivo* models of experimental brain and spinal cord trauma. In: Salzman SK, Faden IA (eds) The neurobiology of central nervous system trauma. Oxford University Press, New York, pp 3–11

2. McIntosh TK, Smith DH, Meaney DF, Kotapka MJ, Gennarelli TA, Graham DI (1996) Neuropathological sequelae of traumatic brain injury: relationship to neurochemical and biomechanical mechanisms. Lab Invest 74: 315–342

3. Marmarou A, Montasser A, Foda A-E, van den Brink W, Campbell J, Kita H, Demetriadou K (1994) A new model of diffuse brain injury in rats. Part I: Pathophysiology and biomechanics. J Neurosurg 80: 291–309

4. Montasser A, Foda A-E, Marmarou A (1994) A new model of diffuse brain injury in rats. Part II: Morphological characterization. J Neurosurg 80: 301–313

Correspondence: Koen Engelborghs, M.D., University Hospital Antwerp, Department of Neurosurgery, Wilrijkstraat 10, B-2650 Edegem, Belgium.

Acta Neurochir (1997) [Suppl] 70: 126–129
© Springer-Verlag 1997

Hypertonic/Hyperoncotic Saline Reliably Reduces ICP in Severely Head-Injured Patients with Intracranial Hypertension

R. Härtl[1], **J. Ghajar**[1], **H. Hochleuthner**[2], and **W. Mauritz**[2]

[1] The Aitken Neuroscience Institute and Cornell University Medical College, New York, NY, U.S.A., and
[2] Trauma Hospital "Lorenz-Böhler", Vienna, Austria

Summary

Hypertonic saline (HS) has been shown to decrease intracranial pressure (ICP) and cerebral water content in experimental models of traumatic brain injury (TBI). The purpose of the present study was to test the efficacy of administration of HS (7,5%) combined with 6% hydroxyethyl starch (molecular weight 200.000/0.60–0.66; HHES) for the treatment of therapy-resistant intracranial hypertension in patients with severe TBI. Six patients with severe TBI (GCS < 8) who met the inclusion criteria (therapy resistant ICP > 25 mmHg, cerebral perfusion pressure (CPP) < 60 mmHg, plasma-Na^+ < 150 mOsm and > 4 hours since the last HS/HHES treatment) were prospectively enrolled in the study and received between one and ten bolus infusions of maximal 250 ml HS/HHES at a rate of 20 ml/min. A total of 32 infusions were given.

Administration of HS/HHES significantly lowered ICP by 44% and improved CPP by 38% to well above 70 mmHg at 30 min without affecting arterial blood pressure or blood gases. Plasma sodium normalized within 30 min. Experimental studies from our laboratory indicate that the ICPlowering effect is primarily due to dehydration of brain tissue and that cerebral blood volume remains largely unaffected by HS.

In summary, HS/HHES reduces otherwise therapy-resistant intracranial hypertension and improves cerebral perfusion even after repeated administration without negatively affecting blood pressure or causing a rebound ICP increase.

Keywords: Head injury; hypertonic saline; small-volume resuscitation; colloids; intracranial pressure.

Introduction

Optimal management of severely head-injured patients with brain edema and intracranial hypertension (IH) is still controversial. Guidelines by the Neurotrauma and Critical Care Joint AANS/CNS Section present a critical pathway for the treatment of established IH [4]. Arterial blood pressure sufficiently high to keep the cerebral perfusion pressure (CPP) above 70 mmHg is regarded as one of the keystones of intracranial pressure (ICP) management to prevent secondary ischemic insults to the brain. Unfortunately, most maneuvers currently used for ICP treatment bear the risk of further reducing perfusion of the brain either by lowering mean arterial blood pressure (MAP) and CPP (mannitol, barbiturates), or by causing cerebral vasoconstriction (hypocapnia). This underlines the need for a therapeutic tool that effectively reduces ICP while preserving or improving CPP.

Treatment of therapy-resistant IH with small volumes of hypertonic saline (HS) has been reported in the past and was associated with a reduction of ICP [5, 13, 28]. The effect of repeated administration of HS over the course of several days, however, has not been investigated. Concerns regarding the possible ICP "rebound" phenomenon, similar to the one observed after repetitive mannitol infusions, have been expressed and would discourage an introduction of this potentially viable treatment modality into clinical practice.

Against this background the present study was conducted in order to test the hypothesis that repeated administration of a new infusion containing HS and hyperoncotic hydroxyethyl starch (HHES) decreases otherwise refractory IH and improves CPP in severe TBI.

Patients and Methods

Six consecutive patients (1 female, 5 males; mean age 32, range 22–47 yrs) with severe TBI (GCS < 8) were enrolled prospectively.* ICP was monitored using an epidural Spiegelberg device. Routine treatment of IH included elevation of head, mild hyperventilation to a pCO_2 of 30–35 mmHg, administration of mannitol, opioids and sedatives. Patients received the study medication if the routine treatment failed to prevent IH and the inclusion criteria were met.

---

* Approval for the study protocol was obtained from the Ethics Committee of the Lorenz-Böhler Trauma Hospital.

Table 1. *Systemic Parameters Before and After Bolus Infusion of 171 ± 74 ml 7.5% NaCl / 6% HES 200.000 in Six Patients, 32 Applications in Total*

	Na$^+$ [mmol/l]	K$^+$ [mmol/l]	CL$^-$ [mmol/l]	Osmolality [mmol/l]	paO$_2$ [mmHg]	paCO$_2$ [mmHg]	pH
Baseline	143.38	4.04	115.03	300.44	128.41	31.94	7.45
SD	5.66	0.51	5.89	12.05	28.65	5.59	0.07
30' after HS/HHES	144.13	4.00	115.16	304.41	124.56	32.66	7.44
SD	5.87	0.51	5.74	12.14	28.07	5.20	0.06

SD Standard deviation.

Inclusion Criteria

- ICP > 25 mmHg;
- CPP < 70 mmHg;
- serum Na$^+$ < 150 mOsm;
- serum osmolality < 320 mOsm;
- > 4 hours since last administration of study medication.

Study Medication

HYPERHAES™, Leopold Inc., Austria. This infusion contains NaCl 7,5% (HS) plus hydroxyethyl starch 6% with a mean molecular weight of 200.000 Dalton/0,60–0,66 (HHES) and has recently been approved for small-volume resuscitation of polytraumatized patients in Austria. The properties of the study drug (sodium concentration 1282 mmol/l, osmolality 2500 mOsm/l, oncotic pressure 62 mmHg) require administration via a central vein.

The HS/HHES infusion was given at a rate of 20 ml/min and was terminated as soon as ICP dropped below 25 mmHg, CPP increased above 70 mmHg or 250 ml HS/HHES had been administered. The intervention was repeated if the patient met the inclusion criteria. The six patients received a total of 32 HS/HHES bolus infusions, between one and ten applications per patient, all within ten days after admission to the ICU. Heart rate (HR), MAP, ICP, and CPP were documented before, 10 and 30 min after HS/HHES infusion. Plasma sodium, potassium, chloride, osmolality and blood gases (pO$_2$, pCO$_2$, pH) were determined before and 30 min after infusion.

Data are depicted as means ± standard deviation. CPP was calculated as MAP minus ICP. The paired t-test was used for statistical comparisons; a p-value < 0.05 was considered significant.

Experimental Study

Parallel to this clinical study experiments were performed in our laboratory (Aitken Neuroscience Institute and Cornell University Medical College, New York) investigating the effect of hypertonic saline / dextran on post-traumatic cerebral blood volume changes in pigs. Seven anesthetized minipigs underwent a 2.5 atm. fluid-percussion TBI and were followed for 5.5 h.* At 4 h the animals received a bolus of 4 ml/kg b.w. 7.5% NaCl/10% Dextran 60 (HSD). Parameters measured included ICP (Codman, Johnson & Johnson) and cerebral blood volume (CBV) using Technetium-99m (^{99m}Tc) labeled red blood cells [11]. Briefly, 10 ml of whole blood was labeled with ^{99m}Tc and reinfused. Regional CBV was measured directly by 4 gamma collimators placed over both cerebral hemispheres. The collimators employed a 20% window over the 140-keV photopeak of ^{99m}Tc. Two additional collimators were

positioned over the animals' lower extremities in order to correct for systematic changes in hematocrit and for the natural decay of the isotope. This allowed us to determine relative changes of CBV over time.

Results

An average of 171 ± 74 ml (range 80–250 ml) HS/HHES were infused per treatment. Heart rate remained unchanged (baseline 93 ± 23 vs. 91 ± 19 at 10 min and 97 ± 24 beats/min at 30 min after HS/HHES infusion). The effects on MAP, ICP and CPP are demonstrated in Fig. 1. MAP remained unchanged while ICP decreased significantly from 45 ± 15 to 25 ± 14 mmHg and CPP increased significantly from 52 ± 18 to 72 ± 16 mmHg. There was no significant difference between the values found at 10 and 30 minutes after infusion of HS/HHES. The administration of HS/HHES did not have any adverse effects on electrolytes, blood gases or plasma osmolality (Table 1). At 30 min after infusion plasma sodium and osmolality were within baseline values.

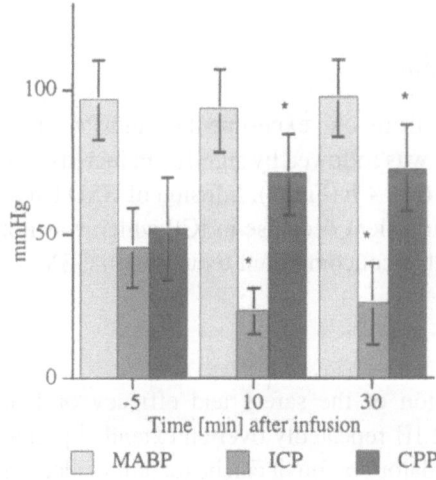

Fig. 1. Response of MAP, ICP and CPP to bolus infusion of 171 ± 74 ml 7.5% NaCl / 6% HES 200.000 in six patients, 32 applications in total (mean ± standard deviation). * p < 0.05 vs. baseline (–5 min)

---

* The experimental study was approved by the Cornell University Medical College Animal Use Committee.

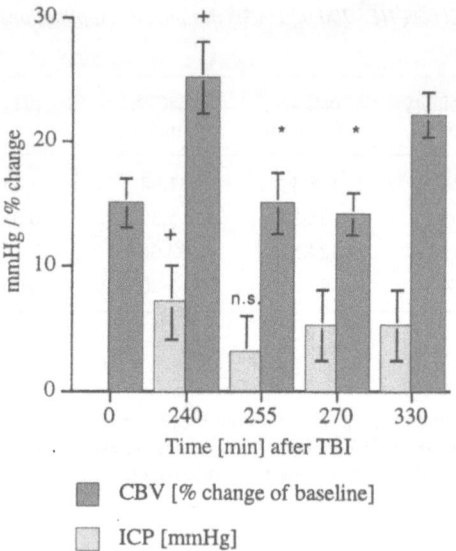

Fig. 2. Cerebral blood volume (CBV) and ICP after traumatic brain injury (TBI) in pigs. Seven anesthetized minipigs underwent a 2.5 atm. fluid-percussion TBI at 0 min and were followed for 5.5 h. At 4 h the animals received a bolus of 4 ml/kg b.w. 7.5% NaCl/10% Dextran 60 (HSD). CBV was determined using Technetium-99m-labeled red blood cells. Dehydration of brain tissue as the main factor responsible for ICP reduction is supported by the finding that post-traumatically increased CBV was largely unaffected by HSD administration. * $p < 0.05$ vs. pre-infusion values at 240 min; + $p < 0.05$ vs. baseline at 0 min; *n.s.* not significant vs. baseline at 0 min

Repeated treatment was *always* followed by a decrease in ICP and did not require the infusion of greater volumes of HS/HHES.

At six months after injury four patients had a good outcome (Glasgow Outcome Score, GOS, 5), one was mildly disabled (GOS 4) and one had died due to uncontrollable IH (GOS 1).

Experimental Study

The results from our experimental study demonstrate that TBI was followed by significant increases in ICP and CBV over 4 h (Fig. 2). Infusion of HSD led to a prompt but transient decrease in ICP which was not associated with a concommitant reduction in CBV.

Discussion

Demonstration of the safety and efficacy of HS/HHES to treat IH repeatedly over an extended period of time is mandatory before it can be recommended for clinical use. The present findings suggest that HS/HHES administration in IH is safe and improves CPP without affecting MAP. This is important because

most conventional ICP-lowering maneuvers bear the risk of further reducing perfusion to the brain by either decreasing blood pressure and CPP (mannitol, barbiturates) or by causing cerebral vasoconstriction (induced by hypocapnia). Other potential side-effects such as critical increases in plasma osmolality or blood gas alterations were not observed in our study. Repeated treatment was always followed by a decrease in ICP and did not require the infusion of greater volumes of HS/HHES. Also, we did not observe transient blood pressure changes during HS/HHES infusion (data not shown), probably because the rate of infusion (20 ml/min) was rather slow. Nervertheless, MAP and plasma osmolality should be carefully monitored.

What is the Mechanism of Action of Hypertonic/Hyperoncotic Saline?

Substantial experimental data have been gathered on the effects of hypertonic fluid resuscitation on the central nervous system after injury [1–3, 6–10, 16–19, 25–27, 29]. A reduction of increased ICP has been observed after administration of HS and is generally attributed to the dehydration of non-injured brain tissue with an intact blood-brain barrier (BBB) [1, 20]. One of us (R.H.) recently reported that treatment with 4 ml/kg 7.2% NaCl/10% dextran 60 after cryogenic brain injury in rabbits decreased brain water content even in areas adjacent to the trauma where the BBB was disrupted [9]. Dehydration of brain tissue as the main factor responsible for ICP reduction is further supported by the finding that in our pig fluid-percussion experiments post-traumatically increased CBV was largely unaffected by HSD. Mannitol, on the other hand, presumably decreases ICP through an improvement of blood rheology leading to autoregulatory vasoconstriction of cerebral blood vessels and a reduction of CBV [14, 15]. This difference might account for the therapeutic efficacy of HS in cases such as the ones presented in this paper, where mannitol was not effective.

The present data in conjunction with other clinical studies and reports of beneficial effects of HS alone, HS /hydroxyethylstarch or HS/dextran in severe TBI with and without IH [5, 12, 13, 21–24, 28] strongly encourage further investigation of this drug in the clinical setting. In contrast to mannitol, HS appears to improve cerebral perfusion mainly by dehydrating brain tissue without affecting cerebral blood volume. Hypertonic/hyperoncotic saline could become an important addition to the therapeutic armamentarium for

ICP management due to its ability to decrease ICP and improve cerebral perfusion without affecting MAP.

Acknowledgements

The experimental study was supported by the Annie Laurie Aitken Charitable Trust Fund. The authors wish to thank Dr. Robert Hariri for his advice and support in conducting the animal experiments.

The clinical work was done at the Trauma Hospital "Lorenz Böhler", Vienna, Austria. The experiments were conducted at the Aitken Neuroscience Institute, Cornell University Medical College, New York.

References

1. Battistella F, Wisner D (1992) Cerebral dehydration following hypertonic saline resuscitation. Circ Shock 37: 16
2. Battistella FD, Wisner DH (1991) Combined hemorrhagic shock and head injury: effects of hypertonic saline (7.5%) resuscitation. J Trauma 31: 182–188
3. Berger S, Schürer L, Härtl R, et al (1995) Reduction of post-traumatic intracranial hypertention by hypertonic/hyperoncotic saline/dextran and mannitol. Neurosurgery 37: 98–108
4. Bullock R, Chesnut R, Clifton G, et al (1995) Guidelines for the management of severe head injury. J.S.o.N.a.C.C. AANS Brain Trauma Foundation, New York
5. Fisher B, Thomas D, Peterson B (1992) Hypertonic saline lowers raised ICP in children after head trauma. J Neurosurg Anesth 4: 4–10
6. Gunnar WP, Merlotti GJ, Barrett J, et al (1986) Resuscitation from hemorrhagic shock. Alterations of the intracranial pressure after normal saline, 3% saline and dextran –40. Ann Surg 204: 686–692
7. Härtl R, Cohen D, Medary M, et al (1995) Effect of hypertonic saline/dextran on intracranial pressure, cerebral blood volume and brain edema after traumatic brain injury in pigs. J Neurotrauma 12: 416 (Abstract)
8. Härtl R, Schürer L, Dautermann C, et al (1993) Effect of hypertonic-hyperoncotic solutions (HHS) on increased ICP after a focal brain lesion and inflation of an intracranial balloon. In: Avezaat CJJ (ed) Intracranial pressure VIII. Springer, Berlin Heidelberg New York Tokyo, pp 612–614
9. Härtl R, Schürer L, Goetz C, et al (1995) The effect of hypertonic fluid resuscutation on brain edema in rabbits subjected to brain injury and hemorrhagic shock. Shock 3: 274–279
10. Kreimeier U, Brueckner UB, Schmidt J, et al (1990) Instantaneous restoration of regional organ blood flow after severe hemorrhage: effect of small-volume resuscitation with hypertonic-hyperoncotic solutions. J Surg Res 49: 493–503
11. Kuhl DE, Alavi A, Hoffman EJ, et al (1980) Local cerebral blood volume in head-injured patients. Determination by emission computed tomography of ^{99m}Tc-labeled red cells. J Neurosurg 52: 309–320
12. Mattox KL, Maningas PA, Moore EE, et al (1991) Prehospital hypertonic saline/dextran infusion for post-traumatic hypotension. The U.S.A. Multicenter Trial. Ann Surg 213: 482–491
13. Meier-Hellmann A, Hannemann L, Kuss B, et al (1990) Treatment of therapy resistant ICP by application of hypertonic saline. Eur Surg Res 22: 303–304
14. Muizelaar JP, Lutz HA, Becker DP (1984) Effect of mannitol on ICP and CBF and correlation with pressure autoregulation in severely head-injured patients. J Neurosurg 61: 700–706
15. Muizelaar JP, Wei EP, Kontos HA, et al (1983) Mannitol causes compensatory cerebral vasoconstriction and vasodilation in response to blood viscosity changes. J Neurosurg 59: 822–828
16. Prough DS, Whitley JM, Taylor CL, et al (1991) Regional cerebral blood flow following resuscitation from hemorrhagic shock with hypertonic saline. Influence of a subdural mass [see comments]. Anesthesiology 75: 319–327
17. Schürer L, Dautermann C, Härtl R, et al (1992) Treatment of hemorrhagic hypotension with hypertonic/hyperoncotic solutions: effects on regional cerebral blood flow and brain surface oxygen tension. Eur Surg Res 24: 1–12
18. Shackford SR, Norton CH, Todd MM (1988) Renal, cerebral, and pulmonary effects of hypertonic resuscitation in a porcine model of hemorrhagic shock. Surgery 104: 553–560
19. Shackford SR, Schmoker JD, Zhuang J (1994) The effect of hypertonic resuscitation on pial arteriolar tone after brain injury and shock. J Trauma 37: 899–908
20. Shackford SR, Zhuang J, Schmoker J (1992) Intravenous fluid tonicity: effect on intracranial pressure, cerebral blood flow, and cerebral oxygen delivery in focal brain injury. J Neurosurg 76: 91–98
21. Vassar MJ, Fischer RP, O'Brien PE, et al (1993) A multicenter trial for resuscitation of injured patients with 7.5% sodium chloride. The effect of added dextran 70. The Multicenter Group for the Study of Hypertonic Saline in Trauma Patients. Arch Surg 128: 1003-1011
22. Vassar MJ, Perry CA, Gannaway WL, et al (1991) 7.5% sodium chloride/dextran for resuscitation of trauma patients undergoing helicopter transport. Arch Surg 126: 1065–1072
23. Vassar MJ, Perry CA, Holcroft JW (1990) Analysis of potential risks associated with 7.5% sodium chloride resuscitation of traumatic shock [published erratum appears in Arch Surg 1991 126 (1): 43]. Arch Surg 125: 1309–1315
24. Vassar MJ, Perry CA, Holcroft JW (1993) Prehospital resuscitation of hypotensive trauma patients with 7.5% NaCl versus 7.5% NaCl with added dextran: a controlled trial. J Trauma 34: 622–632
25. Walsh JC, Zhuang J, Shackford SR (1991) A comparison of hypertonic to isotonic fluid in the resuscitation of brain injury and hemorrhagic shock. J Surg Res 50: 284–292
26. Wisner D, Busche F, Sturm J, et al (1989) Traumatic shock and head injury: effects of fluid resuscitation on the brain. J Surg Res 46: 49–59
27. Wisner DH, Schuster L, Quinn C (1990) Hypertonic saline resuscitation of head injury: effects on cerebral water content. J Trauma 30: 75–78
28. Worthley LI, Cooper DJ, Jones N (1988) Treatment of resistant intracranial hypertension with hypertonic saline. Report of two cases. J Neurosurg 68: 478–481
29. Zornow MH, Scheller MS, Shackford SR (1989) Effect of a hypertonic lactated Ringer's solution on intracranial pressure and cerebral water content in a model of traumatic brain injury. J Trauma 29: 484–488

Correspondence: Roger Härtl, M.D., Department of Neurosurgery, Virchow-Klinikum, Humboldt Universität Berlin, Augustenburger Platz 1, D-13353 Berlin, Federal Republic of Germany.

Acta Neurochir (1997) [Suppl] 70: 130–133
© Springer-Verlag 1997

Topical Application of Insulin Like Growth Factor-1 Reduces Edema and Upregulation of Neuronal Nitric Oxide Synthase Following Trauma to the Rat Spinal Cord

H. S. Sharma[1–3], **F. Nyberg**[2], **T. Gordh**[3], **P. Alm**[4], and **J. Westman**[1]

Laboratory of Neuroanatomy, [1] Department of Anatoma, [2] Department of Pharmaceutical Biosciences, Biomedical Centre, and [3] Department of Anaesthesiology, University Hospital, Uppsala University, Uppsala, and [4] Department of Pathology, University Hospital Lund, Lund, Sweden

Summary

The neuroprotective effects of insulin like growth factor-1 (IGF-1) on spinal cord injury induced edema formation, cell changes and profound upregulation of constitutive isoform of neuronal nitric oxide synthase (cNOS) was examined in a rat model. A focal spinal cord injury produced by making a lesion (about 2 mm deep and 5 mm long) of the right dorsal horn of the T10–11 segment resulted in a marked edema formation, cell injury and upregulation of cNOS following 5 h after trauma. In separate groups application of IGF-1 (0.1 μg/μl) topically on the exposed spinal cord (T10–11) starting from 30 min before injury (20 μl), immediately before injury followed by 30 min, 60 min and thereafter every 1 h after injury until sacrifice resulted in significant attenuation of edema formation and cell changes. Immunohistochemistry showed a less pronounced expression of cNOS in the T9 and T12 segments of the cord in IGF treated rats compared to untreated traumatised controls. These results for the first time show that IGF treatment is neuroprotective and this effects of the IGF appears to be mediated via inhibition of NOS upregulation.

Keywords: Spinal cord injury; insulin like growth factor; nitric oxide synthase; edema.

Introduction

Insulin-like growth factors (IGF) have numerous actions on neuronal and glia cell functions *in vitro*. However, its role in the CNS *in vivo* situation still remains unknown [4–7]. Brain and spinal cord contains relatively high levels of IGF-1 and there are recent evidences which suggest that the content of IGF is reduced following spinal cord injury [5, 12]. On the other hand human cases of amyotrophic lateral scierosis (ALS) showed upregulation of IGF-1 binding in the gray matter of spinal cord [1]. There are reports indicating that various growth factors like IGF-1, nerve growth factors (NGF) and ciliray neurotrophic factor (CNTF) can rescue motor neuron atrophy in Alz-

heimer's diseases, Parkinson diseases, multiple sclerosis and Huntington's diseases [4, 6, 7, 13, 14]. These evidences strongly point out a neuroprotective effect of growth factors in the diseases of nervous system.

Recently the involvement of nitric oxide, a gaseous molecule, in the pathophysiology of cell injury has been suggested [2, 3]. Previous observation from our laboratory showed a marked upregulation of nitric oxide synthase (constitutive and neuronal type, cNOS) following a focal trauma to the rat spinal cord [11]. The number of cNOS positive neurons correlates well with the edematous expansion of the spinal cord and blockade of such activity with cNOS antiserum exhibits neuroprotection indicating an involvement of NO in the pathophysiology of spinal cord edema and cell injury. There are recent evidences indicating that IGF is neuroprotective in ischemic brain injury and experimental autoimmune encephalomyelitis [7, 13]. This investigation was undertaken to examine whether pretreatment with IGF-1 can influence cell changes and edema formation following a focal spinal cord injury in our rat model. Furthermore, in order to clarify the mechanisms of IGF-1 induced neuroprotection we examined the upregulation of cNOS following spinal cord injury using immunohistochemical techniques.

Materials and Methods

Animals

Experiments were carried out on 30 male Wistar rats (body weight 200–300 g) kept under controlled ambient conditions (21 ± 1°C) with 12 h light and 12 h dark schedule. The rat food and tap water were supplied *ad libitum*.

Spinal Cord Injury

Spinal cord injury was inflicted under Equithesin (3 ml/kg, i.p.) anaesthesia by making a longitudinal incision (about 2 mm deep and 5 mm long) into the right dorsal horn of the T10–11 segments [8–10]. The wound was covered with a cotton soaked in 0.9% saline. The rats were allowed to survive 5 h after injury. This experimental condition is approved by the Ethical Committee of Uppsala University.

Treatment with Insulin-like Growth Factor

In a separate group of traumatised rats, IGF-1 (0.1 µg/µl, Kabi Pharmacy, Stockholm) was applied topically on the exposed spinal cord (T10–11) starting from 30 min before injury (20 µl), immediately before injury followed by 30 min, 60 min and thereafter every 1 h after injury until sacrifice.

Spinal Cord Edema

Spinal cord edema was examined using water content of the spinal cord [9, 10]. For this purpose, the spinal cord segments from the T9, T10–11 and T12 were excised, weighed immediately and the placed in an oven maintained at 90°C for 72 h or until the last three measurements of the dry weight were constant. The water content was calculated from the differences between wet and dry weight of the cord.

Nitric Oxide Synthase Immunohistochemistry

For the purpose of NOS immunostaining, the animals were perfused with about 150 ml of 4% paraformaldehyde containing 1.5% glutaraldehyde in 0.1 M phosphate buffer (pH 7.4) at room temperature after a brief washout of the intravascular blood by 0.1 M phosphate buffer (50 ml) at 90 torr perfusion pressure. After perfusion, the animals were wrapped in an aluminium foil and kept overnight at 4°C in a refrigerator. On the next day, the spinal cord samples were dissected out and placed in the same fixative at 4°C. The c-NOS immunoreactivity was examined on free floating vibratome sections (60 µm thick) using antiserum directed against constitutive isoform of neuronal nitric oxide synthase as described earlier [11].

Experimental Protocol

Spinal cord injury (n = 20) was inflicted on the right dorsal horn of the T10–11 segments by making an incision. In one group of animals (n = 10) IGF-1 (0.1 µg/10 µl in phosphate buffer saline) was applied topically 30 min before injury on the exposed spinal cord followed by repeated doses of IGF-1. Normal animals (n = 10) were used as controls. Spinal cord edema was examined in control (n = 5), spinal cord traumatised (n = 5) and IGF treated traumatised (n = 5) rats while NOS immunohistochemistry was done in separate groups of normal (n = 5), spinal cord injured (n = 5) and IGF-1 treated injured (n = 5) rats. Thereafter application of IGF-1 was carried out at every 1 h interval until sacrifice.

Statistical Analysis

The data were analysed statistically using ANOVA followed by Dunnett's test. A p-value less than 0.05 were considered significant.

Results

Spinal Cord Edema

Rats subjected to 5 h spinal cord trauma exhibited profound increase in the spinal cord edema in all the three segments examined. This is apparent with a significant increase in the water content of the T9 (from 66.76 ± 1.23 to 70.23 ± 1.24%, P < 0.001), T10–11 (from 66.87 ± 0.34 to 72.17 ± 0.56%, P < 0.001) and T12 (from 67.04 ± 0.89 to 71.06 ± 0.89%, P < 0.01) segment compared to the control group. Pretreatment with IGF-1 significantly thwarted the edema development in the spinal cord following 5 h after injury. Thus, the water content in the T9 (68.23 ± 0.46%, P < 0.05), T10-11 (69.38 ± 0.56%, P < 0.05) and T12 (68.81 ± 0.38%, P < 0.05) segments was significantly lower compared to the untreated traumatised group (P < 0.05).

Spinal Cord NOS Immunostaining

The control rats showed only a few cNOS positive neurons unevenly distributed in the gray matter of the spinal cord of the T9, T10–11 and T12 segments. A focal trauma to the cord significantly upregulated the NOS immunostaining in the traumatised spinal cord after 5 h. This increase in the NOS immunostaining was most marked in the ipsi-lateral side of the cord compared to the contralateral side. The immunostaining can be seen in the cell cytoplasm and occasionally nucleus of the neurons were densely stained.

Pretreatment with IGF-1 markedly attenuated the cNOS immunostaining in the spinal cord. Thus only a few NOS positive neurons can be seen in the IGF treated traumatised rats. Few NOS neurons showed elongated axons within 5 h period, a feature not observed in untreated rats (Fig. 1).

Examination of NOS immunostaining at ultrastructural level showed that the immunostained material is mainly confined within the cell boarders and located within the cytoplasm attached with endoplasmic reticulum as dark black particies (Fig. 2). This increase in immunostaining at ultrastructural level was much less evident in animals received IGF-1 treatment before injury.

Spinal Cord Pathology

Light microscopy of spinal cord injured rats showed profound swelling and edematous expansion of the cord in the T9, T10–11 and the T12 segments of the cord. The neurons were mainly distorted and the distinction between the gray and white matter of the cord in injured animals was not clear. On the other hand, spinal cord general expansion was considerably reduced and the neurons were less distorted in rats re-

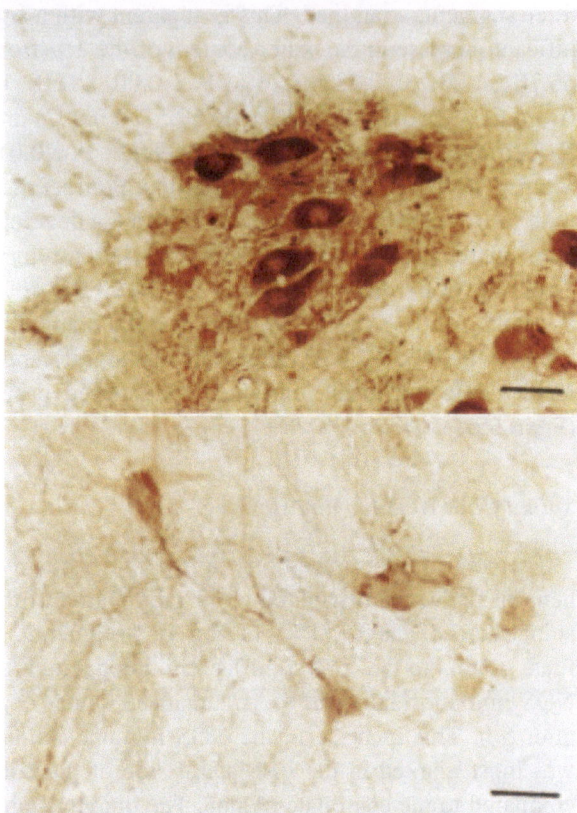

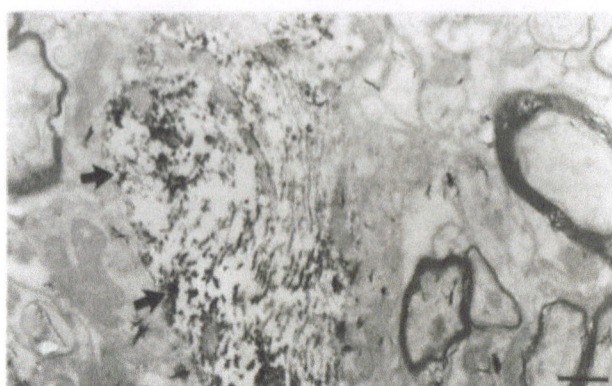

Fig. 2. cNOS immunostaining; T9 ventral horn. Low power electron micrograph shows NOS immunostaining in the cytoplasm of one nerve cell (arrows) attached to the endoplasmic reticulum (dark black particles) following 5 h spinal cord injury in the dorsal horn of the T9 segment (bar = 1 μm)

Fig. 1. 5 h spinal cord injury; T9 ventral horn. Light micrograph of cNOS upregulation in the T9 segment of one spinal cord injured rat and its modification with IGF-1 pretreatment (bar = 50 μm). Pretreatment with IGF-1 markedly attenuated the number of NOS positive neurons after spinal cord injury. Upper: untreated; lower: IGF-1 treated

ceived IGF-1 compared to the untreated injured group. The gray and white matter were distinctly separated and the neuropil appears quite preserved.

Discussion

The most salient new finding of the present study is that repeated application of IGF-1 on the traumatised cord significantly attenuated the edematous swelling and reduced the cell changes of the cord, a feature not reported earlier. Our results are the first to show a significant neuroprotective effects of IGF-1 in *in vivo* situation following acute spinal cord injury.

The spinal cord is very rich in IGF levels and spinal cord injury reduces the IGF content [5, 7]. Our results showed a marked cell injury in the spinal cord of untreated animals. This suggests that a possible decrease in the IGF-1 level following spinal cord injury deprives the needed growth factors to neurons resulting in atrophy or cell death [6, 7, 13, 14]. In the present

study, topical application of IGF-1 apparently protects the nerve cell changes and further suggests that if the growth factors are applied exogenously following trauma, they can induce neuroprotection. The probable mechanisms of IGF induced neuroprotection is unclear. However, it may be that loss of the endogenous growth factor can be restored with exogenous application of the IGF-1. To further confirm this measurement of the growth factor in untreated and IGF-1 treated rats are needed, which may be the subject for additional investigation. Another possibility of the neuroprotective mechanisms of IGF-1 could be due to its effect on attenuation of the trauma-induced stress reaction in the neurons by making an enriched microenvironment and thereby reducing the signs of cell damage [7, 14].

The second most important finding from this study is that IGF-1 has the capacity to thwart cNOS upregulation following spinal cord injury. This observation suggest that growth factors may mediate their neuroprotective effects via inhibition of NOS regulation. This study is the first to provide immunohistochemical evidences that NOS upregulation following spinal cord injury are reduced by repeated topical applications of the IGF-1. The possible mechanisms underlying IGF-1 induced neuroprotection is not known in all its details [7, 13, 14]. However, a possibility exists that the beneficial effects of IGF-1 in spinal cord injury is mediated via inhibition of NOS upregulation [2, 3].

The mechanisms by which IGF induced downregulation of cNOS following spinal cord injury is unclear from this study. It may be that IGF-1 influences the intracellular cascade following trauma by modifying signal transduction and intracellular accumulation of

Ca^{2+} and thus influencing NOS upregulation [2, 3], a feature which require additional investigation. Another possibility is that IGF somehow attenuates the intensity of cellular stress caused by trauma [7], a feature which require additional investigation using specific markers of stress reaction such as heat shock protein and heme oxygenease in IGF-1 treated traumatised rats.

Acknowledgements

This study is supported by grants from Swedish Medical Research Council nrs. 2710, 9459, 9710, 11205, Göran Gustafsson Foundation, Torsten and Ragner Söderberg Foundation, Sweden; Alexander von Humboldt Foundation, Bonn, Germany; The University Grants Commission, New Delhi, India. The technical assistance of Kärstin Flink, Ingamarie Olsson, Inga Hjörte, Ulla Johansson; photographic assistance of Frank Bittkowski and the secretarial assistance of Aruna Misra and Gun Britt Lind are highly appreciated.

References

1. Adem A, Ekblom J, Gillberg PG (1994) Growth factor receptors in amyotrophic lateral sclerosis. Mol Neurobiol 9: 225–231
2. Chiueh CC, Gilbert DL, Colton CA (1994) The neurobiology of NO and OH. Ann NY Acad Sci 738: 1–471
3. Choi DW (1993) Nitric oxide: foe or friend to the injured brain. Proc Natl Acad Sci USA 90: 9741–9743
4. Hefti F (1994) Neurotrophic factor therpay for nervous system degenerative diseases. J Neurobiol 25: 1418–1435
5. Folli F, Bonfanti L, Renard E, Kahn CR, Merighi A (1994) Insulin receptor substrate-1 (IRS-1) distribution in the rat central nervous system. J Neurosci 14: 6412–6422
6. Li L, Oppenheim RW, Lei M, Houenou LJ (1994) Neurotrophic agents prevent motoneuron death following sciatic nerve sections in the neonatal mouse. J Neurobiol 25: 759–766
7. Schwab ME, Bartholdi D (1966) Degeneration and regeneration of axons in the lesioned spinal cord. Physiol Rev 76: 319–370
8. Sharma HS, Olsson Y, Westman J (1995) A serotonin synthesis inhibitor, p-chlorophenylalanine reduces the heat shock protein response following trauma to the spinal cord. An immunohistochemical and ultrastructural study in the rat. Neurosci Res 21: 241–249
9. Sharma HS, Olsson Y, Cervós-Navarro J (1993) Early perifocal cell changes and edema in traumatic injury of the spinal cord are reduced by indomethacin, an inhibitor of prostaglandin synthesis. Acta Neuropathol (Berlin) 85: 145–153
10. Sharma HS, Olsson Y, Dey PK (1990) Early accumulation of serotonin in rat spinal cord subjected to traumatic injury. Relation to edema and blood flow changes. Neuroscience 36: 725–730
11. Sharma HS, Westman J, Olsson Y, Alm P (1996) Involvement of nitric oxide in acute spinal cord injury: an immunocytochemical study using light and electron microscopy in the rat. Neurosci Res 24: 373–384
12. Tsitouras PD, Zhong YG, Spungen AM, Bauman WA (1995) Serum testosterone and growth hormone/insulin-like growth factor-l in adults with spinal cord injury. Horm Metab Res 27: 287–292
13. Yao DL, Liu X, Hudson LD, Webster HD (1995) Insulin-like growth factor I treatment reduces demyealination and up-regulates gene expression of myelin-related proteins in experimental autoimmune encephalomyelitis. Proc Natl Acad Sci USA 92: 6190–6194
14. Yin QW, Johnson J, Prevette D, Oppenheim RW (1994) Cell death of spinal motoneurons in the chick embryo following deafferentation: rescue effects of tissue extracts, soluble proteins, and neurotrophic agents. J Neurosci 14: 7629–7640

Correspondence: Hari Shanker Sharma, Ph.D., Laboratory of Neuroanatomy, Department of Anatomy, Post Box 571, Biomedical Centre, Uppsala University, S-75123 Uppsala, Sweden.

Acta Neurochir (1997) [Suppl] 70: 134–137
© Springer-Verlag 1997

Prostaglandins Modulate Constitutive Isoform of Heat Shock Protein (72 kD) Response Following Trauma to the Rat Spinal Cord

H. S. Sharma and **J. Westman**

Laboratory of Neuroanatomy, Department of Anatomy, Biomedical Centre, Uppsala University, Uppsala, Sweden

Summary

The influence of prostaglandins on the constitutive isoform of heat shock protein (HSP 72 kD) response following a focal trauma to the rat spinal cord was examined using immunohistochemistry. A focal trauma to the spinal cord by making a longitudinal incision into the right dorsal (about 2 mm deep and 5 mm long) of the T10–11 segments, markedly enhanced the upregulation of HSP immunoreactivity in the traumatised as well as in the perifocal T9 and T12 segments. This upregulation of HSP was significantly reduced by pretreatment with indomethacin (10 mg/kg, i.p., 30 min before injury) an inhibitor of prostaglandin synthesis. These results show that blockade of PG synthesis prior to trauma has an inhibitory influence on the upregulation of HSP response, not reported earlier.

Keywords: Prostaglandins; spinal cord trauma; heat shock protein 72 kD.

Introduction

Heat shock proteins (HSP) originally associated with thermal stress is now known to be a universal response following a wide variety of noxious stimuli to the central nervous system (CNS) [14]. Increased expression of HSP in the CNS is a common feature of ischemic, metabolic or traumatic insults [1, 4, 5, 8, 14]. However, the functional significance of this reaction is not well understood. Recent reports suggest that induction of HSP response is associated with the magnitude of cellular stress and can be used as a sensitive and reliable indicator cell injury [11, 13, 14]. There are evidences which suggest that HSP response can be induced by local administration of kainic acid into the brain which can be prevented by pretreatment with NMDA receptor blocker MK-801 [5, 13]. This observation suggest that upregulation of cellular HSP is somehow mediated by neurochemicals probably via specific receptors [13, 14].

Our earlier works suggest that inhibition of prostaglandin synthesis with indomethacin is neuroprotective [6, 7]. Prostaglandins are known as the first mediators of stress [3, 9] and are released following a wide variety of noxious, metabolic, ischemic or hypoxic insults [1, 2, 12]. However, the involvement of prostaglandins in trauma induced stress response is still unknown. To our knowledge, there are no previous report regarding the involvement of prostaglandins in HSP response in the CNS following ischemic, hypoxic or traumatic injury. Therefore, in this investigation we examined the influence of a potent prostaglandin synthesis inhibitor, indomethacin on the spinal cord trauma induced upregulation of constitutive isoform of HSP response in our rat model.

Materials and Methods

Animals

The experiments were carried out on 20 male Wistar rats weighing between 300–350 g under urethane anaesthesia (1.5 g/kg, intraperitoneally, i.p.). The animals were housed at controlled ambient temperature ($22 \pm 1°C$) with a 12 h light and 12 h dark schedule. Food and tap water were supplied *ad libitum*.

Infliction of Spinal Cord Trauma

A dorsal laminectomy was performed at the level of T10–T11 segments of the cord. Spinal cord injury was performed by making an incision into the right dorsal horn (about 2 mm deep and 5 mm long) using a sterile scalpel blade [6, 8]. This experimental procedure was approved by the ethical committee of Uppsala University.

HSP-Immunohistochemistry

Five hours after trauma, the animals were perfused with 100 ml of fixative containing 2.5% glutaraldehyde, 2% paraformaldehyde in 0.1 M sodium phosphate buffer (37°C, pH 7.4) at 100 mmHg preceding a washout with about 50 ml of 0.1 M phosphate buffer saline at room temperature. After fixation, the injured (T10–11) as well as the adjacent cranial (T9) and the caudal (T12) segments were dissected out. The HSP-immuno-histochemistry was done on free floating vibratome (60 μm thick) sections using antibodies directed against constitutive isoform of HSP-70 kD (Amersham,

England) as described earlier [8]. In brief, the sections were then transferred to the primary antibody solution, consisting of a primary antibody (monoclonal HSP 72 kD antiserum, Amersham, UK) diluted 1 : 500 and normal swine serum diluted 1 : 30 in phosphate buffer saline (PBS) and incubated free floating under agitation for 36 h at room temperature [8]. Following six 10-min rinses in PBS and Tris-HCl (pH 7.6), the sections were transferred to the secondary antibody solution (swine anti mouse 1:30 in PBS) and incubated for 60 min at room temperature under agitation. Thereafter, the sections were incubated in the PAP complex solution (1 : 20 in PBS) under the same conditions, with intervening rinses in PBS. Immuno-complexes were localised by incubating the sections for 6–7 min in a solution containing 75 mg of DAB and 30 µl of 30% H_2O_2/ 100 ml of Tris-HCl buffer. The reaction was terminated by transferring the sections to Tris-HCl buffer. The sections were washed in 0.15 M sodium cacodylate buffer and post-fixed for 20 min in 2% OsO_4 dissolved in cacodylate buffer. They were then dehydrated in a graded series of ethanol, embedded in epon between acetate foils and polymerised at 60°C for 48 h [8]. Sections obtained from control, 5 h spinal cord traumatised, indomethacin pretreated controls and spinal cord traumatised animals were processed in parallel. After embedding, the sections were examined in a light microscope for evaluation of the immuno-labelling. For comparison, one section in each group was not osmicated in order to see the labelled neurons against a light background. The non-osmicated sections were examined under light microscope and photographed.

Electron Microscopy

For ultrastructural investigation of labelled neurons, osmicated sections were used. One half of the spinal either left or right side of the T9 or T12 was attached to an Epon block and part of the spinal cord containing labelled neurones was trimmed out. Semi thick sections were stained with toluidine blue and examined under light microscopy and photographed. Ultrathin sections were cut using a diamond knife (LKB, Ultramicrotome, Sweden), collected on one hole grid and stained with uranyl acetate and lead citrate. Some of the sections were unstained and examined under a Phillips 300 transmission electron microscope [8].

Indomethacin Treatment

Separate groups of rats (n = 10) were treated with indomethacin (10 mg/kg i.p., Sigma Chemical Co., USA) 30 min before trauma [6, 7]. These animals were allowed to survive for 5 h after injury. This dose and time schedule inhibits effectively the prostaglandin synthesis in the central nervous system for several hours [12].

Statistical Evaluation

The number of immunostained cell bodies in the T9 and T12 segments were counted in control (n = 5), spinal cord traumatised (n = 5), indomethacin treated controls (n = 5) and drug treated traumatised (n = 5) rats in a blind fashion. The values were expressed as mean ± SD. Student's unpaired t-test was applied to evaluate statistical significance of the data obtained. A p-value less than 0.05 was considered to be significant.

Results

Spinal Cord Pathology

Spinal cord segments after 5 h injury showed signs of tissue destruction and haemorrhages extended deeply into the region corresponding to Rexed's lamina VIII. The dorsal and ventral horns were spongy in appearance and the neurons have distorted cell bodies; some were slightly swollen and others were shrunken. The perifocal segments T9 and T12 exhibited marked expansion of the grey matter which was most pronounced in the ipsilateral side. The white matter was also distorted and vesiculation of myelin sheaths was very common. Pretreatment with the prostaglandin synthesis inhibitor, indomethacin markedly diminished the trauma induced expansion of the cord. The nerve cell changes were much less pronounced than those seen in the untreated group of injured rats.

HSP Immunohistochemistry

The spinal cord of normal rats did not show any evidence of HSP immunoreactivity. However, 5 h after injury, there was a marked upregulation of HSP response in the dorsal and ventral horn of the T9, T10–11 and T12 segments. Thus the traumatised segment revealed more than 30 HSP positive neurons whereas the rostral (T9) and caudal (T12) segments showed about 15 to 20 HSP immunostained nerve cells. The immunolabelling of HSP was seen in the nucleus as well as in the neuronal cytoplasm of the nerve cells (Fig. 1). This response was most marked in the ipsilateral side of the cord. In traumatised rats, dark immunoreaction product of HSP can be seen at ultrastructural level within the cytoplasm of nerve cell bodies and dendrites. One example of two labelled dendrites from the dorsal horn

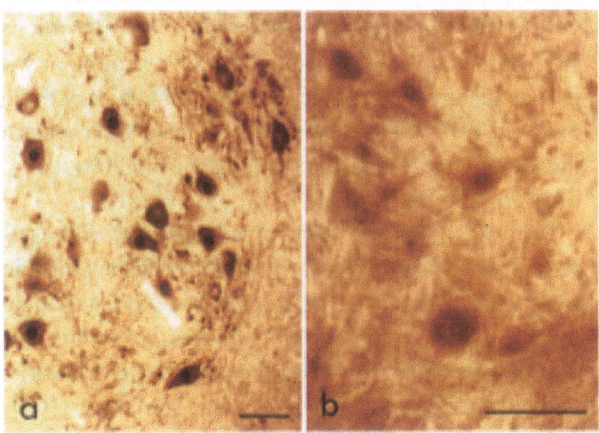

Fig. 1. HSP (72 kd) immunostaining. T9 ventral horn. 5 h spinal cord injury. Low power light micrograph of the non-osmicated vibratome section of HSP-immunostained sections from the ventral horn of T9 segment of one untreated injured rat (a) and one indomethacin pretreated (b) injured animal. In untreated rat, immunoreactivity of HSP seen as brown reaction product is evident in neuronal cytoplasm and in nucleus of the nerve cells. On the other hand, no immunostaining of HSP is present in animals which received indomethacin before injury (bar = 50 µm)

of a T9 segment of the untreated injured rat is shown in Fig. 2. Pretreatment with indomethacin significantly attenuated this increase in HSP response after trauma (Fig. 1b). Thus in indomethacin treated rats, the traumatised (T10–11) segments showed only 6 to 8 positive neurons and the adjacent rostral (T9) and caudal (T12) segments exhibited less than 5 HSP positive nerve cells in the cord. However, indomethacin pretreatment alone did not influence the HSP immunostaining.

Discussion

The present study for the first time shows that the immunoreactivity of the constitutive isoform of HSP 70 kD occurring in neurons around a spinal cord injury can be prevented by pretreatment of rats with indomethacin. This observation suggest that prostaglandins are somehow involved in the cellular stress response following spinal cord injury, not reported earlier. Our observation is in line with the hypothesis that a reduction in the magnitude of cellular stress following injury is primarily responsible for attenuation of the HSP immunostaining [5, 6, 13, 14].

The detailed mechanisms of induction of HSP response following trauma to the spinal cord are not known. It seems quite likely that neurons in the perifocal T9 and T12 and in the injury zone are exposed to wide variety of immunological, chemical, vascular and ionic disturbances caused by secondary injury mechanisms [1, 2, 12]. These factors alone or in combination will produce an adverse effects on the cellular microenvironment [1, 6]. An altered microenvironment will induce disturbances in the molecular machinery of the exposed cells. These exposed cells may then react to the altered microenvironment by abnormal production of stress proteins [1, 2, 6, 8, 11, 12].

Prostaglandins are known mediators of increased vascular permeability and formation of vasogenic edema in the cord [2, 6, 7]. Inhibition of prostaglandin synthesis with indomethacin significantly reduces the vascular permeability disturbances, edema formation and occurrence of cell changes in the spinal cord [6, 7]. Thus it appears that inhibition of prostaglandin synthesis prior to trauma will result in a less disturbed microenvironment of neurons in the spinal cord of injured and perifocal segments. As a result, the neurons within and in the vicinity of the traumatised zone of the spinal cord will feel considerably less stress compared to the untreated injured animals [8]. This may be one important reason for less pronounced HSP response in the

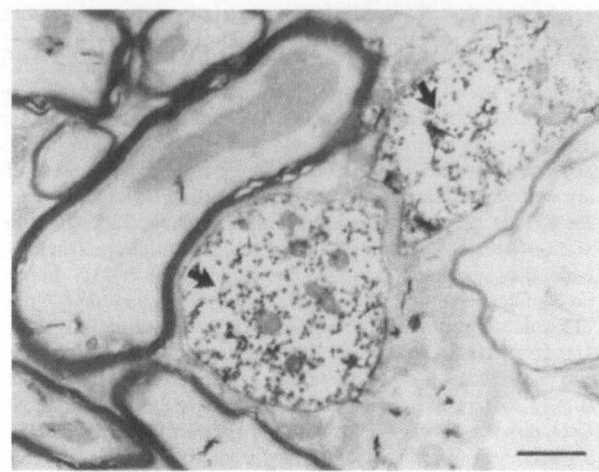

Fig. 2. HSP (72 kd) immunostaining. T9 ventral horn. 5 h spinal cord injury. Low power electron micrograph of two HSP immunolabelled (arrows) dendrites in cross sections obtained from the dorsal horn of T9 segment of an untreated injured rat. This ultrathin section is uncontrasted. A few black crystal like profiles represent non-specific background staining (bar = 1 μm)

indomethacin treated traumatised rats. Alternatively indomethacin may have some direct inhibiting action on the synthesis of the stress proteins.

Recently, various receptors to prostaglandins are identified in the spinal cord [1, 2], thus it would be interesting to find out if a particular prostaglandin receptor is involved in the HSP response following trauma. However, to further clarify this additional investigations with various prostaglandin receptor blockers are needed.

In conclusion, it appears that the HSP response elicited in neurons of the spinal cord after trauma can be prevented by prior treatment with a potent inhibitor of prostaglandin biosynthesis, indomethacin. This indicates that prostaglandins are involved in cellular stress caused by trauma and further suggests that prostaglandins has the capacity to induce HSP response either by direct receptor mediated effects or by their capacity to influence other neurochemical events. Alternatively indomethacin may have some inhibitory influence on the traumatic stress induced expression of constitutive isoform of HSP response after cell injury.

Acknowledgements

This investigation was supported by grants from the Swedish Medical Research Council projects no. 2710, Göran Gustafssons stiftelse, and Torsten and Ragnar Söderburgs stiftelse, Sweden. The skilful technical assistance of Mrs. Kärstin Flink, Ingmarie Olsson and the secretarial assistance of Mrs. Gun Britt Lind and Aruna Misra are acknowledged with thanks.

References

1. Faden AI (1993) Experimental neurobiology of central nervous system trauma. Crit Rev Neurobiol 7: 175–186
2. Faden A, Salzman S (1992) Pharmacological strategies in CNS trauma. TiPS 13: 29–35
3. Hanukoglu I (1977) Prostaglandins as first mediators of stress. New Eng J Med 296: 1414–1415
4. Kato H, Liu Y, Kogure K, Kato K (1994) Induction of 27-kDa heat shock protein following cerebral ischemia in a rat model of ischemic tolerance. Brain Res 634: 235–244
5. Planas A, Soriano MA, Ferrer I, Farré ER (1995) Kainic acid-induced heat shock protein-70, mRNA and protein expression is inhibited by MK-801 in certain brain regions. Eur J Neurosci 7: 293–304
6. Sharma HS, Olsson Y, Nyberg F, Dey PK (1993) Prostaglandins modulate alterations of microvascular permeability, blood flow, edema and serotonin levels following spinal cord injury: an experimental study in the rat. Neuroscience 57: 443–449
7. Sharma HS, Westman J, Nyberg F, Cervós-Navarro J, Dey PK (1994) Role of serotonin and prostaglandins in brain edema induced by heat stress. An experimental study in the rat. Acta Neurochir (Wien) [Suppl] 60: 65–79
8. Sharma HS, Olsson Y, Westman J (1995) A serotonin synthesis inhibitor, p-chlorophenylalanine reduces the heat shock protein response following trauma to the spinal cord. An immunohistochemical and ultrastructural study in the rat. Neurosci Res 21: 241–249
9. Sharma HS, Nyberg F, Westman J, Cervós-Navarro J, Dey PK (1996) Probable involvement of serotonin in the increased permeability of the blood-brain barrier by forced swimming. An experimental study using Evans blue and ^{131}I-sodium tracers in the rat. Behav Brain Res 72:189–196
10. Sloviter RS, Lowenstein DH (1992) Heat shock protein expression in vulnerable cells of the rat hippocampus as an indicator of excitation-induced neuronal stress. J Neurosci 12: 3004–3009
11. Tanon H, Nockels RP, Pitts LH, Noble LJ (1993) Immunolocalization of heat shock protein after fluid percussive brain injury and relationship to breakdown of the blood-brain barrier. J Cereb Blood Flow Metabol 13: 116–124
12. Tator CH, Fehlings MG (1991) Review of the secondary injury theory of acute spinal cord trauma with emphasis on vascular mechanisms. J Neurosurg 75: 15–26
13. Udelsman R, Blake, MJ. Stagg CA, Holbrook NJ (1994) Endocrine control of stress-induced heat shock protein 70 expression *in vivo*. Surgery 115: 611–616
14. Welch WJ (1992) Mammalian stress response: cell physiology, structure/function of stress proteins, and implications for medicine and disease. Physiol Rev 72: 1063–1081

Correspondence: Hari Shanker Sharma, Ph.D., Laboratory of Neuroanatomy, Department of Anatomy, Post Box 571, Biomedical Centre, Uppsala University, S-75123 Uppsala, Sweden.

Acta Neurochir (1997) [Suppl] 70: 138–140
© Springer-Verlag 1997

The Effect of Endothelins on Ion Transport Systems in Cultured Rat Brain Capillary Endothelial Cells

N. Kawai, R. M. McCarron, and **M. Spatz**

Stroke Branch, National Institute of Neurological Disorders and Stroke, National Institutes of Health, Bethesda, MD, U.S.A.

Summary

Brain capillary endothelial cells regulate the movement of ions and water across the blood-brain barrier via specific ion transport systems. Disturbances in these ion transport systems are involved in the formation of ischemic brain edema. This study describes the effects of endothelins (i.e., ET-1 and ET-3) on ion transport systems in cultured rat brain capillary endothelial cells using $^{86}Rb^+$ and $^{22}Na^+$ as markers for K^+ and Na^+, respectively. ET-1 stimulated K^+ uptake and efflux with EC_{50} values of 0.6 nM and 0.5 nM, respectively. The potencies of ET-3 on these responses were considerably lower. Both ET-1 and ET-3 stimulated Na^+ uptake through a Na^+/H^+ exchange system with similar potencies (i.e., EC_{50} = 0.80 nM and 1.89 nM, respectively). ET-stimulated K^+ uptake, K^+ efflux, and Na^+ uptake activities were all inhibited by BQ123 (selective ET_A receptor antagonist). ET-1-stimulated K^+ uptake and efflux, in contrast to Na^+ uptake, were also reduced by protein kinase C inhibitors and by an intracellular Ca^{2+} chelator. The results suggest that ETs can affect the activities of ion and water transport at the blood-brain barrier through different signal transduction mechanisms.

Keywords: Blood-brain barrier; capillary endothelium; ion transport; endothelins.

Introduction

The maintenance of ionic homeostasis in the brain is attributed to ion transport systems (e.g., Na^+,K^+-ATPase, Na^+/H^+-exchange and Na^+-K^+-Cl^- cotransport) that control ion and water fluxes between blood, extracellular spaces and cerebrospinal fluid (CSF). The endothelium of the cerebral capillaries, the principle cellular element of the blood-brain barrier (BBB), has been recognized as important multifunctional cell type which possesses he above-mentioned ion transport systems [3, 7]. Although disturbances of these ion transport systems have been implicated in the formation of ischemic brain edema [2], the mechanisms and factors responsible for this process are unclear. Endothelins (ET-1, ET-2, and ET-3) are potent vasoactive peptides originally isolated from cultured porcine aortic endothelial cells [13]. In the central nervous system, vascular endothelial cells, glial cells and neurons are known to produce ETs (see review [7]). Since brain capillary endothelial cells also express ET-receptors [13], they exhibit the capacity to respond to ETs in a paracrine or autocrine manner. Recent studies described ET_A-like receptors expressed on cultured brain capillary endothelial cells that are linked to ion transport systems, such as the Na^+-K^+-Cl^- cotransport [5, 12], Na^+,K^+-ATPase [5, 7], and K^+ channels [12]. In addition, ET-1 and ET-3-stimulated Na^+/H^+ exchange activity is mediated by atypical ET_A-like receptors in cultured rat brain capillary endothelial cells (RBEC) [6, 11]. The detection of increased ET levels in CSF of stroke and subarachnoid hemorrhage patients [4, 10], as well as in brain and CSF of experimental ischemic animals [1, 9], suggests that ETs may modulate BBB functions seen in ischemic brain. This report summarizes published and unpublished studies concerned with the effect of ET-1 and ET-3 on ion transport systems expressed on cultured RBEC [5, 6].

Materials and Methods

RBEC derived from adult rats were isolated and cultivated by a modified technique originally described by Spatz *et al.* [8]. K^+ uptake, K^+ efflux and Na^+ uptake activities were measured in RBEC grown in 96-well microtiter plates by using $^{86}Rb^+$ and $^{22}Na^+$ as tracers for K^+ and Na^+, respectively, as previously described [5, 6]. For the K^+ uptake study, RBEC were incubated with $^{86}Rb^+$ (0.2 μCi/well) at room temperature for 10 min. Ouabain (2 mM)-sensitive and bumetanide (20 μM)-sensitive K^+ uptakes were defined as Na^+, K^+-ATPase and Na^+-K^+-Cl^- cotransport activities, respectively. K^+ uptake (expressed as nmol/mg protein/min) was based on the rate of $^{86}Rb^+$ uptake and the K^+ content in the incubation buffer. For the K^+ efflux study, RBEC loaded with $^{86}Rb^+$ (0.1 μCi/well, 2 h) were incubated with ETs or vehicle for indicated periods of time. The amount of $^{86}Rb^+$ released into supernatant during indicated period (expressed as percentage of total $^{86}Rb^+$ originally loaded) was considered as K^+ efflux activity. For the Na^+ uptake study, RBEC were washed and allowed to equilibrate in 40 μl of Na^+ free uptake buffer [10 mM Tris-HCl buffer (pH 7.4) containing 5.3 mM KCl, 1.8 mM $CaCl_2$, 0.8 mM $MgSO_4$, 5.6 mM glucose, 250 mM sucrose, and 0.1% BSA] for 15 min at 37°C. Subsequently, 1 mM ouabain and indicated concentrations of ETs were added and RBEC were incubated with $^{22}Na^+$ (0.3 μCi/well, Amersham) with 3 mM NaCl for 5 min at room temperature. The rate of Na^+ uptake (nmol/mg protein/min) was based on the ratio of $^{22}Na^+$ uptake and the Na^+ content in the buffer. Where indicated, RBEC were pretreated with the intracellular Ca^{2+} chelator, BAPTA/AM (25 μM in M199) for 10 min and washed prior to the addition of ETs.

Results and Discussion

ET-1 and ET-3 stimulated K^+ uptake into RBEC from two- to three-fold with half-maximal effective concentrations (EC_{50}) of 0.6 ± 0.2 nM and 21.5 ± 4.1 nM, respectively. ET-1 or ET-3-stimulated K^+ uptake was inhibited by ouabain (30–40%) or bumetanide (60–70%), indicating the stimulation of both Na^+,K^+-ATPase and Na^+-K^+-Cl^- cotransport. ET-1 or ET-3 also increased the rate of K^+ efflux up to two-fold with EC_{50} values of 0.5 ± 0.1 nM and 14.9 ±1.5 nM, respectively. These responses were abolished by 300 μM quinine, indicating the involvement of Ca^{2+}-activated K^+ channels. ET-1 stimulation of K^+ uptake through both Na^+, K^+-ATPase and Na^+-K^+-Cl^- cotransport were significantly reduced by the presence of quinine, suggesting an intimate relationship between uptake and efflux of K^+. Moreover, it was observed that the ET-1-stimulation of K^+ efflux occurred immediately (< 30 sec) after the administration of ET-1, whereas the increase in the rate of K^+ uptake became significant only after 90 sec. The data suggests that ET-1 may initially stimulate K^+ efflux through Ca^{2+}-activated K^+ channels, while the K^+ uptake activity is secondarily stimulated by the loss of intracellular K^+. In addition, it was shown that treatment with 5-ethyl-5-isopropyl-amiloride (EIPA, 20 μM) abolished

the two-fold increased Na^+ uptake induced by ET-1 or ET-3, indicating involvement of the Na^+/H^+ exchange system in these responses. The EC_{50} values of ET-1 and ET-3 for the Na^+ uptake were similar (0.8 ± 0.1 nM and 1.9 ± 0.4 nM, respectively).

ET-1 or ET-3-stimulated K^+ uptake, K^+ efflux, or Na^+ uptake activity were all completely inhibited by the selective ET_A antagonist, BQ123 (300 nM) but were not affected by the selective ET_B antagonist, BQ788 (300 nM). These findings indicate that all of these ion-transport responses are mediated by ET_A- but not ET_B-receptors. The signal transduction systems involved in ET-stimulated ion-transport activities were evaluated by using a protein kinase C (PKC) activator, phorbol myristate acetate (PMA), a PKC inhibitor, bisindolylmaleimide (BISI), an intracellular Ca^{2+} chelator, BAPTA/AM, and a potent protein-tyrosine kinase inhibitor, genistein (Table 1). The results showed that ET-stimulation of K^+ uptake and efflux activities were stimulated by PMA and were inhibited by BISI (200 nM), BAPTA/AM (10 μM), or genistein (50 μM). ET-stimulation of Na^+ uptake activity was not affected by PMA, BISI or BAPTA/AM, but was significantly reduced by genistein.

Conclusion

The data demonstrate that RBEC exposed to ETs showed increased activities of ion transport systems including Na^+,K^+-ATPase, Na^+-K^+-Cl^- cotransport, Ca^{2+}-activated K^+ channels, and Na^+/H^+ exchange systems. All of these responses were mediated by ET_A (and not ET_B) receptors. Different signal transduction pathways such as PKC, intracellular Ca^{2+}, and protein-tyrosine phosphorylation are involved in these responses. These results suggest that ETs can affect ion and water transport at the BBB, and may, therefore, play an important role in the pathomechanism of ischemic brain edema.

Table 1. *Summary of ET_A Receptor-Mediated Ion Transport Responses to Endothelin*

Movement of ions	Ion transport systems	IC_{50} (nM) ET-1/ET-3	Signal transductions
K^+ influx	Na^+-K^+-Cl^- cotransport Na^+,K^+-ATPase	0.6/21.5	Protein kinase C Ca^{2+} mobilization Protein-tyrosine kinase (?)
K^+ efflux	Ca^{2+}-activated K^+ channels	0.5/14.9	Protein kinase C Ca^{2+} mobilization Protein-tyrosine kinase (?)
Na^+ influx	Na^+/H^+ exchange	0.8/1.9	Protein-tyrosine kinase (?)

Acknowledgement

The authors wish to acknowledge Ms. Devera Schoenberg, M.S., for her expert editorial assistance in the preparation of this manuscript.

References

1. Barone FC, Globus MY-T, Price WJ, White RF, Storer BL, Feuerstein GZ, Busto R, Ohlstein EH (1994) Endothelin levels increase in rat focal and global ischemia. J Cereb Blood Flow Metab 14: 337–342
2. Betz AL, Keep RF, Beer ME, Ren X (1994) Blood-brain barrier permeability and brain concentration of sodium, potassium, and chloride during focal ischemia. J Cereb Blood Flow Metab 14: 29–37
3. Eisenberg HM, Suddith RL (1979) Cerebral vessels have the capacity to transport sodium and potassium. Science 206: 1083–1085
4. Ehrenreich H, Lange M, Near KA, Anneser F, Schoeller LA, Schmid R, Winkler PS, Kehrl JH, Schmiedek P, Goebel FD (1992) Long term monitoring of immunoreactive endothelin-1 and endothelin-3 in ventricular cerebrospinal fluid, plasma, and 24-hr urine of patients with subarachnoid hemorrhage. Res Exp Med 192: 257–268
5. Kawai N, McCarron RM, Spatz M (1995a) Endothelins stimulate sodium uptake into rat brain capillary endothelial cells through endothelin A-like receptors. Neurosci Lett 190: 85–88
6. Kawai N, Yamamoto T, Yamamoto H, McCarron RM, Spatz M (1995b) Endothelin 1 stimulates Na^+, K^+-ATPase and Na^+-K^+-Cl^- cotransport through ET_A receptors and protein kinase C-dependent pathway in cerebral capillary endothelium. J Neurochem 65: 1588–1596
7. Spatz M, Stanimirovic D, McCarron RM (1996) Endothelin as a mediator of blood-brain barrier function. In: Greenwood J (ed) New concepts of blood-brain barrier. Plenum, Amsterdam, pp 47–61
8. Spatz M, Bembry J, Dodson RF, Hervonen H, Murray MR (1980) Endothelial cell culture derived from isolated cerebral microvessels. Brain Res 191: 577–582
9. Spatz M, Stanimirovic D, Strasser A, McCarron RM (1995) Nitro-L arginine augments the endothelin-1 content of cerebrospinal fluid induced by cerebral ischemia. Brain Res 684: 99–102
10. Suzuki H, Sato S, Suzuki Y, Takekoshi K, Ishihara N, Shimoda S (1990) Increased endothelin concentration in CSF from patients with subarachnoid hemorrhage. Acta Neurol Scand 81: 553–554
11. Vigne P, Desmarets J, Guedin D, Frelin C (1996) Properties of an endothelin-3 sensitive ET_A-like endothelin receptor in brain capillary endothelial cells. Biochem Biophys Res Comm 20: 839–842
12. Vigne P, Farre AL, Frelin C (1994) Na^+-K^+-Cl^- cotransporter of brain capillary endothelial cells. J Biol Chem 269: 19925–19930
13. Yanagisawa M, Kurihara H, Kimura S, Tomobe Y, Kobayashi, M, Mitsui Y, Yazaki Y, Goto K, Masaki T (1988) A novel potent vasoconstrictor peptide produced by vascular endothelial cells. Nature (Lond) 332: 411–415

Correspondence: Maria Spatz, M.D., Stroke Branch, NINDS, National Institutes of Health, 36 Convent Drive, MSC 4128, Bethesda, MD 20892-4128, U.S.A.

Acta Neurochir (1997) [Suppl] 70: 141–143
© Springer-Verlag 1997

Neurotoxicity of Serum Components, Comparison Between CA1 and Striatum

E. Kadota[1], K. Nonaka[1], M. Karasuno[1], K. Nishi[1], K. Teramura[2], and S. Hashimoto[2]

[1] Division of Pathology, Kishiwada City Hospital, Osaka, and [2] 2nd Department of Pathology,
Kinki University School of Medicine, Osaka, Japan

Summary

In vasogenic brain edema, the neurotoxicity of extravasated serum components may contribute to neuronal damage. In the hippocampal CA1 sector and striatum, the neurotoxicity of serum was investigated. Rat serum was prepared as follows:

Serum-1: whole serum, Serum-2: ultrafiltrated through a membrane with cut-off at molecular weight (MW) 100,000, Serum-3: through a membrane with cut-off at MW 20,000, and Serum-4: through a membrane with cut-off at MW 5,000. The infusion edema model was utilized for infusion of autologous serum into the brain. The brain tissue was histologically evaluated. The level of glutamate, total protein, and albumin was also measured in the sera used for infusion. The following results were obtained: 1) CA1 neurons were more vulnerable to all infused sera than striatal neurons, 2) there was a strong cellular response in the striatal site of infusion, but only a minimal in the CA1-sector, 3) the severity of damage of CA1 correlated with the glutamate concentrations of the infused sera, 4) further, there was a relationship between the degree of striatal neuronal loss and the amount of protein and albumin present in the infusate. It is, therefore, concluded that the neurotoxic properties of vasogenic edema fluid are also affected by specific features of the brain region of its extravasation. In addition, the pathological mechanisms associated with irreversible damage of neurons might be different in the CA1-sector and the striatum.

Keywords: Vasogenic brain edema; neurotoxicity of serum; hippocampal CA1 region; striatum.

Introduction

In vasogenic brain edema the neurotoxic properties of extravasated serum components may contribute to neuronal damage. In this study, we have simulated an increasing severity of blood-brain barrier (BBB) breakdown by intracerebral infusion of autologous sera, which were ultrafiltrated through membranes with various molecular weight cut-offs. Neurotoxicity was investigated in the hippocampal CA1-sector and the striatum.

Material and Methods

Rat (Wistar, male, 250–340 g body weight) sera were prepared as follows: Serum-1: whole serum, Serum-2: ultrafiltrated through a membrane with cut-off at MW 100,000, Serum-3: through a membrane with cut-off at MW 20,000, and Serum-4: through a membrane with cut-off at 5,000. The rat infusion brain edema model was utilized. The auto-sera were diluted twice with physiological saline and infused (25 µl / 25 min) into the CA1-sector and striatum by stereotactic control in ketamine anesthesia (100 mg/kg). In a control group, 25 µl of physiological saline were infused within 25 min. The rats were sacrificed 4 days after infusion, and the brain was histologically evaluated. For quantitative assessment, the maximum width of the CA1 lesion was measured in frontal sections, and the maximum diameter of the striatal lesion was measured in coronal sections. The glutamate levels in the sera were analyzed by HPLC, als well as the concentrations of total protein and albumin.

Results

The morphometrically assessed size of the focus of infusion was markedly larger in the CA1-sector than in the striatum in all experiments (Fig. 1). Infusion of all sera caused extensive neuronal death in CA1. On the other side, only Serum-1 and -2 resulted in statistically significant increased striatal lesions as compared to control (saline only). There were also histologically qualitative differences between these groups and the controls. Striatal lesions were characterized by marked cellular responses, such as gliosis, polymorphonuclear leukocyte infiltration, and mitosis (Fig. 2A), while the CA1 foci showed almost no inflammatory reactions (Fig. 2B). The concentration of glutamate, total protein, and albumin present in the infused serum is shown in Fig. 1.

Discussion

It is currently shown that the hippocampal CA1-sector is more vulnerable than the striatum to serum

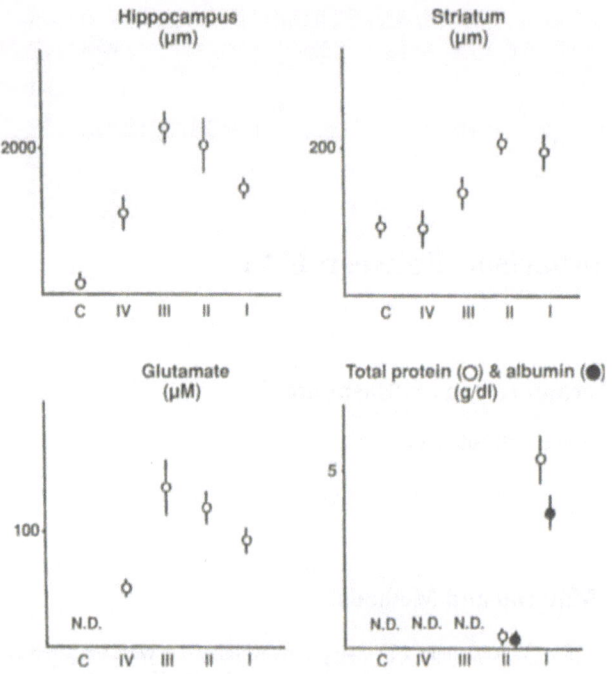

Fig. 1. Morphometric evaluation of lesion diameter (μm) in hippocampus and striatum and concentrations of glutamate, total protein, and albumin. *N.D.* Not detectable. Serum-I: whole serum, II: M.W. 100,000 cut-off, III: 20,000 cut-offs, and IV: 5,000 cut-off. *C* Control (physiological saline). Mean ± SEM

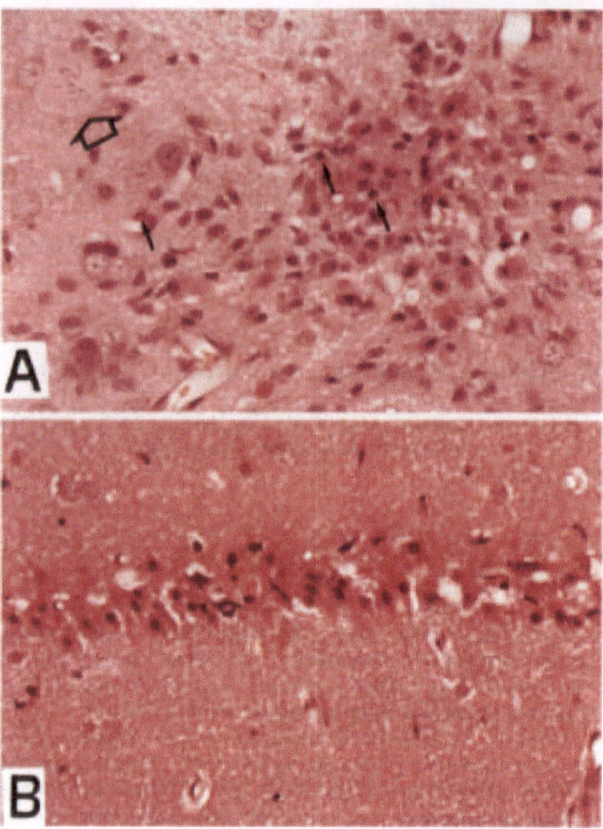

Fig. 2. Microphotographs of striatum (A) and CA1 (B). (A) The striatal lesions were accompanied by a marked cellular response, such as gliosis, polymorphonuclear leukocyte infiltrations (arrow) and mitoses (open arrow). (B) The CA1 foci showed pyknosis, karyorrhexis, and parenchymatous homogenization, but almost no inflammatory reactions (HE stain)

constituents, and that even the small-molecular components of serum cause extensive changes in the CA1-sector. In addition, histological differences were also observed between these two regions. The striatal lesions seemed necrotic, while the cell changes of the CA1-sector appeared to be apoptotic [4]. It is, therefore, suggested that the pathological mechanisms causing neuronal death were different in striatum and CA1.

Since glutamate receptors are densely distributed in the CA1[6]-sector, and glutamate plays an important role in CA1 neuronal damage, we have measured the glutamate concentration in the different serum preparations. As seen, the level of glutamate was well correlated with the morphological findings indicating CA1 injury. Further, the high-molecular weight substance(s) present in the sera led to neuronal reactions accompanied with marked cellular changes [3] in the striatum. We have, therefore, investigated the relationship between the histological alterations in the striatum and the level of total protein and albumin in the serum infusates. Again, both were relatively well correlated. Based on these results it is suggested that the glutamate- and total protein- and albumin content in serum is associated with the CA1- and striatal damage, respectively.

It may be questionable, however, to attribute the neurotoxicity of serum in the CA1-sector only to the presence of glutamate. Serum-4 contained 49.9 μM of glutamate, the total amount of glutamate infused was therefore 1.25 nM in animals with Serum-4 injection, which had a considerable neuronal loss. The foci of damage were more extensive than those observed in Benveniste's experiments, where a total amount of 10 nM glutamate was infused [1]. It is further questionable to attribute the serum neurotoxicity found in striatum only to the presence of proteins and albumin. In spite of an absence of differences of the histological findings between Serum-1 injected and Serum-2 injected animals, it must be emphasized that the protein- and albumin content was significantly higher in Serum-1 than Serum-2.

There are other studies on the neurotoxicity of serum with regard to a combined and/or additive effect of the various serum components. For example, insulin [5] or albumin [2] may enhance the neurotoxicity of glutamate. It was, therefore, suggested that not only glutamate but also other serum constituent(s) contribute to the

CA1 neuronal death. Similarly, the neurotoxicity of serum in the striatum should be studied with regard to factors other than protein and albumin.

In conclusion, we suggest that serum components are causing different forms and degrees of tissue damage in the CA1-sector and striatum. Investigations should be performed in the future to elucidate details of this toxicity, and the contribution of serum to brain damage from ischemia.

References

1. Benveniste H, Jorgensen MB, Sandberg M, Christensen T, Hagberg H, Diemer NH (1 989) Ischemic damage in hippocampal CA1 is dependent on glutamate release and intact innervation from CA3. J Cereb Blood Flow Metab 9: 629–639
2. Bjorner H, Evy GI, Frode F (1994) Neurotoxicity of albumin *in vivo*. Neurosci Lett 167: 29–32
3. Lawrence MK, John NB (1983) Serum factor supporting long-term survival of rat central neurons in culture. Science 220: 1394–1396
4. Majno G, Joris I (1995) Apoptosis, oncosis, and necrosis. An overview of cell death. Am J Pathol 146: 3–15
5. Martin S, Sandor LE (1991) Development of glutamate neurotoxicity in cortical cultures: induction of vulnerability by insulin. Develop Brain Res 62: 293–296
6. Monaghan DT, Holets VR, Toy DW, Cotman CW (1983) Anatomical distributions of four pharmacologically distinct 3H-L-glutamate binding sites. Nature 306: 176–179

Correspondence: Eiji Kadota M.D., Division of Pathology, Kishiwada City Hospital, 2, Gakuhara-Cho, Kishiwada City, Osaka 596, Japan.

Acta Neurochir (1997) [Suppl] 70: 144–147
© Springer-Verlag 1997

Role of Calcium Ions in Acidosis-Induced Glial Swelling

F. Ringel[1], N. Plesnila[1], R. C. C. Chang[1], J. Peters[1], F. Staub[2], and A. Baethmann[1]

[1] Institute für Surgical Research, Klinikum Grosshadern, Ludwig-Maximilians-University, Munich, and
[2] Department of Neurosurgery, University of Cologne, Federal Republic of Germany

Summary

Tissue acidosis occurring in cerebral ischemia and traumatic brain injury is a mediator of cytotoxic brain edema. *In vitro*, extracellular lactacidosis induces swelling of glial cells in a dose dependent manner. pH-regulatory membrane transporters and channels have been identified which are involved in the increase of the glial cell volume. Underlying mechanisms of their activation are poorly understood, however. We have, therefore, addressed the question, whether and how Ca^{2+}-ions play a role in acidosis-induced glial swelling and intracellular acidification. For that purpose C6 glioma cells were suspended and the pH in the medium was lowered from 7.4 (baseline) to 6.2 by isotonic lactic acid. Cell volume and intracellular pH (pH_i) were assessed by flow cytometry. In the presence of Ca^{2+}-ions the cell volume reached a maximum of 125.1% from acidosis. In experiments using a calcium-free suspension medium, cell swelling from acidosis was inhibited by 74%. Additional buffering of intracellular calcium (Ca^{2+}_i) had no further inhibitory effect on acidosis-induced cell swelling, while buffering of Ca^{2+}_i by BAPTA-AM alone did not affect the glial volume increase secondary to administration of lactic acid. pH_i which was decreasing from acidosis was not affected by the experimental modifications of the Ca^{2+}-concentration in the medium or cytosol. The present data indicate that lactacidosis-induced glial swelling depends on the presence of extracellular Ca^{2+}-ions, while release of Ca^{2+}-ions from intracellular stores does not seem to be involved.

Keywords: Cerebral ischemia; traumatic brain injury; glial swelling; lactacidosis; calcium ions.

Introduction

Cerebral ischemia and traumatic brain injury are associated with an enhanced anaerobic metabolism leading to intra- and extracellular lactacidosis [6, 10]. Accumulation of lactic acid most likely is involved in the manifestation of secondary brain damage following a primary insult. Lactacidosis may contribute to the death of neurons and glia and lead to the formation of cytotoxic brain edema [7, 8, 16, 17]. Lactic acid accumulating in the intracellular compartment may spill over from necrotic or severely damaged cells in an ischemic or traumatic focus into the surrounding perifocal tissue resulting in extracellular acidosis. It has been shown *in vitro* that administration of lactic acid causes glial swelling in a dose-dependent manner together with intracellular acidification [18]. Our present understanding of mechanisms underlying the acidosis-induced glial swelling favors an activation of pH-regulatory membrane channels, such as the Na^+/H^+- or Cl^-/HCO_3^--antiporters [4, 5, 18]. Further information, however, on activating or modulating mechanisms of these membrane transport processes is currently not available. It is conceivable that Ca^{2+}-ions known to play an important role in many physiological and pathophysiological cellular processes including cell volume regulation [9, 13, 15], are involved in the acidosis-induced glial swelling. E.g., the intracellular Ca^{2+}-overload occurring in cerebral ischemia or trauma in nerve- and glial cells might be operative also in the cell swelling process elicited by acidosis. Flow cytometric studies were currently performed *in vitro* to explore the influence of calcium-ions on swelling and intracellular acidification of glial cells from acidosis.

Material and Methods

The basic experimental model has been frequently described [5, 18]. Briefly, C6 glioma cells were cultured under standard conditions (37°C, humidified air with 5% CO_2) using Dulbecco's Modified Eagle Medium containing 25 mM bicarbonate as buffer. The medium was supplemented with 10% fetal calf serum (FCS) and 100 IU/ml of penicillin G and 50 µg/ml streptomycin. Subcultivation was carried out daily. The cells were harvested from culture upon reaching confluency by addition of 0.05% trypsin / 0.02% EDTA in phosphate buffered saline and resuspended in FCS-free medium. The cell suspension was transferred to a Plexiglas incubation chamber equipped with electrodes for continuous monitoring of the medium pH, temperature and pO_2. The suspension was supplemented with a humidified mixture of O_2, N_2 and CO_2 by a membrane oxygenator. A magnetic stirrer prevented sedimentation of the cells. For the experiments cells in the 70th to 90th passage of subcultivation were used.

The cell volume was determined by flow cytometry using an advanced Coulter system with hydrodynamic focussing [1]. Flow cytometry was also employed for measurements of the intracellular pH (pH_i) utilizing the pH-sensitive fluorescence indicator BCECF. The fluorescence emission of BCECF was measured at a pH-sensitive and pH-insensitive wavelength. The fluorescence values were plotted against each other and the slope of the resulting regression line used as a measure of the intracellular pH. pH_i of the glial cells was calibrated by clamping medium and pH_i at eight different pH values, ranging from 5.0 to 8.5 utilizing nigericin and a high K^+-level in these suspension media.

The experiments were performed following incubation of the cells with BCECF for 20 min, calibration of pH_i and a 60 minute control period, used to assess the cell volume, pH_i and the medium osmolarity under baseline conditions. Subsequently, acidosis of pH 6.2 was induced by addition of isotonic lactic acid. Cell volume and pH_i were monitored for 60 minutes during lactacidosis and for 30 min after neutralization of the medium to pH 7.4 by NaOH.

In order to study the role of Ca^{2+}-ions in the acidosis-induced glial swelling, experiments were performed in normal medium and after omission of Ca^{2+}-ions. For that purpose Ca^{2+}-free isotonic medium was supplemented with 0.5 mM of the pH-independent calcium-chelator BAPTA. The cells were washed three times in this medium to remove residual Ca^{2+}-ions and transferred then to the incubation chamber. Calcium-ions released from intracellular stores were buffered in the cytosol by incubating the cell suspension with 0.1 mM of the membrane permeable acetoxymethylester derivative of BAPTA (BAPTA-AM) for 30 min at 37°C in a glass chamber. In a third group glial cells suspended in Ca^{2+}-free medium were incubated with BAPTA-AM in addition, for cytosolic calcium buffering in the absence of extracellular calcium-ions.

Results

The volume response of C6 glioma cells to lactacidosis in the presence and absence of Ca^{2+}-ions in the suspension medium is summarized in Table 1.

All obtained parameters remained constant during baseline conditions. Cell volume started to increase immediately after acidification reaching a maximum volume of 125.1 ± 2.5 (% of baseline; mean ± SEM; n = 9) at 60 min exposure to acidosis. Upon neutralization of the medium to pH 7.4, the cell volume was shrinking back to 105.4 ± 1.8 (% of baseline; mean ± SEM; n = 9) within 30 min.

The acidosis-induced glial swelling was inhibited by 74% when the experiments were conducted under omission of extracellular Ca^{2+}-ions. The maximum volume increase reached a level of only 106.4 ± 1.9 (% of baseline; mean ± SEM; n = 5; p < 0.05 vs. control). After neutralization of pH in the suspension, the glial volume returned to a near baseline value.

Additional buffering of cytosolic Ca^{2+}-ions by BAPTA-AM in a Ca^{2+}-free suspension medium had no further effect on glial swelling from acidosis. The maximum of cell swelling in the absence of extracellular Ca^{2+}-ions and buffering of cytosolic Ca^{2+}-ions by BAPTA-AM was 108.9 ± 2.1 (% of baseline; mean ± SEM; n = 5; p < 0.05 vs. control) which was not different from the corresponding volume increase in experiments with Ca^{2+}-free medium alone.

Moreover, when the cells were incubated with 0.1 mM BAPTA-AM for buffering the release of Ca^{2+}-ions from intracellular stores but suspended in medium with a normal Ca^{2+}-level, the extent of cell swelling upon acidification with lactic acid was not different from that in the control group. A maximum swelling of 120.9 ± 1.8 was attained in this group at 60 min (% of baseline; mean ± SEM; n = 5; n.s. vs. control).

pH_i of glial cells suspended in normal medium was 7.15 under baseline conditions but was decreasing promptly to 6.27, once the medium pH was lowered to

Table 1. *Volume Response of C6 Glioma Cells to Lactacidosis of pH 6.2.* The cells were suspended in normal (control) or calcium-free medium with addition of the pH-independent calcium chelator BAPTA (0.5 mM). Buffering of cytosolic Ca^{2+}-ions released from intracellular stores was achieved by incubation with 0.1 mM of the cell permeant Ca^{2+}-chelator BAPTA-AM

Time	PH_e	Cell volume			
		Control (n = 9)	Ca^{2+}-free medium + BAPTA (n = 5)	Ca^{2+}-free medium + BAPTA + BAPTA-AM (n = 5)	Ca^{2+}-containing medium + BAPTA-AM (n = 5)
−15 min	7.4	100.73 ± 0.42	99.99 ± 0.38	99.83 ± 0.70	100.21 ± 0.07
−10 min	7.4	99.99 ± 0.32	99.43 ± 0.68	99.55 ± 0.67	100.17 ± 0.14
1 min	6.2	107.43 ± 0.74	103.57 ± 0.89[a]	102.89 ± 1.17[a, b]	106.38 ± 0.92
10 min	6.2	116.33 ± 1.29	105.78 ± 1.21[a]	105.41 ± 1.24[a, b]	111.61 ± 0.64
30 min	6.2	120.95 ± 1.46	106.27 ± 1.82[a]	106.74 ± 1.58[a, b]	117.20 ± 1.15
60 min	6.2	125.12 ± 2.45	105.67 ± 2.19[a]	108.92 ± 2.14[a, b]	120.93 ± 1.76
70 min	7.4	110.44 ± 1.57	97.26 ± 1.74[a]	102.27 ± 1.35	112.71 ± 1.63
90 min	7.4	105.38 ± 1.82	98.18 ± 2.32	104.71 ± 3.37	110.28 ± 1.64

Mean ± SEM. [a] p < 0.05 vs. control, [b] n.s. vs. Ca^{2+}-free medium only (Kruskal-Wallis and Dunn's post hoc test).

6.2. The level of intracellular acidification was not further changed during the 60 min period with exposure to lactacidosis. Following neutralization of the medium, pH$_i$ returned to baseline values. None of the groups with intracellular buffering of Ca^{2+}-ions and/or omission of Ca^{2+}-ions from the suspension medium was found to have a different response of pH$_i$, neither under baseline conditions nor in acidosis.

Discussion

The present findings demonstrate that glial swelling from lactic acid exposure depends markedly on the presence of extracellular calcium ions. On the other side a release of Ca^{2+}-ions from intracellular stores, e.g. mitochondria or the endoplasmatic reticulum, does not seem to play a role in the processes underlying acidosis-induced glial swelling. As seen, the buffering of cytoplasmic Ca^{2+}-ions by BAPTA-AM alone did not affect acidosis-induced cell swelling. Even buffering of intracellular Ca^{2+}-ions in the absence of Ca^{2+}-ions in the suspension medium had no additional inhibitory potential as compared to the experiments in Ca^{2+}-free medium alone. It is not clear yet, whether the involvement of extracellular Ca^{2+}-ions in acidosis-induced cell swelling is attributable to (i) a net-influx of Ca^{2+}-ions through the cell membrane or to (ii) a function of extracellular Ca^{2+} for activation of membrane transport proteins.

The response of the intracellular calcium level to extracellular acidosis varies between different cell types in the CNS. While primary cultured neurons are increasing their intracellular calcium concentration during acidosis [12, 14], primary cultured astrocytes do not [11]. Therefore, an extra-to-intracellular influx of Ca^{2+}-ions as underlying mechanism might not necessarily be involved in acidosis-induced cell swelling. Lohr *et al.* [2] have shown that the regulatory volume decrease after hypotonic swelling in C6 glioma cells is markedly dependent on the presence of extracellular Ca^{2+}-ions. However, an increase of the intracellular Ca^{2+}-concentration was not detectable. It might be possible that extracellular calcium ions are needed for activation of membrane transport proteins without their net-influx through the cell membrane. To elucidate respective details of the involvement of Ca^{2+}-ions, further investigations are necessary.

The present findings suggest in addition that the membrane channels and transporters taking part in the acidosis induced glial swelling are not exclusively involved in the regulation of pH$_i$. This conclusion is based on the observation that omission of Ca^{2+}-ions from the medium had no influence on the pH$_i$ of glial cells, neither under baseline conditions nor during acid exposure. We propose, therefore, that the response of the cell volume and of the pH$_i$ to acidosis are in part distinct processes, however, which are difficult to reconcile with the present understanding of acidosis-induced glial swelling.

Acknowledgments

The excellent technical assistance of Ingrid Kölbl and Susanne Guretzky is gratefully acknowledged. The project was supported by a grant from Deutsche Forschungsgemeinschaft to Dr. F. Staub (Sta: 406/2-1). Raymond C. C. Chang was supported by the Deutscher Akademischer Austauschdienst.

References

1. Kachel V, Glossner E, Kordwig G, Ruhenstroth-Bauer G (1977) Fluvo-metricell, a combined cell volume and cell fluorescence analyzer. J Histochem Cytochem 25: 804–812
2. Lohr JW, Yohe LA (1994) Mechanisms of hypoosmotic volume regulation in glioma cells. Brain Res 667: 263–268
3. Duffy S, MacVicar BA (1996) *In vitro* ischemia promotes calcium influx and intracellular calcium release in hippocampal astrocytes. J Neurosci 16: 71–81
4. Kempski O, Staub F, Jansen M, Schödel F, Baethmann A (1988) Glial swelling during extracellular acidosis *in vitro*. Stroke 19: 385–392
5. Kempski O, Staub F, v Rosen F, Zimmer M, Neu A, Baethmann A (1988) Molecular mechanisms of glial swelling *in vitro*. Neurochem Pathol 9: 109–125
6. Kraig RP, Pulsinelli WA, Plum F (1985) Heterogenous distribution of hydrogen and bicarbonate ions during complete brain ischemia. In: Kogure K, Hossmann K-A, Siesjö BK, Welsh FA (eds) Progress in brain research, Vol 63. Elsevier, Amsterdam, pp 155–166
7. Kraig RP, Petito CK, Plum F, Pulsinelli WA (1987) Hydrogen ions kills brain at concentrations reached in ischemia. J Cereb Blood Flow Metab 7: 379–386
8. Kimelberg HK (1995) Current concepts of brain edema. Review of laboratory investigations. J Neurosurg 83: 1051–1059
9. McCarty NA, O'Neil RG (1992) Calcium signalling in cell volume regulation. Physiol Rev 72: 1037–1061
10. Nakai H, Yamamoto YL, Diksic M, Worsley KJ, Takara E (1988) Triple-tracer autoradiography demonstrates effects of hyperglycemia on cerebral blood flow, pH, and glucose utilization in cerebral ischemia of rats. Stroke 19: 764–772
11. Neary JT, Fu Q, Bender AS, Norenberg MD (1993) Effect of external acidosis on basal and ATP-evoked calcium influx in cultured astrocytes. Brain Res 603: 211–216
12. Nedergaard M (1995) Intracellular Ca^{2+} transients evoked by lactic acid in cultured mammalian neurons. Am J Physiol 268: R506–R513
13. O'Connor E, Kimelberg HK (1993) Role of calcium in astrocyte volume regulation and in the release of ions and amino acids. J Neurosc 13: 2638–2650
14. OuYang YB, Mellergard P, Kristián T, Kristiánova V, Siesjö BK (1994) Influence of acid-base changes on the intracellular

calcium concentration of neurons in primary culture. Exp Brain Res 101: 265–271

15. Pierce SK, Politis AD (1990) Ca^{2+}-activated cell volume recovery mechanisms. Ann Rev Physiol 52: 27–42

16. Siesjö BK (1988) Acidosis and ischemic brain damage. Neurochem Pathol 9: 31–88

17. Siesjö BK, Katsura K, Mellergard P, Ekholm A, Lundgren J, Smith M-L (1993) Acidosis-related brain damage. In: Kogure K, Hossmann K-A, Siesjö BK (eds) Progress in brain research, Vol 96. Elsevier, Amsterdam, pp 23–48

18. Staub F, Baethmann A, Peters J, Weigt H, Kempski O (1990) Effects of lactacidosis on glial cell volume and viability. J Cereb Blood Flow Metab 10: 866–876

19. Szatkowski M, Attwell D (1994) Triggering and execution of neuronal death in brain ischemia: two phases of glutamate release by different mechanisms. TINS 17: 359–365

Correspondence: Nikolaus Plesnila, M.D., Institute for Surgical Research, Klinikum Grosshadern, University of Munich, Marchioninistrasse 15, D-81366 München, Federal Republic of Germany.

Acta Neurochir (1997) [Suppl] 70: 148–151
© Springer-Verlag 1997

Glutamate Induced Astroglial Swelling – Methods and Mechanisms

E. Hansson[1], F. Blomstrand[1], S. Khatibi[2], T. Olsson[2], and L. Rönnbäck[1]

[1] Institute of Neurobiology and Institute of Clinical Neuroscience, Department of Neurology, Göteborg University, and
[2] Department of Applied Electronics, Chalmers University of Technology, Göteborg, Sweden

Summary

Glutamate (Glu) plays an important role in the early development of brain injuries caused by ischemia, i.e. stroke, or brain trauma. Glu induces a rapid astroglial swelling which, in turn, deranges the composition of neuroactive substances in the extracellular space. We report that Glu can induce astroglial cell swelling by interaction with metabotropic Glu receptors (mGluRs). Furthermore, the Na^+-K^+-$2Cl^-$ cotransporter, a Na^+-K^+ ATPase, and the Na^+-dependent electrogenic Glu carrier seem to be involved in this Glu-induced astroglial cell swelling. Two methods for studying cell swelling are described. One is based on variations in the signal emitted by the fluorescent probe fura-2/AM when excited at its isosbestic point. These variations were shown to be directly proportional to variations in intracellular volume. Relative changes in cell volume and intracellular calcium concentration could be detected simultaneously in single astroglial cells. The other method used permits the cell volume to be calculated in relative terms with the aid of image processing techniques.

Keywords: Astrocyte; cell volume; Ca^{2+}; glutamate; cell volume quantification.

Introduction

Astrocytes constitute a prominent part of the brain cells both in terms of number and in terms of volume. These cells are responsible for the homeostasis of ions and amino acids in the extracellular (e.c.) space. They control the ionic and amino acid concentrations there both by expression and activation of ion channels for instance Ca^{2+}, Na^+ and K^+ and by expression and regulation of uptake systems with high capacity and high affinity for glutamate (Glu), γ aminobutyric acid (GABA) and taurine [3, 6, 9, 12]. The cells also have high capacity for controlling their own cell volume. As the e.c. space in the brain is small compared with the cell volume, moderate changes in astroglial cell volume may influence the e.c. milieu substantially [7]. This is, in fact, one important event in the early development of brain injuries caused by a stroke or brain trauma. The excitatory neurotransmitter Glu is one of the more important individual factors in the initial cell swelling [13]. Below we describe some methods for determining variations in cell volume at the single cell level.

Materials and Methods

Cell Cultures

Primary cultures were prepared from newborn rat cerebral cortex, using a previously described method with some modifications [4].

Volume Measurements

The relative changes in cell volume and the parallel intracellular (i.c.) calcium concentrations ($[Ca^{2+}]_i$) were examined in single cells using a Spex Fluoromax System. The measurements were performed as previously described [4], except for the use of three instead of two excitatory wavelengths. The cells were loaded with the highly fluorescent, intracellular Ca^{2+} sensitive probe fura-2/AM. Volume measurements were carried out at the isosbestic point (358 nm), where the probe is ion insensitive and the emitted fluorescent signals are related only to the i.c. dye concentration [2, 4]. By switching the excitation wavelengths between the isosbestic point and the Ca^{2+} sensitive wavelengths 340 nm and 380 nm, we detected simultaneously relative volume changes and $[Ca^{2+}]_i$ changes after Glu stimulation. Using fluo-3/AM in an imaging system Ca^{2+} transients were also observed in many cells simultaneously.

A computerized 3-dimensional (3-D) imaging system for the quantification of cell volume is under development. A series of images are produced from the microscope by focusing up and down through the specimen. Owing to the large depth of field in light microscopes [11], each point of the specimen becomes a divergent double cone (the 3-D analogue of the Airy disc) which contaminates all the collected 2-D images. Thus each image contains both in-focus information from the focal plane and out-of-focus information from the neighbouring planes (Fig. 2), in the form of a blurring effect on the image. The out-of-focus removal (deblurring) is accomplished by traditional image analyses. Developing a suitable deblurring method is a significant part of our work. Furthermore important is that trends caused by bleaching of normal and swollen glial cells can be detected and compensated for by the system. The characteristics of an optical system can be described by its point spread function (PSF). This function can be computed (theoretically) or estimated (experimentally). We applied both methods to obtain the best possible results with our system.

Results and Discussion

Comments on the Methods of Quantifying Changes in Cell Volume

The techniques developed to estimate volume changes at the single cell level are now believed to be reliable enough to allow detailed studies of swelling phenomena. An important advantage of our photometric method is that rapid and simultaneous changes in cell volume and $[Ca^{2+}]_i$ can be measured on intact cells in a monolayer (Fig. 1). Furthermore, the experiments are easy to perform and the amount of equipment required is relatively limited. A disadvantage is

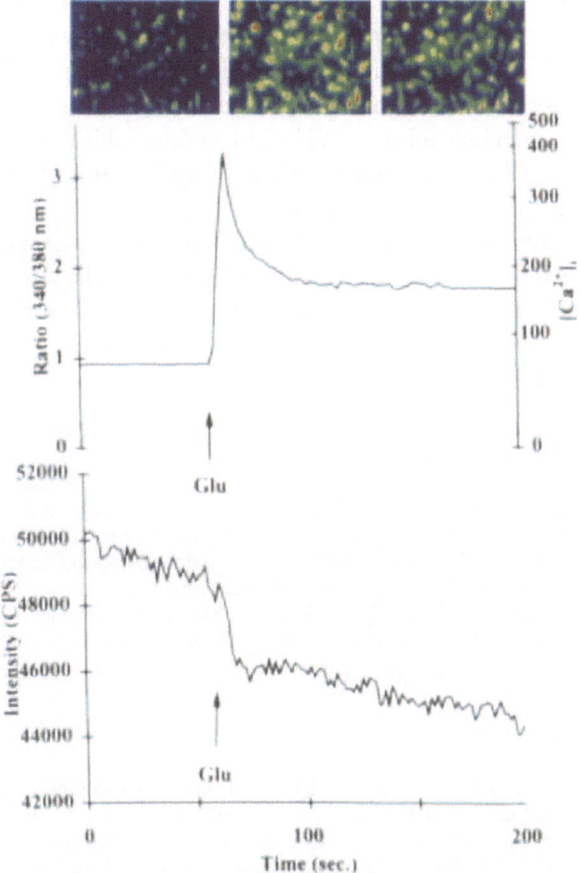

Fig. 1. Typical recordings of simultaneous $[Ca^{2+}]_i$ increase (using 340/380 nm ratio, top) and cell swelling (using 358 nm excitation, bottom) after addition of 100 µM Glu. The cells were loaded with fura-2/AM and studied in a photometric system. Colored figures correspond to Ca^{2+} transients seen in several cells simultaneously after addition of 100 µM Glu. The cells were loaded with fluo-3/AM. Pseudocolors show normal (blue and green), increased (yellow) and highly increased (red) $[Ca^{2+}]_i$

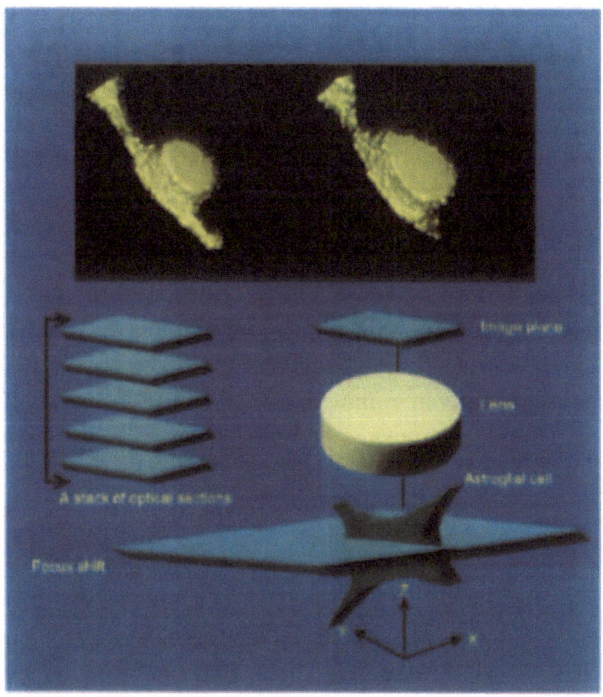

Fig. 2. Simplified principle of the optical sectioning (bottom, right). The 3-D image of the astroglial cell is generated from a stack of 2-D images (bottom, left). The 3-D cell reconstructions on top represents a normal (left) and a swollen (right) astroglial cell

that the method assumes that the cells swell in a similar way. If some cells increase in size relatively more upward than laterally, then even more fluorescent molecules might accumulate in the delimited zone. Thus, if the cells do not increase in size in a similar way, then the changes in fluorescence intensity will not be proportional to the degree of swelling for all cells. A safer method to register volume changes would be to determine cell volume in 3 dimensions. Therefore, we developed a method to be applied to 3-D optical section images of fluorescently labeled single cells (Fig. 2). The 3-D images produced using this system are comparable to those obtained using confocal microscopy. In fact, our system has an advantage over confocal microscopy, namely that a widefield light microscope, with an image intensifier camera, has a substantially higher sensitivity than early commercial confocal microscopes. Furthermore, the light exposure of the cells can be several orders of magnitude less with such a camera system than with a confocal microscope. Thus photo bleaching and photo damage to the cells are reduced, which is crucial in the estimation of volume changes in the glial cells. The system also permits registration of volume changes in several cells at the same time (which is possible also with the photometric system when using imaging). Among the drawbacks of the 3-D imaging system is that it requires heavy computational power and that the analyses are time-consuming.

Molecular Mechanisms Underlying Glu-Induced Astroglial Swelling

It has been suggested that astroglial swelling is caused by a transmembrane transport of Glu coupled to the uptake of Na^+ ions which, in turn causes an osmotically driven volume increase [13]. The uptake of Glu into the astrocytes occurs in the presence of a steep i.c. to e.c. concentration difference, which is energy consuming, and the transport is driven by the electrochemical gradient for Na^+. The net increase of i.c. osmolality caused by the influx of Na^+ and Glu has been proposed as one mechanism responsible for glial swelling [13]. The Na^+-K^+-$2Cl^-$ cotransporter and the opening of Cl^- channels have also been implicated [15]. Ca^{2+} has also been shown to be involved in the Glu-induced cell swelling [8, 10].

One hypothesis that we have suggested is that Glu interacts with mGluRs, which causes cell swelling. The mGluRs activate phospholipase C (PLC) to produce inositol 1,4,5-trisphosphate (IP_3), which in turn mobilizes i.c. Ca^{2+}. Thereafter, there might be an influx of Ca^{2+} through the plasma membrane. Glu also interacts with those mGluRs which inhibit adenylate cyclase and decrease the cyclic AMP production. This inhibition of cyclic AMP formation might cause an opening of L-Ca^{2+} channels and activation of $G_{i\alpha}$ might cause an opening of inward rectifying K^+ channels. Based on knowledge of other cell systems, it has been suggested that the Ca^{2+}-dependent outward rectifying K^+ channels are activated to compensate for the K^+ required for the Na^+-K^+-$2Cl^-$ cotransport [1]. The Na^+-K^+-ATPase is activated, and subsequently also an electrogenic Na^+-dependent Glu carrier. The astroglial swelling induced by Glu is not exclusively the result of these processes. It requires another, as yet unidentified mechanism, probably some ketamine sensitive, ion channel complex for K^+ outflow and probably also for Na^+ influx [4, 5].

Aspects Relating to Glu-Induced Physiological Astroglial Swelling

As is clear from the above, the Glu-induced rapid astroglial swelling is of utmost importance in the pathophysiology of the earliest stage of a brain injury.

However, Glu-induced astroglial swelling may also be of importance in normal brain physiology. Thus, the concentrations and transport capacities of neuroactive substances in the e.c. space might be influenced by astroglial swelling and a secondary reduction of the e.c. volume. Our finding that the astroglial cell volume can be altered by receptor stimulation, e.g. via different mGluRs, raises the question of whether volume changes in the astroglial network could be one physiological mechanism for control of the e.c. fluid volume. If this is the case, the concentrations of ions, neuroactive and trophic substances in the e.c. space could be regulated within local brain regions. Alternatively, rapid volume changes within the astroglial syncytium, with secondary pulsating changes of the e.c. space, could regulate transport pathways for e.c. substances. Thereby glial mGluRs activation could induce changes in the transport and concentration of e.c. messengers. Another possibility is that astroglial swelling leads to a narrowing of the astroglial cell membranes in the synaptic regions, resulting in morphologically closer interaction between neurons and glia, and economization of the signaling substances [14]. In addition, this mechanism could quite simply shield synaptic regions from substances in the e.c. space.

Further studies are needed to clarify the causes and the role of astroglial swelling, and to explore the possibilities of therapy to prevent or attenuate this astrocytic response, which may be detrimental to neuronal survival.

Acknowledgements

This work was supported by grants from the Swedish Medical Research Council (grant no 12X-06812), from the Swedish Work Environment Fund (Grant no 94-0214), from the Swedish Council for Work Life Research (Grant no 95-0231) and from The Swedish National Board for Industrial and Technical Development (NUTEK, Grant, no 9304274). The skilful work of Ulrika Johansson is greatly appreciated.

References

1. Blatz AL, Magleby KL (1987) Calcium-activated potassium channels. Trends Neurosci Sci 10: 463–467
2. Eriksson PS, Nilsson M, Wågberg M, Rönnbäck L, Hansson E (1992) Volume regulation of single astroglial cells in primary culture. Neurosci Lett 143: 195–199
3. Hansson E (1988) Astroglia from defined brain regions as studied with primary cultures. Progr Neurobiol 30: 369–397
4. Hansson E (1994) Metabotropic glutamate receptor activation induces astroglial swelling. J Biol Chem 269: 21955–21961
5. Hansson E, Rönnbäck L (1995) Astrocytes in glutamate neurotransmission. FASEB J 9: 343–350

6. Hertz L (1979) Functional interactions between neurons and astrocytes I. Turnover and metabolism of putative amino acid neurotransmitters. Progr Neurobiol 13: 277–323

7. Kimelberg HK (1991) Swelling and volume control in brain astroglial cells. In: Gilles R, et al (eds) Advances in comparative and environmental physiology, vol 9. Springer, Berlin Heidelberg New York Tokyo, pp 81–117

8. Koyoama Y, Baba A, Iwata H (1991) L-Glutamate induced swelling of cultured astrocytes is dependent on extracellular Ca^{2+}. Neurosci Lett 122: 210–212

9. Murphy S, Pearce B (1987) Functional receptors for neurotransmitters on astroglial cells. Neuroscience 22: 381–394

10. O'Connor ER, Kimelberg HK (1993) Role of calcium in astrocyte volume regulation and in the release of ions and amino acids. J Neurosci 13: 2638–2650

11. Sheppard CJR (1987) Depth of field in optical microsopy. J Microsc 149: 73–75

12. Sontheimer H (1992) Astrocytes, as well as neurons, express a diversity of ion channels. Can J Physiol Pharmacol 70: S223–S238

13. Schneider GH, Baethmann A, Kempski O (1992) Mechanisms of glial swelling induced by glutamate. Can J Physiol Pharmacol 70: S334–S343

14. Smith SJ (1992) Do astrocytes process neural information? In: Yu ACH, Hertz L, Norenberg MD, Syková E, Waxman SG (eds) Progr Brain Res, vol 94. Elsevier, Amsterdam, pp 119–136

15. Staub F, Peters J, Kempski O, Schneider G-H, Schürer L, Baethmann A (1993) Swelling of glial cells in lactacidosis and by glutamate: significance of Cl$^-$-transport. Brain Res 610: 69–74

Correspondence: Dr. Elisabeth Hansson, Institute of Neurobiology, Göteborg University, Medicinaregatan 5, S-41390 Göteborg, Sweden.

Acta Neurochir (1997) [Suppl] 70: 152–154
© Springer-Verlag 1997

Impaired Learning of Active Avoidance in Water-Intoxicated Rats

M. Yamaguchi[1], T. Yamada[1], I. Kinoshita[1], S. Wu[2], T. Nagashima[2], and N. Tamaki[2]

[1] Faculty of Health Science and [2] Department of Neurological Surgery, Kobe University School of Medicine, Kobe, Japan

Summary

Brain edema is an important clinical condition. Pathophysiological findings on behavioral changes may be helpful for a comprehensive understanding of brain edema. However, only few reports on behavioral studies of brain edema have so far appeared. Experiments using psychological techniques on animals are rather time-consuming and may not be suitable for the study of transient conditions, as brain edema caused by trauma, vascular accidents, or others. We have developed a method for avoidance learning of rats using a running wheel apparatus with computer assistance. This model was employed in studies on brain edema from water intoxication in rats. As a result, avoidance learning was significantly impaired by water intoxication. Either direct overhydration of the brain or indirect effects, as a decrease in cerebral blood flow, or both, are suggested as mechanisms underlying the impairment of behavior.

Keywords: Water intoxication; avoidance learning; neuropsychology.

Introduction

Brain edema may produce mental dysfunction. Studies of underlying mechanisms on a neuropsychological basis may provide valuable information for neurology, neurosurgery, and rehabilitation. Since experimental brain edema induced in rats by water intoxication is a simple and reproducible model, we have evaluated avoidance learning of these animals with overhydration by using a simple shuttle box method [5]. Thereby, we have found a decrease in blood flow of the edematous brain following water intoxication [6]. Since a sophisticated computer assisted apparatus is available in our laboratory, we would like to present recently obtained data of high quality on impaired learning of active avoidance of water-intoxicated rats.

Materials and Methods

Male Fisher strain rats of 120 to 210 gm body weight were used in the experiments because of their excellent learning ability when compared with other strains [3]. Using the method of Wasterlain and Posner [4], distilled water in a dosis of 10% body weight was intraperitoneally injected. To avoid any influence on the learning ability, vasopressin was not given. The water content of the brain was determined according to the method of Elliot and Jasper [2]. Two hours after water loading, active avoidance learning was started utilizing the running wheel method of Iso *et al.* [3]. The learning program was as follows: a rat placed in the apparatus must turn the wheel by running for at least 45 degrees within 15 seconds after a lamp was turned on. Unless the task was performed sufficiently, an electric shock (ES) was administered instantly by the floor grid of the aluminum bar of the wheel as punishment. The ES was produced by a scrambled AC current with an intensity of about 1 mA.

Learning of active avoidance was evaluated in the following manner: During the 1st trial, learning for 10 min under light and 5 min rest in dark was repeated 3 times. The rats were returned then to their home cages. After 60 min, the 2nd trial was carried out in the same manner as before. A 3rd trial followed after another 60 min interval. The 60 min interval method of learning proved to be effective for acute experiments as the behavioral study in water intoxication brain edema [7]. The average numbers of ES's in the 1st trial of each animal were compared with those of the 2nd or 3rd trials using the paired t-test. A significant decrease in the number of ES's between the 1st and the subsequent trials was considered as active avoidance learning.

In the control group 0.9% saline was used instead of distilled water given to the animals with water-intoxication. The learning task was applied in the same manner and the results were compared.

Results

A significant increase in water content of the brain tissue was observed at 2 hours after water loading (Fig. 1). The learning experiment was, therefore, started at this time point as described above.

In preliminary experiments, we have confirmed that the water loading does not disturb the running ability in the wheel cage, as long as the volume of distilled water was limited to 10% of the body weight.

The average numbers of ES's in the 1st trial of water-intoxicated animals were compared with those of the 2nd or 3rd trial, whereby non-significant differ-

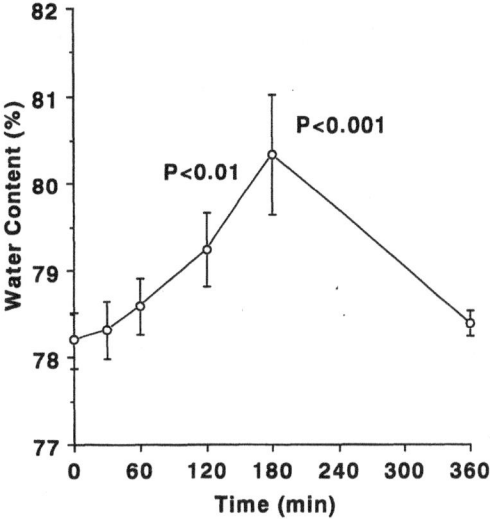

Fig. 1. Time course of water content

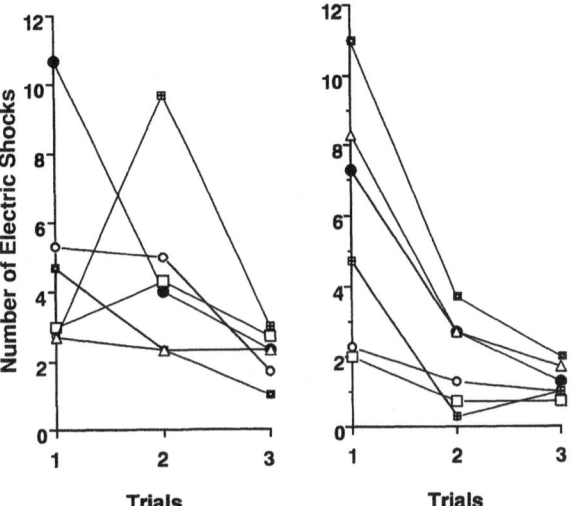

Fig. 2. Avoidance learning after intraperitoneal injection of distilled water or 0.9% saline (volume load = 10% of body weight). Each symbol represents one individual rat of the group of rats with water-intoxication (left) or saline administration (right)

ences were observed as indicated in Fig. 2. However, the average numbers of ES's in the control group showed a significant decrease in the 2nd and 3rd trial when compared with the 1st trial (P < 0.05 and 0.005, respectively).

Discussion

A transient reversible state of impaired neurological or mental function caused by brain edema is considered to be a distinct symptom as compared to the permanent disruptive state of the central nervous system function in clinical practice. To better understand this pathophysiological state, behavioral studies of animals with experimental reversible brain edema may contribute to the progress of the clinical diagnostic assessment. As brain edema caused by water-intoxication is a simple and reproducible model in experimental animals, we are reporting a behavioral study [5] using this condition.

Only few experimental reports using psychological analysis have appeared concerning brain edema. Clasen et al. [1] reported investigations on experimental brain edema based on behavioral studies in animals with lead encephalopathy. Behavioral analyses, however, almost always require a longer period to complete when compared to investigations using biochemical, physiological, or morphological techniques. Some psychological experiments, e.g. using a maze task in food deprived animals, or forced swimming in the water maze system are not suitable for a behavioral study under rapidly changing conditions as acute brain edema.

In previous work using the shuttle box method, significantly increased numbers of ES's were observed in water-intoxicated rats when compared with the controls [5]. This method requires, however, an excellent technique of animal handling. Rough handling of rats by untrained examiners or an insufficient period of habituation in the experimental apparatus might interfere with the experimental results. Further, the length of time necessary to complete learning might vary.

We have recently developed a rapid (240 min, in total) method of avoidance learning of rats [7] based on a computer assisted running wheel task, which was applied in animals with water intoxication. The transient yet significant increase in brain water content was studied by this method of experimental psychology.

References

1. Clasen RA, Hoeppner TJ, Hartman JF, et al (1985) Electron microscopic and behavioral studies in experimental lead encephalopathy. In: Inaba Y, Klatzo I, Spatz M (eds) Brain edema VI. Springer, Berlin Heidelberg New York Tokyo, pp 48–58
2. Elliot KAC, Jasper H (1949) Measurement of experimentally induced brain swelling and shrinkage. Am J Physiol 157: 122–129
3. Iso H, Brush FR, Fujii M, et al (1988) Running wheel avoidance learning in rat (Rattus norvegicus): effect of contingencies and comparison of different strains. J Comp Psych 102: 350–371

155

154

4. Wasterlain CG, Posner JB (1969) Cerebral edema in water intoxication. I. Arch Neurol 19: 71–78
5. Yamaguchi M, Kinoshita I, Sobue I (1990) Mental dysfunction in water intoxication brain edema. Advances in neurology, vol 52. Raven, New York, p 561
6. Yamaguchi M, Wu S, Ehara K, *et al* (1994) Cerebral blood flow of rats with water-intoxicated brain edema. Acta Neurochir (Wien) [Suppl] 60: 190–192
7. Yamaguchi M, Yamada T (1996) A successful running wheel method of active avoidance learning for 240 minutes on Fisher-strain rats. Bull Allied Med Sci Kobe 12: 187–192

Correspondence: Michio Yamaguchi, M.D., Faculty of Health Science, Kobe University School of Medicine, 7-10-2 Tomogaoka, Suma, Kobe 65401, Japan.

Acta Neurochir (1997) [Suppl] 70: 155–158
© Springer-Verlag 1997

Topical Application of 5-HT Antibodies Reduces Edema and Cell Changes Following Trauma of the Rat Spinal Cord

H. S. Sharma[1, 2], **J. Westman**[1], and **F. Nyberg**[2]

[1] Laboratory of Neuroanatomy, Department of Anatomy, and [2] Department of Pharmaceutical Biosciences, Biomedical Center, Uppsala University, Uppsala, Sweden

Summary

Involvement of serotonin in the early microvascular reactions and cell changes following trauma of the spinal cord was examined using topical application of serotonin antibodies to the traumatised cord in a rat model. A focal trauma of the spinal cord was produced by making an incision into the right dorsal horn of the T10-11 segments (about 2 mm deep and 5 mm long); the animals were allowed to survive 5 h after injury. Monoclonal 5-HT antibodies (1:20) were applied (25 µl in 10 sec) to the traumatised spinal cord 2 min after injury. There was a significant reduction in the breakdown of the blood-spinal cord barrier, edema formation, and cell changes in the traumatised rats which received 5-HT antiserum compared to the injured rats given saline. These results show that 5-HT is an important mediator involved in the early pathophysiological responses of spinal cord injury.

Keywords: Spinal cord injury; 5-HT; edema; blood-spinal cord barrier; cell changes; immunohistochemistry.

Introduction

Spinal cord injury is a serious clinical problem and the factors responsible for the trauma induced edema and cell changes are still not known in all details [3, 9]. Serotonin (5-hydroxytryptamine, 5-HT) is an important mediator of vasogenic edema formation and of disturbances of the microvascular permeability in the central nervous system (CNS) [2, 14]. This amine influences the signal transduction cascade in many neuronal pathways including gene expression [1, 2]. The involvement, however, of 5-HT in the disease processes of the brain and spinal cord is not well understood, and its role in traumatic injuries of the CNS is still controversially discussed [1–3, 8–10].

Earlier work of our laboratory has shown that plasma- and spinal cord levels of serotonin increase profoundly following a focal spinal cord injury and that inhibition of the serotonin biosynthesis by p-chlorophenylalanine (p-CPA) markedly attenuates edema formation and cell changes in the traumatised cord [11–13]. These observations may indicate an important role of 5-HT in the pathophysiology of spinal cord injuries.

Subsequent studies of other laboratories using 5-HT receptor blocking drugs, however, have shown controversial results [3, 8, 9]. This discrepancy can be easily understood, because serotonin has more than seven types of receptors and multiple receptor sub-types. Thus, analysis of 5-HT by using a few selective receptor blocking drugs in a traum model may not provide unequivocal results. In addition, the dose response and time schedule of any drug treatment may influence the final outcome. Thus, novel studies using more selective receptor antagonists of serotonin are needed to improve its understanding in traumatic injuries of the CNS.

Molecular modelling and receptor recognition studies have recently shown that application of antibodies against a particular protein or neurotransmitter is a most powerful tool to antagonise the physiological functions of a ligand, when the antibody has the capacity to bind with specific receptor proteins *in vivo* [4–7, 17, 18]. Antibodies applied at the surface of the spinal cord penetrate deeply into the tissue within 10 min neutralising there the physiological effects of the natural ligands [4, 5]. Thus, in order to further elucidate the involvement of serotonin in spinal cord injury we have administered serotonin antiserum to the traumatised spinal cord to examine edema formation, microvascular permeability changes, and early cell reaction in our rat model.

Materials and Methods

Animals

Experiments were carried out in 30 male Wistar rats (body weight 200–300 g) under Equithesin (3 ml/kg, i.p.) anaesthesia. The rats were housed at a controlled ambient temperature (21 ± 1°C) with a 12 h light and 12 h dark schedule. The rat feed and tap water were supplied ad libitum.

Spinal Cord Injury

Spinal cord injury was inflicted by making a longitudinal incision of the right dorsal horn (about 2 mm deep and 5 mm long) of the T10–11 segments [11, 13]. The animals were allowed to survive 5 h after injury. The experimental protocol was approved by the Ethical Committee of the Uppsala University.

Application of 5-HT Antiserum

In separate group of rats, commercial monoclonal 5-HT antiserum (DAKO, Hamburg, Germany) (1:20) was administered (25 μl in 10 sec) to the traumatised spinal cord 2 min after injury [15, 16]. The animals were allowed to survive 5 h after injury. Separate groups of untreated traumatised rats or animals treated with normal rabbit serum after trauma were used as controls.

Spinal Cord Edema

Spinal cord edema was examined by measurement of the tissue water content [11, 12]. In brief, 5 h after injury, the animals were decapitated and the spinal cord was quickly removed. The T9, 10–11 and T12 segments were excised, weighed and placed in an oven at 90°C for 72 h. The water content of the cord was determined by using the wet and dry weight of the spinal cord.

Blood-Spinal Cord Barrier Permeability

The microvascular permeability was measured by using uptake of Evans blue and radiolabelled iodine into the tissue [12, 13]. For this purpose, Evans blue (2% solution, 0.3 ml/100 g) and ^{131}I-sodium (10 μCi/100 g) were injected into the right femoral vein 5 h after injury. The tracers were allowed to circulate for 5 min. Intravascular tracer was washed out by a brief saline rinse and the spinal cord was taken out. The total blood radioactivity was measured in a

sample collected by heart puncture immediately before perfusion. Extravasation of the radiotracer was expressed as percent of the blood radioactivity. Evans blue content of the cord was measured colorimetrically [12, 13].

Spinal Cord Pathology

For histology, animals were perfused through the heart (at 100 torr) with a solution of 4% paraformaldehyde containing 1.5% glutaraldehyde in 0.1 M phosphate buffer, pH 7.4 at room temperature which was preceded by a brief saline wash. After perfusion tissue pieces of the T9 and T12 segment were taken out and embedded in epon for routine light- and electron microsopy. The cell changes were examined by light- and electron microscopy in the T9 and T12 segments using toloidine blue staining [15, 16].

Statistical Analysis

The data obtained were analysed by using ANOVA followed by Dunnett's test for statistical significance. A p-value less than 0.05 was considered significant.

Results

Spinal Cord Edema

The focal spinal cord trauma resulted in a profound increase in the tissue water content in all segments examined. Administration of 5-HT antiserum to the dorsal surface of the traumatised spinal cord 2 min after injury significantly reduced edema formation (Fig. 1). This effect was absent in animals which received normal rabbit serum in an identical manner.

Blood-Spinal Cord Barrier Permeability

Untreated rats had a profound increase in extravasation of Evans blue and ^{131}I-sodium into the T9 and T12 segment of the cord. The increase in tracer extravasa-

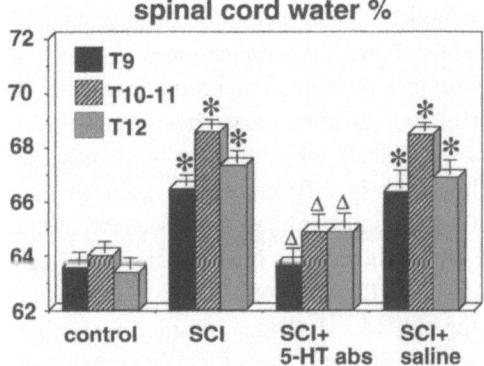

Fig. 1. Spinal cord water content in control and traumatised rats and its modification by 5-HT antiserum or saline. Treatment with 5-HT antiserum markedly attenuated the increase of the spinal cord water content after 5 h injury. * P < 0.001 compared to control; Δ P < 0.05 compared to SCI

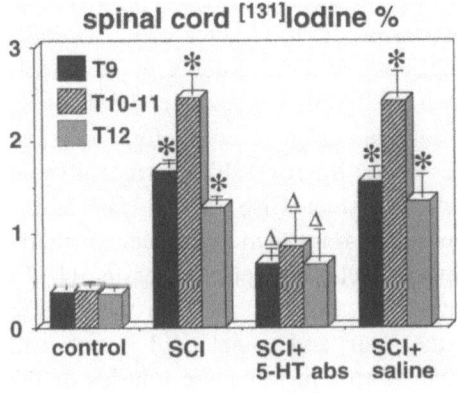

Fig. 2. Extravasation of [131] iodine across the blood-spinal cord barrier in control and traumatised rats and its modification by 5-HT antiserum or saline. Pretreatment with 5-HT antiserum significantly reduced extravasation of the radiotracer into the spinal cord. * P < 0.001 compared to control; Δ P < 0.05 compared to SCI

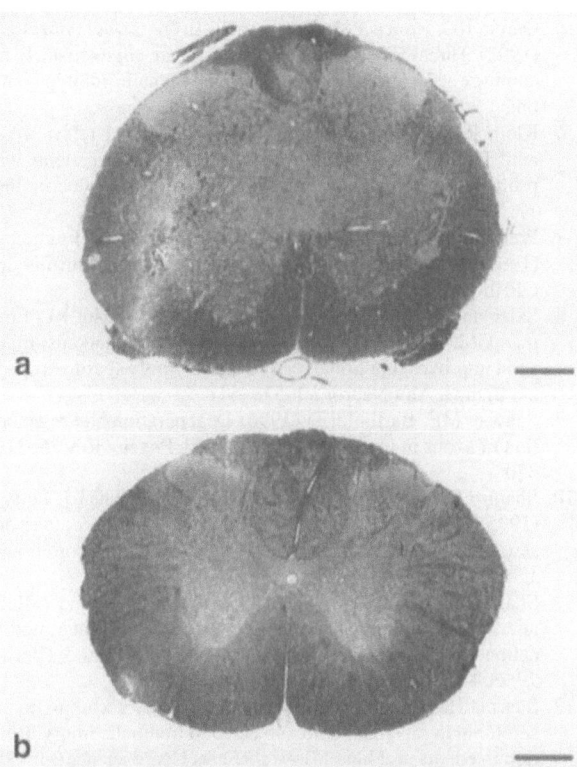

Fig. 3. Histological section of the T9 segment of an untreated (a) and a 5-HT antiserum treated (b) animal 5 h after trauma. Treatment with 5-HT antiserum markedly reduced general swelling of the cord and attenuated cell injury (bar = 250 μm)

tion in the spinal cord was markedly reduced in rats receiving 5-HT antiserum (Fig. 2).

Spinal Cord Pathology

Light microscopy of untreated traumatised spinal cord segments confirmed marked swelling, edema and cell changes 5 h after injury (Fig. 3 a). The T9 and T12 segment contained many distorted neurons, and demonstrated general sponginess of the white and grey matter, along with distortion of the myelin sheaths. In the 5-HT antiserum treated rats, however, the spinal cord was less swollen as compared to the untreated traumatised group (Fig. 3 b).

Discussion

Our results using 5-HT antiserum for the first time provide strong evidence for the conclusion that serotonin is involved in the pathophysiology of spinal cord injury. This is supported by the findings that pretreatment with 5-HT antiserum attenuated edema formation, the microvascular permeability disturbances and

the occurrence of cell changes following focal trauma of the spinal cord.

It appears therefore that application of 5-HT antiserum neutralises the pathophysiological effects of the trauma induced release of 5-HT. Strong evidences is available that antibodies may mimic the biological function of physiological ligands [17, 18]. The ability of certain antibodies to mimic both the chemical and biological functions of ligands or receptors has received solid experimental support in numerous studies [4–7]. It has been shown that antireceptor-antibodies mimic ligands structurally better when only a small segment of the ligand is involved in receptor recognition [5, 17]. That application of 5-HT antiserum antagonises the physiological function of 5-HT *in vivo* is in line with our previous observation on topical application of antibodies to dynorphin-A or nitric oxide synthase, which were neuroprotective and able to prevent the trauma induced upregulation of dynorphin or nitric oxide synthase, respectively [15, 16].

Although the mechanisms of the 5-HT induced edema and cell changes are not yet clear, it seems quite likely that 5-HT induces a breakdown of the blood-spinal cord barrier [11–13]. This is in agreement with the finding that 5-HT induces breakdown of the blood-brain barrier, edema, and cell changes in normal mice and rats infused with small amounts intravenously [14]. The vasoactive effect of 5-HT causes vasoconstriction in microvascular beds of the nervous system [2, 12, 13] leading to a reduction of cerebral blood flow [2, 14]. This effect appears to be mediated by serotonin 5-HT1a and 5-HT2 receptors [1, 2].

The fact that 5-HT plays an important role in the pathobiology of spinal cord trauma is also confirmed by the observation that mianserin, a potent antagonist of 5-HT1c and 5-HT2 receptors reduces the adverse neurological outcome following spinal cord injury [3, 8, 10]. This effect of the compound, however, is dose related.

A low dosage may have beneficial effects while a higher dose adverse effects. Our previous observations have shown hat high doses of cyproheptadine (a 5-HT2 receptor antagonist) worsen the spinal cord evoked responses and edema following injury by a similar trauma model in rats [11, 12]. Pretreatment with ketanserin in normal rats or mice prior to 5-HT infusion, however, results in attenuation of BBB breakdown and vasogenic edema [14]. Hence, the receptor mediated effects of 5-HT are still contradictory.

Recently, more than seven types of 5-HT receptors were identified in the CNS [1, 2]. Each 5-HT receptor is further classified in multiple receptor subtypes according to ligand binding. The physiological action of these individual receptor subtypes is not well known. Yet, compounds exhibiting properties of a pure receptor antagonist or its subtype without having any effect on other receptor subtypes are still lacking. Thus, the specific inhibition of a particular 5-HT receptor or its subtypes *in vivo* is not achieved so far [1, 2]. Therefore, the role of a particular receptor or its subtypes mediating effects of 5-HT in trauma is still not clear.

Our results using antiserum against 5-HT do not shed any light on the nature of particular receptors involved mediating the 5-HT effects on microvascular permeability, edema formation, or cell changes. These observations strongly suggest, however, that 5-HT is involved in the pathophysiology of spinal cord injury.

In conclusion, our observations using 5-HT antiserum show for the first time that 5-HT antibodies have the capacity to attenuate trauma induced alterations of the microvascular permeability, edema formation, and cell changes. Obviously, a reduction of microvascular permeability disturbances and vasogenic edema formation most likely is responsible for attenuation of adverse cell reactions. These observations support strongly an involvement of 5-HT in the pathophysiology of early spinal cord injury.

Acknowledgements

This study is supported by grants from Swedish Medical Research Council nrs. 2710, 9459, Göran Gustafsson Foundation, Torsten and Ragner Söderberg Foundation, Sweden; Alexander von Humboldt Foundation, Bonn, Germany; The University Grants Commission, New Delhi, India. The technical assistance of Kärstin Flink, Ingamarie Olsson, Margaretta Einarson, Madeliene Thörnwall, Gunilla Tibling; photographic assistance of Frank Bittkowski and secretarial assistance of Gunilla Åberg and Gun Britt Lind are highly appreciated.

References

1. Chaouloff F (1993) Physiopharmacological interactions between stress hormones and central serotonergic systems. Brain Res Rev 18: 1–32
2. Essman W (1978) Serotonin in health and diseases, vol I–V. Spectrum, New York
3. Faden AI (1993) Experimental neurobiology of central nervous system trauma. Crit Rev Neurobiol 7: 175–186
4. Frelinger AL 3rd, Cohen I, Plow EF, Smith MA, Roberts J, Lam SC-T, Ginsberg MH (1990) Selective inhibition of integrin function by antibodies specific for ligand-occupied receptor conformers. J Biol Chem 265: 6346–6352
5. Garcia KC, Ronco PM, Verroust PJ, Brünger AT, Amzel LM (1992) Three-dimensional structure of an angiotensin II-fab complex at 3A: hormone recognition by an anti-idiotypic antibody. Science 257: 502–507
6. Klein R, Bansch M, Berg PA (1992) Clinical relevance of antibodies against serotonin and gangliosides in patients with primary fibromyalgia syndrome. Psychoneuroendocrinology 17: 593–598
7. Prammer KV, Boyer J, Ugen K, Shattil SJ, Kieber-Emmons T (1994) Bioactive Arg-Gly-Asp conformations in anti-integrin GPIIb-IIIa antibodies. Receptor 4: 93–108
8. Salzman SK, Puniak MA, Liu ZJ, Maitland-Heriot RP, Freeman GM, Agresta CA (1991) The serotonin antagonist mianserin improves functional recovery following experimental spinal trauma. Ann Neurol 30: 533–541
9. Schwab ME, Bartholdi D (1996) Degeneration and regeneration of axons in the lesioned spinal cord. Physiol Rev 76: 319–370
10. Shapiro S, Kubek M, Siemers E, Daly E, Callahan J, Putty T (1995) Quantification of thyrotrophin-releasing hormone and serotonin content changes following graded spinal cord injury. J Surg Res 59: 393–398
11. Sharma HS, Olsson Y (1990) Edema formation and cellular alterations following spinal cord injury in rat and their modification with p-chlorophenylalanine. Acta Neuropathol (Berlin) 79: 604–610
12. Sharma HS, Olsson Y, Dey PK (1990) Early accumulation of serotonin in rat spinal cord subjected to traumatic injury. Relation to edema and blood flow changes. Neuroscience 36: 725–730
13. Sharma HS, Olsson Y, Nyberg F, Dey PK (1993) Prostaglandins modulate alterations of microvascular permeability, blood flow, edema and serotonin levels following spinal cord injury: and experimental study in the rat. Neuroscience 57: 443–449
14. Sharma HS, Olsson Y, Dey PK (1995) Serotonin as a mediator of increased microvascular permeability of the brain and spinal cord. Experimental observations in anaesthetised rats and mice. In: Greenwood J, Begley D, Segal M, Lightman S (eds) New concepts of a blood-brain barrier. Plenum, New York, pp 75–80
15. Sharma HS, Olsson Y, Nyberg F (1995) Influence of dynorphin-A antibodies on the formation of edema and cell changes in spinal cord trauma. In: Nyberg F, Sharma HS, Wissenfeld-Halin Z (eds) Prog Brain Res 104. Elsevier, Amsterdam, pp 401–416
16. Sharma HS, Westman J, Olsson Y, Alm P (1996) Involvement of nitric oxide in acute spinal cord injury: an immunocytochemical study using light and electron microscopy in the rat. Neurosci Res 24: 373–384
17. Shattil SJ, Weisel JW, Kieber-Emmons T (1992) Use of monoclonal antibodies to study the interaction between an integrin adhesion receptor, GP IIb-IIIa, and its physiological ligand, fibrinogen. Immunomethods 1: 53–63
18. Taub R, Gould R J, Garsky VM, Ciccarine TM, Hoxie J, Friedman PA, Shattil SJ (1989) A monoclonal antibody against platelet fibrinogen receptor contains a sequence that mimics a receptor recognition domain in fibrinogen. J Biol Chem 264: 259–265

Correspondence: Hari Shanker Sharma, Ph.D., Laboratory of Neuroanatomy, Department of Anatomy, Box 571, Biomedical Centre, Uppsala University, S-75123 Uppsala, Sweden.

Acta Neurochir (1997) [Suppl] 70: 159–161
© Springer-Verlag 1997

Steroids Decrease Uptake of Carboplatin in Rat Gliomas – Uptake Improved by Intracarotid Infusion of Bradykinin Analog, RMP-7

K. Matsukado[1], S. Nakano[1], R. T. Bartus[2], and K. L. Black[1]

[1] Jonsson Comprehensive Cancer Center, Division of Neurosurgery, UCLA Medical Center, Los Angeles, CA, and
[2] Alkermes, Inc., 64 Sidney Street, Cambridge, MA, U.S.A.

Summary

This study sought to determine whether dexamethasone (DXN) treatment of rats with intracranial gliomas would 1) further impair delivery of carboplatin to brain tumors, and 2) whether intracarotid infusion of the bradykinin analog, RMP-7, would improve delivery during concurrent DXN treatment. In DXN pretreated animals, 3 mg/kg/day of DXN was administered intraperitoneally for 3 days prior to Ki determinations. Ki of [^{14}C] carboplatin into DXN-treated tumors and brain surrounding tumor (BST) was significantly lower compared to non-DXN treated tumors and BST (3.30 ± 0.91 vs. 4.47 ± 1.80, $p < 0.05$, and 0.94 ± 0.84 vs. 2.18 ± 0.79, $p < 0.05$, respectively). Intracarotid infusion of RMP-7 significantly increased the Ki for carboplatin in DXN-treated tumors (6.35 ± 3.10 vs. 3.30 ± 0.91, $p < 0.01$), however, RMP-7 increased Ki to a greater extent in tumors not pretreated with DXN (12.07 ± 3.60 vs. 4.47 ± 1.80, $p < 0.0001$). Dexamethasone decreases transport of carboplatin into brain tumors. Intracarotid infusion of RMP-7 selectively increases carboplatin transport to tumors.

Keywords: Blood-brain barrier; bradykinin; brain tumor; carboplatin; glucocorticoid; RG2 glioma.

Introduction

Previous studies have demonstrated that a BTB limits adequate delivery of antitumor agents to tumors and the immediately adjacent brain [1, 3, 8]. Intracarotid infusion of bradykinin or its analog, RMP-7, was recently shown to selectively increase delivery of carboplatin and other compounds to brain tumors [5–7, 9].

Importantly, many patients with brain tumors are treated with the glucocorticoid, dexamethasone (DXN), which may further impair delivery of antitumor drugs across the BTB [12–14]. This study sought therefore to determine, using an experimental rat glioma model, whether pretreatment with DXN further decreased transport of carboplatin to brain and/or tumor tissue and to determine whether RMP-7 retained the ability to selectively open the BTB after pretreatment with DXN.

Materials and Methods

Intracerebral Inoculation of RG2 Cells

Female Wistar rats were anesthetized and RG2 glioma cells ($1 \times 10^5/5\ \mu l$) were implanted into the right basal ganglia stereotactically.

Dexamethasone Treatment of Animals

From seven days after tumor implantation, rats received either 3 mg/kg of DXN diluted in PBS to a final volume of 0.5 ml/animal or the same volume of PBS once per day for 3 days. Rats were divided into four groups: Group 1: no DXN pretreatment prior to intracarotid infusion of 0.1 μg/kg/min of RMP-7 (n = 7); Group 2: no DXN pretreatment prior to intracarotid saline infusion (n = 7); Group 3: DXN pretreatment prior to intracarotid RMP-7 infusion (n = 7); and Group 4: DXN pretreatment prior to intracarotid saline infusion (n = 7).

Permeability for [^{14}C] Carboplatin

At 10 days after tumor implantation, a polyethylene (PE-10) catheter was inserted retrograde through the external carotid artery to the common carotid artery bifurcation ipsilateral to the tumor. RMP-7 or saline was infused into the right carotid artery at a rate of 53.3 μl/min for 15 minutes.

Autoradiography

Twenty μm coronal brain sections were cut with a cryotome. Autoradiograms were generated by coexposing the sections with tissue-calibrated ^{14}C standards for 2 weeks. The sequential section was stained with hematoxylin and eosin and the cross-sectional area of tumors was measured. The regional radioactivity was measured in tumor, brain surrounding tumor (BST; areas within a 2 mm distance from the border of the tumor), right cortex (Rt. Cortex), left cortex (Lt. Cortex), right white matter (Rt. WM), left WM (Lt. WM), right basal ganglia (Rt. BG), and left BG (Lt. BG). Mean tumor size was determined by measuring tumor dimensions along the long axis of the tumor and across the tumor at the widest point perpendicular to the long axis, and substituting the valves into the following equation:

$$\text{Mean tumor size (cu mm)} = [\text{length (mm)} \times \text{width (mm)}] / 2$$

Ki Value and Blood Volume Calculation

The regional permeability in the brains and tumor tissues were expressed by the unidirectional transfer constant, Ki value (µl/g/min), and were calculated using the following equation of Ohno and Ziylan [10, 15]:

$$Ki = \frac{Cbr - VoCbl}{\int_0^T Cpl \cdot dt}$$

Cbr is the brain or tumor concentration of the tracer at the end of experiment (dpm/g), *Cbl* is the blood concentration of the tracer at the end of experiment (dpm/g), *T* is the duration of the experiment (min), and *Cpl* is the arterial plasma concentration (dpm/ml). *Vo* is the regional cerebral blood volume in the tissue (µl/g).

Results

Tumor Size

DXN therapy resulted in a lower mean tumor size compared to the saline injected group (3.93 ± 0.71 vs. 2.22 ± 0.93, p < 0.01). DXN also appeared to reduce the vascular density assessed by laminin immunohistochemistry in RG2 gliomas (data not shown).

Regional Permeability for [14C] Carboplatin

DXN pretreatment for 3 days significantly decreased the Ki of [14C] carboplatin into tumors by 26%, and into BST by 57% compared to non DXN pretreated tumors and BST, respectively. In tumors not pretreated with DXN, intracarotid RMP-7 infusion significantly increased carboplatin transport into tumors by 170%. In contrast, in DXN pretreated animals, intracarotid infusion of RMP-7 significantly increased carboplatin transport into tumors by 92%. DXN nor RMP-7 changed carboplatin transport in normal brain tissue in this study (Fig. 1).

Discussion

Patients with brain tumors are frequently treated with DXN or other glococorticoids to reduce brain swelling and mass effect related to brain tumors [2, 4, 13, 14]. Although DXN treatment may result in a temporary symptomatic improvement in patients, DXN may also reduce tumor permeability, which may further impair drug delivery to tumors [11, 15]. Previ-

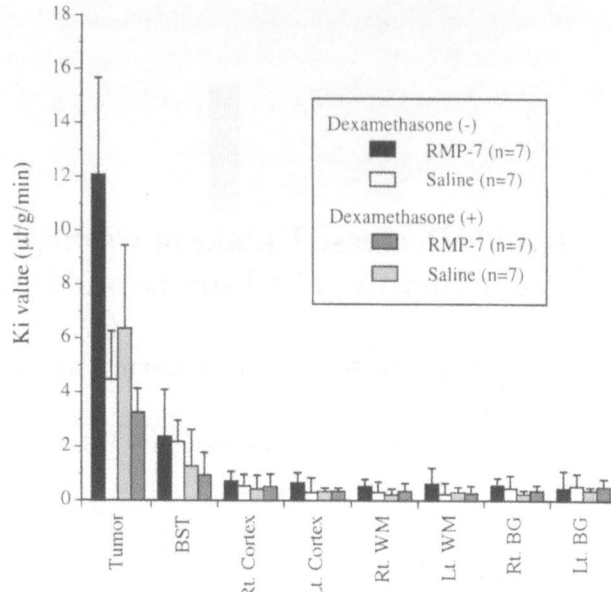

Fig. 1. Quantitative determination of permeability in PBS and DXN pretreated groups. Each bar indicates mean ± SD. DXN pretreatment for 3 days significantly decreased the Ki of [14C] carboplatin into tumors by 26%, and into BST by 57% compared to non DXN pretreated tumors and BST, respectively. In tumors not pretreated with DXN, intracarotid RMP-7 infusion significantly increased carboplatin transport into tumors by 170%. In contrast, in DXN pretreated animals, intracarotid infusion of RMP-7 significantly increased carboplatin transport into tumors by 92%. DXN nor RMP-7 changed carboplatin transport in normal brain tissue in this study

ous studies have demonstrated intracarotid infusions of RMP-7 selectively increases transport of carboplatin to experimental RG2 gliomas and significantly increases survival in rats with intracranial gliomas [7]. Patients with malignant gliomas and metastatic brain tumors are being treated in clinical trials with intracarotid or intravenous RMP-7 and carboplatin. DXN could influence the ability of RMP-7 to increase transport of carboplatin to tumor tissue in these patients. The present study, using an experimental glioma model in rats, show that intracarotid infusion of RMP-7 results in a significant increase in carboplatin transport despite DXN pretreatment for 3 days. However, without DXN pretreatment, RMP-7 increased carboplatin transport by 170%, in contrast, with DXN pretreatment, RMP-7 increased carboplatin transport by only 92% in this model. We believe that the present findings have important implications in how DXN should be utilized in patients receiving RMP-7 treatment for brain tumors. This study suggested that for maximal delivery of compounds across microvessels into brain tumors, use of DXN should be minimized.

References

1. Fenstermacher JD, Cowles AL (1977) Theoretic limitations of intracarotid infusion in brain tumor chemotherapy. Cancer Treat Rep 61: 519–526
2. Fishman RA (1982) Steroids in the treatment of brain edema [editorial]. N Engl J Med 306: 359–360
3. Groothuis DR, Fischer JR, Lapin G, Bigner DD, Vick NA (1982) Permeability of different experimental brain tumor models to horseradish peroxidase. J Neuropathol Exp Neurol 41: 164–185
4. Gutin PH (1975) Corticosteroid therapy in patients with cerebral tumors: benefits, mechanisms, problems, practicalities. Semin Oncol 2: 49–56
5. Inamura T, Black K (1994) Bradykinin selectively opens blood-tumor barrier in experimental brain tumors. J Cereb Blood Flow Metab 14: 862–870
6. Inamura T, Nomura T, Bartus R, Black K (1994) Intracarotid infusion of RMP-7, a bradykinin analog: a method for selective drug delivery to brain tumors. J Neurosurg 81: 752–758
7. Matsukado K, Inamura T, Nakano S, Fukui M, Bartus R, Black K (1996) Enhanced tumor uptake of carboplatin and survival in glioma-bearing rats by intracarotid infusion of bradykinin analog, RMP-7. Neurosurgery 39: 125–134
8. Neuwelt EA, Barnett PA, Bigner DD, Frenkel EP (1982) Effects of adrenal cortical steroids and osmotic blood-brain barrier opening on methotrexate delivery to gliomas in the rodent: the factor of the blood-brain barrier. Proc Natl Acad Sci USA 79: 4420–4423
9. Nomura T, Inamura T, Black KL (1994) Intracarotid infusion of bradykinin selectively increases blood-tumor permeability in 9L and C6 brain tumors. Brain Res 659: 62–66
10. Ohno K, Pettigrew KO, Rapoport ST (1978) Lower limits of cerebrovascular permeability to nonelectrolytes in the conscious rat. Am J Physiol 253: H299–H307
11. Reichman HR, Farrell CL, Del Maestro RF (1986) Effects of steroids and nonsteroid anti-inflammatory agents on vascular permeability in a rat glioma model. J Neurosurg 65: 233–237
12. Warnke PC, Molnar P, Lapin GD, Kuruvilla A, Groothuis DR (1995) The effects of dexamethasone on transcapillary transport in experimental brain tumors: II. Canine brain tumors. J Neurooncol 25: 29–38
13. Weinstein JD, Toy FJ, Jaffe ME, Goldberg HI (1973) The effect of dexamethasone on brain edema in patients with metastatic brain tumors. Neurology 23: 121–129
14. Yamada K, Ushio Y, Hayakawa T, Arita N, Yamada N, Mogami H (1983) Effects of methylprednisolone on peritumoral brain edema. A quantitative autoradiographic study. J Neurosurg 59: 612–619
15. Ziylan YZ, LeFauconnier JM, Bernard G, Bourre JM (1988) Effect of dexamethasone on transport of alpha-aminoisobutyric acid and sucrose across the blood-brain barrier. J Neurochem 51: 1338–1342

Correspondence: Keith L. Black, M.D., Division of Neurosurgery, 17-382 NPI, UCLA Medical Center, Los Angeles, CA 90095-7039, U.S.A.

Acta Neurochir (1997) [Suppl] 70: 162–164
© Springer-Verlag 1997

Effect of Glycerol on Blood Flow Distribution in Tumoral and Peritumoral Brain Tissue

M. Niwa[1], H. Oyama[3], M. Furuse[1], S. Takada[1], T. Kawai[1], Y. Ishikawa[2], H. Kuchiwaki[4], S. Inao[4], K. Ichimi[1], and M. Shibayama[4]

Department of [1] Neurosurgery and [2] Radiology, Nakatsugawa General Municipal Hospital, [3] Department of Neurosurgery, Chyukyou Hospital, and [4] Department of Neurosurgery, Nagoya University School of Medicine, Japan

Summary

To evaluate the effect of glycerol, thirty-two patients with brain tumor were directed to the study, including 17 gliomas and 15 meningiomas. Blood flow before and after the administration of glycerol were measured with Xe CT. Glioma was significantly hypo-perfused. The peritumoral edema of glioma and meningioma were also hypo-perfused. On the other hand, Meningioma was significantly hyper-perfused. After the administration of glycerol, blood flows were increased except for glioma. We suggested that, vascular responses to glycerol was different in the two tumor types. The steal phenomena of blood flow might occur in glioma.

Keywords: Peritumoral edema; blood flow; glycerol; Xe CT.

Introduction

Glycerol has been used for the therapy of brain tumor. It causes reduction of brain edema by osmotic difference, and improves blood flow. Effect of glycerol on blood flow for brain tumor has not enough been studied so far. We measured blood flow in the tumor and the peritumoral edema to evaluate the effect of glycerol intravenous administration on blood flow. Further, difference in flow distribution between glioma and meningioma was evaluated.

Materials and Methods

Thirty-two patients with brain tumor were directed to the study, including 17 gliomas (15 glioblastoma, 2 astrocytomas) and 15 meningiomas (13 meningothelial, 2 malignant). Pathologies of all patients were confirmed by surgical operation. Blood flow was measured with stable Xe CT (inhalation of 25% stable Xe for 3 minutes and exhaustion for 5 minutes). ROIs (region of interest) were set on tumor, peritumoral edema and control (contralateral brain corresponding to the edema) regions. Entire hemispheres of the tumor side and the non tumor side were also studied. To decide the region, we referred enhanced CT image and T1 weighted MRI for the tumor, and T2 weighted MRI for the peritumoral edema in addition to plain CT image. After the first blood flow measurement with Xe CT, 200 ml of 10% glycerol was infused for 15 minutes. The second measurement was carried out immediately after the administration of glycerol. Data were analyzed using t-test. Statistical significance was set at $p < 0.05$.

Results

In glioma cases, the values of blood flow before the administration of glycerol were 36.4 ± 3.9 ml/100 g/min (mean $\pm$ S.E.) in the tumor, 37.5 ± 3.6 ml/100 g/min in the edema, 55.6 ± 3.0 ml/100 g/min in the control, 52.1 ± 5.0 ml/100 g/min in the hemisphere of tumor side and 56.9 ± 3.4 ml/100 g/min in the hemisphere of non tumor side. In meningioma cases, these were 73.7 ± 6.1 ml/100 g/min in the tumor, 33.8 ± 4.0 ml/100 g/min in the edema, 54.0 ± 5.4 ml/100 g/min in the control, 53.5 ± 3.9 ml/100 g/min in the hemisphere of tumor side and 52.4 ± 3.8 ml/100 g/min in the hemisphere of non tumor side (Fig. 1). There were no significant difference between the blood flows in entire hemispheres of tumor side and non tumor side in both cases of glioma and meningioma. The tumor part of glioma was significantly hypo-perfused in blood flow. The peritumoral edema of glioma and meningioma were also hypo-perfused. On the other hand, Meningioma was significantly hyper-perfused. After the administration of glycerol, blood flows were increased except for glioma. In glioma cases, relative values of blood flow after the administration of glycerol were $86.9 \pm 6.3\%$ in the tumor, $119.7 \pm 4.8\%$ in the edema, $125.1 \pm 5.4\%$ in the control, $111.8 \pm 4.0\%$ in the hemisphere of tumor side and $116.3 \pm 5.3\%$ in the hemisphere of non tumor side. In meningioma cases, these were $109.2 \pm 6.0\%$ in the tumor, $108.8 \pm 5.3\%$ in the edema, $121.9 \pm 5.4\%$ in the control, $109.5 \pm 6.1\%$ in

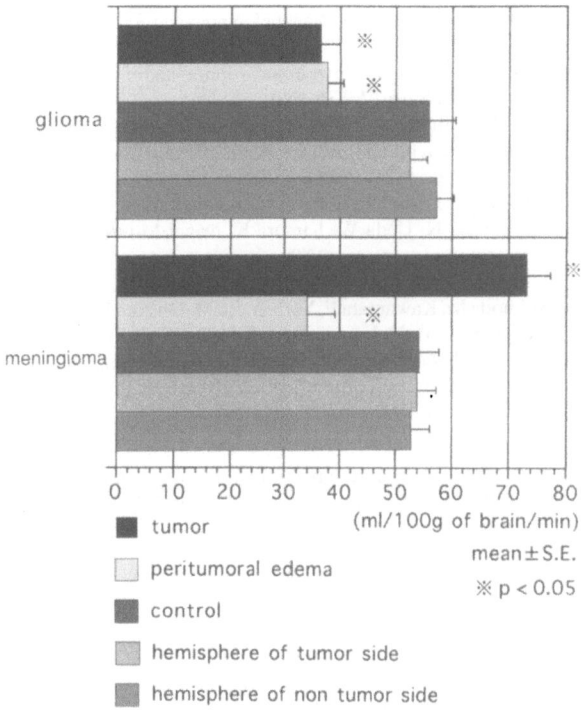

Fig. 1. The values of blood flow before the administration of glycerol. Glioma was significantly hypo-perfused. The peritumoral edema of glioma and meningioma were also hypo-perfused. On the other hand, meningioma was significantly hyperperfused

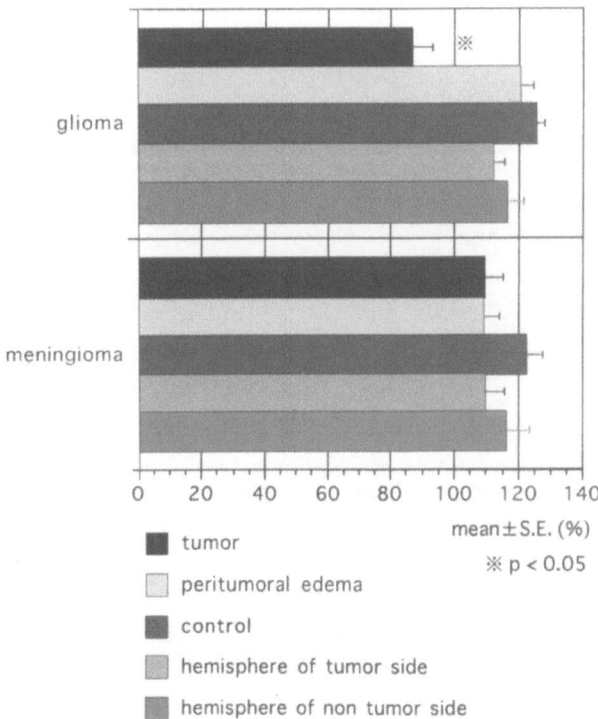

Fig. 2. Relative values of blood flow (after/before the administration of glycerol). Blood flows were increased except for glioma

the hemisphere of tumor side and $116.1 \pm 7.6\%$ in the hemisphere of non tumor side (Fig. 2). Only we observed decreased blood flow in glioma. Increase rates of blood flow after the administration of glycerol in the tumor and the peritumoral edema of meningioma were relatively low, compared with the control. However, there were no significant difference among them.

Discussion

Blood flow in brain tumor is various. It seems to be decided by vascularity, degree of cell damage and so on. Ronald et al. [1] reported that mean tumor blood flow was less than that in the same automatic region of the contralateral hemisphare using CD Fischer rats with RT-9 brain tumor. Still, he suggested that it related to tumor size, location and presence of necrosis. Kida et al. [4] measured blood flow for brain tumors and analysed that meningioma was hyper-perfused and metastatic tumor was hypoperfused. Nakamura et al. [5] described that gliomas and metastatic tumors were hypo-perfused. In our cases, glioma was hyper-perfused and meningioma was hypo-perfused. That differences may be due to pathological type or/and vascularity. We discussed blood flow in the tumor, but it was doubtful. Because blood flow should be measured only in brain tissue but tumoral tissue. However, we dealt tumoral tissue as brain tissue. Regarding the peritumoral edema, there are numerous report that it is hypoperfused [4, 6]. However, it does not interfere with blood flow or flow resulation as long as intracranial pressure is normal [2]. In our cases, blood flows were hypo-perfused in the peritumoral edema both in glioma and meningioma. Although we did not measure intracranial pressure, it might be high.

Effect of glycerol for brain tumor was less evaluated. Shimoda et al. [6] reported that blood flows in all the regions except for the tumor increased after the administration of glycerol. Blood flow in the tumor did not change. Ishikawa et al. [3] measured blood flow in hemisphere including meningioma following the administration of glycerol. Blood flows in all the regions increased by about 20%. In our study, blood flows in all the regions except for glioma increased after the administration of glycerol. Blood flow in glioma decreased. We supposed that in glioma blood brain barrier (BBB) was destroyed, while BBB was preserved in the peritumoral edema to some degree. Glycerol did not improve blood flow in the tumor. Blood flow in the peritumoral edma increased after the administration of glycerol. It seems to be caused by steal of blood flow from the tumor to the peritumoral brain tissue. Meningioma was hyper-perfused. Glycerol effected both on the tumor and the peritumoral edema. In meningioma cases, increase rates of blood flow in the tumor and the peritumoral edema after the administration of glycerol were relatively low compared with that of cotrol. Glycerol effects on brain tumors variously. We should use glycerol for a patient with brain tumor more carefully.

References

1. BIasberg R, Molnar P, Horowitz M, Kornblith P, Pleasants R, Fenstermacher J (1983) Regional blood flow in RT-9 brain tumors. J Neurosurg 58: 863–873
2. Hossmann KA, Bloink M, Wilmes F, Wechsler W (1980) Experimental peritumoral edema of the cat brain. Adv Neurol 8: 323–340
3. Ishikawa M, Kikuchi H, Nagata I, Yamagata S, Taki W, Kobayashi A, Yonekura Y, Nishizawa S (1989) The effect of glycerol on regional blood flow, blood volume and oxygen metabolism. Neurol Surg 17: 635–640
4. Kida Y, Ishiguri H, Ichimi K, Kobayashi T (1992) Evaluation of the regional blood flow in and around brain tumors by means of Xe-enhanced CT. Progress CT 14: 25–31
5. Nakamura O, Nomura K, Segawa H, Takakura K, Nakagome T, Yoshimasu N, Ueda W, Kimura K, Nagai M (1983) rCBF in brain tumors as measured by Xenon enhanced CT. Neurol Surg13: 37–43
6. Shimoda M, Kawamata F, Yamamoto M, Ohsuga H, Hidaka M, Oda S, Shibuya N, Yamamoto I, Sato O (1989) The evaluation of cerebral hemodynamics in patients with intracranial tumors by stable Xenon CT: the effect of glycerol administration on regional blood flow. Progress CT 11: 161–168

Correspondence: Masahiro Niwa, M.D., Department of Neurosurgery, Nakatsugawa General Municipal Hospital, 1522-1 Komamba, Nakatsugawa-shi, Gifu-ken 508, Japan.

Acta Neurochir (1997) [Suppl] 70: 165–166
© Springer-Verlag 1997

Assessment of Vasoreactivity in Brain Edema by Acetazolamide Activation SPECT and PET

S. Inao[1], H. Kuchiwaki[1], K. Ichimi[1], M. Shibayama[1], J. Yoshida[1], K. Itoh[2], T. Katoh[2], M. Nishino[2], N. Narita[2], and S. Gambhir[2]

[1] Department of Neurosurgery and [2] Department of Radiology, Nagoya University School of Medicine, Nagoya, Japan

Summary

Our study was performed to find out cerebrovascular reactivity post acetazolamide administration in patients with peritumoral edema.

Adult patients (n = 9) underwent CBF measurement by 99mTc-HMPAO SPECT pre and post 1 gram I.V. acetazolamide. In all patients, this procedure was repeated once again within 10 days of performing tumor removal. Five of these patients also underwent CBF measurement pre and post 1 gram I.V. acetazolamide post surgery only using oxygen-15 labeled H_2O PET. Asymmetry index (AI) was calculated as ratio of ROI counts in the peritumoral edematous area and symmetrical ROI on the contralateral normal hemisphere. The AI increased after acetazolamide in edematous gray matter post operatively though the resting AI remained almost same post operatively. AI in edematous white matter showed non-significant increase post operatively both at rest and after acetazolamide. Good linear correlation of AI between PET and SPECT was observed both in gray and white matter. The improvement of vascular reactivity in edematous gray matter after tumor removal suggests that mass effect not only reduces CBF but also suppresses vascular reactivity. White matter vascular reactivity in early post operative period is little improved, possibly due to factors other than mass effect i.e. excess water accumulation in white matter perivascular space.

Keywords: Peritumoral edema; cerebrovascular reactivity; acetazolamide.

Introduction

Although both the experimental and clinical brain edema has been studied on its pathophysiological aspect, only few [2, 4] were studied on the vascular reactivity of the edematous brain tissue by changing either CO_2 or blood pressure (autoregulation). We focused on the peritumoral brain edema pre and post surgery, and measured both cerebral blood flow and the vascular reactivity by acetazolamide administration to clarify the characteristic change of the peritumoral brain edema between with mass and without mass.

Subject and Method

We studied 9 adult patients (age 30 to 72, mean 52.9 years) with unilateral spratentorial brain tumors including 5 meningiomas, 3 malignant gliomas, 1 metastatic brain tumor. They had a peritumoral edema limited within ipsilateral hemisphere to the tumor. In all patients, CBF measurements were performed by Tc-99m HMPAO SPECT before and after 1 gram of acetazolamide administration. After they were operated and the tumor was totally removed, post operative CBF measurement by the same protocol and technique were undergone within 10 days after the surgery. Five of these patients also underwent CBF measurement pre and post 1 gram i.v. acetazolamide post surgery only using oxygen-15 labeled H_2O PET.

A circular region of interest (ROI) was placed over the cortical and white matter areas in the peritumoral zone in the transverse slice showing the most pronounced abnormality which was trained in neuroanatomy with reference to the patient's CT or MR images. An equal sized ROI was placed over the corresponding region of the contralateral cerebral hemisphere. Regional radioactivity count densities were obtained for a total of 8 pair of bilateral regions. Asymmetry index (AI) was calculated as ratio of ROI counts in the peritumoral edematous area and symmetrical ROI on the contralateral normal hemisphere (AI = edematous brain / contralateral brain). Separate ROI's were drawn for gray and white matter. This index was used for comparison.

Result

The AI increased after acetazolamide in edematous gray matter post operatively, from 0.76 ± 0.05 to 0.88 ± 0.06 ($P < 0.05$), though the resting AI remained almost same post operatively (0.88 ± 0.05 to 0.87 ± 0.02). The AI in non-edematous gray matter at rest and post acetazolamide were 0.99 ± 0.03 and 1.01 ± 0.02 respectively. AI in edematous white matter showed non-significant increase post operatively both at rest and after acetazolamide. Good linear correlation of AI between PET and SPECT was observed both in gray ($r = 0.66$) and white matter ($r = 0.45$).

Discussion

The effect of brain edema on CBF has been reported by many authors, and the results were inconclusive. It remains unclear whether or not CBF is altered by brain edema. In our previous experiment [3], we found that the excess water accumulation of water in brain tissue by itself did not decrease CBF even when the driving pressure of edema fluid was present. However, in the clinical setting, there are many evidences that CBF is decreased in edematous area when the tumor exists [1]. One of our aim was to investigate whether or not CBF is still decreased in the edematous area after the tumor is already removed. Our present data indicated that CBF in the edematous gray and white matter is still decreased within 10 days after tumor removal when the edematous legion was apparent on CT or MRI.

The vascular reactivity in the affected gray matter improved after tumor removal, suggesting that this edematous gray matter had been affected mainly by the compression due to the mass. The vascular reactivity in the edematous white matter is impaired till 10 days after tumor removal, indicating that its impaired reactivity is due to causes other than mass effect, possibly due to excess water accumulation in the perivascular space.

Although our study is preliminary and the patients number is limited, the remaining perifocal brain edema after the surgery is still under the ischemic condition and loss of vascular reactivity, so that it should be medically treated for the protection of neural tissue.

References

1. Hino A, Imahori Y, Tenjin H, Mizukawa N, Ueda S, Hirakawa K, Nakahashi H (1990) Metabolic and hemodynamic aspects of peritumoral low-density areas in human brain tumor. Neurosurgery 26: 615–621
2. Hossmann K-A, Blöink M, Wilmes F, Wechsler W (1980) Experimental peritumoral edema of the cat brain. In: Cervós-Navarro J, Ferszt R (eds) Advances in neurology, vol 28. Raven, New York, pp 323–340
3. Inao S, Kuchiwaki H, Sugita K (1993) Microcirculation in experimental brain oedema assessed by laser-Doppler flowmetry. Neurol Res 15: 264–268
4. Marmarou A, Takagi H, Walstra G, Shulman K (1980) The role of brain tissue pressure in autoregulation of CBF in areas of brain edema. In: Shulman K, Marmarou A, Miller JD, Becker DP, Hockwald GM, Brock M (eds) Intracranial pressure IV. Springer, Berlin Heidelberg New York, pp 257–267

Correspondence: Suguru Inao, M.D., Department of Neurosurgery, Nagoya Univeristy School of Medicine, 65 Tsurumai-cho, Showa-ku, Nagoya 466, Japan.

Acta Neurochir (1997) [Suppl] 70: 167–169
© Springer-Verlag 1997

Tumor Specific Contrast Enhancement Study of Mn-Metalloporphyrin (ATN-10) – Comparison of Rat Brain Tumor Model, Cytotoxic and Vasogenic Edema Models

H. Fujimori[1], A. Matsumura[1], T. Yamamoto[1], Y. Shibata[1], T. Yoshizawa[1], K. Nakagawa[1], Y. Yoshii[1], T. Nose[1], I. Sakata[2], and S. Nakajima[3]

[1] Department of Neurosurgery, University of Tsukuba, [2] Toyo Hakka Co. Ltd, and [3] Asahikawa Medical College, Japan

Summary

ATN-10, Mn-metalloporphyrin, has been developed as a tumor selective contrast agent for magnetic resonance (MR) imaging. To investigate the tumor specificity of ATN-10, we produced three experimental *in vivo* models; rat bran tumor (9L glioma) model, vasogenic (cold injury) and cytotoxic brain edema (24-hour MCA occlusion) models. The time course of contrast enhancement was compared after intravenous injection of ATN-10 or Gd-DTPA, measuring the signal intensity of the region of interest. After ATN-10 administration, the 9L glioma model showed early (5 min) and delayed (24 hr-) peak enhancement whereas the cold injury model showed only early enhancement and the 24-hour MCA occlusion model did not show significant enhancement. After Gd-DTPA administration, all three models showed similar pattern of only early enhancement. As a contrast agent for MR imaging, ATN-10 showed different behavior than Gd-DTPA in demonstrating the blood-brain barrier disruption and moreover ATN-10 showed selective enhancement in experimental brain tumors.

Keywords: Brain neoplasms; porphyrin; vasogenic edema; cytotoxic edema; magnetic resonance imaging.

Introduction

Due to its high resolusion and ability for evaluating tissue characteristics, magnetic resonance (MR) imaging is one of the most useful methods for brain tumor diagnosis. The application of Gd-DTPA is valuable for the detection of brain tumors. However, it is difficult to distinguish brain tumors from another intracerebral pathologic conditions with BBB disruption. Especially in a clinical setting, the imaging of the brain tumor which was modified after some therapies has become more complicated. Porphyrins have been known to accumulate in malignant tumors and some porphyrin derivatives without phototoxicity have been developed as potential tumor selective MR imaging contrast

agents [8]. ATN-10, Mn-metalloporphyrin, which applied phase I trial as ^{111}In-labeled scintigraphic agent accumulates in malignant tumors and besides has T1 shortning effect in MR imaging [6]. In this study, we compared the behavior of ATN-10 as a tumor selective contrast agent with Gd-DTPA as a BBB tracer in rat brain tumor model and vasogenic and cytotoxic brain edema models.

Materials and Methods

Animal Preparation

Thirty adult male Fisher rats (weighing 290–400 g) were devided into three experimental models.

1) *Brain tumor model* (n = 10): 9L glioma cells ($1 \times 10^4/10$ μl) were inoculated stereotactically into the basal ganglia of the right hemisphere of the rats under pentobarbital anesthesia. Two weeks after operation, the animals were reanesthetized with pentobarbital for MR imaging.

2) *Vasogenic brain edema model* (n = 10): The vasogenic brain edema model was induced by cold injury. The animals were anesthetized by injection of pentobarbital intraperitoneally. A 4 mm diameter cyrindrical copper rod, cooled to $-73°C$ in a mixture of dry ice and acetone, was applied to the intact dura through the burr hole for 60 seconds.

3) *Cytotoxic brain edema model* (n = 10): The right middle cerebral artery (MCA) was occluded permanently using a modification of the intraluminal technique described by Longa *et al.* [10]. The animals were anesthetized with 1–1.5% halothane with 70% N_2O and 30% O_2 during the operation. After 24 hours of permanent MCA occlusion, the animals were reanesthetized with pentobarbital for MR imaging.

MR Imaging Procedure and Data Analysis

A Biospec 2.35T system (Bruker) was used. T2 and T1-weighted spin-echo (SE) coronal images were obtained with 2040 / 80 and 512 / 28 ms (repetition time / echo time), 4.6 cm field of view, 1.6 mm slice thickness, 128×128 matrix and 2 times signal averaging. After these baseline sequences were obtained, the animals recieved 0.2 mmol/kg of Gd-DTPA or 0.02 mmol/kg of ATN-10 via the tail vein. The imagings were performed before and 5, 30 minutes, 1, 2, 3, 6, 12 and 24 hours after injection of the contrast agents. All T1-weighted images were displayed to ensure registration of the region of interest (ROI) placement for each portion of the cortex. The time course of contrast enhancement was compared, measuring the signal intensity (SI) ratio; SI of ROI in the lesion / SI of ROI in the contralateral normal brain.

Results

1) Gd-DTPA

In 9L glioma, Gd-DTPA lead to a peak SI ratio at 5 minutes after intravenous injection. And within 30 minutes, SI ratio decreased again to half of its maximal value. The contrast enhancement in cold injury and in 24-hour MCA occlusion reached maximal SI ratios at 30 minutes after administration. And within 2 hours, SI ratios decreased to half of their maximal values (Fig. 1). Then after 6 hours, SI ratios in all three models maintained their precontrast levels.

2) ATN-10

In 9L glioma, ATN-10 lead to a peak SI ratio at 5 minutes after intravenous injection. And SI ratio of the tumors increased again after 3 hours and remained high value at 24 hours after administration (Fig. 2). The contrast enhancement in cold injury reached maximal SI ratio at 5 minutes after administration and decreased to its control level within 2 hours (Fig. 2). No significant contrast enhancements were observed in the 24-hour MCA occlusion model after ATN-10 administration (Fig. 1).

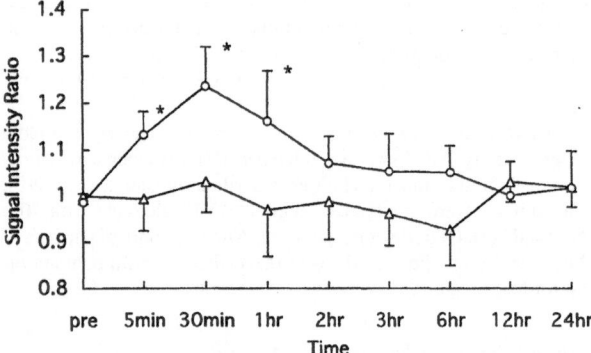

Fig. 1. The time course of enhancement in the 24-hour MCA occlusion model following administration of Gd-DTPA (○) and ATN-10 (△). Statistical significance: * $p < 0.01$ different from ○ and △ by Student's t test

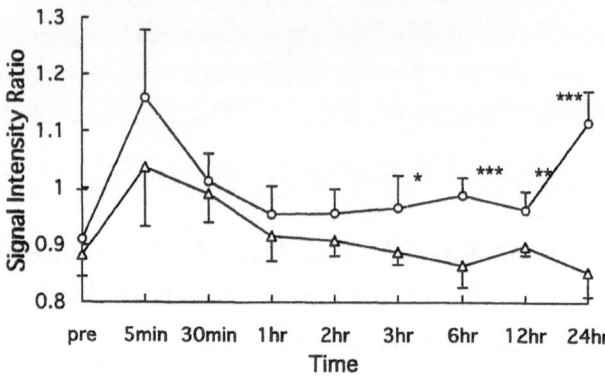

Fig. 2. The time course of enhancement in 9L glioma (○) and in cold injury (△) following administration of ATN-10. Statistical significance: * $p < 0.05$, ** $p < 0.01$, *** $p < 0.001$ different from ○ and △ by Student's t test

Discussion

The time course of enhancement after ATN-10 administration showed quite different pattern in each model. In the 9L glioma model, biphasic contrast enhanced pattern was revealed whereas only trancient enhancement in the cold injury model and no significant enhancement in the 24-hour MCA occlusion model were shown. On the other hand, after Gd-DTPA administration, all three models showed similar pattern of only early transient enhancement.

Our study indicated two major results. The first one is that Gd-DTPA caused increase of SI in the 24-hour MCA occlusion model but ATN-10 didn't (Fig. 1). For Gd-DTPA has been known as a BBB disruption tracer, the 24-hour MCA occlusion model has not any longer been pure cytotoxic edema model. It should contain the early stage of BBB disruption. According to the previous studies, the BBB opens only to micromolecules at the time of 24 hours after permanent MCA occlusion of rats, so that few macromolecules such as serum proteins cross even the damaged BBB [2, 4]. However ATN-10 caused no increases of SI like Gd-DTPA did, although the molecular weights of Gd-DTPA (743) and ATN-10 (1088) are not quite different. Some investigators have described the strong binding of porphyrin to lipoproteins such as low-density-lipoprotein (LDL) and transferrin [1, 7]. Therefore it was surpposed that ATN-10 was not extravasated in the 24-hours MCA occlusion model because of binding to lipoproteins. But as BBB distruption progress, the macromolecules including ATN-10 which was binding to lipoproteins should start to leak out from intravascular space [3]. Actually in 72-hours MCA occlusion which presented the BBB permeability to proteins [2], ATN-10 showed early significant enhancement like in the cold injury model (unpublished data).

The second point is re-enhancement of ATN-10 in the 9L glioma model (Fig. 2). It indicates selective accumulation of ATN-10 in tumor cells. However the mechanism of porphyrin-tumor affinity is unclear. In malignant tumor cells, the uptakes of LDL [5] and transferrin [9] via receptors mediated endocytosis are increased for cell proliferation. And it is expected that Mn-metalloporphyrin binding to LDL or transferrin in plasma, accumulates into the tumor cells indirectly by increased uptakes of LDL and transferrin. As a contrast agent for MR imaging, ATN-10 behaves like a protein tracer in the brain edema, besides it accumulates actively through LDL- or transferrin-receptor mediated mechanism in tumor cells. ATN-10 may be used as a tumor-specific contrast agent and may also characterize the activity of the tumor after various clinical treatment procedures.

References

1. De Smidt PC, Versluis AJ, van Berkel TJC (1993) Properties of incorporation, redistribution, and integrity of porphyrin-low density lipoprotein complexes. Biochemistry 32: 2916–2922

2. Gotoh O, Asano T, Koide T, Takakura K (1985) Ischemic brain edema following occlusion of the middle cerebral artery in the rat. I: The time courses of the brain water, sodium and potassium contents and blood-brain barrier permeability to ^{125}I-albumin. Stroke 16: 101–109

3. Hatashita S, Hoff JT (1990) Brain edema and cerebrovascular permeability during cerebral ischemia in rats. Stroke 21: 582–588

4. Menzies SA, Betz AL, Hoff JT (1993) Contribution of ions and albumin to the formation and resolution of ischemic brain edema. J Neurosurg 78: 257–266

5. Murakami M, Ushio Y, Mihara Y, Karatsu J, Horiuchi S, Morino Y (1990) Cholesterol uptake by human glioma cells via receptor-mediated endocytosis of low-density lipoproteins. J Neurosurg 73: 760–767

6. Nakajima S, Yamauchi H, Sakata I, Hayashi H, Yamazaki K, Maeda T, Kubo Y, Samejima N, Takemura T (1993) ^{111}In-labeled Mn-metalloporphyrin for tumor imaging. Nucl Med Biol 20: 231–237

7. Nakajima S, Takemura T, Sakata I (1995) Tumor-localizing of porphyrin and its affinity to LDL and transferrin. Cancer Lett 92: 113–118

8. Nelson JA, Schmiedl U (1991) Porphyrins as contrast media. Magn Reson Med 22: 366–371

9. Recht L, Torres GO, Smith TW, Raso V, Griffin TW (1990) Transferrin receptor in normal and neoplastic brain tissue: implications for brain-tumor immunotherapy. J Neurosurg 72: 941–945

10. Zea Longa E, Weinstein PR, Carlson S, Cummins RW (1989) Reversible middle cerebral artery occlusion without craniectomy in rats. Stroke 20: 84–91

Correspondence: Hiroyuki Fujimori, M.D., Biomedizinische NMR Forschungs GmbH, Max-Planck-Institut für biophysikalische Chemie, Am Fassberg 11, D-37077 Göttingen, Federal Republic of Germany.

Acta Neurochir (1997) [Suppl] 70: 170–172
© Springer-Verlag 1997

Apparent Diffusion Coefficient (ADC) and Magnetization Transfer Contrast (MTC) Mapping of Experimental Brain Tumor

K. Ikezaki[1], M. Takahashi[2], H. Koga[1], J. Kawai[2], Z. Kovács[1], T. Inamura[1], and M. Fukui[1]

[1] Department of Neurosurgery, Neurological Institute, Faculty of Medicine, Kyushu University, and
[2] Research Department, Contrast Media Laboratory, Nihon Shering KK, Japan

Summary

Brain tumor tissue contains different pathological areas, such as tumor cell rich parts, necrotic tissues, and cyst. Furthermore, both neovascularization and edema formation progress along with the tumor progression. In this study we employed diffusion weighted (DW) and magnetization transfer contrast (MTC) imaging to chronologically investigate the biological characteristics of a rat glioma. RG-2 glioma cells were implanted stereotactically into the right hemisphere of male Wistar rats. MR images were taken 1, 2 and 3 weeks after inoculation. Apparent diffusion coefficient (ADC) and MTC values were calculated as follows; ADC = −1n (SI-DW / SI-T2) / 1096, MTC = 1 − SI-MTon / SI-MToff. Each mapping image was made based on the calculated average values of four pixels. The spatial signal changes and the real values were compared to the histological findings. The apparent increase of ADC was noted in the parenchyma adjacent to tumor suggesting the progression of edema. The tumor itself had similar or slightly increased ADC. Cystic and necrotic components appeared 2 weeks after implantation and they showed significantly higher ADC than those calculated in the contralateral putamen. On the other hand, MTC was slightly decreased in the parenchyma adjacent to the tumor, markedly within the tumor, and maximally in the cystic and necrotic area suggesting accumulation of macromolecules such as growth factors, cytokines, and serum albumin.

Keywords: Brain neoplasm; diffusion weighted image; magnetization transfer contrast; magnetic resonance imaging.

Introduction

Diffusion-weighted magnetic resonance imaging (DWI), which is based on the translational movement or diffusion of water [4, 6]. Extensive studies, especially in stroke, has been reported using this techniques [3–5, 8]. The calculated apparent diffusion coefficient (ADC) is able to provide a quantitative analysis of water diffusibility and has been applied in the early detection of cerebral stroke and the evaluation of brain edema. On the other hand, magnetization transfer contrast technique has become a focus of interest for many

sites [1]. This technique depends on the exchange of two pools of proton: a free (mobile) pool, and a bound (less mobile in proteins and macromolecules) pool. Because the magnitude of the magnetization effect depends on the presence of the bound pool, the change is tissue specific, allowing differentiation of tissues by the degree and complexity of their macromolecule structures [2, 7]. In brain tumors, these techniques have not been studied extensively. In this study, we attempted to analyze the biochemical changes quantitatively in a brain tumor *in vivo* by calculating ADC and MTC values and producing ADC and MTC mapping images.

Materials and Methods

Animal Experiments

Exponentially growing RG2 glioma cells (1×10^5 / 5 μl) were implanted stereotactically into the right hemisphere of 15 male Wistar rats under pentobarbital anesthesia. After 1, 2, and 3 weeks, five rats in each group were anesthetized with pentobarbital and urethane. Magnetic resonance (MR) images were taken sequentially. Rats were decapitated following the gadolinium enhancement study, and the brains were removed and immersed in formaldehyde solution for histological (hematoxilin-eosin) study.

MR Imaging

Imaging experiments were performed on a 4.7 T animal imager (Omega CSI-II, GE NMR Instruments, CA) equipped with self-shielded gradients in combination with a homemade bird-cage coil. T2WI (TR/TE = 1500/80 msec) multislice sequence giving four 2.5 mm thick coronal images of the brain was used to localize the lesions. Diffusion weighted images were obtained in the spin echo sequences with motion probe gradient (b = 1096 sec/mm²). MTC-off images were taken in the gradient echo sequence (TR / TE = 100 / 8 msec). To obtain MTC-on images an additional saturation pulse was applied to the signal from bound proton before the gradient echo sequence. Other parameters were FOV = 60, and 128 × 128 matrix zero filled to 256 × 256 matrix. To obtain ADC and MTC mapping images, the signal intensities (SI) in every four voxels were used for calculation. ADC (mm²/sec) = –1n (SI-DW / SI-T2) / 1096, MTC = 1-SI-MTC / SI-MToff. The Gadolinium enhanced T1 weighted images were taken finally using the spin echo method (TR / TE = 600 / 24.5 msec). Each of SI was related to the SI of a simultaneously measured external standard, consisting of a cylindrical plastic tube that contained water. The SI was likewise determined by a region-of- interest technique in the external standard, the tumor tissue, the ipsilateral cortex, the contralateral caudate-putamen and the cortex.

Results

Image Analysis

The representative ADC and MTC mapping images, reproduced on a 64 × 64 matrix are shown in Fig. 1 (a, b). The increase of ADC was noted in the tissue adjacent to the tumor. The white matter also has higher ADC. The tumor tissue had same or slightly increased (average 10%) ADCs when compared to ADC in the contralateral caudate putamen. On the other hand, MTC in the tumor was decreased markedly (average 30%) when compared to that in the contralateral putamen. The tissues adjacent to the tumor also showed decreased MTCs.

The chronological changes of ADC and MTC in each anatomical structure are presented in Fig. 2. There was no significant change of ADC within the tumor tissue. However, 2 weeks after implantation, the tumor contained cystic and necrotic components and started to show significantly higher ADC (p < 0.05, maximally 50%) than that in the contralateral putamen. The ADC in the tissue-adjacent to the tumor also increased along with the edema formation. On the other hand, MTC in tumor was lower (average 20%) than that in the contralateral caudate putamen at 1 week. The difference increased at 2 and 3 week (up to 30%). In the cystic and necrotic area of tumor and adjacent brain tissue, MTC decreased maximally (66% of the control).

Discussion

Since ADC represents the translational movement of water diffusion, and the changes in membrane permeability by failure of energy metabolism, it can be used to analyze ischemic lesion quantitatively and differentiate penumbra from necrotic tissue [3–5, 7, 8]. On the other hand, MTC works based on the interaction of bulk water protons with protons of tissue macromolecules and can generate high contrast between tissues with different macromolecule compositions [1, 2, 7].

The present study tried to reveal the potential of ADC and MTC mapping images to evaluate biochem-

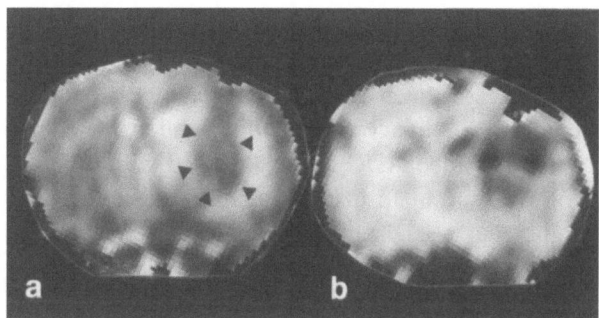

Fig. 1. (a) An ADC mapping image 2 weeks post-inoculation of RG-2 glioma cells. The tumor tissue (encircled by arrow heads) has iso- to hypo-signal intensities. The surrounding tissue shows increased ADC (approximately 2-fold higher than ADC in the contra lateral hemisphere). (b) The MTC mapping image of the same slice. The tumor tissue shows decreased MTC values. There is an apparent delineation of the tumor from the surrounding tissue. The adjacent tissue also shows decreased MTC values when compared to the contra lateral hemisphere

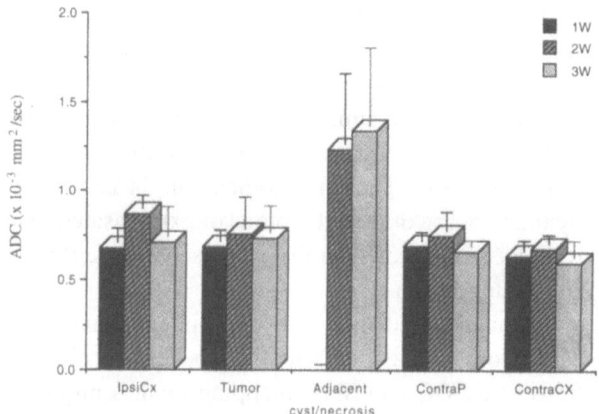

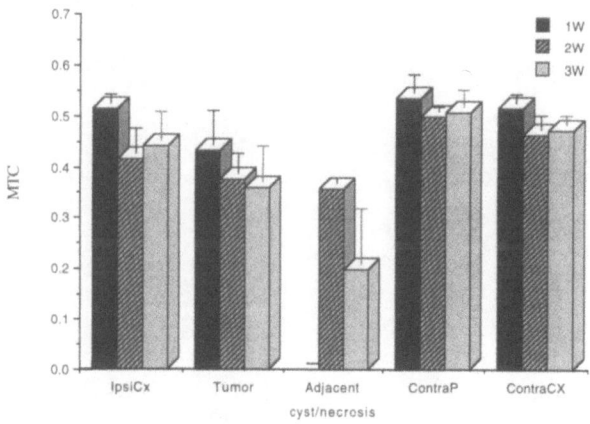

Fig. 2. Upper: Chronological changes of ADC in the various tissues. The tumor tissue has normal or slightly increased ADC. ADC in the adjacent tissue and in the degenerative portion of tumor shows increased ADCs; 2 weeks after tumor cell inoculation. Lower: The chronological changes of MTC in the various tissues. The tumor has reduced MTC. The adjacent tissue and the ipsilateral cortex also shows a decrease of MTC

ical changes in tumor and surrounding tissue. The histopathology of tumor alters according to the evolving processes such as increasing cellularity, tumorangiogenesis, hyper permeability, and degenerative changes. Varied ADC were calculated within the tumor. We speculate that the increase of cell density might reduce ADC. On the other hand, necrosis or cyst formation and increased permeability due to tumorangiogenesis might contribute to the increase of ADC.

In contrast, a decrease of MTC was observed in the tumor from 1 week to 3 weeks. The increase of cell density, the extravasated macromolecules due to hyper permeability, the secreted macromolecules such as growth factors and cytokines are all factors that might might increase the number of bound protons. In tumor surrounding tissue and also the white matter, the T2WI showed marked edema formation. The increased ADC might represent a bulk flow of water (vasogenic edema). Hypoxic condition might also affect on ADC since a decreased regional blood flow and increased cerebrovascular volume has been pointed out in these areas (ischemic penumbra). Interestingly, a chronological decrease of MTC was observed in the tumor surrounding tissue. These phenomena might be affected by the increase of bound protons of extravasated macromolecules rather than the increase of bulk flow of free water proton.

Further detailed analysis of these phenomena is necessary to correlate them with the biochemical changes, however, ADC and MTC mapping images might become useful clinical tools when considering tumor characteristics and the effects of chemotherapeutic agents.

Acknowledgments

This work was supported partly by the grant from the Ministry of Education, Science and Culture, Japan. We thank Ms. Terasaki for her assistance preparing histological sections.

References

1. Balaban RS, Ceckler TL (1992) Magnetization transfer contrast in magnetic resonance imaging. Magn Reson Q 8:116–137
2. Barker GJ, Tofts PS, Gass A (1996) An interleaved sequence for accurate and reproducible clinical measurement of magnetization transfer ratio. Magn Reson Imaging 14: 403–411
3. Hasegawa Y, Fisher M, Latour LL, Dardzinski BJ, Sotak CH (1994) MRI diffusion mapping of reversible and irreversible ischemic injury in focal brain ischemia. Neurology 44: 1481–1490
4. Hossmann KA, Hoehn-Berlage M (1995) Diffusion and perfusion MR imaging of cerebral ischemia. Cerebrovasc Brain Metab Rev 7: 187–217
5. Kohno K, Hoehn-Berlage M, Mies G, *et al* (1995) Relationship between diffusionweighted MR images, cerebral blood flow, and energy state in the experimental brain infarction. Magn Reson Imaging 13: 73–80
6. Le Bihan D, Breton E, Lallemand D, Grenier P, Cabanis E, Laval-Jeantet M (1986) MR imaging of intravoxel incoherent motions: application to diffusion and perfusion in neurogenic disorders. Radiology 161: 401–407
7. Prager JM, Rosenblum JD, Huddle DC, *et al* (1994) The magnetization transfer effect in cerebral infarction. AJNR 15: 1497–1500
8. Takahashi M, Fritz-Zieroth B, Chikugo T, Ogawa H (1993) Differentiation of chronic lesions after stroke in stroke-prone spontaneously hypertensive rats using diffusion weighted MRI. Magn Reson Med 30: 485–488

Correspondence: Kiyonobu Ikezaki, M.D., Ph.D., Department of Neurosurgery, Neurological Institute, Faculty of Medicine, Kyushu Universty 60, Fukuoka 812-82, Japan.

Acta Neurochir (1997) [Suppl] 70: 173–175
© Springer-Verlag 1997

The Origin of Lactate in Peritumoral Edema as Measured by Proton-Magnetic Resonance Spectroscopic Imaging

K. G. Go[1], **A. P. Krikke**[2], **R. L. Kamman**[2], and **M. A. A. M. Heesters**[3]

Departments of [1] Neurosurgery, [2] Diagnostic Radiology, and [3] Radiotherapy, University Hospital Groningen, The Netherlands

Summary

Using *in vivo* proton-magnetic resonance spectroscopy (^{1}H-MRS), which allows the measurement of metabolites of adequate tissue concentration, the origin of lactate in peritumoral edema has been assessed by comparison with lactate levels in the central and marginal areas of the tumor in 18 patients with cerebral gliomas. In the majority of cases lactate content in the area of peritumoral edema was lower than that in the tumor margin or tumor center, which is consistent with the assumption that the tumor is the source of lactate, which then reaches the surrounding area of edema by diffusion. In 3 of the 18 cases the amount of lactate in the peritumoral edematous tissue was higher than in the tumor, indicating that the lactate is locally produced on account of ischemia due to regional elevation of tissue pressure in the edematous area.

Keywords: Proton-magnetic resonance spectroscopy; peritumoral edema; cerebral lactate; tissue perfusion.

Introduction

In patients with brain tumors, peritumoral edema has been implicated in causing symptomatology on account of deficient perfusion (ischemia) due to elevation of regional tissue pressure. This has been indicated by earlier studies showing decreased energy charge potential and elevated lactate in biopsies of peritumoral edema [2, 3]. Currently, lactate may be assessed *in vivo* by the technique of proton magnetic resonance spectroscopy (^{1}H-MRS). In addition, ^{1}H-MRS allows the assessment of other metabolites of adequate tissue concentration, such as mobile choline metabolites, including phosphocholine and glycerophosphorylcholine, the creatine pool including creatine and phosphocreatine, and N-acetylaspartate (NAA), a marker of neurons. The metabolites appear as readily discernible peaks in the spectrum. The place of a peak on the abscissa denotes the specific chemical shift of resonance frequency exhibited by the metabolite or a certain protoncontaining group it contains, based on the specific molecular environment of the proton delivering the signal (Fig. 1). With respect to normal tissue, brain tumors exhibit an increased choline peak, which pertains to increased membrane biosynthesis, a more or less severely reduced NAA peak indicating replacement of the neuronal population by neoplastic cells, and often the appearance or increase of lactate [1]. The lactate may derive from tumor-specific aerobic glycolysis, and tends to occur in malignant gliomas. Therefore, lactate in the peritumoral edematous area may be of dual origin; it may have come from the tumor by diffusion or bulk flow, or the lactate in peritumoral edema may be a consequence of decreased tissue perfusion due to elevation of local tissue pressure.

Material and Methods

The study was conducted on 18 patients with primary gliomas, 9 of which were glioblastomas or high-grade astrocytomas, 6 were astrocytomas of intermediate or low grade, and 3 were oligodendrogliomas. In patients 1-dimensional as well as 2-dimensional ^{1}H-MRS was performed with a Philips Gyroscan whole body system of 1.5 T, using the PRIME sequence for localization, with water suppression by means of a selective inversion method, and data acquisition started at the zero crossing point of water. One-dimensional ^{1}H ± MRS comprised measuring a row of 9 ml voxels (TR 2000; TE 272; with 16 FID accumulations in 32 phase encoding steps), whereas in 2D[1]H-MRS a 32×32 matrix of 1 cm^3 voxels was acquired. For spectroscopic imaging (MRSI) (Fig. 2), signal intensity of each metabolite was projected voxel by voxel over an MR image, obtained from the peak areas, defined between the chemical shifts of 3.1–3.3 ppm for choline, 3.1–2.9 ppm for creatine, 1.9–2.1 ppm for N-acetyl aspartate, and 1.2–1.4 ppm for lactate. The lactate peak areas in the tumor margin, the peritumoral edema, and in normal tissue were expressed as percentages of the lactate peak area in the tumor center. The area of edema was defined as the area of increased signal intensity on the T$_2$-weighted MRI, but contrary to tumor, with neither choline increase, nor NAA decrease. In addition, the amount of edema was graded as 0: no, 1: scanty, 2: obvious and 3: massive; and signs of tissue compression or displacement were noted.

Results and Discussion

In 3 (cases 85, 96, and 98) of the 18 cases the amount of lactate in the peritumoral edematous tissue was higher than in the tumor (Fig. 3). These cases all showed evidence of tissue compression, although the edema was of grade 2 in two cases, and of grade 1 in the other. It is conceivable that in these few cases the higher lactate content in peritumoral edema is locally produced on account of ischemia due to regional elevation of tissue pressure in the edematous area.

In the total of 18 cases the signs of tissue compression occurred in 9 cases, grade 3 edema in 3, grade 2 edema in 10, and grade 1 edema in 5 cases. There was no correlation between the amount of edema and evidence of tissue compression, probably because not only the edema, but also the tumor itself may be responsible for tissue compression. The lactate content in the edematous tissue tended to be higher in the cases

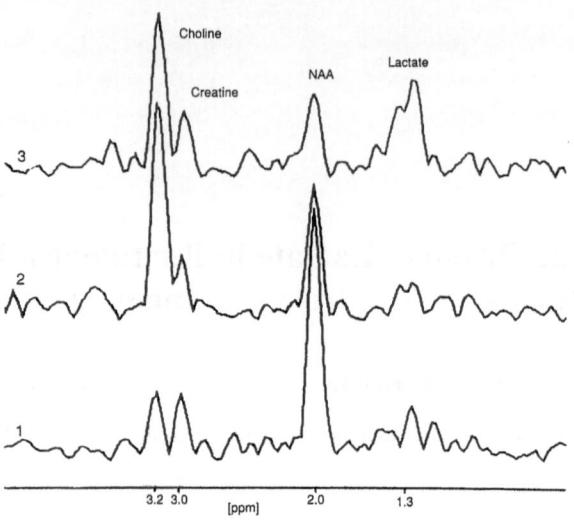

Fig. 1. Proton magnetic resonance spectrum of a high-grade astrocytoma. *1* Normal tissue with low choline, high NAA, and low lactate peaks; *2* and *3* tumor with increased choline and lactate, and decreased NAA peaks

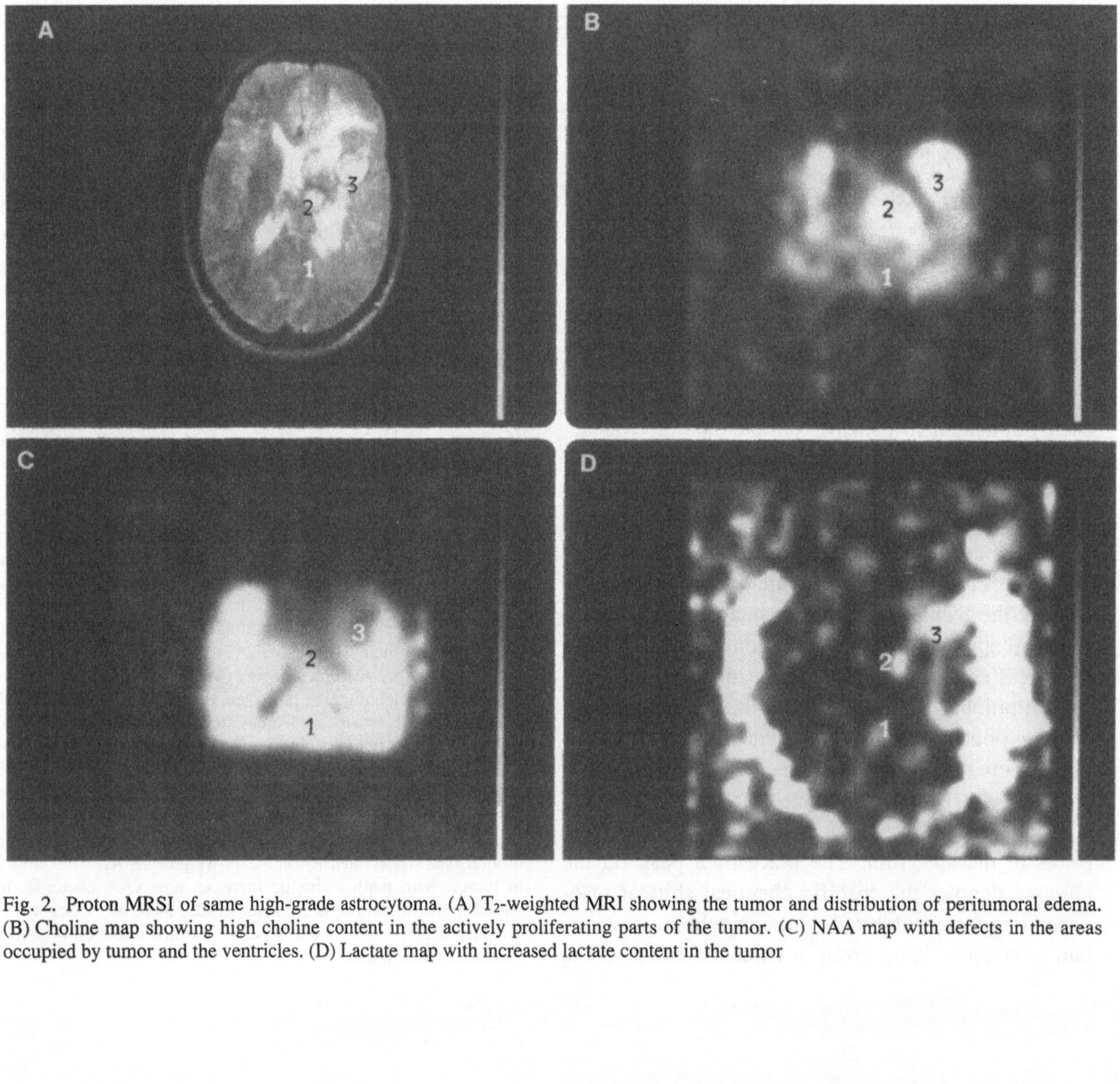

Fig. 2. Proton MRSI of same high-grade astrocytoma. (A) T$_2$-weighted MRI showing the tumor and distribution of peritumoral edema. (B) Choline map showing high choline content in the actively proliferating parts of the tumor. (C) NAA map with defects in the areas occupied by tumor and the ventricles. (D) Lactate map with increased lactate content in the tumor

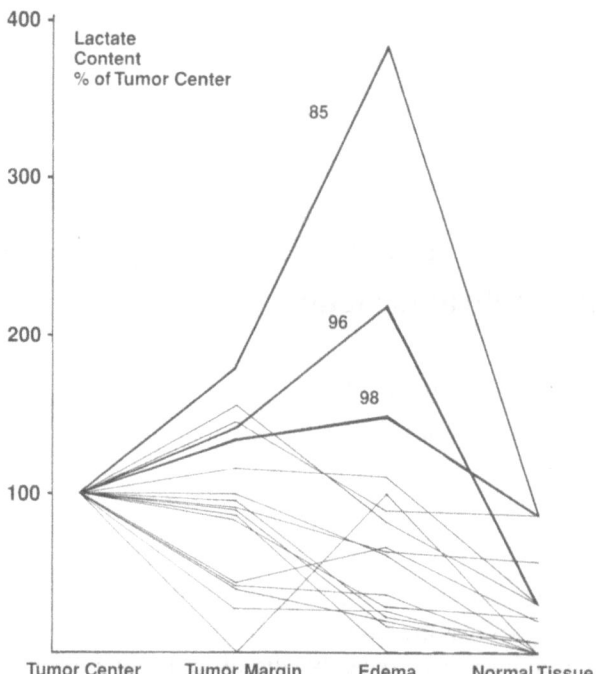

Fig. 3. Graph showing lactate content in tumor center, tumor margin, area of edema, and normal tissue expressed in % of lactate content in tumor center. Except in cases 85, 96 and 98, lactate content in the area of edema is lower than in the tumor center

then reaches the surrounding area of edema by diffusion. The production of lactate by gliomas may pertain to the preference of many tumors for aerobic glycolysis [4]. This also explains an increased glucose consumption rate of some tumors, although no correlation has yet been found between increased ^{18}F-fluoro-2-deoxyglucose on the PET-scan and elevated lactate on the ^{1}H-MRS [1]. The amount of lactate seemed higher in the center than in the margin of the tumor, but the difference was not significant in this series. In a previous series the lactate content (expressed with respect to creatine content), was higher in the center of high-grade gliomas [1], where ischemic conditions may also prevail due to inadequate vascularization.

References

1. Go KG, Kamman RL, Mooyaart EL, Heesters MAAM, Pruim J, Vaalburg W, Paans AMJ (1995) Localised proton spectroscopy and spectroscopic imaging in cerebral gliomas, with comparison to positron emission tomography. Neuroradiology 37: 198–206
2. Reulen HJ, Medzihradsky F, Enzenbach R, Marguth F, Brendel W (1969) Electrolytes, fluids and energy metabolism in human cerebral edema. Arch Neurol 21: 517–525
3. Schmiedek P, Baethmann A, Sippel G, Oettinger W, Enzenbach R, Marguth F, Brendel W (1974) Energy state and glycolysis in human cerebral edema. The application of a new freeze-stop technique. J Neurosurg 40: 351–364
4. Warburg O (1956) On the origin of cancer cells. Science 123: 309–314

Correspondence: K. G. Go, M.D., Department of Neurosurgery, University Hospital Groningen, Hanzeplein 1, Groningen 9721 TP, The Netherlands.

with evidence of tissue compression than in those without, although the difference was not significant (p = 0.075).

In the majority of cases in which lactate content in the area of peritumoral edema was lower than that in the tumor (margin or center) (Fig. 3), it may be assumed that the tumor is the source of lactate, which

Acta Neurochir (1997) [Suppl] 70: 176–178
© Springer-Verlag 1997

Neuroprotective Properties of a Novel Antioxidant (U-101033E) with Improved Blood-Brain Barrier Permeability in Focal Cerebral Ischemia

R. Schmid-Elsaesser[1], S. Zausinger[2], E. Hungerhaber[2], A. Baethmann[2], and H.-J. Reulen[1]

[1] Department of Neurosurgery, and [2] Institute für Surgical Research, Klinikum Grosshadern, Ludwig-Maximilians-University, Munich, Federal Republic of Germany

Summary

Many efforts have been undertaken to develop antioxidants against free radical induced brain damage. 21-aminosteroids, although accumulating in the cell membrane, thus protecting vascular endothelium from peroxidative damage hardly penetrate the blood-brain barrier. A novel group of antioxidants, the pyrrolopyrimidines, has a markedly improved ability to enter the brain parenchyma. In our current study the neuroprotective potential of the 21-aminosteroid U-74389G was compared with that of the pyrrolopyrimidine U-101033E in a rat model of reversible focal cerebral ischemia. Sprague-Dawley rats were subjected to unilateral occlusion of the middle cerebral artery with assignment to one of three treatment arms (n = 10 each), receiving either vehicle, U-74389G, or U-101033E. Regional CBF was recorded bilaterally by laser Doppler flowmetry. In addition, neurological examination was performed daily, with assessment of infarct volume at day seven. U-101033E reduced the infarct volume significantly by 51%, whereas U-74389G afforded non-significant attenuation only. U-101033E was found to improve neurological recovery promptly; animals with U-74389G began to recover only at the end of the experimental observation period. Differences in the regional CBF were not found in the contralateral hemispheres for either treatment group. We conclude that antioxidative compounds which cross the blood-brain barrier are more effective in focal cerebral ischemia than agents which predominantly act on the endothelium of cerebral microvessels.

Keywords: Focal cerebral ischemia; free radicals; lipid peroxidation; 21-aminosteroid; pyrrolopyrimidine.

Introduction

Oxygen free radicals are postulated to have a critical role in acute postischemic neuronal damage. 21-aminosteroids (e.g. tirilazad) are potent inhibitors of free radical-induced lipid peroxidation. U-74389G is another 21-aminosteroid, which is structurally related to tirilazad mesylate, having similar pharmacodynamic and pharmaeokinetic properties [5]. Both have a high affinity for the endothelial cell membrane and may, thus, protect vascular endothelium against peroxida-

tive damage. However, 21-aminosteroids are not expected to cross the blood-brain barrier (BBB). Pyrrolopyrimidines are recently discovered antioxidants, which have a significantly greater potential to enter the brain parenchyma [6]. Both brain parenchyma and its vascular endothelium can generate free radicals, but it is unclear which of these tissues constitutes the major source of radical production and thereby requiring specific therapeutic protection preferentially [10, 13, 14]. We have presently compared the neuroprotective properties of a 21-aminosteroid (U-74389G) that primarily acts on vascular endothelium with that of a pyrrolopyrimidine (U-101033E), which penetrates the BBB.

Materials and Methods

Thirty-two male Sprague-Dawley rats (250–300 g) were intubated and ventilated with 0.8% halothane and a mixture of 70% N_2O and 30% O_2. The temporalis muscle and rectal temperature were maintained at 37°C throughout the experiment. Physiological variables as blood pressure, blood gases, hemoglobin, hematocrit, glucose were monitored and kept within normal limits without differences between groups. Three groups of rats were studied (n = 10 each): Control animals receiving vehicle only (0.02 M citric acid) and experimental animals subjected to treatment with either U-74389G or U-101033E (3 × 3.0 mg/kg) before ischemia, at reperfusion, and one hour later. All rats were subjected to middle cerebral artery occlusion (MCAO) by insertion of an intraluminal silicone-coated 4-0 nylon thread for 90 min [17]. Regional cerebral blood flow (rCBF) was measured by laser Doppler flowmetry (LDF) during ischemia and for 60 min during reperfusion. Two burr holes were drilled bilaterally 0.5 mm posterior and 5 mm lateral of the bregma. Bent flow probes were placed above the exposed dura using a micromanipulator. Animals with a marked decrease of contralateral blood flow observed by laser Doppler flowmetry shortly after insertion of the filament were excluded from the study since this finding indicates subarachnoid hemorrhage [1]. The development of and recovery from neurologic deficits were assessed by daily examinations using a grading scale of 0 to 5 according to

Bederson *et al.* [16]. Seven days after the initial ischemia insult the brain was subjected to perfusion fixation and coronally cut in 400 µm intervals. The sections were stained with HE for planimetrical determination of the spread of infarction. Statistical comparisons were made using the Kruskal-Wallis ANOVA on Ranks followed by comparison of all groups versus control (Dunnett's Method). Differences were considered significant at $p < 0.05$. Results are presented as means ± SEM.

Results

The experimental groups did not differ with respect to the pre-, intra- or postischemic blood pressure or arterial blood gases. All animals remained normothermic during surgery and the postoperative observation period. Administration of U-101033E afforded immediate and significant improvement of the neurological function compromized by MCA-occlusion, while neurological recovery was delayed in animals receiving U-74389G. A significantly improved neuro-score was observed only at the end of the experimental observation period at day six. Moreover U-101033E afforded significant ($P < 0.05$) inhibition of infarct formation, i.e. by 51% from 65.1 ± 9.5 mm^3 in the untreated controls to 32.1 ± 6.2 mm^3 (mean ± SEM). Attenuation of infarct formation by U-74389G was statistically not significant. Spread of infarction amounted to 47.8 ± 9.9 mm^3 in this group (Table 1).

No significant rCBF differences were found in the various experimental groups. Insertion of the vessel filament resulted in a reduction of the cerebral blood flow to 20% of baseline in tissue areas supplied by the middle cerebral artery in all groups. Upon reperfusion, postischemic hyperemia was observed for 15 to 20 min, while blood flow fell then to about 70% of baseline until 1 hour after onset of reperfusion. The regional CBF of the contralateral hemisphere remained unchanged throughout the experiment.

Discussion

U-101033E exhibits marked neuroprotective properties as indicated by improvement of neurological function post ischemia and by inhibition of infarct formation, i.e. by 51% compared to only 24% afforded by the 21-aminosteroid. The findings support the hypothesis that antioxidants, which are able to cross the blood-brain barrier are therapeutically more effective for cerebral ischemia than those that do not. Hall *et al.* [6] have reported that U-101033E inhibits infarct growth by 27% in mice with permanent MCA-occlusion contrary to tirilazad, which was only minimally effective. Inhibition of infarct formation by the pyrrolopyrimidine most likely is due to a better access to the ischemic brain parenchyma. In transient ischemia, subsequent reperfusion might be expected to enhance the drug concentration in postischemic brain, whereas in permanent vessel occlusion drugs may be delivered only to tissue with sufficient collateral flow.

The marked difference in efficacy of the 21-aminosteroid and the pyrrolopyrimidine in transient focal ischemia as currently demonstrated raises the question where the generation of free radicals and radical-induced injury takes place. Both brain parenchyma and the vascular endothelium have the potential for producing radicals [10, 13, 14]. Findings on the therapeutic efficacy of radical scavengers suggest that antioxidants or other agents, which are able to cross the BBB are most effective for cerebral protection [12]. This may be explained by the lipophilicity of these compounds providing access to neuronal cell membranes where lipid peroxidation is particularly active [14]. For example, agents, which pass through the blood-brain barrier may accumulate in mitochondria and prevent free radical damage of components of the respiratory chain there. Other blood-brain barrier permeable antioxidants including allopurinol, LY-178002, and dimethylthiourea (DMTU) have been found to have neuroprotective properties in animals with transient forebrain ischemia or permanent focal ischemia [3, 8, 11], while antioxidative agents with poor barrier permeability were not effective or were minimally so [4, 7, 9].

Although many free radical scavengers are only moderately effective as inhibitors of infarct formation, e.g. by 25–35% [13], more convincing results have

Table 1. *Total Infarct Volume Given in Cubic mm* (mean ± SEM)

	Group		
	Controls (n = 10)	U-74389G (n = 10)	U-101033E (n = 10)
Infarct volume (mm^3)	65.1 ± 9.5	47.8 ± 9.9	32.1 ± 6.2[a]

[a] $p < 0.05$ versus vehicle-treated controls (Kruskal-Wallis ANOVA on Ranks).

been realised with administration of the spin trapping agent α-phenyl-N-tert-butyl nitrone (PBN) [2, 15]. Nitrone-based spin traps are able to penetrate the BBB readily at high concentrations and to react with transient free radicals leading to the formation of stable spin adducts. The reported 50% inhibition of infarct spread in focal reversible ischemia in rats with pretreatment by PBN [15] corresponds to our results obtained with U-101033E. This may reflect accumulation of these compounds in cellular organelles and membranes indicating that a protective therapeutic agent should be able to reach the sitc of free radical formation and damage.

Our current results do not provide evidence that either U-101033E or U-74389G affect rCBF during ischemia or during one hour of reperfusion. Consequently the beneficial effects of these antioxidants must be independent from improvement of CBF.

How brain-permeable antioxidants as the pyrrolopyrimidines or PBN protect the ischemic brain remains unclear. More information is required to improve our understanding of radical-mediated cell injury. Since both vascular endothelium and the brain parenchyma may contribute to this process in ischemia, it is conceivable that a combination of antioxidative agents, one with regional endothelial activity, the other penetrating the BBB, may afford antioxidation plus radical scavenging in blood vessels and the brain parenchyma. Such a combination could be superior to the currently employed monotherapy.

Acknowledgements

This work was supported by the Deutsche Forschungsgemeinschaft (Schm 1067/2–1). The authors wish to thank Dr. Ed Hall of Upjohn-Company for the generous gift of U-74389G and U-101033E.

References

1. Bederson JB, Germano IM, Guarino L (1995) Cortical blood flow and cerebral perfusion pressure in a new noncraniotomy model of subarachnoid hemorrhage in the rat. Stroke 26: 1086–1091
2. Cao XH, Phillis JW (1994) Alpha-phenyl-tert-butyl-nitrone reduces cortical infarct and edema in rats subjected to focal ischemia. Brain Res 644: 267–272
3. Clemens JA, Ho PP, Panetta JA (1991) LY178002 reduces rat brain damage after transient global forebrain ischemia. Stroke 22: 1048–1052
4. Clemens JA, Panetta JA (1994) Neuroprotection by antioxidants in models of global and focal ischemia. Ann NY Acad Sci 738: 250–256
5. Hall ED, McCall JM, Means ED (1994) Therapeutic potential of the lazaroids (21-aminosteroids) in acute central nervous system trauma, ischemia and subarachnoid hemorrhage. Adv Pharmacol 28: 221–268
6. Hall ED, Andrus PK, Smith SL, Oostveen JA, Scherch HM, Lutzke BS, Raub TJ, Sawada GA, Palmer JR, Banitt LS, Tustin JS, Belonga KL, Ayer DE, Bundy GL (1996) Neuroprotective efficacy of microvascularly-localized versus brain-penetrating antioxidants. Acta Neurochir (Wien) [Suppl] 66: 107–113
7. Haun SE, Kirsch JR, Helfaer MA, Kubos KL, Traystman RJ (1991) Polyethylene glycol-conjugated superoxide dismutase fails to augment brain superoxide dismutase activity in piglets. Stroke 22: 655–659
8. Itoh T, Kawakami M, Yamauchi Y, Shimizu S, Nakamura M (1986) Effect of allopurinol on ischemia and reperfusion-induced cerebral injury in spontaneously hypertensive rats. Stroke 17: 1284–1287
9. Karlsson BR, Loberg EM, Grogaard B, Steen PA (1994) The antioxidant tirilazad does not affect cerebral blood flow or histopathologic changes following severe ischemia in rats. Acta Neurol Scand 90: 256–262
10. Kumar M, Liu GJ, Floyd RA, Grammas P (1996) Anoxic injury of endothelial cells increases production of nitric oxide and hydroxyl radicals. Biochem Biophys Res Commun 219: 497–501
11. Martz D, Rayos G, Schielke GP, Betz AL (1989) Allopurinol and dimethylthiourea reduce brain infarction following middle cerebral artery occlusion in rats. Stroke 20: 488–494
12. Moore LE, Traystman RJ (1994) Role of oxygen free radicals and lipid peroxidation in cerebral reperfusion injury. Adv Pharmacol 31: 565–576
13. Siesjö BK, Agardh CD, Bengtsson F (1989) Free radicals and brain damage. Cerebrovasc Brain Metab Rev 1: 165–211
14. Traystman RJ, Kirsch JR, Koehler RC (1991) Oxygen radical mechanisms of brain injury following ischemia and reperfusion. J Appl Physiol 71: 1185–1195
15. Zhao Q, Pahlmark K, Smith ML, Siesjö BK (1994) Delayed treatment with the spin trap a-phenyl-N-tert-butyl nitrone (PBN) reduces infarct size following transient middle cerebral artery occlusion in rats. Acta Physiol Scand 152: 349–350
16. Bederson JB, Pitts LH, Tsuji M, Nishimura MC, Davis RL, Bartkowski H (1996) Rat middle cerebral artery occlusion: evaluation of the model and development of aneurologic examination. Stroke 17: 472–476
17. Koizumi J, Yoshida Y, Nakazawa T, Ooneda G (1986) A new experimental model of cerebral embolism in rats in which recirculation can be introduced in the ischemic area. Jpn J Stroke 8: 1–8

Correspondence: Robert Schmid-Elsaesser, M.D., Department of Neurosurgery, Ludwig-Maximilians-University, Klinikum Grosshadern, Marchioninistrasse 15, D-81377 Munich, Federal Republic of Germany.

Acta Neurochir (1997) [Suppl] 70: 179–181
© Springer-Verlag 1997

Effect of α-Trinositol on Swelling and Damage of Glial Cells by Lactacidosis and Glutamate

F. Staub[1], **J. Peters**[2], **N. Plesnila**[2], **R. C. C. Chang**[2], and **A. Baethmann**[2]

[1] Department of Neurosurgery, University of Cologne, Köln, and [2] Institute for Surgical Research, Klinikum Grosshadern, University of Munich, München, Federal Republic of Germany

Summary

The therapeutic efficacy of α-trinositol (D-myo-inositol-1,2,6-trisphosphate), an isomer of the intracellular messenger IP_3, was analized for cytotoxic swelling and damage of glial cells *in vitro* from lactacidosis or glutamate. Lactacidosis and the interstitial accumulation of glutamate are prominent sequelae in ischemic or traumatic brain tissue. C6 glioma cells harvested from culture and suspended in a physiological medium were either exposed to pH 5.0 by administration of lactic acid, or to 1 mM glutamate at normal pH. Cell swelling and viability were quantified by blood flow cytometry. Addition of α-trinositol (3 mM) under control conditions at pH 7.4 resulted in transient cell shrinking to $96.5 \pm 1.3\%$ of control within 3 min ($p < 0.05$). Lactacidosis of pH 5.0 led to an increase in cell volume to $139.7 \pm 1.3\%$ within 20 min, whereas α-trinositol reduced the swelling response by approximately 25% ($p < 0.01$). In addition, cell viability was severely affected at pH 5.0 amounting to only $53.8 \pm 3.1\%$ after 60 min. α-Trinositol was found to markedly improve cell viability; at 60 min $70.2 \pm 1.6\%$ of the cells were still viable ($p < 0.01$). Addition of glutamate (1 mM) led to a steady increase in cell size, reaching 110% of control after 120 min, irrespective of wether α-trinositol was present or not. The attenuation of cell swelling may be attributed to an interference with pH-regulatory mechanisms, such as the Na^+/H^+-antiporter, while protection of cell viability might be caused be effects of α-trinositol on Ca^{2+}-overload. On the other hand, the increase in cell volume by glutamate associated with its intracellular uptake was not influenced by α-trinositol.

Keywords: α-Trinositol; cell swelling; lactacidosis; glutamate; cytotoxic brain edema.

Introduction

Swelling of glial- and nerve cells, i.e. cytotoxic brain edema, is a common finding in cerebral ischemia, trauma, metabolic disorders, and in association with vasogenic brain edema [1]. In ischemia or severe head injury tissue homeostasis is severely affected. There is a massive release of excitatory transmitters, such as glutamate, development of tissue acidosis, accumulation of K^+-ions in the extracellular space, or of Ca^{2+}-ions in the intracellular compartment as well as formation of autacoids, such as free radicals among others [2, 13]. In previous studies the significance of acidosis for cell swelling and irreversible cell damage was explored on a quantitative basis using C6 glioma cells or astrocytes from primary culture [14]. Cell swelling from acidosis occurred once the pH was lowered to 6.8 or below, whereas cell viability started to decline at pH 5.6. Another objective of the present study addresses the property of glutamate to induce swelling. The excitatory neurotransmitter is released in large amounts in ischemic and traumatized brain tissue [2]. It was found to induce glial and nerve cell swelling *in vivo* and *in vitro* [12].

Since both, acidosis and the release of glutamate must be considered as key factors for cytotoxic cell swelling and damage from cerebral ischemia and trauma, specific inhibition of these mechanisms might be therapeutically beneficial. The purpose of the present study was to investigate the therapeutic potential of α-trinositol (D-myo-inositol-1,2,6-trisphosphate) an isomer of the intracellular second messenger IP_3 (D-myo-inositol-1,4,5-trisphosphate). α-Trinositol was studied in cytotoxic brain edema *in vitro*, induced in suspended glial cells by the administration of lactic acid or glutamate, respectively.

Materials and Methods

C6 glioma cells were cultivated as monolayers in Petri dishes using Dulbecco's modified minimal essential medium (DMEM) buffered with 25 mM bicarbonate. The medium was supplemented with 10% fetal calf serum (FCS) and 100 IU/ml penicillin G and 50 μg/ml streptomycin. The cells were grown in a humidified atmosphere of 5% CO_2 and room air at 37°C. The cells were harvested with 0.05% trypsin-0.02% EDTA in phosphate-buffered saline and washed twice thereafter. After resuspension in serum-free medium the glial cells were transferred to a plexiglas incubation chamber supplied with electrodes for control of pH, temperature, and pO_2. A gas-permeable silicon rubber tube in the chamber provided the cell suspension with a mixture of O_2, CO_2, and N_2 [9]. The volume of the glial cells was determined by flow cytometry using an advanced coulter system with hydrodynamic focusing [8]. The technique was also employed for measurement of cell viability by exclusion of the fluorescence dye propidium iodide (final concentration: 40 µg/ml) [14]. The experiments were preceded by a 30 min control period for measurement of cell volume, viability, and medium osmolality under normal conditions. In the control group (n = 5) effects of α-trinositol (3 mM; Perstorp Pharma, Perstorp, Sweden) were tested on volume and viability of the glial cells under normal conditions, i.e. pH 7.4 and pO_2 of 80–100 mmHg. For induction of lactacidosis the pH of the medium was lowered from 7.4 (control) to 5.0 by addition of isotonic lactic acid (300 mosmol/l) at the end of the control period (n = 5). Cell volume and viability were monitored for 60 min during lactacidosis. In further studies at normal pH, the cell suspension was added with 1 mM glutamate (final concentration) and the cell volume and viability were measured over 120 min (n = 5). Inhibition of cell swelling from acidosis or glutamate was studied by addition of α-trinositol (3 mM) prior to induction of lactacidosis (n = 5) or administration of glutamate to the suspension (n = 5).

Results

The average volume of C6 glioma cells during the control period at pH 7.4 was 901.2 ± 7.3 µm³; $94.3 \pm 0.2\%$ of the cells were viable. The addition of α-trinositol (3 mM) to the cell suspension under control conditions did not influence cell viability during an observation period of 60 minutes. On the other hand, cell volume decreased to $96.5 \pm 1.3\%$ of control within 3 minutes after administration of the inhibitor ($p < 0.05$). Cell shrinking by α-trinositol was only transient, however, since cell volume returned to normal after 10 minutes.

As in previous studies, addition of lactic acid to the suspension led to an increase in volume of the C6 glioma cells [14]. At pH 5.0 cell volume expandes within 1 minute to $119.2 \pm 2.8\%$ of control followed by further swelling to $139.7 \pm 1.3\%$ after 20 minutes. Subsequently, cell swelling leveled off and the cell volume was constant during the remaining observation period. In the presence of α-trinositol, swelling of C6 glioma cells at pH 5.0 was significantly attenuated during the whole observation period ($p < 0.01$). The increase in cell size was reduced by approximately 25%, reaching only 113.3 ± 1.0 after 1 minute or $131.1 \pm 1.1\%$ after 20 minutes. In addition to cell swelling, cell viability was severely affected at pH 5.0 [14]. After 30 minutes, viability of the cells had fallen to $60.6 \pm 4.7\%$, whereas only $53.8 \pm 3.1\%$ of the cells were viable at 60 minutes. α-Trinositol was found to markedly attenuate the decrease of cell viability by

lactacidosis at pH 5.0. After 30 minutes $75.1 \pm 2.3\%$ and after 60 minutes $70.2 \pm 1.6\%$ of the cells were found viable ($p < 0.01$).

Addition of glutamate to the glial suspension at a final concentration of 1 mM in the medium led to an almost linear increase in cell size over time, irrespective of whether α-trinositol was present or not. The increase in cell volume amounted to $106.0 \pm 1.1\%$ of control after 60 minutes and to $106.6 \pm 0.4\%$ when α-trinositol was administered. After 120 minutes, cell swelling was $109.7 \pm 1.2\%$ without α-trinositol as compared to $110.1 \pm 0.7\%$ in the presence of the compound. Viability of the C6 glioma cells was not affected by glutamate [12].

Discussion

Several inositol phosphates are found intracellularly in animal cells, where the 1,4,5-isomer is involved in release of Ca^{2+}-ions from intracellular stores [4]. The 1,2,6-isomer α-trinositol does not seem to be naturally occuring in animal tissue, but has been shown to have several pharmacologic effects. α-Trinositol acts as an antagonist to the vasoconstrictor effect of the sympathetic co-transmitter neuropeptide-Y (NPY) and may thus influence tissue blood flow in situations with intense sympathetic stimulation [7]. As shown in the present experiments as well as in work by other groups, α-trinositol appears to have effects on several kind of edema and inflammation. The substance was found to decrease lung edema formation after smoke inhalation in sheep and to suppress edema generation and albumin extravasation in thermally injured skin in rats [11]. α-Trinositol may exert these beneficial effects on a cellular level by antagonization of an increased microvascular permeability, stabilization of the tissue and cell membranes and reduction of gap-opening between endothelial cells [11]. Concerning formation of brain edema, it was recently shown that α-trinositol attenuates vasogenic brain edema from a focal lesion in rabbits [3]. The results of this study suggest in addition, that the substance has a therapeutic effect on cytotoxic brain edema induced by acidosis. Since the compound was shown to interact with membrane transporters like Na^+/K^+-ATPase [5], it is conceivable that it also interferes with the Na^+/H^+-antiporter which is activated during acidosis-induced glial swelling [14].

Furthermore, α-trinositol was found to protect cell viability at pH 5.0. Information is available that acidosis among others activates lipid peroxidation simultaneously inhibiting respiratory activity of brain mitochondria [13]. Both mechanisms causing damage to the cell membrane and energy failure facilitate cellular influx of Ca^{2+}-ions and its adverse sequelae, including Ca^{2+}-overload of mitochondria and activation of proteases, endonucleases and lipases. α-Trinositol might preserve cell viability by antagonization of these processes, as it was shown to attenuate iron- and H_2O_2-stimulated lipid peroxidation in rat liver microsomes or bovine brain liposomes [6]. In addition, the protection of cell viability in lactacidosis might be attributed to interference of α-trinositol with intracellular Ca^{2+}-fluxes. It has been reported that intravenous administration of α-trinositol attenuated the influx of ^{45}Ca into vascular smooth muscle cells stimulated by NPY- or ATP-induced contraction [15].

Administration of 1 mM glutamate to the cell suspension led to a steady cell volume increase to 110% of control within 120 minutes and that swelling was not inhibited by α-trinositol, contrary to cell swelling caused by lactacitosis. It was previously shown that glutamate-induced glial swelling is associated with a decrease of the glutamate level in the medium [12]. Evidence is available that swelling of glial cells by glutamate is based on an active intracellular accumulation of the amino acid [10]. The glutamate uptake occurs against a steep intra- to extracellular concentration difference. and is fueled by a concurrent influx of Na^{2+}-ions along their electrochemical gradient [10]. The intracellular accumulation of glutamate together with Na^+-ions raises cell osmolality as the ultimate mechanism of swelling. The present findings indicate that α-trinositol is not involved in glial swelling from glutamate as well as its clearance by the cells.

The present results demonstrate therapeutic properties of α-trinositol against the swelling and damage of glial cells by lactacidosis, making further studies worthwhile on its potential to influence brain edema from ischemia or trauma *in vivo*.

References

1. Baethmann A, Maier Hauff K, Kempski O, Unterberg A, Wahl M, Schürer L (1988) Mediators of brain edema and secondary brain damage. Crit Care Med 16: 972–978

2. Baethmann A, Maier Hauff K, Schürer L, Lange M, Guggenbichler C, Vogt W, Jacob K, Kempski O (1989) Release of glutamate and of free fatty acids in vasogenic brain edema. J Neurosurg 70: 578–591

3. Berger S, Staub F, Stoffel M, Eriskat J, Schürer L, Baethmann A (1994)Therapeutical efficacy of a novel chloride-transport blocker and an IP_3-analogue in vasogenic brain edema. In: Ito U, Baethmann A, Hossmann KA, Kuroiwa T, Marmarou A, Reulen HJ, Takakura K (eds) Brain edema IX. Acta Neurochir (Wien) [Suppl] 60: 534–537

4. Berridge MJ, Irvine RF (1984) Inositol trisphosphate, a novel second messenger in cellular signal transduction. Nature 312: 315–321

5. Carrington AL, Calcutt NA, Ettlinger CB, Gustafsson T, Tomlinson DR (1993) Effects of treatment with myo-inositol or its 1,2,6-trisphosphate (PP56) on nerve conduction in streptozotocin-diabetes. Eur J Pharmacol 237: 257–263

6. Claxson A, Morris C, Blake D, Siren M, Halliwell B, Gustafsson T, Löfkvist B, Bergelin I (1990) The anti-inflammatory effects of D-myo-inositol-1,2,6-trisphospate (PP56) on animal models of inflammation. Agents Actions 29: 68–70

7. Edvinsson L, Adamsson M, Jansen I (1990) Neuropeptide Y antagonistic properties of D-myo-inositol-1,2,6-trisphosphate in guinea pig basilar arteris. Neuropeptides 17: 99–105

8. Kachel V, Glossner E, Kordwig E, Ruhenstroth-Bauer G (1977) Fluvo-metricell, a combined cell volume and cell fluorescence analyzer. J Histochem Cytochem 25: 804–812

9. Kempski O, Chaussy L, Groß U, Zimmer M, Baethmann A (1983) Volume regulation and metabolism of suspended C6 glioma cells: an *in vitro* model to study cytotoxic brain edema. Brain Res 279: 217–228

10. Kimelberg HK, Pang S, Treble DH (1989) Excitatory amino acid-stimulated uptake of $^{22}Na^+$ in primary astrocyte cultures. J Neurosci 9: 1141–1149

11. Nakazawa H, Gustafsson TO, Traber LD, Herndon DN, Traber DL (1994) α-Trinositol decreases lung edema formation after smoke inhalation in an ovine model. J Appl Physiol 76: 278–282

12. Schneider GH, Baethmann A, Kempski O (1992) Mechanisms of glial swelling induced by glutamate. Can J Physiol Pharmacol 70 [Suppl]: S334–343

13. Siesjö BK (1992) Pathophysiology and treatment of focal cerebral ischemia. Part 1: Pathophysiology. J Neurosurg 77: 169–184

14. Staub F, Baethmann A, Peters J, Weigt H, Kempski O (1990) Effects of lactacidosis on glial cell volume and viability. J Cereb Blood Flow Metab 10: 866–876

15. Wahlestedt C, Reis DJ, Yoo H, Adamsson M, Andersson D, Edvinsson L (1992) A novel inositol phosphate selectively inhibits vasoconstriction evoked by the sympathetic co-transmitter neuropeptide Y (NPY) and adenosine triphosphate (ATP). Neurosci Lett 143: 123–126

Correspondence: Frank Staub, M.D., Department of Neurosurgery, University of Cologne, Joseph Stelzmann Str. 9, D-50924 Köln, Federal Republic of Germany.

Acta Neurochir (1997) [Suppl] 70: 182–184
© Springer-Verlag 1997

Effects of Lecithinized SOD on Contusion Injury in Rats

M. Yunoki[1], **Y. Noguchi**[1], **S. Nishio**[1], **Y. Ono**[1], **M. Kawauchi**[1], **S. Asai**[1], **T. Ohmoto**[1], **M. Asanuma**[2], and **N. Ogawa**[2]

[1] Department of Neurological Surgery, Okayama University Medical School, and [2] Department of Neuroscience, Institute of Molecular and Cellular Medicine, Okayama University Medical School, Okayama, Japan

Summary

To analyze the effect of lecithinized superoxide dismutase (SOD) on superoxide accumulation after traumatic injury, the expression of Cu,Zn-SOD mRNA was examined after contusion in rat using Northern blotting. As determined by specific gravity, lecithinized SOD decreased brain edema. The expression of Cu,Zn-SOD mRNA increased at the core, peripheral and contralateral hemisphere of injury. These increases were then suppressed by lecithinized SOD. Our results support the hypothesis that superoxide may play an important role in edema formation after contusion, and that lecithinized SOD appears to prevent brain edema through a protective effect against superoxide injury.

Keywords: Contusion; superoxide dismutase (SOD); free radicals.

Introduction

We have previously reported an increase in SOD activity [5] and the increased expression of Cu,Zn-SOD mRNA [4] after brain contusion, indicating that superoxide may play an important role in traumatic brain injury [4, 5, 9]. On the other hand, the therapeutic application of SOD has been limited because of its low cell membrane affinity and its rapid metabolism [6]. To overcome these problems, several chemically modified preparations of SOD, including polyethylene glycol-conjugated SOD [17] and pyran SOD [14], have been investigated. However, these have not been approved for clinical use because of their insufficient pharmacological potency. Recently, increased potency of lecithinized SOD, in which a lecithin derivative was covalently bound to recombinant human SOD, has been reported [5, 6]. In this study, we analyzed endogenous Cu,Zn-SOD mRNA expression and specific gravity to examine the effect of lecithinized SOD on brain contusion.

Methods

Twenty male SD rats (weighing 250–300 g) were divided into four groups. In the first group, a burr hole six mm in diameter was made in the right parietal potion, and one ml of saline was administered intravenously (sham group: n = 5). The second group underwent sham operation, and lecitinized SOD (Seikagaku Co., Tokyo, Japan) (3000 units/kg) was administered (sham + SOD group: n = 5). In the third group, one ml of saline was administered intravenously one minute before traumatic insult. The contusion was made by dropping a 20 g weight from a height of 30 cm onto the exposed dura of the right parietal region (contusion group: n = 5). In the fourth group, lecithinized SOD (3000 units/kg) was administered one minute before the same insult (contusion + SOD group: n = 5). Six hours after each operation, each rat was decapitated and the cortex was dissected from the injured portion (core), 4 mm anterior to the injured portion (peripheral), and from the contralateral hemisphere (distal). The water content of each portion of the cortex was measured using the specific gravity method [11]. The expression of Cu,Zn-SOD mRNA in each portion was analyzed using Northern blotting. The total RNA fraction was prepared from each portion according to the single-step method of Chomczynski [1]. The integrity of RNA preparations and the consistency of sample loading were verified by the loading of 5 μg total RNA stained with ethidium bromide. The probe used for hybridization was 48-mer oligonucleotide of rat Cu,Zn-SOD cDNA (base 468–512) [2]. The optical densities (O.D.) of the hybridization signal were analyzed using a computerized image-analysis system (RAS 1000, Amersham). Data were presented as the mean ± S.D. Stasitical analysis of the data was performed using the one-way ANOVA followed by the posthoc Duncan's multiple comparison test or the Mann-Whitney U test.

Results

The results of specific gravity measurements are shown in Table 1. The specific gravity in all three portions of the sham and sham + SOD groups showed no change (data not shown). In the contusion group, specific gravity was low in the core and peripheral portion compared with the distal portion. This tendency was also observed in the contusion + SOD group,

Table 1. *The Results of Specific Gravity Measurement in the Contusion and Contusion + SOD Group*

Group	Core	Peripheral	Distal
Contusion	1.036 ± 0.002	1.039 ± 0.001	1.047 ± 0.001
Contusion + SOD	1.036 ± 0.003	1.043 ± 0.002	1.048 ± 0.002

* p < 0.05, ** p < 0.01.

but the contusion group had a lower specific gravity than the contusion + SOD group in the periphery (p < 0.05). In contrast, there was no significant difference in the core between the contusion and the contusion + SOD group. Table 2 shows the Cu,Zn-SOD mRNA expression in each portion. In all three portions of the contusion group, Cu,Zn-SOD mRNA expression increased compared with the sham group. This increase was suppressed in the contusion + SOD group. In contrast, there were no significant differences in all three portions of the sham + SOD group compared with the sham group.

Discussion

SOD is normally present in cells at a sufficient level to scavenge intracellular superoxide [10]. Although extracellular SOD was reported as a protector in the extracellular space and endothelial cell surface, the activity of extracellular SOD is low [7]. This suggests that exogenous SOD may be used clinically by scavenging excess superoxide at the cell membrane. However, its rapid metabolic clearance and low affinity to cell membranes limit its clinical application [6]. Incorporation of SOD into a drug delivery system may overcome such a disadvantage. Several chemically modified preparations of SOD, including polyethylene glycol-conjugated SOD [17] and pyran SOD [14], have been investigated to overcome these problems, but

these have not been approved for clinical use because of their insufficient pharmacological potency. Igarashi et al. have synthesized lecithinized SOD, in which a lecithin derivative is covalently bound to recombinant human SOD, and have reported that it has higher cellular affinity, delayed plasma disappearance, and 10 times higher brain distribution than unmodified SOD [6]. On the other hand, we have already indicated that SOD gene expression increases following traumatic injury [4]. This increase has not been proven to lead to SOD protein synthesis [12, 16], but can be seen as an indicator of the severity of superoxide injury [16]. In the current study, we have investigated the change of SOD gene expression after lecithinized SOD administration. At the core, the increased gene expression in the contusion group was suppressed in the contusion + SOD group, but water content showed no significant difference between the two groups. In contrast, both increased gene expression and edema were suppressed by lecithinized SOD at peripheral regions.

We believe the reason why lecithinized SOD did not decrease edema at the core of injury is that some factors other than superoxide may play a role in edema formation. However, this suggests that the protective gene expression against superoxide is preserved, and superoxide injury is decreased by lecithinized SOD in the core and periphery. Indeed, Kinouchi et al. have observed the protective effects of increased endogenous SOD against ischemic brain injury in transgenic mice overexpressing SOD transgenes [8] and our results have demonstrated the effectiveness of exogenous SOD. Our results also showed the increased SOD gene expression at the contralateral hemisphere of contusion. Although the reason why is uncertain, bilateral increases in total tissue calcium and calcium flux in the cortex after contusion injury have been reported [3]. Cellular calcium influx is also associated with cortical spreading depression [15]. Furthermore, Raghupathi et al. have reported the induction of an immediate early gene at the contralateral hemisphere of contusion inju-

Table 2. *Cu,Zn-SOD mRNA Expression of the Cortex in Three Portions* (counts/mm²)

Group	Core	Peripheral	Distal
Sham	2245.1 ± 591.9	2764.4 ± 718.0	1633.6 ± 684.3
Sham + SOD	2058.7 ± 819.4	2226.8 ± 845.7	1643.8 ± 363.3
Contusion	3226.0 ± 895.3	3677.0 ± 1266.0	3688.3 ± 968.7
Contusion + SOD	1808.3 ± 714.2	2087.2 ± 575.4	1379.5 ± 690.9

* p < 0.05, ** p < 0.01.

ry [15]. Cortical spreading depression may be responsible for the increased SOD gene expression at the contralateral hemisphere. Further study in this area is needed.

References

1. Chomczynski P, Sacchi N (1987) Single-step method of RNA isolation by acid guanidium thiocyanate-phenol-chloroform extraction. Anal Biochem 162: 156–159
2. Delabar JM, Nicole A, D'Auriol L, Jacob Y (1987) Cloning and sequencing of rat CuZn superoxide dismutase cDNA. Correlation between CuZn superoxide dismutase mRNA level and enzyme activity in rat and mouse tissue. Eur J Biochem 166: 181–187
3. Fineman I, Hovda DA, Smith M, Yoshino A, Becker DA (1993) Concussive brain injury is associated with a prolonged accumulation of calcium: a ^{45}Ca autoradiographic study. Brain Res 624: 94–102
4. Fukuhara T, Nishio S, Ono Y, Kawauchi M, Asari S, Ohmoto T (1994) Induction of Cu,Zn-superoxide dismutase after cortical contusion injury during hypothermia. Brain Res 657: 333–336
5. Fukuhara T, Gotoh M, Kawauchi M, Asari S, Ohmoto T (1994) Superoxide scavenging activity in the extracellular space of the brain in forming edema. Neurosurgery 35: 924–929
6. Igarashi R, Hoshino J, Ochiai A, Morizawa Y, Mizushima Y (1994) Lecithinized superoxide dismutase enhances its pharmacological potency by increasing its cell membrane affinity. J Pharmacol Exp Ther 271: 1672–1677
7. Karlsson K, Marklund SL (1989) Binding of human extracellular- superoxide dismutase C in cultured cell line and blood cells. Lab Invest 60: 659–666
8. Kinouchi H, Epstein CJ, Mizui T, Carlson E, Chen SF, Chan PH (1991) Attenuation of focal cerebral ischemic injury in transgenic mice overexpressing Cu,Zn superoxide dismutase. Proc Natl Acad Sci USA 88: 11158–11162
9. Kontos HA, Wei EP (1986) Superoxide production in experimental brain injury. J Neurosurg 64: 803–807
10. Marklund SL (1984) Extracellular superoxide dismutase in human tissue and human cell lines. J Clin Invest 74: 1398–1403
11. Marmarou A, Poll W, Shulman K, Bhagavan H (1978) A simple gravimetric technique for measurement of cerebral edema. J Neurosurg 49: 530–537
12. Matsuyama T, Michishita H, Nakamura H, Tsuchiyama M, Shimizu S, Watanabe K, Sugita M (1993) Induction of cooper-Zinc superoxide dismutase in gerbil hippocampus after ischemia. J Cereb Blood Flow Metab 13: 135–144
13. Nilsson P, Hillered L, Olsson Y, Sheardown MJ, Hansen AJ (1993) Resional changes in interstial K$^+$ and Ca^{2+} levels following cortical compression contusion trauma in rats. J Cereb Blood Flow Metab 13: 183–192
14. Oda T, Akaike T, Hamamoto T, Suzuki F, Hirano T, Maeda H (1989) Oxygen radicals in influenza-induced pathogenesis and treatment with pyran polymer-conjugated SOD. Science 244: 974–976
15. Raghupathi R, Mcintosh TK (1996) Regionally and temporally distinct patterns of induction of c-fos, c-jun and junB mRNAs following experimental brain injury in rat. Molecular Brain Res 37: 134–144
16. Uyama O, Matsuyama T, Michishita T, Nakamura H, Sugita M (1992) Protective effects of human recombinant superoxide dismutase on transient ischemic injury of CA1 neurons in gerbils. Stroke 23: 75–81
17. Veronese FM, Boccu E, Schiavon O, Velo G (1983) Anti-inflammatory and pharmacokinetic properties of superoxide dismutase devatized with polyethylene glycol via active esters. J Pharm Pharmacol 35: 757–758

Correspondence: Masatoshi Yunoki, M.D., Department of Neurological Surgery, Okayama University Medical School, 12-5-1 Shikata-cho, Okayama 700, Japan.

Acta Neurochir (1997) [Suppl] 70: 185–187

Extracellular Changes of Taurine in the Peri-Infarct Zone: Effect of Lubeluzole

D. Scheller[1], **M. de Ryck**[2], **G. Clincke**[2], and **F. Tegtmeier**[1]

[1] Janssen-Cilag GmbH, Drug Discovery, Neuss, Federal Republic of Germany, and [2] Janssen Research Foundation, Beerse, Belgium

Summary

Lubeluzole is a neuroprotective compound that has been shown to stereoselectively rescue sensorimotor function and reduce infarct size in a photochemical stroke model in rats. Tissue swelling, which occurs in the peri-infarct zone, is accompanied by a compensatory taurine release. Therefore, using a microdialysis technique, we aimed at measuring changes of extracellular concentrations of taurine in the peri-infarct zone and the effects of lubeluzole and its R-isomer. Lubeluzole blocked the increase of taurine in tissue immediately surrounding a photochemically induced thrombotic neocortical infarct. By contrast, the R-isomer was completely inactive. We hypothesize that lubeluzole may reduce osmoregulatory stress in peri-infarct tissue.

Keywords: Taurine; microdialysis; lubeluzole; photochemical stroke; nitric oxide.

Introduction

The sulfur-containing amino acid taurine has been shown to rise subsequent to hypoosmotic stimuli in the extracellular space [3]. Taurine is suggested to play an important role during enhanced osmoregulatory activity [8]. Within a transition zone surrounding the irreversibly damaged core of an infarct ('penumbra', 'peri-infarct zone'), cell swelling has been described as one of the earliest events preceding cell damage, as detected histologically [10]. Thus, taurine might be expected to rise within that zone due to upregulated osmoregulation. Therefore, we aimed at determining extracellular changes of taurine in the peri-infarct zone of a focal, Rose Bengal-induced, thrombotic infarct in the neocortex of rats.

Posttreatment with labelazole, a novel neuroprotective compound aimed at treatment of acute stroke [2] has been shown to stereoselectively rescue sensorimotor function after photochemical neocortical infarcts in rats [1]. Lubeluzole also reduced infarct size in the photochemical as well as middle cerebral artery occlusion stroke models [1]. Therefore, using a neuroprotective dose of lubeluzole, we investigated its effect on the peri-infarct taurine response and, with corresponding controls, we compared lubeluzole to the R-isomer.

Methods

A light fibre was positioned in front of a burr hole in the parietal bone of anaesthetised male Wistar rats (230 to 270 g, Urethane 1.55 to 1.95 g/kg; body temperature kept at 37°C). A microdialysis (MD) probe (2 mm, Carnegie Medicin, Stockholm, perfusate: CSF; flow rate: 2 µl/min) was implanted into the supposed peri-infarct area at an angle of about 30° from caudal to frontal. Probe position was verified histologically afterwards. Direct current (DC) was registered by a microelectrode inserted into the cortex in the vicinity of the MD probe. After equilibration, Rose Bengal was given i.v. (70 mg/kg). Illumination lasted for 5 min. Lubeluzole or its R-isomer (1.25 mg/kg each) was infused 10 min after light offset. Controls received equal amounts of vehicle solution (10% cyclodextrine). Amino acids were determined using HPLC with fluorescence detection after automated precolumn derivatization with o-phthaldialdehyde. Statistics were performed using ANOVA for repeated measures ('split-plot model') based on SAS algorithms.

Result

As shown in Fig. 1, extracellular taurine started to rise after onset of illumination at about the occurrence of the first spreading depression (SD). In control rats (control 1, performed in parallel to the lubeluzole treatment), taurine started from a level of 2.77 ± 0.74 prior to illumination to reach a final level of 10.75 ± 3.77 µmol/l (n = 8). As illustrated in Fig. 2, treatment with lubeluzole (n = 9) prevented the rise of taurine (basal level: 3.01 ± 0.73; final levels: 6.02 ± 4.34 µmol/l; p = 0.04). In another control group (controls 2, performed in parallel to treatment with the R-isomer), taurine rose from 2.18 ± 1.08 to 9.13 ± 3.15 µmol/l

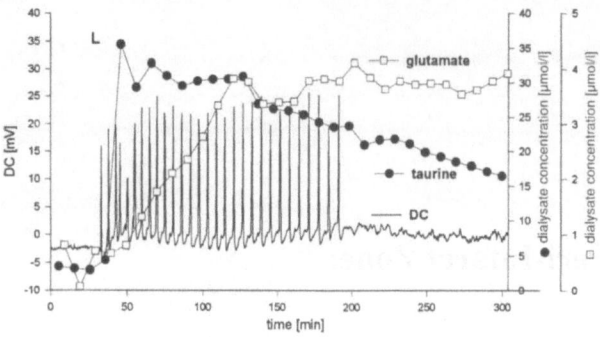

Fig. 1. Time course of dialysate taurine concentration determined within the peri-infarct zone of a photothrombotic neocrotical infarct in relation to dialysate glutamate and spreading depressions. *L* Onset of illumination

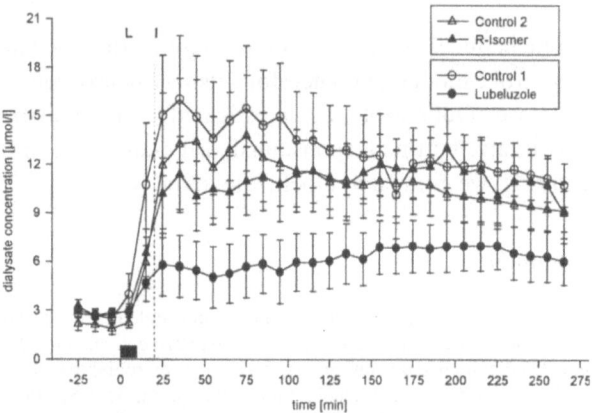

Fig. 2. Course of dialysate concentrations of taurine before and after photochemical induction of a neocortical infarct in rats. *L* Onset of illumination; *I* injection of i.v. bolus at 10 min after offset of illumination. (○, ●) Vehicle versus lubeluzole (1.25 mg/kg i.v.); (□, ■) vehicle versus R-isomer (1.25 mg/kg i.v.)

(n = 6) at 6 h after infarction. Treatment with the R-isomer had no effect on peri-infarct changes in extracellular taurine (basal level: 3.27 ± 1.07; final level: 9.01 ± 5.62 µmol/l, n = 9, p = 0.98) (Fig. 2).

Discussion

Posttreatment with lubeluzole, but not its R-isomer, blocked the extracellular rise of taurine in the peri-infarct zone of a thrombotic neocortical infarct in rats. This agrees with other stereoselective effects of lubeluzole. For instance, lubeluzole stereoselectively rescues sensorimotor function and reduces infarct size in a photochemical stroke model in rats [1]. In the same model, lubeluzole blocks peri-infarct extracellular rise of glutamate, whereas its R-isomer is virtually ineffective [1]. *In vitro*, prolonged pretreatment with lubeluzole prevented glutamate-induced neuronal death in

hippocampal neuronal cultures, whereas its R-isomer was nine times less active. Under those conditions, lubeluzole decreased glutamate-stimulated intracellular cGMP production, i.e., downregulated glutamate-induced activation of the nitric oxide synthase pathway, whereas its R-isomer was seven times less active [4]. Following co-administration with nitric oxide donors (SIN-1 or sodium nitroprusside), only lubeluzole, but not its R-isomer, blocked neuronal death in a concentrationdependent manner [5]. Therefore, lubeluzole blocks nitric oxide-induced neurotoxicity in a stereoselective manner. Downregulation of the nitric oxide synthase pathway and antagonism of nitric oxide neurotoxicity could lead to downregulation of neurotransmitter release, as nitric oxide may be involved in NMDA-receptor mediated glutamate release [6]. Whether such a mechanism is responsible for lubeluzole's stereoselective blockade of taurine release remains to be further investigated. Alternatively, blockade of the peri-infarct taurine response by lubeluzole could be due to reduction of (possibly glutamate-mediated) osmoregulatory stress in the peri-infarct tissue. However, the mechanism of such a protective principie is not yet understood. In addition to antagonizing NO-induced neurotoxicity, lubeluzole blocks sodium currents in isolated hippocampal neurons [7]. However, contrary to its stereoselective effects on NO-induced neurotoxicity and on the peri-infarct taurine and glutamate responses [9], lobeluzole's blockade of the sodium current is not stereoselective: both lubeluzole and its R-isomer block sodium currents equipotently [7]. Because cellular swelling may constitute an important stage in the cascade leading to cell death, prevention of the excessive energy expenditure required for volume regulation in the peri-infarct tissue, may also contribute to improved neurological outcome as evidenced by lubeluzole.

References

1. De Ryck M, Keersmaekers R, Duytschaever H, Claes C, Clincke G, Janssen M, Van Reet G (1996) Lubeluzole protects sensorimotor function and reduces infarct size in a photochemical stroke model in rats. J Pharmacol Exp Therap 279 (2)
2. Diener HC, Hacke W, Hennerici M, Radberg J, Hantson L, De Keyser J (1996) Lubeluzole in acute ischemic stroke – a double blind, placebo controlled phase II trial. Stroke 27: 76–81
3. Lehmann A, Carlström C, Nagelhus EA, Ottersen OP (1991) Elevation of taurine in hippocampal extracellular fluid and cerebrospinal fluid of acutely hypotonic rats: contribution by influx from blood? J Neurochem 56: 690–697
4. Lesage A, De Loore KL, Osikovska-Evers B, Peeters L, Leysen JE (1994) Lubeluzole, a novel neuroprotectant, inhibits

the glutamate-activated NOS pathway. Soc Neurosci Abstr 20: 185

5. Maiese K, TenBroeke M, Kue I (1996) Neuroprotection of lubeluzole is mediated through the signal transduction pathways of nitric oxide. J Neurochem

6. Montague PR, Ganceyco CD, Winn MJ, Marchase RB, Friedlander, MJ (1994) Role of NO production in NMDA receptor-mediated neurotransmitter release in cerebral cortex. Science 263: 973–977

7. Osikowska-Evers B, Wilhelm D, Nebel U, Hennemann P, Scheufler E, Tegtmeier F (1995) The effects of the novel neuroprotective compound lubeluzole on sodium current and veratridine induced sodium load in rat brain neurons and synaptosomes. J Cereb Blood Flow Metab 15 [Suppl 1]: S380

8. Pasantes-Morales H, Schousboe A (1988) Volume regulation in astrocytes: a role for taurine as an osmoeffector. J Neurosci Res 20: 505–509

9. Scheller D, Kolb J, Szathmary S, Zacharias E, de Ryck M, van Reempts J, Clincke G, Tegtmeier F (1995) Extracellular changes of glutamate in the peri-infarct zone. Effect of lubeluzole. J Cereb Blood Flow Metab 15 [Suppl 1]: S379

10. Van Reempts J, Borgers M (1994) Histopathological characterization of photochemical damage in nervous tissue. Histol Histopath 9: 185–195

Correspondence: Dr. D. Scheller, Janssen-Cilag GmbH, Drug Discovery, Raiffeisenstrasse 8, D-41470 Neuss, Federal Republic of Germany.

Acta Neurochir (1997) [Suppl] 70: 188–190
© Springer-Verlag 1997

Effect of Tromethamine (THAM) on Infarct Volume Following Permanent Middle Cerebral Artery Occlusion in Rats

K. L. Kiening, G. H. Schneider, A. W. Unterberg, and **W. R. Lanksch**

Department of Neurosurgery, Virchow Medical Center, Humboldt University of Berlin, Berlin, Federal Republic of Germany

Summary

This study investigates the influence on tromethamine (THAM) on ischemic volume induced by permanent middle cerebral artery occlusion (MCAO) in rats.

14 male Sprague Dawley rats underwent left sided permanent MCAO by electro coagulation. Animals were treated either by 3-M THAM given intravenously in a single dosage of 0.6 mmol/kg body weight (THAM group: n = 7) 10 min following MCAO and again 1, 2, 3, 4 and 5 hours later or by NaCl 0.9% (placebo group: n = 7) in the same mode. Mean arterial blood pressure (MABP) was monitored for 30 min post MCAO and arterial blood gases were taken 10 min after the first injection. The extent of ischemia volume was assessed by planimetry of coronal sections stained with triphenyl-tetrazolium chloride (TTC) and with hematoxilin/eosin (HE). Tests for significance were accomplished by ANOVA on ranks. A difference of $p < 0.05$ was considered significant.

The THAM group showed an insignificant decrease in MABP 1 min after injection (THAM: 75 ± 11 mmHg, placebo: 86 ± 10 mmHg). Arterial pH was significantly different (THAM: 7.46 ± 0.04; placebo: 7.32 ± 0.03). In TTC staining, the ischemia volume – given in absolute values and percentage of the total left volume – was significantly reduced in the THAM group (THAM: 43.9 ± 8.3mm³ / 7.0 ± 1.3%; placebo: 95.2 ± 13.8 mm³ / 14.2 ± 2.0%). In HE staining, the reduction of ischemia, volume did not reach statistical significance (THAM: 49.1 ± 9.9 mm³ / 9.6 ± 1.8%; placebo: 66.3 ± 14.5 mm³ / 13.1 ± 2.8%).

Based on these results, a moderate neuroprotective effect of THAM in experimental cerebral infarction could be demonstrated.

Keywords: Focal ischemia; THAM; neuroprotection.

Introduction

Intracellular cerebral acidosis as a result of anaerobic metabolism is supposed to be a major driving force for the development of cytotoxic edema after focal ischemia. This is due to an increase in intracellular osmotic load due to lactate accumulation and an increased exchange of intracellular H^+ and HCO_3^- against extracellular Na^+ and Cl^-. Both mechanisms lead to an increase in intracellular water content and cell swelling [8]. Consequently, the ischemic penumbra can progress to infarction which worsens neurological outcome. Tromethamine (THAM), a buffer for intracellular acidosis, may prevent cytotoxic edema and preserve the penumbra.

In the past, application of THAM in experimental head trauma and in patients presenting with severe head injury revealed positive effects, namely reduction of raised intracranial pressure, control of cerebral edema, and EEG improvement [2, 6, 7]. Its efficacy on reduction of infarct volume in the setting of experimental cerebral ischemia, however, has been pursued in cats only [5]. The purpose of this study was to investigate the influence of THAM on ischemia volume induced by permanent middle cerebral artery occlusion (MCAO) in rats.

Material and Methods

During anesthesia (ketamine 50 mg/kg and xylazine 10 mg/kg IM), permanent occlusion of the left middle cerebral artery (MCA) by electro coagulation from the origin of the lateral striate arteries to the inferior cerebral vein was performed using the Tamura [10] technique in male Sprague-Dawley rats (n = 14, weighing 450 g in average). Animals were allowed to breathe spontaneously. Cannulation of the tail artery [monitoring of mean arterial blood pressure (MABP); blood gas sampling] and of the external jugular vein (i.v.-injections) was performed.

Body temperature was maintained at 37°C. Seven animals were injected intravenously with a 3-M solution of THAM in a single dosage of 0.6 mmol/kg b.w. 10 min following MCAO and again 1, 2, 3, 4 and 5 hrs later. Respective controls (n = 7) received NaCl 0,9% as placebo. Mean arterial blood pressure was monitored after MCAO up to 30 min after the first injection. Arterial blood gas analyses were taken 10 min after the first injection.

Animals were sacrificed 24 hrs after MCAO. The brains were removed and cut in seven coronal 2 mm thick slices which were immediately immersed in a 2% solution of 2,3,5-triphenyltetrazolium chloride (TTC) [1, 4]. TTC slices were photographed from both sides and the stained and non-stained areas of the opposing surfaces of two consecutive TTC slices were planimetrically quantified and averaged.

Afterwards, a representative 20 μm slice was cut out from each 2 mm-slice, stained with hematoxilin/eosin (HE). Planimetric measurements were performed separately for stained and non-stained areas.

Infarct volumes from both stain techniques were calculated and depicted in absolute values (mm³) as well as in percentage of total left hemispheral volume (%). Results are given as mean ± standard error of mean (SEM). Statistical significance was accomplished using ANOVA on ranks. A difference of $p < 0.05$ was considered to be significant. Values are given as mean ± standard error of mean (SEM).

Results

Application of THAM caused an immediate mild decrease of MABP (n.s.) for 1 min compared to placebo (THAM: 75 ± 11 mmHg; placebo: 86 ± 10 mmHg). In arterial blood gas analyses, a significant difference in pH only (THAM: 7.46 ± 0.04; placebo: 7.32 ± 0.03; $p < 0.01$) was seen.

In TTC staining, there was a significant reduction ($p < 0.05$) of about 50% in THAM treated animals in both absolute (Fig. 1) and percentage infarct volume (THAM: 43.9 ± 8.3 mm³ / $7.0 \pm 1.3\%$) (placebo: 95.2 ± 13.8 mm³ / $14.2 \pm 2.0\%$). In HE staining, an infarct volume reduction by THAM administration was also seen but did not reach significance (THAM: $49,1 \pm 9.9$ mm³ / $9.6 \pm 1.8\%$) (placebo: 66.3 ± 14.5 mm³ / $13.1 \pm 2.8\%$) (Fig. 2).

Discussion

In cerebral ischemia, there is an increased intracellular H^+ concentration resulting in intracellular acidosis. Staub [8] reported that acidification below pH of 6.8 caused immediate swelling of glial cells and cell viability decreased in relation to the severity of acidosis. Hillered [3] reported inhibited mitochondrial respiration which was correlated with a decrease in pH. Hence, amelioration of intracellular acidosis may reduce ischemic brain damage, especially in the penumbra where cells are at high risk for death. Treatment of intracellular acidosis can be performed by application of THAM of which at least 30% of a single dosage accumulates intracellulary [7]. In this study, both staining techniques – TTC and HE – showed a reduction of infarct volume in the THAM group although not significantly with HE. These results are in accordance with Kitaoka [5] who also described a reduction on infarct volume of 50% in MCAO in cats. In the study of Kitaoka [5], only TTC staining was performed.

The difference in ischemic volume in both staining techniques raises questions. While some authors could not find substantial differences in ischemia volume either with TTC or HE staining, others report that infarction volume is smaller in HE staining compared to TTC [1, 4]. However, differences tend to vanish when brains are removed at a later time point, e.g. 24 hrs after occlusion [1]. Our finding of a markedly lower ischemic volume in HE staining was therefore unexpected. A further reason for the difference in infarct size of TTC vs. HE might be due to the presence of edema. Edema was shown to increase ischemia volume substantially [3]. This source of error, however, could be attenuated by comparing ischemia, and non-ischemia volumes by expressing the data as "percentage of total left hemispheral volume" [9]. This was done in our study leading to the same results as found with absolute measurements. In TTC staining,

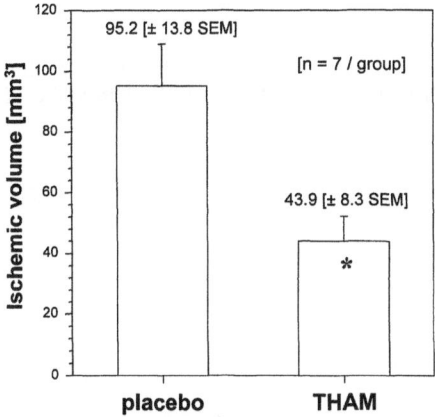

Fig. 1. Absolute ischemia volume of left cerebral hemispheres after MCAO in rats. In TTC staining, THAM applications induces a significant reduction of 53.9% in infarction

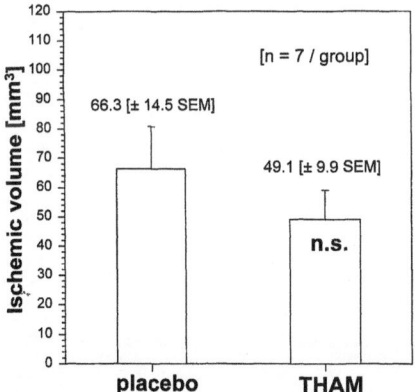

Fig. 2. Absolute ischemia volume of left cerebral hemispheres after MCAO in rats. In HE staining, the THAM group showed reduction of infarction by 25.9% (not significant)

ischemia volume reduction was 53.9% [absolute values (mm³)] and 50.7% [percentage of total left hemisphere volume (%)], whereas in HE staining, reduction was 25.9% [absolute values (mm³)] and 26.7% [percentage of total left hemisphere volume (%)].

From our results and Kitaokas [5] findings, application of THAM may reduce infarction size in permanent MCAO, presumably by reduction of intracellular acidosis. Further studies, e.g. with a higher dosage of THAM and a larger number of animals, are needed to substantiate these results. Results of therapeutic studies in MCAO relying on a single staining technique only should be interpreted cautiously.

References

1. Bederson JB, Pitts LH, Germano, SM, *et al* (1986) Evaluation of 2,3,5-triphenyltetrazolium chloride as a stain for detection and quantification of experimental cerebral infarction in rats. Stroke 17: 1304–1308
2. Gaab MR, Seegers K, Smedema RJ, *et al* (1990) A comparative analysis of THAM (Tris-buffer) in traumatic brain oedema. Acta Neurochir (Wien) [Suppl] 51: 320–323
3. Hillered L, Ernster L, Siesjö BK (1984) Influence of *in vitro* lactic acidosis and hypercapnia on respiratory activity of isolated rat brain mitochondria. J Cereb Blood Flow Metab 4: 430–437
4. Isayama, K, Pitts LH, Nishimura MC (1991) Evaluation of 2,3,5-triphenyltetrazolium chloride staining to delineate rat brain infarcts. Stroke 22: 1394–1398
5. Kitaoka T, Nagao S, Kuyama H, *et al* (1994) The effect of THAM on experimental focal cerebral ischemia and clinical outcome in severe head injury. In: Nagai H, Kamiya K, Ishii S (eds) Intracranial pressure IX. Springer, Berlin Heidelberg New York Tokyo
6. Muizelaar JP, Marmarou A, Ward JD, *et al* (1991) Adverse effect of prolonged hyperventilation in patients with severe head injury: a randomized clinical trial. J Neurosurg 75: 731–739
7. Rosner MJ, Becker DP (1984) Experimental brain injury: successful therapy with the weak base, thromethamine. J Neurosurg 60: 961–971
8. Staub F, Baethmann A, Peters J, *et al* (1990) Effects of lactacidosis an volume and viability of glial cells. Acta Neurochir (Wien) [Suppl] 51: 3–6
9. Swanson RA, Sharp FR (1994) Infarct measurement methodology (letter to editor). J Cereb Blood Flow Metab 14: 697
10. Tamura A, Graham D, McCulloch J (1981) Focal cerebral ischemia in the rat: description of technique and early neuropathological consequences following middle cerebral artery occlusion. J Cereb Blood Flow Metab 1: 53–60

Correspondence: Karl L. Kiening, M.D., Department of Neurosurgery, Virchow Medical Center, Humboldt University of Berlin, Augustenburger Platz 1, D-13353 Berlin, Federal Republic of Germany.

Acta Neurochir (1997) [Suppl] 70: 191–193
© Springer-Verlag 1997

Antioxidant, OPC-14117, Attenuates Edema Formation and Behavioral Deficits Following Cortical Contusion in Rats

T. Kawamata[1], **Y. Katayama**[1], **T. Maeda**[1], **T. Mori**[1], **N. Aoyama**[1], **T. Kikuchi**[2], and **Y. Uwahodo**[2]

[1] Department of Neurological Surgery, Nihon University School of Medicine, Tokyo, and
[2] Third Tokushima Institute of New Drug Research, Otsuka Pharmaceutical Co. Ltd., Tokushima, Japan

Summary

Oxygen free radicals may contribute to tissue injury processes in the central nervous system following ischemia or trauma. Recent studies have suggested that inhibition of free radicals improves the outcome in experimental models involving such conditions, and antioxidant therapy appears promising. In the present study, behavioral changes and edema formation in a rat cortical contusion model were investigated, and the effects of a superoxide radical scavenger, OPC-14117, were tested. Wistar rats were anesthetized with halothane inhalation. Cortical contusion was induced in the parietal cortex employing a controlled cortical impact device. Immediately following injury induction, OPC-14117 was administered (300 mg/kg, p.o.). Edema formation was assessed in the center and peripheral areas of the contusion by the specific gravity method. Behavioral changes were evaluated by the Morris water maze test and the habituation of exploratory activity. The results revealed that the vehicle-administered control showed progressive edema formation and behavioral deficits following the injury. These changes were significantly attenuated by the OPC-14117 treatment ($p < 0.05$). Further, OPC-14117 reduced the size of contusional necrosis ($p < 0.05$). These findings suggest that superoxide free radicals are involved in contusion-induced edema formation, necrosis formation, and behavioral deficits, and that OPC-14117 has a therapeutic potential to prevent secondary cell damage following traumatic brain injury.

Keywords: Cerebral contusion; brain edema; free radical scavenger.

Introduction

Severe head injury is often complicated by complex secondary or delayed pathophysiological events leading to catastrophic damage to the central nervous system. One of these events is massive edema formation in the tissue surrounding the cerebral contusion. It is important to elucidate the pathophysiology underlying such contusion induced edema formation, since a principle goal of treatments for traumatic brain injury is to prevent the occurrence of secondary damage following injury.

Oxygen free radicals may contribute to various kinds of tissue injury in the central nervous system following ischemia or trauma. Recent studies have suggested that inhibition of free radicals improves secondary neural tissue damage in experimental models involving such conditions, and antioxidant therapy appears promising [7, 8].

In an attempt to clarify whether or not oxygen free radicals contribute to secondary cellular damage following cerebral contusion, we investigated edema formation and behavioral changes in a rat cortical contusion model. The effects of the superoxide radical scavenger, OPC-14117, were also tested [2, 5].

Materials and Methods

Surgical Procedure and Injury Induction

Male Wistar rats (200–250 g) were anesthetized with a gas mixture of 66% nitrous oxide, 33% oxygen and 1% halothane. The head of each animal was secured in a stereotaxic apparatus and an 8-mm diameter craniectomy (centered 3 mm caudal to the bregma, 3 mm lateral to the midline) was performed on the left side of the parietal cranium. The dura was left intact. Cortical contusion was induced by a controlled cortical impact device, as described in detail elsewhere [1]. A 5-mm diameter injury tip, 6-m/sec impact velocity and 3-mm penetration depth were employed for the injury induction. These parameters were chosen to provide a moderate level of cortical contusion.

Drug Administration

Immediately following the injury, the superoxide radical scavenger, OPC-14117, was administered trans-orally (300 mg/kg). This dose was chosen on the basis of previous experiments in which it had been found to be the most effective [2, 5]. Vehicle-administered animals and sham-operated animals were employed as non-treated controls and normal controls respectively.

Behavioral Assessments

Cognitive deficits were evaluated by the Morris water maze test (days 6–12 post-injury) and the habituation of exploratory activity (days 22 and 23 post-injury) [4, 6].

Evaluation of Brain Edema

Edema formation was assessed by tissue specific gravity at 1, 3, 6, and 24 hours after the injury induction (n = 5, respectively). The specific gravity of the brain tissue was determined by the method of Marmarou *et al.* [3]. Small amounts of cortical tissue were sampled from the center of the contusion and from peripheral areas 3 mm distant from the center. The samles were dropped into a linear gradient column of bromobenzene and kerosene. Tissue specific gravity was calculated from the standard curve calibrated using anhydrous K_2SO_4 solutions of known specific gravity.

Histological Evaluations

After completion of the behavior testing, the animals were transcardially perfused with saline solution followed by modified Karnovsky's paraformaldehyde-glutaraldehyde fixative under deep anesthesia. The brain was then removed and placed in Karnovsky's fixative for at least 48 hours. Coronal sections were cut at a thickness of 10 μm and stained with hematoxylin and eosin (HE). The histology was evaluated under a light microscope, and the size of the contusion was determined at the center of the contusion using a computerized image analyzing system.

Results

The non-treated/injured rats exhibited significant deficits in their Morris water maze performance and in their habituation of exploratory activity, as compared to those of the sham-operated rats, indicating that the cortical contusion caused cognitive dysfunction (Fig. 1). Administration of OPC-14117 displayed no statistically significant effect but there was a tendency for the water maze performance to be improved. The impairment of the habituation of exploratory activity

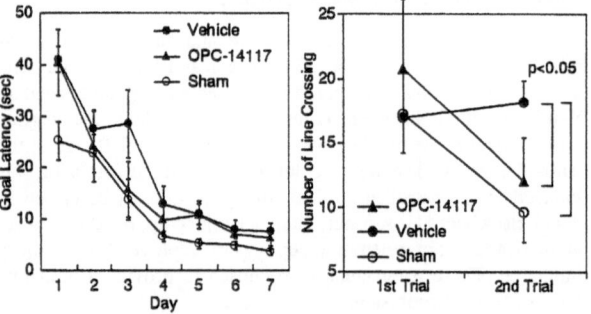

Fig. 1. Cortical contusion-induced deficits in Morris water maze performance (left) and in the habituation of exploratory activity (right), as compared to those of sham-operated animals. OPC-14117 treatment showed no statistically significant effect but there was a tendency for the water maze performance to be improved. The impairment of the habituation of exploratory activity was significantly attenuated by the OPC-14117 treatment (p < 0.05) (mean ± S.E.)

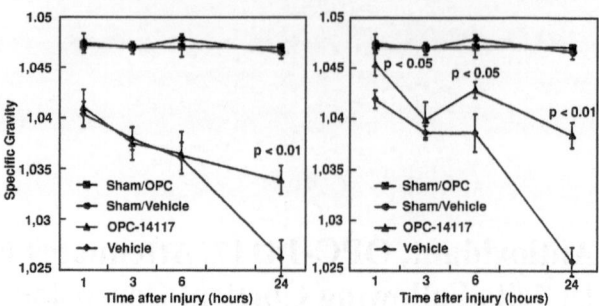

Fig. 2. Changes in specific gravity following contusion demonstrating that cerebral contusion induces progressive edema formation both in the center (left) and in the peripheral areas (right) of the contusion. Such edema formation was significantly attenuated by OPC-14117 administration. The effects of OPC-14117 were more evident in the peripheral areas than in the center of the contusion, suggesting that superoxide radicals may contribute to edema formation especially in the peripheral areas of the contusion (mean ± S.E.)

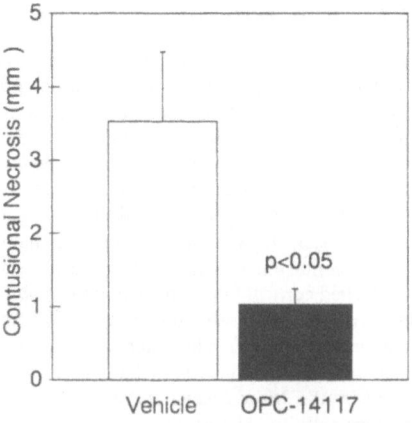

Fig. 3. The size of contusion-induced necrotic cavity was significantly reduced by OPC-14117 administration (p < 0.05) (mean ± S.E.)

was significantly attenuated by the OPC-14117 treatment (p < 0.05).

The changes in specific gravity suggested that cerebral contusion induced progressive edema formation both in the center and in the peripheral areas of the contusion. Such edema formation was significantly attenuated by OPC-14117 administration, especially in the peripheral areas (Fig. 2).

The histological evaluations revealed contusional necrosis measuring 3.53 ± 1.89 mm^2 in the non-treated/injured animals and 1.02 ± 0.46 mm^2 in the treated/injured animals, indicating that OPC-14117 significantly reduced the contusion size (p < 0.05) (Fig. 3).

Discussion

The results of the present study demonstrate that experimental cortical contusion can produce significant impairments of cognitive functions and progressive formation of brain edema. Further, OPC-14117 administration immediately after injury induction can reduce each of these injury-related deficits, as well as the size of contusional necrosis.

Previous studies have shown that the superoxide radical scavenger, OPC-14117, can reduce hydrogen peroxide (H_2O_2) generation and lipid peroxidation, improve survival under hypoxic conditions, and enhance recovery after cerebral concussion [2, 5]. The present findings indicate that OPC-14117 is also beneficial for the treatment of experimental contusion injury, and that superoxide radicals are involved in the process of secondary cell damage associated with cerebral contusion.

It has been reported that free radicals, such as superoxide, are produced in large amounts following brain injury [7, 8]. Oxygen free radicals are highly toxic products of molecular oxygen of H_2O_2, which can induce cellular injury by oxidizing lipids, proteins or nucleic acids. Lipid membranes, particularly of the microvasculature, are vulnerable to the action of free radicals because of their high content of phospholipid-containing polyunsaturated fatty acids. This type of free radical-mediated process may contribute to breakdown of the BBB and subsequent edema formation in some pathological conditions [7]. The generation of free radicals in such membranes gives rise to extensive cellular damage by inducing lipid peroxidation in chain reactions, through which the lipids produce additional free radicals. OPC-14117 may act to terminate these chain reactions by scavenging free radicals before they can cause too much damage. Inhibition of such oxygen radical-mediated destructive events at the earliest possible moment in the injury process could

provide greater sparing of neuronal cells, thus resulting in more complete behavioral recovery.

In conclusion, the results of the present study indicate that oxygen free radicals are involved in contusion-induced edema formation, necrosis formation, and cognitive deficits, and the superoxide radical scavenger, OPC-14117, has a powerful therapeutic potential to prevent secondary cell damage following traumatic brain injury.

References

1. Dixon CE, Clifton GL, Lighthall JW, *et al* (1991) A controlled cortical impact model of traumatic brain injury in the rat. J Neurosci Meth 39: 1–10
2. Fisher M, Arpano MM (1992) Inhibition of stimulated human leukocyte hydrogen peroxide generation by a novel antioxidant, OPC-14117. J Neurolog Sci 109: 107–110
3. Marmarou A, Poll W, Shulman K, *et al* (1978) A simple gravimetric technique for measurement of cerebral edema. J Neurosurg 49: 530–537
4. Morris RGM (1984) Development of a watermaze procedure for studying spatial learning in the rat. J Neurosci Meth 11: 47–60
5. Oshiro Y, Sakurai Y, Tanaka T, *et al* (1991) Novel cerebroprotective agents with central nervous system stimulating activity. J Med Chem 34: 2004–2013, 2014–2023
6. Platel A, Porsolt RD (1982) Habituation of exploratory activity in mice: a screening test for memory enhancing drugs. Psychopharmacology 78: 346–352
7. Roof RL, Duvdevani R, Braswell L, *et al* (1994) Progesteron facilitates cognitive recovery and reduces secondary neuronal loss caused by cortical contusion injury in male rats. Exp Neurol 129: 64–69
8. Smith DH, Okiyama K, Thomas MJ, *et al* (1991) Evaluation of memory dysfunction following experimental brain injury using the Morris water maze. J Neurotrauma 8: 259–269

Correspondence: Tatsuro Kawamata, M.D., Ph.D., Department of Neurological Surgery, Nihon University School of Medicine, 30-1 Oyaguchi-Kamimachi Itabashi-ku, Tokyo 173, Japan.

Acta Neurochir (1997) [Suppl] 70: 194–197
© Springer-Verlag 1997

OPC-21268, an Orally Effective, Nonpeptide Arginine Vasopressin V₁ Receptor Antagonist Reduces Vasogenic Brain Edema

I. Bemana, E. Takahashi, T. Nakamura, H. Kuyama, and **S. Nagao**

Department of Neurological Surgery, Kagawa Medical University, Kagawa, Japan

Summary

We examined the effect of orally administered OPC-21268, a nonpeptide Arginine Vasopressin V_1 receptor antagonist, on cold induced vasogenic brain edema in rat. Cold brain injury was induced by applying a copper rode cooled with liquid nitrogen for one minute. To mimic clinical use, one hour after induction of the cold lesion, rats were treated with orally administered OPC-21268 at doses of 100 mg, 200 mg, and 300 mg/kg every 8 hr for 24 hours. Two percent Evans blue in saline, in a volume of 1 ml/kg was given intravenously prior to cold injury. Twenty four hours after induction the cold lesion, brain water, brain tissue electrolytes, and plasma osmolality and electrolytes were measured. Quantitative evaluation of BBB permeability was performed using the Evans blue fluorescence method. The injury resulted in significant increases in the brain water and brain tissue sodium, and Evans blue concentration in both the lesioned and contralateral hemispheres ($p < 0.01$). OPC-21268 at doses of 200 mg and 300 mg/kg significantly decreased brain water and Evans blue concentrations in both the lesioned and contralateral hemispheres ($p < 0.01$). Brain tissue sodium content was significantly reduced at a dose of 300 mg/kg in the lesioned side ($p < 0.05$). There were no significant changes in other parameters throughout the experiments. Our results indicate that OPC-21268 exerts a protective effect in areas where the maximal amount of BBB breakdown occurs.

Keywords: Vasogenic brain edema; OPC-21268; rat; blood-brain barrier.

Introduction

Accumulating evidence derived from animal experiments suggests that centrally released Arginine vasopressin (AVP) plays an important role in the permeability of brain capillaries to water [2, 9], in the regulation of cerebrospinal fluid production [4], the intracranial pressure [7], and in the pathogenesis of brain edema [3, 10], and that these effects are mediated via the AVP V_1 receptor [5, 12]. The existence of V_1 receptor in the brain has been reported [8]. An AVP V_1 receptor antagonist has also been reported to reduce brain edema in cats and rats [11, 13]. Recent work from our laboratory has shown that the intraventricular administration of AVP V_1 receptor antagonist reduced cold induced vasogenic brain edema in rat [6]. Vasopressin antagonists developed for therapeutic use so far are all peptide analogs and, therefore, do not have high enough bioavailability when given orally [15]. In this study we report the effect of OPC-21268, a nonpeptide AVP V_1 receptor antagonist on cold induced vasogenic brain edema in the rat. Furthermore, we assessed the vascular protein leakage by the quantitative evaluation of BBB permeability using the Evans blue fluorescence method.

Materials and Methods

One hundred seventy three adult male Sprague-Dawley rats weighing 300–400 g each were anesthetized with an intraperitoneal injection of pentobarbital sodium (25 mg/kg), supplemented by diethyl ether anesthesia. The scalp was incised along the sagittal midline, and the left parietal bone was exposed. Cold lesion was induced by application of a copper rode (5 mm in diameter) cooled with liquid nitrogen to the exposed parietal bone for one minute. After the induction of the lesion, the skin incision was closed with sutures, the anesthetic was discontinued, the animals were allowed to recover, returned to their cages and given free access to food and water.

The animals were divided into three groups. Group A (n = 16) sham operated rats. Group B (n = 17) saline treated rats with cold lesion. Group C (n = 55) OPC-21268 treated rats with cold lesion. In group C, rats were treated with orally administered OPC-21268, a nonpeptide AVP V_1 receptor antagonist (Otsuka Pharmaceutical Co., Japan) at doses of 100 mg/kg (n = 20), 200 mg/kg (n = 20), and 300 mg/kg (n = 15) every, 8 hr for 24 hours (starting one hr after the induction of cold lesion). Blood pressure of the animals was intermittently measured by the tail-cuff method (Programmable Sphygmomanometer, Riken Kaihatsu, Japan), before and 1, 3, 6, 12, and 24 hours after cold injury and p.o. administration of OPC-21268. After 24 hours blood was taken from the femoral artery for the determination of plasma osmolality and electrolytes. The rats were then sacrificed by decapitation and their brains removed and divided into the injured and contralateral hemispheres. Specimens were immediately weighed to obtain the wet weight (WW).The tissues were then dried in an oven at 110°C for 24 hours and weighed again to obtain the dry weight (DW). The formula (WW − DW) / WW × 100 was used to calculate the water content expressed as the percentage of wet weight. The dehydrated samples were digested in 10 ml of 2N nitric acid for 48 hours to release the ions into the solution. Sodium and potassium contents were measured using atomic absorption spectrophotometry. Ion content was expressed in mmol/kg dry weight.

Quantitative Evaluation of Blood-Brain Barrier Permeability

Two percent Evans blue in physiological saline (1 ml/kg) was given intravenously as a BBB permeability tracer prior to cold injury, to sham operated rats (n = 15), to cold injury with saline treated rats (n = 15), and to cold injury with OPC-21268 treated rats 100 mg/kg (n = 15), 200 mg/kg (n = 20), 300 mg/kg (n = 20). After 24 hours cardiac perfusion was performed with 200 ml of physiological saline to clear the cerebral circulation of Evans blue. The brains were then rapidly removed and examined for evidence of Evans blue.They were then divided into the injured and contralateral hemispheres and weighed. The extraction of Evans blue dye was performed according to Uyama *et al.* [14]. Evans blue concentration was expressed as μgm/gm of wet weight calculated against a standard curve.

All values reported are mean ± standard error. Statistical analysis was carried out by analysis of variance (ANOVA) using the Bonferroni-Dunn t test for multiple comparisons. Statistical significance was accepted for $p < 0.05$.

Results

Twenty four hours after the cold injury there were significant increases in brain water content to 80.50 ± 0.05% and 79.46 ± 0.05% in the lesioned and contralateral hemispheres respectively compared to 78.50 ± 0.4% in the sham operated group ($p < 0.01$) (Table 1). Brain tissue Na^+ content was also significantly increased to 326.05 ± 5.36 and 276.27 ± 7.79 mmol/kg dry weight in the lesioned and contralateral hemispheres compared to 228.45 ± 22.65 mmol/kg dry weight in the normal group ($p < 0.01$).The brain tissue K^+ decreased but did not reach the level of significance. Quantitative Evans blue determination revealed a significant rise of extravasated Evans blue to 14.25 ± 0.87 and 4.41 ± 0.57 μg/gm wet weight in the lesioned and non-lesioned hemispheres compared to 0.44 ± 0.04 μg/gm wet weight in the sham operated animals ($p < 0.01$). P.o. administration of OPC-21268 at the doses of 200 mg and 300 mg/kg every 8 hr for 24 hours significantly reduced brain water and Evans blue extravasation both in the lesioned and contralateral hemispheres $p < 0.01$ (Table 1). At the dose of 100 mg/kg there was a trend to decrease the brain water content in the lesioned side, but it was not statistically significant.

Table 1. *Changes in the Brain Water, Brain Tissue Sodium and Potassium and Evans Blue Concentrations Following Cold Injury and p.o. Administration of OPC-21268.* Values are mean ± standard error of the mean

	Brain water (%)		Na+ (mmol/kg dry weight)		K+ (mmol/kg dry weight)	
	LS	NLS	LS	NLS	LS	NLS
Normal (n = 15)	78.50 ± 0.4		228.45 ± 22.65		506.80 ± 16.94	
C.L. group (n = 15)	80.50 ± 0.05[a]	79.46 ± 0.05[a]	326.05 ± 5.36[a]	276.27 ± 7.79[a]	481.83 ± 5.07	487.72 ± 6.30
OPC-21268 treated						
100 mg/kg (n =20)	80.29 ± 0.05	79.23 ± 0.05	335.86 ± 9.68	277.00 ± 6.2	491.50 ± 8.19	485.21 ± 10.1
200 mg/kg (n = 20)	79.61 ± 0.05[b]	78.79 ± 0.07[b]	311.27 ± 6.26	278.24 ± 6.8	492.18 ± 7.05	495.33 ± 5.58
300 mg/kg (n = 15)	79.55 ± 0.1[b]	78.86 ± 0.1[b]	292.14 ± 10.68[c]	263.39 ± 8.79	493.28 ± 7.66	491.37 ± 7.25

		LS	NLS
Evans blue (μgm/gm wet weight)			
Normal group (n = 15)		0.44 ± 0.04	
C.L. group (n = 15)		14.25 ± 0.87[a]	4.41 ± 0.57[a]
OPC-21268 treated	100 mg/kg (n = 15)	10.39 ± 0.63[b]	2.26 ± 0.19
	200 mg/kg (n = 20)	6.62 ± 0.44[b]	1.83 ± 0.15[b]
	3300 mg/kg (n = 20)	5.21 ± 0.38[b]	1.35 ± 0.17[b]

p.o. Per oral; *CL* cold lesion; *LS* lesion side; *NLS* non-lesion side.
[a] P < 0.01 compared to normal group.
[b] P < 0.01 compared to cold lesion (non-treated) group.
[c] P < 0.05 compared to lesion side in cold lesion group.

However, the same dose significantly reduced the Evans blue extravasation in the lesioned hemispheres. Brain tissue Na$^+$ content was also significantly decreased at a dose of 300 mg/kg of OPC-21268 ($p < 0.05$) (Table 1). There were no significant changes in the systemic arterial blood pressure, and plasma electrolytes and osmolality throughout the experiments among the three groups.

Discussion

Our study has demonstrated that increases in brain water content induced by a cold lesion were significantly inhibited after P.O. administration of OPC-21268, a nonpeptide AVP V$_1$ receptor antagonist. This suggests that AVP increases the water permeability of the brain mainly via the V$_1$ receptor. Our results are consistent with other reports [6, 11, 13], that intraventricular administration of AVP V$_1$ receptor antagonist reduces vasogenic brain edema.

OPC-21268 (1-{1-[4-(3-acetyl-aminopropexy)benzoyl]-4-piperidyl}-3,4-dihydro-2(1H)-quinolinone) is a nonpeptide AVP V$_1$ receptor antagonist. The drug is well absorbed after oral and intraperitoneal administration. It selectively antagonises binding to the V$_1$ subtype of AVP receptors in a competitive manner [15]. Changes in brain tissue sodium content are also significantly suppressed following p.o. administration of OPC-21268. In focal ischemia model using Brattleboro rats, Dickinson and Betz [1] suggested that AVP does not selectively alter sodium transport, but induces generalised increases in the permeability of solutes and water at the blood-brain barrier by opening transcellular pathways to solute influx. OPC-21268 may have reduced the permeability of sodium in the present study.

Cold injury for one min also resulted in significant leakage of serum proteins into the brain parenchyma as evidenced by increased Evans blue concentration. This protein leakage was significantly decreased following OPC-21268 treatment. The extravasation of serum proteins is one of the major causes of vasogenic brain edema. However, to date it has not been determined whether centrally released AVP facilitates the extravasation of serum proteins in pathological conditions. AVP has been reported to alter the blood-brain barrier permeability to amino acids, however [1].

In our experiment, reduction of blood-brain barrier permeability to Evans blue following oral administration of OPC-21268, indicate that AVP might also facilitate the extravasation of serum proteins under pathological conditions.

Because brain water, tissue sodium contents, and Evans blue concentration were all lower in the lesioned hemispheres of the OPC-21268 treated animals, vasogenic brain edema may have been attenuated by a protective effect of V$_1$ receptor antagonist on brain capillaries which resulted in the maintenance of the endothelial blood-brain barrier. The reduction of brain edema in the contralateral hemispheres was thought to be caused by a decrease in spillover of edema fluid from the lesioned to the contralateral side through the corpus callosum.

Our finding that cold induced vasogenic brain edema is significantly reduced 24 hours after the oral administration of OPC-21268, a nonpeptide AVP V$_1$ receptor antagonist, indicate that OPC-21268 predominantly exerts a protective effect in areas where maximal BBB breakdown occurs. Our data also support the hypothesis that AVP influences the brain capillary permeability and contributes to edema formation under pathological conditions. Finally AVP V$_1$ receptor antagonists are useful in the treatment of vasogenic brain edema.

Acknowledgments

The authors are grateful to the Otsuka Pharmaceutical Co. Ltd. Japan, for the gift of OPC-21268.

References

1. Dickinson LD, Betz AL (1992) Attenuated development of ischemic brain edema in vasopressin-deficient rats. J Cereb Blood Flow Metab 12: 681–690
2. Doczi T, Szerdahelyi P, Gulya K, *et al* (1982) Brain water accumulation after the central administration of vasopressin. Neurosurgery 11: 402–407
3. Doczi T, Laszlo FA, Szerdahelyi P, Joo F (1984) Involvement of vasopressin in brain edema formation: further evidence obtained from the Brattleboro diabetes insipidus rat with experimental subarachnoid hemorrhage. Neurosurgery 14: 436–441
4. Faraci FM, Mayhan WG, Farrell WJ, Heistad DD (1988) Humoral regulation of blood flow to choroid plexus: role of arginine vasopressin. Circ Res 63: 373–379
5. Faraci FM, Mayhan WG, Heistad DD (1990) Effect of vasopressin on production of cerebrospinal fluid: possible role of vasopressin (V$_1$) receptors. Am J Physiol 258: R94–R98
6. Kagawa M, Nagao S, Bemana I (1996) Arginine vasopressin receptor antagonists for the treatment of vasogenic brain edema: an experimental study. J Neurotrauma 13: 273–279
7. Noto T, Nakajima T, Saji Y, Nagawa Y (1978) Effect of vasopressin on intracranial pressure of rabbit. Endocrinol Jpn 25: 591–596
8. Phillips PA, Abrahams JM, Kelly J, Paxinos G, Grzonka Z, Mendelssohn FAO, Johnston CI (1988) Localization of vasopressin binding sites in rat brain by *in vitro* autoradiography

using a radioiodinated V_1 receptor antagonist. Neuroscience 27: 749–761

9. Raichle ME, Grubb RL Jr (1978) Regulation of brain water permeability by centrally-released vasopressin. Brain Res 143: 191–194

10. Reeder RF, Nattie EE, North WG (1986) Effect of vasopressin on cold-induced brain edema in cats. J Neurosurg 64: 941–950

11. Rosenberg GA, Estrada E, Kyner WT (1988) The effect of arginine vasopressin and V_1 receptor antagonist on brain water in cat. Neurosci Lett 95: 241–245

12. Rosenberg GA, Estrada E, Kyner WT (1990) Vasopressin-induced brain edema is mediated by the V_1 receptor. Adv Neurol 52: 149–154

13. Rosenberg GA, Scremin O, Estrada E, Kyner WT (1992) Arginine vasopressin V_1 antagonist and atrial natriuretic pep-tide reduce hemorrhagic brain edema in rats. Stroke 23: 1767–1774

14. Uyama O, Okamura N, Yanase M, Narita M, Kawabata K, Sugita M (1988) Quantitative evaluation of vascular permeability in the gerbil brain after transient ischemia using Evans blue fluorescence. J Cereb Blood Flow Metab 8: 282–284

15. Yamamura Y, Ogawa H, Chihara T, Kondo K, Onogawa T, Nakamura S, Mori T, Tominaga M, Yabuuchi Y (1991) OPC-21268, an orally effective, nonpeptide vasopressin V_1 receptor antagonist. Science 252: 572–574

Correspondence: Iraj Bemana, M.D., Department of Neurological Surgery, Kagawa Medical University, 1750-1 Ikenobe, Miki-cho, Kita-Gun, Kagawa 761-07, Japan.

Acta Neurochir (1997) [Suppl] 70: 198–201
© Springer-Verlag 1997

Treatment of Acute Intracranial Hypertension with RU 51599, a Selective Kappa Opioid Agonist

S. Nagao, I. Bemana, E. Takahashi, T. Nakamura, and **H. Kuyama**

Department of Neurological Surgery, Kagawa Medical University, Kagawa, Japan

Summary

RU 51599, a selective kappa opioid agonist which is a potent aquaretic, was studied for its effect on acute intracranial hypertension. In ketamine anesthetized cats acute intracranial hypertension was induced by progressive inflation of an epidural balloon with physiological saline at a constant rate of 0.5 ml/hr for three hours. In the control group (n = 8), the balloon was maintained inflated for another an hour after which it was deflated. In the post deflation period monitoring was continued for one hour. In the treatment group (n = 8), cats were treated by an intravenous (i.v.) injection of RU 51599, at a dose of 1 mg/kg every hour at the beginning of balloon inflation, during balloon inflation, at the completion of inflation, and after deflation. Changes in intracranial pressure (ICP), mean arterial blood pressure (MAP), cerebral perfusion pressure (CPP), blood gases, serum electrolytes and osmolality, and brain water content were studied in both groups. In the control group, epidural brain compression resulted in significant increases in the mean ICP up to 80.7 ± 9.8 mmHg at 3 hrs (during balloon inflation), 68.6 ± 8.3 after complete inflation, and 62.1 ± 11.4 mmHg after deflation ($P < 0.01$), and significant decreases in CPP to 55.5 ± 14.0 mmHg at 3 hrs (during balloon inflation), 43.0 ± 11.2 mmHg after inflation, and 36.3 ± 9.9 mmHg after deflation ($P < 0.01$). In the treatment group there were significant decreases in the mean ICP to 35.2 ± 6.8 mmHg at 3 hrs (during balloon inflation), 32.3 ± 7.9 after inflation, and 16.1 ± 3.6 mmHg after deflation ($P < 0.01$), and significant increases in CPP to 103.2 ± 6.1 mmHg at 3 hrs (during balloon inflation), 109.0 ± 8.8 mmHg after inflation, and 102.7 ± 8.2 mmHg after deflation ($P < 0.01$). Brain water content was also significantly reduced ($P < 0.05$). There were no significant changes in the serum electrolytes and osmolality throughout the experiments. Our results suggest that, the mechanism by which RU 51599 reduces ICP is related to reduction in the brain water content.

Keywords: Intracranial pressure; cerebral perfusion pressure; RU 51599; brain water content.

Introduction

It has recently been reported that kappa opioid receptor agonists inhibit antidiuretic hormone secretion and promote water excretion in animals and humans [4, 8]. RU 51599 (niravoline) is a selective kappa opioid receptor agonist which has been shown in animals [10], and healthy male volunteers [1, 11] to have potent aquaretic activity, characterised by pure water diuresis without associated electrolyte excretion. The objective of this study was to determine the effects of RU 51599 on acute intracranial hypertension induced by epidural balloon compression in cat, and to define the possible mechanism responsible for this action.

Materials and Methods

Thirty one unselected adult cats were anesthetized with intramuscular injection of ketamine hydrochloride (30 mg/kg). The animals were paralyzed with pancuronium bromide (1 mg/kg), and ventilated with room air. A femoral artery and vein were cannulated for continuous monitoring of arterial blood pressure, collection of blood samples, and for the administration of medications. A small burr hole was made in the left parietal region for the placement of an epidural balloon to induce brain compression, and a plate type pressure transducer for continuous measuring of intracranial pressure was introduced in the right parietal epidural space. Body temperature was maintained at 37 ± 0.5°C by the use of a heating pad. Each cat received 5 ml/kg/hr of Ringer's lactate solution as maintenance fluid throughout the experiment.

The animals were divided into three groups. Group A was the brain compression (control) group (n = 8). Using an infusion pump, brain compression was induced by progressive inflation of an epidural balloon with physiological saline at the constant rate of 0.5 ml/hr for 3 hours. After 3 hours balloon inflation was stopped (but remained inflated). Monitoring was continued for another one hour, after which the balloon was deflated. In the post deflation period monitoring was continued for one hour, then the imal was sacrificed. Group B (n = 8) included animals treated during brain compression with RU 51599. An intravenous (i.v.) injection of RU 51599 (Roussel Uclaf, France) was given at a dose of 1 mg/kg every one hour, starting at the beginning of balloon inflation, during balloon inflation, at completion of inflation, and after deflation (5 doses). In sham operation animals (group C, n = 5), the effect of RU 51599 on physiological parameters was studied for 4 hours. Brain water content was evaluated in the sham operated and RU 51599 treated and non-treated animals (5 each) at the end of 3 hours brain compression. Changes in intracranial pressure (ICP), mean arterial blood pressure (MAP), cerebral perfusion pressure (CPP)

(CPP), blood gases and PH, serum electrolytes and osmolality, and body weight were studied in all animals throughout the experiments. The brain water content was determined by the specific gravimetric method after sacrifice.

Statistical Analysis: All values reported are mean ± standard error. Statistical analysis was carried out using statistical analysis system (SAS). Statistical significance was accepted for p < 0.05.

Results

In the baseline observation prior to balloon inflation the mean ICP and CPP were 7.5 ± 0.7 mmHg and 135.3 ± 7.0 mmHg in the control, and 5.6 ± 0.7 mmHg and 132.8 ± 8.7 mmHg in the RU 51599 treated group respectively. In the control group, progressive epidural brain compression caused significant increases in the mean ICP to 46.6 ± 10.6 at 2 hrs, 80.7 ± 9.8 mmHg at 3 hrs during balloon inflation, 68.6 ± 8.3 after inflation, and 62.1 ± 11.4 mmHg after deflation (P < 0.01) (Fig. 1), and significant decreases in CPP to 92.7 ± 7.3 at 2 hrs, and 55.5 ± 14.0 at 3 hrs during balloon inflation, 43.0 ± 11.2 after inflation, and 36.3 ± 9.9 mmHg after deflation period (P < 0.01) (Table 1). Intravenous injection of RU 51599 at a dose of 1 mg/kg

Table 1. *MAP, CPP, Plasma Electrolytes and Osmolality, and Blood Gases in Sham-Treated, Control, and RU 51599-Treated Cats During Epidural Brain Compression.* Values are the mean ± standard error of the mean

	Baseline	During balloon inflation			Post inflation	Post deflation
		1 hr	2 hrs	3 hrs	1 hr	1 hr
Sham group (n = 5)						
MAP	142.4 ± 9.6	141.4 ± 5.1	142.0 ± 5.9	138.2 ± 4.6	136.0 ± 4.4	–
CPP	135.0 ± 9.6	133.2 ± 5.2	133.0 ± 6.2	129.0 ± 4.8	125.6 ± 4.8	–
Na^+	156.10 ± 2.3	157.50 ± 2.9	157.80 ± 2.8	158.30 ± 2.9	157.80 ± 2.9	–
K^+	2.46 ± 0.28	2.38 ± 0.22	2.56 ± 0.10	2.59 ± 0.07	2.76 ± 0.04	–
Cl^-	120.56 ± 2.5	120.94 ± 3.1	119.16 ± 3.1	119.72 ± 3.3	119.48 ± 3.2	–
osmo	316.80 ± 8.8	319.40 ± 9.2	323.40 ± 9.2	318.60 ± 8.4	317.40 ± 9.0	–
PH	7.37 ± 0.05	7.32 ± 0.07	7.44 ± 0.06	7.44 ± 0.03	7.45 ± 0.02	–
pCO_2	35.54 ± 4.80	38.56 ± 4.89	36.46 ± 4.50	35.28 ± 3.13	34.06 ± 3.23	–
pO_2	103.20 ± 4.92	94.40 ± 7.26	106.0 ± 5.06	101.0 ± 4.42	101.0 ± 5.02	–
Control group (n = 8)						
MAP	142.8 ± 7.3	145.0 ± 7.1	139.3 ± 8.2	136.2 ± 16.5	111.6 ± 9.3[a]	98.5 ± 12.2[b]
CPP	135.3 ± 7.0	129.2 ± 6.7	92.7 ± 7.3	55.5 ± 14.0[d]	43.0 ± 11.2[d]	36.3 ± 9.9[d]
Na^+	152.60 ± 1.0	153.12 ± 0.8	153.11 ± 0.7	155.00 ± 1.9	152.39 ± 0.7	153.01 ± 0.4
K^+	2.40 ± 0.17	2.44 ± 0.1	2.48 ± 0.1	2.67 ± 0.1	2.62 ± 0.2	2.64 ± 0.1
Cl^-	119.17 ± 2.1	119.71 ± 1.5	119.76 ± 1.2	121.62 ± 2.4	119.47 ± 1.4	119.84 ± 2.1
osmo	320.75 ± 3.0	317.12 ± 3.1	316.50 ± 3.9	317.25 ± 3.9	319.25 ± 2.7	320.62 ± 2.9
PH	7.42 ± 0.02	7.41 ± 0.03	7.38 ± 0.04	7.37 ± 0.03	7.35 ± 0.02	7.35 ± 0.04
pCO_2	29.26 ± 2.78	28.96 ± 2.53	33.28 ± 3.71	32.78 ± 2.98	34.04 ± 3.46	31.66 ± 5.22
pO_2	94.28 ± 5.36	91.08 ± 7.93	79.21 ± 7.93	78.52 ± 6.57	80.30 ± 6.02	84.75 ± 10.30
RU 51599 teated (n = 8)						
MAP	138.6 ± 9.1	130.8 ± 10.5	134.3 ± 5.86	138.5 ± 7.0	141.3 ± 9.3[c]	118.8 ± 8.9
CPP	132.8 ± 8.7	120.1 ± 10.5	116.0 ± 5.5	103.2 ± 6.1[e]	109.0 ± 8.8[e]	102.7 ± 8.2[e]
Na^+	151.16 ± 0.6	153.90 ± 0.4	152.99 ± 0.7	153.00 ± 0.9	153.21 ± 0.6	152.55 ± 0.8
K^+	2.83 ± 0.28	2.34 ± 0.18	2.56 ± 0.14	2.77 ± 0.22	3.04 ± 0.27	3.23 ± 0.32
Cl	120.39 ± 1.7	123.79 ± 3.5	121.10 ± 1.6	126.09 ± 4.7	122.64 ± 2.3	122.91 ± 2.4
osmo	320.25 ± 3.2	320.0 ± 4.9	324.87 ± 6.2	322.62 ± 5.4	324.50 ± 5.9	326.50 ± 5.8
PH	7.40 ± 0.03	7.45 ± 0.03	7.45 ± 0.02	7.47 ± 0.03	7.44 ± 0.03	7.41 ± 0.05
pCO_2	32.25 ± 2.80	31.25 ± 3.37	30.56 ± 2.64	26.36 ± 2.49	26.26 ± 1.99	26.99 ± 1.69
pO_2	90.37 ± 6.61	87.71 ± 4.41	85.13 ± 5.37	90.25 ± 4.74	89.13 ± 4.73	90.00 ± 4 95

MAP Mean arterial pressure (mmHg); *CPP* cerebral perfusion pressure (mmHg); *osmo* plasma osmolality (mOsmol/kg). Plasma Na^+, K^+, Cl^- (mEq/l). Blood gases (mmHg).
[a] P < 0.05; [b] P < 0.01 vs. before balloon inflation; [c] p < 0.05 compared to control group in post inflation period; [d] P < 0.01 vs. before balloon inflation; [e] P < 0.01 compared to respective values in the control group.

Table 2. *Changes in the Brain Water Content.* Values are the mean ± standard error of the mean

	Left hemisphere (compression side)			Right hemisphere (contralateral side)		
	gray matter	white matter	basal ganglia	gray matter	white matter	basal ganglia
Sham-treated	80.52 ± 0.40	68.22 ± 0.74	67.77 ± 0.36	79.54 ± 0.27	68.19 ± 1.04	66.83 ± 0.86
Non-treated	80.19 ± 0.34	68.52 ± 0.34	67.42 ± 0.70	80.32 ± 0.35	67.90 ± 0.57	68.04 ± 0.88
RU 51599-treated	79.16 ± 0.15[a]	66.19 ± 0.24[b]	65.29 ± 0.27[a]	78.42 ± 0.05[b]	65.84 ± 0.42[a]	63.65 ± 0.17[b]

Brain water content was determined in the sham operated and RU 51599 treated and non-treated animals (5 each) at the end of 3 hours of epidural brain compression by specific gravimetric method.
[a] $P < 0.05$; [b] $P < 0.01$ compared to respective values in the control group.

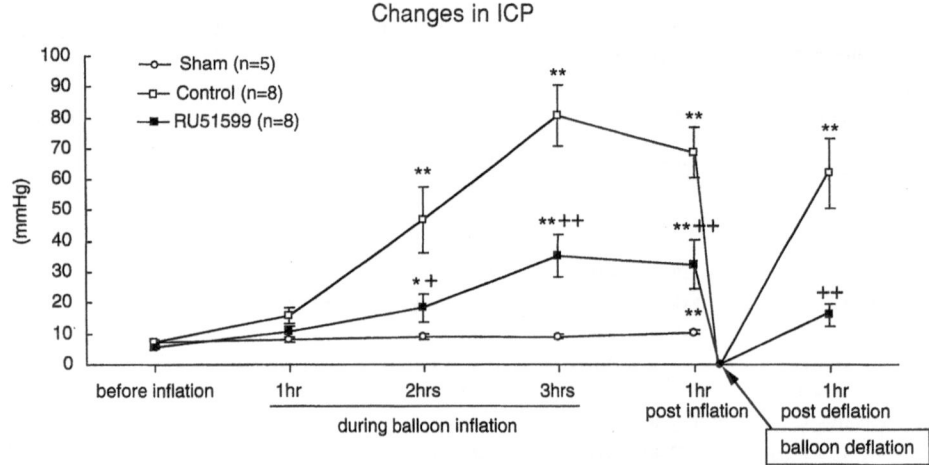

Fig. 1. Changes in the intracranial pressure (mmHg), before epidural balloon inflation, 1, 2, and 3 hrs (during balloon inflation), 1 hr after inflation and 1 hr after deflation in 3 experimental groups. Values are the mean ± standard error of the mean. * $p < 0.05$, ** $p < 0.01$ vs. before epidural balloon inflation. + $p < 0.05$, ++ $p < 0.01$ compare to control group

every hour significantly decreased ICP to 18.3 ± 4.4 at 2hrs ($P < 0.05$), and 35.2 ± 6.8 mmHg at 3 hrs during balloon inflation, 32.3 ± 7.9 after inflation, and 16.1 ± 3.6 mmHg after deflation period ($P < 0.01$) (Fig. 1), and significant increases in CPP to 116.0 ± 5.5 mmHg at 2hrs ($P < 0.05$), 103.2 ± 6.1 mmHg at 3 hrs during balloon inflation, 109.0 ± 8.8 after inflation period, and 102.7 ± 8.2 mmHg after deflation period compared to the control group ($P < 0.01$) (Table 1). No significant changes, were observed in the plasma osmolality and electrolytes, blood gases, and blood pressure (Table 1). RU 51599 treatment also resulted in significant reduction in the brain water content in both the compression and contralateral hemispheres ($P < 0.05$) (Table 2).

Discussion

RU 51599 (niravoline) is a new, highly selective kappa opioid receptor agonist which has been shown in animals and humans to have potent aquaretic activity, characterised by pure water diuresis without associated electrolytes excretion [1, 11]. Binding and autoradiographic studies have demonstrated the presence of κ-opioid receptors in the supraoptic and paraventricular nuclei of hypothalamus and neurohypophysis [3, 7]. It has also been reported that opioid receptors within the blood-brain barrier (BBB) are primarily involved in kappa agonist-induced water diuresis and possibly inhibition of vasopressin (AVP) secretion [2, 13]. Studies on the mechanism of action of RU 51599 suggest it acts via central inhibition of vasopressin secretion [10]. There have been reports of increased AVP secretion during acute intracranial hypertension [9], and of elevated plasma and cerebrospinal fluid levels of AVP in some patients with subarachnoid hemorrhage [14], and stroke [6]. It has also been suggested that increased intracranial pressure is a stimulus to centrally released vasopressin [12]. The above findings indicate that, increased plasma and cerebrospinal fluid AVP might have significant implications for raised intracranial pressure.

Our results have demonstrated that acute intracranial pressure induced by epidural brain compression was significantly reduced during treatment with RU 51599, a selective κ-opioid agonist, which inhibits central AVP secretion. The reduction in the ICP was associated with significant increases in CPP (Fig. 1 and Table 1). The i.v. administration of RU 51599 in this experiment did not induce significant changes in the plasma electrolytes and osmolality indicating that, it is a potential drug for the treatment of raised intracranial pressure, and intracranial diseases associated with hyponatremia, including clinical situations where current medical management is unsatisfactory. Brain water content was also significantly decreased in the RU 51599 treated group during epidural brain compression. This suggests that the mechanism by which RU 51599 reduced ICP is partly via a reduction in the brain water content. Since arginine vasopressin is reported to increase systemic arterial pressure, a decrease in AVP secretion may induce hypotension with a subsequent decrease in CPP. However, in our experiment i.v. administration of RU 51599, which inhibits AVP secretion did not induce significant changes in the MAP throughout the experiments (Table 1).

Our experiment has demonstrated that acute intracranial hypertension induced by progressive epidural brain compression is significantly reduced with i.v. administration of RU 51599, a selective κ-opioid receptor agonist. The reduction in the ICP is accompanied by significant increases in CPP and significant decreases in brain water content without significant changes in plasma osmolality and electrolytes. We suggest that the reduction in the brain water content is one of the mechanisms by which RU 51599 decreased ICP. However, this does not exclude the possible additive effect of this drug on other intracranial compartments, notably cerebrospinal fluid volume.

Acknowledgments

The authors are grateful to the Nippon Hoechst Marion Roussel, Japan, for providing the RU 51599.

References

1. Bellissant E, Denolle T, Sinnassamy P, Lecoz F, Gandon JM (1995) Pharmacodynamics of a new kappa opioid agonist, niravoline in healthy volunteers (abstr.). Clin Pharmacol Ther 57: 142 PI–29
2. Brooks DP, Giardina G, Gellai M, Dondio G, Edwards RM, Petrone G, DePalma PD, Sbacchi M, Jugus M, Misiano P, Wang YX, Clarke GD (1993) Opiate receptors within the blood-brain barrier mediate Kappa agonist-induced water diuresis. J Pharmacol Ther 226: 164–171
3. Bunn SJ, Hanley MR, Wilkin GP (1985) Evidence for a kappa-opioid receptor on pituitary astrocytes: an autoradiographic study. Neurosci Lett 55: 317–323
4. Hamon G, Jouquey S (1990) Kappa agonists and vasopressin secretion. Horm Res 34: 129–132
5. Hamon G, Fortin M, LeMartret O, Jouquey S, Vincent JC, Bichet DG (1994) Pharmacological profile of niravoline, a new aquaretic compound (abst.). J Am Soc Nephrol 5: 272
6. Joynt RJ, Feibel JH, Sladek CM (1981). Antidiuretic hormone levels in stroke patients. Ann Neurol 9: 182–184
7. Mansour A, Khachaturian H, Lewis ME, Akil H, Watson SJ (1988) Anatomy of CNS opioid receptors. Trends Neurosci 11: 308–314
8. Peters GR, Ward NJ, Antal EG, et al (1987) Diuretic actions in man of a selective kappa opioid agonist: U-62,066E. J Pharmacol Exp Ther 240: 128–131
9. Rap ZM, Chwalbinka-Moneta J (1978) Vasopressin concentration in the blood during acute short-term intracranial hypertension in cats. Adv Neurol 20: 381–388
10. Rossi NF (1995) The mechanisms of κ-opioid agonist-induced water diuresis: Central vs. peripheral actions. In: Saito T, Kurokawa K, Yoshida S (eds) Neurohypophysis, recent progress of vasopressin and oxytocin research. Elsevier, Amsterdam, pp 289–299
11. Sinnassamy P, Sultan E, Bichet DG (1994). Aquaretic effect of RU 51599, a kappa opioid agonist in healthy volunteers. J Am Soc Nephrol 5: 373 (Abstract)
12. Sorensen PS, Gjerris F, Hammer M (1984) Cerebrospinal fluid vasopressin and increased intracranial pressure. Ann Neurol 15: 435–440
13. Van de Heijning BJM, Van den Herik IK, Van Wimersma Greidanus TB (1991) Pharmacological assessment of the site of action of opioids on the release of vasopressin and oxytocin in the rat. Eur J Pharmacol 197: 175–180
14. Vang H, Jenkins JS (1981) Vasopressin in plasma and CSF of patients with subarachnoid haemorrhage. J Neurol Neurosurg Psychiatry 44: 216–219

Correspondence: Seigo Nagao, M.D., Department of Neurological Surgery, Kagawa Medical University, 1750-1 Ikenobe, Miki-cho, Kita-gun, Kagawa 761-07, Japan.

Acta Neurochir (1997) [Suppl] 70: 202–205

The Effect of Nitric Oxide Inhibition on Ischemic Brain Edema

Y. Yasuma, A. Strasser, C. Ruetzel, R. M. McCarron, and **M. Spatz**

Stroke Branch, NINDS, National Institutes of Health, Bethesda, MD, U.S.A.

Summary

The involvement of nitric oxide (NO) in the development of ischemic cytotoxic edema was investigated by inhibiting nitric oxide synthase (NOS) activity with Nω-nitro-L-arginine (NLA). Bilateral carotid artery occlusion (15 min) alone or with release (15 and 60 min) served as a model for edema induction. NLA, Nω-nitro-D-arginine methyl ester (D-NAME) or Ringer's solution were administered 4 hr prior to ischemia or sham operation. Treatment with a stable nitroxide radical, 4-hydroxy-2,2,6,6-tetramethylpipe-ridine-L-oxyl (TPL), was used to assess free radical involvement in edema. Accumulation of tissue water was evaluated by measuring specific gravity (SG) of brain cortex and histological examination. There was a greater reduction of cortical SG in early reperfusion (15 min) and a lesser decrease in SG (60 min later) in NLA- than in D-NAME- or Ringer's-treated gerbils. The NLA effect was confirmed by histological examination of the brain tissue. TPL treatment (pre- and postischemic) ameliorated the formation of edema to the same degree as NLA. The findings indicate a biphasic NLA modulation of cytotoxic edema most likely mediated through absence or presence of NO-derived free radicals.

Keywords: Ischemic edema; nitric oxide; free radicals; cytotoxic edema.

Introduction

Brain edema (increase in tissue water content) associated with ischemia consists of cytotoxic and vasogenic components [7]. Basically, the formation of ischemic cerebral edema represents an osmotic phenomenon triggered by biochemical disturbances of cellular membranes. The ischemically induced release of neurotransmitters andlor polyunsaturated fatty acids have been implicated in the development of brain edema [2, 3, 5]. In particular, a reduction in Na$^+$, K$^+$ATPase activity and a close temporal relationship between the altered 5-hydroxytryptamine (5-HT) metabolic pathway and accumulation of water in the tissue was observed during early postischemic reperfusion [11]. Among other factors including reactive oxygen species (ROS), hydrogen peroxide formed during deg-radation of dopamine (DA) by monoamine oxidase (MAO) activity and/or derived from nitric oxide (NO) metabolism has been thought to participate in free radical formation [8, 9, 12]. However, recent data have suggested that the disturbed antioxidative mitochondrial enzyme(s) activity rather than DA metabolism by MAO contributes to free radical tissue injury and edema during early perfusion after global ischemia [8]. The present study explores a possible role of NO in the development of ischemic cytotoxic edema.

Materials and Methods

Separate groups of 3-month-old female Mongolian gerbils (5–8 animals in each) under halothane and N_2O/O_2 (2:1) or pentobarbital (20 mg/kg) (1.5%) anesthesia and spontaneous ventilation were used for the induction of ischemia by bilateral carotid artery occlusion (15 min) alone or with reperfusion (15 or 60 min) as reported previously [8, 14]. Systemic blood pressure (SBP), cerebral blood flow (CBF) and rectal temperature were continuously monitored and maintained at 37–38°C with a thermostatically regulated heating lamp during the entire experimental procedure.

Nω-nitro-L-arginine (NLA), Nω-nitro-D-arginine methyl ester (D-NAME) (40 mg/kg) in Ringer's solution or solvent were injected 4 hr prior to ischemia or sham operation to assess free radical involvement in some experiments. In some experiments 4-hydroxy-2,2,6,6-tetramethylpiperidine-L-oxyl (TPL), a stable nitroxide radical, was injected i.p. (50 mg/kg) before or i.v. (25 mg/kg) 15 min after release of occlusion. The specific gravity (SG) of each brain cortex was measured at the end of designated experimental periods [13]. For histological examination, separate groups of animals were perfused with 4% phosphate-buffered paraformaldehyde.

Results were analyzed using one-way analysis of variance (ANOVA) followed by Fisher's least-squares difference test between particular experimental groups.

Results

None of the treatments affected body or temporal muscle temperature. However, NLA raised the level of SBP 41–59% above control (66.7 ± 3.5 – 75.8 ± 1.8 mmHg) and delayed the initial recovery of CBF.

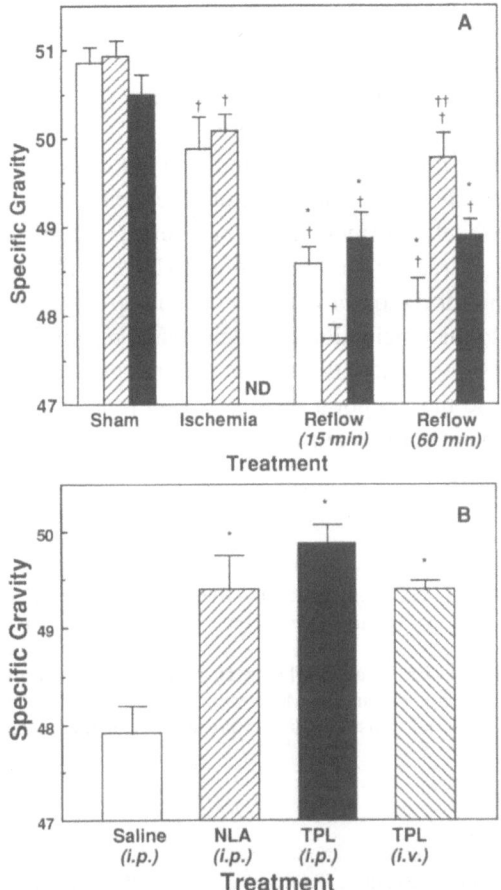

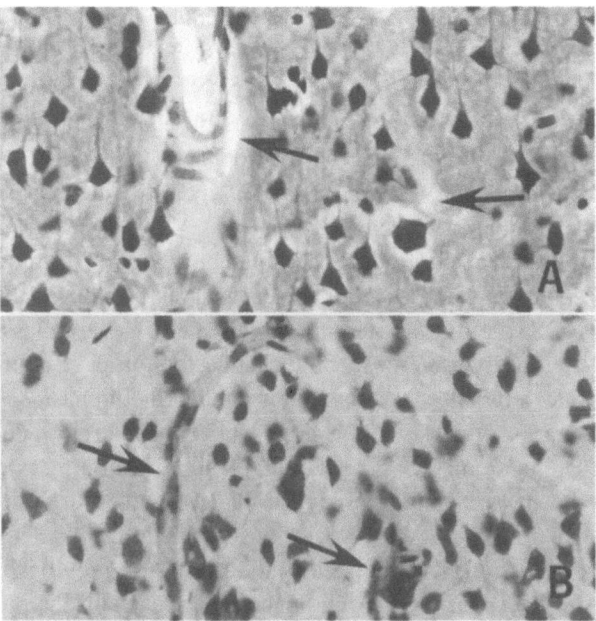

Fig. 2. Light photomicroscopy (cresyl violet stained) of cerebral cortex from D-NAME- (A) and NLA- (B) treated gerbils (×40). (A) Shows widely open lumina of microvessels with prominent vacuolization of the tissue. Arrows indicate vacuolization in the perivascular space and neuropil. (B) Shows constricted microvessels with prominent endothelial lining and occasional vacuolization of the tissue. Arrows indicate microvessels

Fig. 1. (A) The effect of NOS inhibition on cerebral cortical specific gravity. Animals were injected with Saline, NLA, or D-NAME, as described in the Materials and Methods section. The specific gravity data represent the mean ± S.E. (n = 8–17) at indicated time of ischemia/reperfusion. * Significant difference from NLA by ANOVA + F-PLSD (p < 0.05); + significant difference from sham by ANOVA + F-PLSD (p < 0.05); ++ significant difference from 15 min reflow by ANOVA + F-PLSD (p < 0.05); ND not determined. (B) Effect of a stable nitroxide radical on NOS inhibition on cortical specific gravity. NLA Nω-nitro-L-arginine was administered 4 hr whereas TPL (4-hydroxy-2,2,6,6-tetra-methylpiperidine) was injected either i.p before induction of ischemia or i.v. 15 min after reperfusion. The data represent the mean ± S.E. (n = 8–17) value obtained at reperfusion (60 min) after global ischemia (15 min). * Indicate significant differences between saline and NLA- or TPL-treated gerbils (p < 0.01) ANOVA followed by Fisher's protected least squares difference test

As shown in Fig. 1A, ischemia/reperfusion reduced the level of SG in the cortex of Ringer's-, D-NAME- and NLA-injected animals as compared to sham-tested gerbils. In addition, NLA alone decreased cortical SG to a greater degree at 15 min and increased SG levels at 60 min of reflow as compared to the values observed in either Ringer's- or D-NAME-treated gerbils. Both the pre- and postischemic i.p. administration of TPL (as in NLA treatment) prevented the reduction of cortical SG

observed in saline-injected animals at 60 min of reperfusion (Fig. 1B).

Histologically, the brains of Ringer's- or D-NAME-treated animals showed well-perfused open vascular lumina with separated perivascular tissues and diffuse small and large vacuolization of the gray and white matter (Fig. 2A). In contrast, in NLA-treated gerbils all the cerebral vessels were compressed showing barely detectable lumina but prominent microvascular endothelial lining. The gray and white matter revealed only occasional focal vacuoles (Fig. 2B).

Discussion

These findings clearly indicate a biphasic effect of NLA on the cortical accumulation of water during ischemia/reperfusion. The results of the second phase of cytotoxic edema in contrast to the first phase are in agreement with the reported NLA-induced decrease of brain edema and infarct volume after permanent or transient middle cerebral artery occlusion [12]. The observed increased reduction in SG level (= greater accumulation of water in the tissue) in early reperfusion of NLA- vs. Ringer's- and D-NAME-treated animals indicate an initial deleterious effect resulting from a disturbed NO metabolism.

NLA is one of Nω-monosubstituted L-arginine ana-logs widely used as NOS inhibitors which reduce both cNOS and iNOS. The inhibitory NLA effect is irre-versible on brain cNOS but reversible against endothe-lial cNOS and iNOS in macrophages. A single i.p. injection of NLA (50 mg/kg) reportedly decreased neuronal activity by 50% [4].

Based on our findings, it cannot be ascertained which cell type (vascular, glial, or neuronal) and the degree of NOS activity was inhibited by this agent. Nevertheless, the observed stereospecific changes of cortical SG in-duced by NLA treatment indicate that the biphasic al-teration of SG levels are due to NOS inhibition since the D-enantiomer, D-NAME, had no significant effect on the SG level or morphological changes which were sim-ilar to those found in Ringer's-injected gerbils. This conclusion is reinforced by the noted and previously reported vascular reactivities (pre- and postischemic elevation of BP and disturbed postischemic transient recovery of CBF) caused by NLA inhibition of NOS [14]. Thus, these findings strongly suggest involvement of NO in the formation of cytotoxic brain edema. In addition, the temporal postischemic tissue responses to NLA, namely decreased SG values at 15 min and in-creased SG levels at 60 min as compared to those seen in Ringer's- or D-NAME-injected animals, indicate that the NO initially prevents but subsequently contributed to the development of cytotoxic edema.

The findings of this study also indicate that TPL, the stable nitroxide radical which can react with various ROS, ameliorates cortical cerebral edema irrespective of whether it was given prior to the induction of ischemia or after the re-establishment of circulation (15 min) [10,15]. Their low toxicity, membrane perme-ability (including the blood-brain barrier) and biologi-cal activity which mimics superoxide (SOD) activity protects cells from oxidative stress mediated by oxidiz-ing processes *in vitro* and *in vivo*. Its anti-edematous action presented here is in agreement with nitroxide reduction of brain edema observed in closed head injury [1].

The noted temporal causal association of NLA and TPL amelioration of cytotoxic edema at 60 min of reperfusion strongly suggest ROS derivation from NO. The involvement of ROS and/or NO in the formation of ischemic edema and its reduction by SOD and other antioxidants have been reported in various models of cerebral ischemia [2, 3, 5, 6, 9]. However, most of these studies did not address the evolution of edema and/or the temporal role of NO in the formation of cytotoxic edema during reperfusion.

The present findings not only support NO participa-tion in the formation of ROS but also provide an additional factor which may play a role in the second phase of ischemic cytotoxic edema.

In conclusion, ischemically-induced cytotoxic ede-ma represents one of many features resulting from a cascade of cellular (membrane) biochemical changes. The demonstrated biphasic response to NOS inhibition during the formation of cytotoxic edema greatly con-tributes to the elucidation of mechanisms responsible for the development of this type of edema. It also draws attention to the temporal duality of NO function and thus to potential clinical ramifications.

Acknowledgement

This study is dedicated to the memory of Dr. Bogumir B. Mrsulja who originally and greatly contributed to the elucidation of mechanisms involved in the development of ischemic cytotoxic edema.

The authors wish to acknowledge Dr. Nabil Azzam for the preparation of photographs and Ms. Devera Schoenberg, M.S., for her expert editorial assistance in the preparation of this manu-script.

References

1. Beit-Yannai E, Zhang R, Trembovler V, Samuni A, Shohami E (1996) Cerebroprotective effect of stable nitroxide radicals in closed head injury in the rat. Brain Res 717: 22–28
2. Chan PK, Longar S, Fishman (1985) Oxygen-free radicals: Potential edema mediators in brain injury. In: Inaba Y, Klatzo I, Spatz M (eds) Brain edema. Springer, Berlin Heidelberg New York Tokyo, pp 317–335
3. Chan PK, Epstein CJ, Kinuchi H, Imaizumi S, Carbon B, Chen SF (1993) Role of superoxide dismutase in ischemic brain injury, reduction of edema and infarction in transgenic mice following focal cerebral ischemia. Prog Brain Res 96: 97–104
4. Dwayer MA, Brendt DS, Snyder SH (1991) Nitric oxide irre-versible inhibition by L-NGarginine in brain *in vitro* and *in vivo*. Biochem Biophys Res Comm 176: 1136–1141
5. Hall ED, Braughler JM (1989) Central nervous system trauma and stroke. II. Physiological and pharmacological evidence for involvement of oxygen radicals and lipid peroxidation. Free Rad Biol Med 6: 303–313
6. Huang Z, Huang PL, Panahian N, Dalkara T, Fishman MC, Moskowitz MA (1994) Effects of cerebral ischemia in mice deficient in neuronal nitric oxide synthase. Science 265: 1883–1885
7. Klatzo I (1994) Evolution of brain edema concept. Acta Neuro-chir (Wien) [Suppl] 60: 3–6
8. Ishii H, Stanimirovic DB, Chang CJ, Mrsulja BB, Spatz M (1993) Dopamine metabolism and free-radical related mito-chondrial injury during transient brain ischemia in gerbils. Neurochem Res 18: 1193–1201
9. Kumura E, Yoshimine T, Iwatsuki K-I, Yamanaka K, Tanaka S, Hayakawa T, Shiga T, Kosaka H (1996) Generation of nitric oxide and superoxide during reperfusion after focal cerebral ischemia in rats. Am J Physiol 270 (Cell Physiol 39): C748–C752

10. Mitchell JB, DeGraff W, Kaufman D, Krishna MC, Samuni A, Finkelstein E, Ahn MS, Hahn SM, Gamson J, Russo A (1991) Inhibition of oxygen-dependent radiation-induced damage by the nitroxide superoxide dismutase mimic, Tempol. Arch Biochem Biophys 389: 62–70

11. Mrsulja BB, Djuric BM, Crejic V, Mrsulja BJ, Abe K, Spatz M, Klatzo I (1980) Biochemistry of experimental ischemic edema. Adv Neurol 28: 217–230

12. Nagafuji T, Sugiyama M, Matsui T, Muto A, Naito S (1995) Nitric oxide synthase in cerebral ischemia: possible contribution of nitric oxide synthase activation in brain microvessels to cerebral ischemic injury. Mol Chem Neuropathol 26: 107–157

13. Nelson SR, Mantz M-L, Maxwell JA (1971) Use of specific gravity in the measurement of cerebral edema. J Appl Physiol 30: 268–271

14. Strasser A, Yasuma Y, McCarron RM, Ishii H, Stanimirovic D, Spatz M (1994) Effect of nitro-L-arginine on cerebral blood flow and monoamine metabolism during ischemia/reperfusion in the Mongolian gerbil. Brain Res 664: 197–201

15. Samuni A, Godinger D, Aronovitch J, Russo A, Mitchell JB (1991) Nitroxides block DNA scission and protect cells from oxidative damage. Biochemistry 30: 555–561

Correspondence: Maria Spatz, M.D., Stroke Branch, NINDS, NIH, 36 Convent Drive, MSC 4128, Bethesda, MD 20892-4128, U.S.A.

Acta Neurochir (1997) [Suppl] 70: 206–208
© Springer-Verlag 1997

Blood-Brain Barrier Disturbances After rt-PA Treatment of Thromboembolic Stroke in the Rat

E. Busch, K. Krüger, K. Fritze, P. R. Allegrini, M. Hoehn-Berlage, and **K. A. Hossmann**

Max-Planck-Institute für Neurological Research, Department of Experimental Neurology, Köln, Federal Republic of Germany

Summary

We studied the effects of rt-PA (recombinant tissue type-plasminogen activator) treatment on the blood-brain barrier (BBB) after thromboembolic stroke in rat. New MRI methods of diffusion and perfusion imaging to observe the hemodynamic and biophysical effects of thrombolysis were combined with methods for assessment of BBB disturbances. In untreated animals clot embolism produced a rapid drop in MRI perfusion values and the ADC (apparent diffusion coefficient), with subsequent infarction. BBB disturbances, visualised as extravasation of serum proteins on cryostat sections, were manifest in nearly all animals in the borderzone of infarcts. In animals treated with rt-PA 15 min after clot embolism thrombolysis resulted in reperfusion of affected brain regions with subsequent improvement of ADC values. Final lesion size on ADC maps was reduced by 36% relative to untreated animals. However, BBB disturbances were not improved after treatment. To the contrary, rt-PA treated animals showed further regions with serum protein extravasation in the infarcted territories and in distant non-ischemic brain regions. MR imaging with the BBB tracer GdDTPA showed more pronounced and widespread contrast enhancement in the rt-PA treated than in the untreated group. Increased blood-brain barrier disturbances have to be taken into account even when thrombolytic therapy is started very early after the onset of stroke.

Keywords: Blood-brain barrier; thrombolysis; rt-PA; thromboembolic stroke; rat; MRI.

Introduction

Recirculation of the brain after a period of focal ischemia carries the risk of brain edema. Following thrombolytic therapy disturbances of the blood-brain barrier may explain the high incidence of intracerebral hemorrhage of up to 20%, and the rather modest therapeutic improvement in only 10% of the treated patients [3, 7]. The mechanisms responsible for this disturbance after thrombolysis of stroke are poorly understood. With the advent of functional MR imaging, the status of the blood-brain barrier can be correlated with the hemodynamic and biophysical conse-

quences of thrombolytic therapy. To study the effect of rt-PA on the blood-brain barrier after thromboembolic stroke, we combined advanced MR techniques of diffusion and perfusion imaging with the assessment of the blood-brain barrier at the experimental endpoint.

Materials and Methods

Thromboembolic stroke was induced in 17 Wistar rats by intracarotid injection of 12 medium sized fibrin rich autologous clots. All experiments were physiologically fully controlled. One group of animals (n = 9) was treated over 45 min with 10 mg/kg rt-PA, starting 15 min after embolisation. The other group received an infusion of saline. Evolution of the ischemic injury was followed continuously by multislice diffusion MR imaging on a 4.7 T tomograph. ADC maps were calculated to observe the severity of the ischemic impact [4]. Brain tissue perfusion was assessed using an arterial spin tagging technique [5]. At the end of the experimental time, 3.5 hours after embolisation, the permeability of the blood-brain barrier was assessed by gadoliniumDTPA (GdDTPA) enhanced T1-weighted MR imaging. Extravasation of serum proteins was also visualized in cryostat-sections of the brains using the PAP method [9] and compared to metabolic images of ATP-distribution, achieved by bioluminescence imaging [6], from adjacent brain sections.

Results

In untreated animals (n = 8) clot embolism produced instantaneous reduction in blood flow and a rapid fall of ADC which continued to decline throughout the observation time. Treatment with rt-PA (n = 9) resulted in marked improvement of blood flow in 6 animals. ADC began to recover after a time lag of 15 to 80 min indicating reversal of tissue injury. The final ADC lesion volume of untreated animals was 61 ± 7% of ipsilateral hemisphere as compared to 39 ± 8% in the treated group.

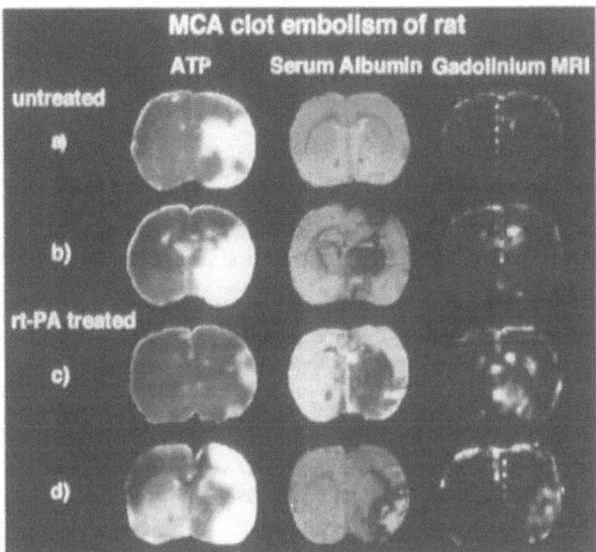

Fig. 1. Local distribution of ATP, the extravasation of serum proteins and the extravasation of GdDTPA in two examples of untreated and rt- PA treated animals 3.5 h after clot embolism. For each animal adjacent cryostat sections and the corresponding MRI slice are shown. The slices of animal a) show a medium sized infarct, defined as area of ATP-depletion, without extravasation of serum albumin or GdDTPA. On the slices of animal b) extravasation of serum albumins can be seen in the borderzone of the infarct. In animal c) treatment with rt-PA resulted in only a small cortical infarct. However, the area with visible serum albumin extends throughout the basalganglia and corresponds well with extravasation of GdDPTA. MRI perfusion measurements demonstrated both ischemia and subsequent reperfusion of this particular brain region during the time course of the experiment. On the images of animal d) blood-brain barrier disturbances within the infarcted territory are detected both by extravasation of serum albumins and GdDPTA

Table 1. *Blood-Brain Barrier Disturbances 3.5 h After Thromboembolic Stroke in Rat*

	Untreated (n = 8) (number of animals)	rt-PA treated (n = 8) (number animals)
In infarct	0	2
In borderzone of infarct	7	7
Distant to infarct	0	3
No BBB disturbance	1	1
Visible on GdDPTA MRI	1	4

Number of animals in each group with extravasation of serum proteins in the territories of infarct, the borderzone of the infarct, in distant brain regions to the infarct or without extravasation. Extravasation of serum proteins was visualised in cryostat-sections using the PAP method. Infarcts were defined as regions with ATP-depletion. Additionally the number of animals with extravasation of GdDPTA as visible on T_1-weighted magnetic resonance images is stated. BBB disturbances occurred in the same number of animals in each group, but within the infarcted territory and in distant brain regions such observations were only made in rt-PA treated animals. On GdDTPA enhanced MR images, blood-brain barrier disturbances were more often visible after thrombolysis. One animal died after thrombolysis due to intracerebral hemorrhage.

Serum protein extravasation was observed in seven of eight animals of both groups. In all of these animals serum proteins were found in the borderzone of infarcts, defined as regions of ATP depletion on adjacent cryostat sections (Fig. 1, Table 1). Although thrombolysis resulted in a significant reduction of infarct size, the areas of serum protein extravasation in the borderzone of infarcts were comparable. In rt-PA treated animals serum protein extravasation was additionally observed within brain infarcts or in distant brain regions (Table 1).

In untreated animals GdDTPA extravasation on MRI images was only found in one animal. In contrast, widespread GdDTPA induced enhancement was detected in four of the treated animals, mainly in the basal ganglia and in one case also in the cortex (Fig. 1). One animal died due to intracerebral hemorrhage after thrombolysis.

Discussion

Thromboembolic stroke consistently produced extravasation of serum proteins indicating blood-brain barrier disturbances. In both groups these disturbances were most pronounced in the borderzone of infarcts. However, blood-brain barrier disturbances after thrombolytic treatment were found to be more widespread and included areas within the infarcts and distant, non-ischemic areas of the brain. The marked gadolinium enhancement after 3.5 hours in thrombolized animals confirms that massive breakdown of the blood-brain barrier could not be prevented, and even seemed to be enhanced, although therapy was initiated already at 15 min after clot embolism. Serum protein extravasation within infarcted areas can be explained by reperfusion to already irreversibly damaged brain tissue. Mechanisms for enhanced BBB disturbances in the borderzone of infarcts might include microembolism [8] and peroxidative events associated with reperfusion injury [2]. The finding of protein extravasation in non-ischemic regions of the brain supports suggestions of a direct effect of rt-PA on the cerebral endothelium [1, 10]. Our findings underline that blood-brain barrier disturbances have to be taken into account even if thrombolytic therapy is initiated very early after onset of stroke. The precise mechanisms of rt-PA induced BBB disturbances should be the subject of further studies.

References

1. Conforti G, Dominguez-Jimeńez C, Ronne E, Hoyer-Hansen G, Dejana E (1994) Cell-surface plasminogen activation causes a retraction of *in vitro* cultured human umbilical vein endothelial cell monolayer. Blood 83: 994–1005
2. Dirnagl U, Lindauer U, Them A, Schreiber S, Pfister H-W, Koedel U, Reszka R, Freyer D, Villringer A (1995) Global cerebral ischemia in the rat: online monitoring of oxygen free radical production using chemiluminescence *in vivo*. J Cereb Blood Flow Metab 15: 929–940
3. Hacke W, Kaste M, Fieschi C, *et al* (1995) Intravenous thrombolysis with recombinant tissue plasminogen activator for acute hemispheric stroke. JAMA 274: 1017–1025
4. Hoehn-Berlage M, Norris DG, Kohno K, Mies G, Leibfritz D, Hossmann K-A (1995) Evolution of regional changes in apparent diffusion coefficient during focal ischemia of rat brain: the relationship of quantitative diffusion NMR imaging to reduction in cerebral blood flow and metabolic disturbances. J Cereb Blood Flow Metab 15: 1002–1011
5. Kerskens CM, Hoehn-Berlage M, Schmitz B, Busch E, Bock C, Gyngell ML, Hossmann K-A (1996) Ultrafast perfusion-weighted MRI of functional brain activation in rats during forepaw stimulation: comparison with T_2*-weighted MRI. NMR Biomed 8: 20–23
6. Kogure K, Furones Alonso O (1978) A pictorial presentation of endogenous brain ATP by a luminescent method. Brain Res 154: 273–284
7. The National Institute of Neurological Disorders and Stroke rt-PA Stroke Study Group (1995) Tissue plasminogen activator for acute ischemic stroke. N Engl J Med 333: 1581–1587
8. Schuier FJ, Vise M, Hossmann K-A, Zülch KJ (1978) Cerebral microembolization. II. Morphological studies. Arch Neurol 35: 264–270
9. Sternberger LA, Hardy PH, Cuculis JJ, Meyer HG (1970) The unlabeled antibody enzyme method of immunohistochemistry. Preparation and properties of soluble antigen-antibody complex (horseradish peroxidase-antihorseradish peroxidase) and its use in identification of spirochetes. J Histochem Cytochem 18: 315–333
10. Vassali JD, Sappino AP, Belini D (1991) The plasminogen activator/plasmin system. J Clin Invest 88: 1067–1072

Correspondence: K.-A. Hossmann, M.D., Max-Planck-Institut für neurologische Forschung, Gleuelerstrasse 50, D-50931 Köln, Federal Republic of Germany.

Acta Neurochir (1997) [Suppl] 70: 209–211

The Effect of Dotarizine (Ca^{2+} Channel Blocker) on Cerebral Vessel Reactivity in Animals Subjected to Hyperventilation and Anoxia

Z. Czernicki[1], N. Kuridze[1], J. Jurkiewicz[1], and **J. Cervós-Navarro[2]**

[1] Department of Neurosurgery, Medical Research Centre, Polish Academy of Sciences, Warsaw, Poland, and
[2] Institute of Neuropathology, Free University, Berlin, Federal Republic of Germany

Summary

Dotarizine – a novel piperazine derivative – belongs to wide spectrum Ca$^+$ channel antagonists. It was reported to have strong vasodilatory and antiserotoninergic activities. Unlike other Ca$^+$ channnel blockers Dotarizine was found to have lower oral toxicity. In the presented study the influence of the oral administration of the novel compound on the blood flow velocity changes in different cerebral arteries – in basilar artery (BA) and middle cerebral artery (MCA) – was investigated under hyperventilation and hypoxic conditions of rabbits. In the first experimental group 25 mg/kg of Dotarizine dissolved in 0,25% agar was administered orally three times at the 10 hours' intervals. The sham group of animals was fed with agar of the same concentration. The results revealed that oral administration of Dotarizine diminished the vasoconstrictive effect of hyperventilation and this was more pronounced in MCA than in BA. During anoxic conditions stronger vasodilatatory effects were observed in both groups of vessels and the low value of pulsatility index (PI) reflected pronounced decrease of the peripheral resistance, in comparison to the control group. Thus, the oral administration of Dotarizine decreases the peripheral resistance of cerebral vessels and therefore seems to have influence on the minute arteries of cerebrovascular system of the brain.

Keywords: Ca^{2+} channel blocker; Dotarizine; cerebrovascular reactivity; hyperventilation; anoxia.

Introduction

Dotarizine (1-(diphenylomethyl)-4-[3-(2-phenyl-1, 3-dioxolan-2-yl)prophyl]-piperazine) – a novel piperazine derivative – is chemically related to Cinnarizine and Flunarizine, which both have been reported to reveal antihistaminic, anti-α-adrenergic and Ca^{2+} antagonistic activities [7, 8]. Dotarizine differs from the latter drugs because it also exhibits a pronounced antiserotonergic activity [1]. It also has been found to have lower oral toxicity [5]. As a vasostabilizing agent, especially for cerebral vessels [2], Dotarizine was reported to increase cerebral blood flow (CBF) and cerebral oxygen consumption [3] in experimental animals.

In the presented study the influence of the oral administration of the compound on the blood flow velocity changes in different cerebral arteries was investigated under hyperventilation and hypoxic conditions.

Materials and Methods

The experiments were carried out on rabbits of both sexes weighing from 3.0 to 3.5 kg. The animals were anaesthetised intravenously with urethane – 10 mg/kg and α chloralose – 80 mg/kg. After tracheotomy was performed the femoral artery and vein were cannulated for arterial and central venous pressure monitoring, blood sampling and drug administration. Mera-PIAP (Poland) pressure transducers with MCK-4011 (TEMED-Poland) electromanometers were used for pressure recording. Data was monitored and computed with an application of a computer program. During all surgical preparation xylocaine (Astra-R, Sweden) was applied for local analgesia. After surgical preparation the animals were paralyzed with Pavulon (Organon) at a dose of 0,2 mg/kg and artificially ventilated. During the experiments the animals were under general anesthesia inhaling nitrous oxide and oxygen in a ratio of 2:1 during normoventilation, in a ratio of 0,5:3 during hyperventilation and during the anoxic conditions respiration was stopped for 3 min. Continuous $P_{Et}CO_2$ monitoring in expired air (Datex Capnograph), and periodical blood gases analysis (CIBA Blood Gas Analyzer) were performed for evaluation of ventilation. The animals were placed in sphinx position with the head in a stereotaxic apparatus. Blood flow velocity (BFV) in middle cerebral artery (MCA) and basilar artery (BA) was recorded during the experiments by using Transcranial Doppler apparatus (Medasonics) (TCD). BFV in the investigated vessels was measured by the PW-2MHz TCD probe which was positioned on the right eyeball of the experimental animal for the MCA investigation, or to the posterior skull for the BA investigation.

Experiments were carried out on the three groups of animals. In the first two groups (10 rabbits) 25 mg/kg of Dotarizine dissolved in 0.25% agar was administered orally three times at the 10 hours' intervals. The sham group of animals (5) was fed with agar of the same concentration according to the same time schedule. In the first group of treated animals the hyperventilation was performed for 15 min ($P_{Et}CO_2$ 18 ± 2 mmHg, PaCO$_2$ in the arterial blood 16 ± 2 mmHg). Data concerning flow velocities in both investigated vessels before hyperventilation and at 15 min of hyperventilation.

In the second group of Dotarizine treated animals the ventilation was stopped for 3 min and all parameters were registered before and after anoxia. The sham group of animals was subjected to the same ventilation conditions as the previous two groups. The data were statistically analysed using paired two-sample t-tests for mean values.

Results

The changes of BFV in MCA in control and drug-treated groups during 15 min hyperventilation are presented on the Fig. 1. In the sham group of animals hyperventilation caused decrease of the initial BFV values to 60%. In the Dotarizine treated group the mean velocity was decreased only to 85% of its initial values.

Figure 1 also presents BFV changes in BA during the same conditions. In this vessel the drug influence on mean velocity was less pronounced, however, a sharp decrease of diastolic velocity in the drug-treated group during hyperventilation could be observed. Comparing the reactivity of MCA and BA during hyperventilation in two groups of experimental animals it can be seen that Dotarizine diminished the vasoconstrictive effect of hyperventilation, and this effect was more pronounced in MCA than in BA (Fig. 1).

In the second group of drug-treated animals, where the ventilation was cut off for 3 min, stronger vasodilatatory effects during anoxic conditions were observed in both groups of vessels when compared to untreated animals. However, the difference in BFV changes during anoxia, between control and drug- treated groups,

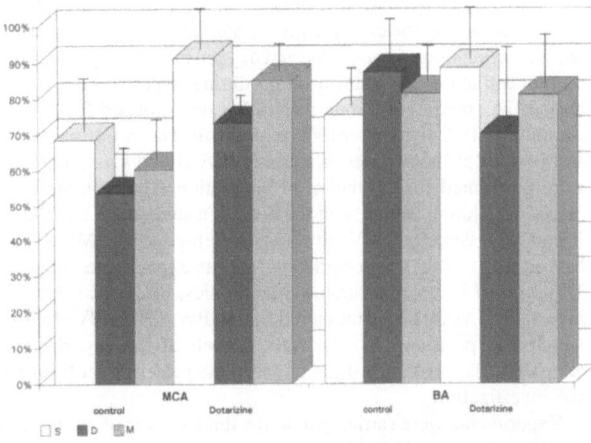

Fig. 1. Blood flow velocity (BFV) changes in middle cerebral artery (*MCA*) and basilar artery (*BA*) during 15 min hyperventilation in control and Dotarizine-treated groups of experimental animals. BFV values are expressed in percentage versus the initial BFV values obtained during normoventilation in control and drug-treated groups respectively. *S* Systolic blood flow velocity, *D* diastolic blood flow velocity, *M* mean blood flow velocity

was more pronounced in BA in comparison to MCA (Fig. 2).

Evaluation of Pulsatility Index (PI) of TCD measuring in MCA and BA revealed a tendency to decrease in Dotarizine-treated animal groups (Fig. 3). This observation suggests a decrease of vascular resistances, as an effect of Dotarizine.

Discussion

The vasodilatative effect of Dotarizine on cerebrovascular reactivity has already been reported by other authors [3, 6]. In our previous study it was also demonstrated that intravenous injection of Dotarizine in a dose of 0,5 mg/kg in cats virtually neutralizes the hypocapnic vasoconstrictive effect on cerebral vessels,

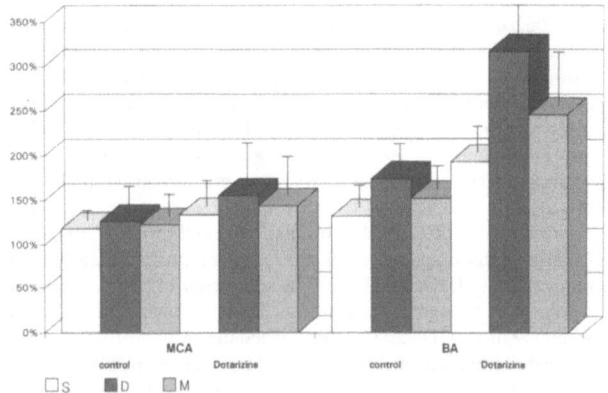

Fig. 2. Blood flow velocity (BFV) changes in middle cerebral artery (*MCA*) and basilar artery (*BA*) during 3 min anoxia in control and Dotarizine-treated groups of animals. BFV values are expressed in percentage versus the initial BFV values obtained during normoventilation in control and drug-treated groups respectively. *S* Systolic blood flow velocity, *D* diastolic blood flow velocity, *M* mean blood flow velocity

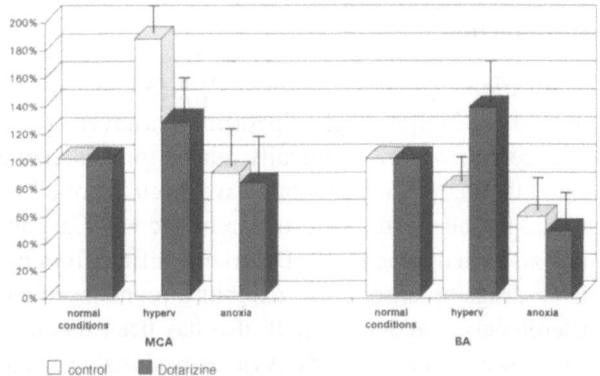

Fig. 3. Changes of pulsatility index (PI) of TCD measuring in MCA and BA in percentage in control and Dotarizine-treated groups of animals during hyperventilation and anoxia

and returns the cerebral blood flow velocity to its initial values [4]. It can be concluded that the oral administration of the piperazine derivative – Dotarizine has different influence on the branches of middle cerebral and of the basilar arteries systems.

Since Dotarizine impairs the vasoconstrictive effect of hyperventilation it seems to have a stabilising effect on cerebrovascular reactivity and diminishes cerebrovascular resistance also. Therefore this compound could be a promising prophylactic drug in the treatment of migraine attacks. Its chronic effect on cerebrovascular reactivity needs to be studied further.

References

1. Agut J, Sacristan A, Oriz JA (1990) Action on 5-HT-2 receptor binding in rat frontal cortex. Eur J Pharmacol 183 (6): 2147
2. Catheuser CF, Braso A, Sacristan A, Ortiz JA (1994) Dotarizine effects on peripheral and pulmonary circulation and cardiac dynamics in dogs. Pharmacology 48: 3
3. Catheuser CF, Gomez F, Sacristan A, Ortiz JA (1993) Effects of Dotarizine on rat cerebral blood flow autoregulatory response to PaCO$_2$ alterations, on cerebral O$_2$ consumption and on electrocorticogram activity. Naunyn Schmiedebergs Arch Pharmacol 347 [Supp]: R 79
4. Chomicki J, Jurkiewicz J, Zabolotny W, Czernicki Z, Cervós-Navarro J (1995) Effect of Dotarizine on CO$_2$–dependent cerebrovascular reactivity. Acta Neurochir (Wien) 136: 186–188
5. Gubert G, Braso A, Sacristan A, Oriz JA (1987) Synthesis of some n-benzhydrylpiperazine derivatives as calcium antagonists. Arzneim Forsch Drug Res 37: 1103–1107
6. Lazarova M, Potkova B, Potkov VD (1995) Effect of Dotarizine on electroconvulsive shock or pentilenotetrazol-induced amnesia and on seizure reactivity in rats. Methods Find Exp Clin Pharmacol 17 (1): 53–58
7. Phillis JW, Delong JK, Towner JK (1985) The effects of Lidoflazine and Flunarizine on cerebral reactive hyperemia. Eur J Pharmacol 112: 323–329
8. Todd PA, Benfield P (1989) Flunarizine. A reappraisal of its pharmacological properties and therapeutic use in neurological disorders. Drugs 38: 481–499

Correspondence: Zbigniew Czernicki, M.D., Ph.D., Department of Neurosurgery, Medical Research Centre, Polish Academy of Sciences, Barska st. 22, 02-315 Warsaw, Poland.

Acta Neurochir (1997) [Suppl] 70: 212–215
© Springer-Verlag 1997

Substance P Endopeptidase Activity in the Rat Spinal Cord Following Injury: Influence of the New Anti-Oxidant Compound H 290/51

M. Thörnwall[1], H. S. Sharma[1], T. Gordh[2], P.-O. Sjöquist[3], and F. Nyberg[1]

[1] Department of Pharmaceutical Biosciences, [2] Biomedical Centre, Department of Anaesthesiology, University Hospital, Uppsala University, Uppsala, and [3] Pharmacology CV, Astra Hässle, Mölndal, Sweden

Summary

The influence of the new antioxidant compound H-290/51 was examined on the substance P endopeptidase (SPE) activity in a rat model of spinal cord injury. This compound (H-290/51) has neuroprotective effects on edema and cell changes in this model. Infliction of trauma to the cord by making an incision into the right dorsal horn of the T10-11 segment resulted in a marked upregulation of SPE in the segments rostral to the lesion. On the other hand, the injured and adjacent caudal segments exhibited a marked downregulation of the enzyme activity. Pretreatment with H 290/51 increased the SPE activity in the T9 segment but downregulated the enzyme activity in the T10-11 and T12 segments. The drug induced enzyme activity change was not further influenced by the trauma of the cord. The results indicate that a focal trauma induces widespread alterations in spinal cord SPE activity which can be influenced by the anti-oxidant drug H 290/51, suggesting that SPE is somehow involved in cell injury.

Keywords: Spinal cord trauma; substance P endopeptidase; oxidative stress; anti-oxidant; neuroprotection.

Introduction

The level of specific neuropeptides and the activity of neuropeptidases known to degrade neuropeptides are altered in various neurological diseases [2, 6, 7, 9–12, 20]. Waters and Davis [18] have reported that substance P and substance P endopeptidase are somehow involved in the pathology of senile dementia of the Alzheimer type. This conclusion is based on the fact that the metabolic half life of substance P is significantly increased in human post-mortem cerebral cortex. The decrease in half life of substance P was correlated with the activity of substance P endopeptidases and significantly related with metalloendopeptidases. The changes were most pronounced in the cerebral cortex, while such a relationship was not apparent in the hippocampus or temporal brain. The alterations in

substance P endopeptidases strongly indicate a role of an altered metabolism as significant factor of nerve cell pathology in senile dementia of Alzheimer's type. An involvement of substance P and its converting enzyme in the brain pathology by trauma to the central nervous system, however, is still poorly understood [12, 13, 17].

Spinal cord injury is a serious clinical situation in which edema and the cell changes dominate the pathological outcome as leading mechanisms of the neurological deficit, such as paresis and paraplegia [5, 7, 9, 17, 20]. The mechanisms and significance of various neurochemicals involved in the pathology of early cell injury are still unknown. A focal injury of the spinal cord may induce a cascade of pathophysiological events, such as release of neurotransmitters, lipid peroxidation, and generation of free radicals leading to cell and tissue damage [5, 13–15, 17]. Neurons, glial cells, and microvessels in segments of the cord around the primary injury are exposed to a wide range of adverse alterations of their microenvironment [9–13]. In order to improve the outcome from focal spinal cord injury, therapeutic trials focus on procedures to reduce secondary injuries and to preserve as many cells as possible in the perifocal region [17, 20].

Previous work of our laboratory has shown that focal spinal cord injury induces marked alterations of the substance P content in the spinal cord of perifocal segments [12]. These segments have marked cell changes and edema [10]. Pretreatment with p-chlorophenylalanine (p-CPA), a serotonin synthesis inhibitor was found to markedly reduce edema and the cell changes of the injured spinal cord and to attenuate changes of substance P indicating an involvement of the peptide in the pathophysiology of spinal cord injury [12]. However, detailed mechanisms of the substance P induced pathology of the spinal cord are still unclear.

Receptors for substance P are present in the spinal cord [6], and recent experimental evidence suggests that the peptide induces a release of glutamate, probably via neurokinin 1 (NK1) receptors [3]. Observations in human astrocytoma cells have shown that substance P inhibits the glutamate uptake and stimulates the glutamate efflux from astrocytes thereby causing glutamate toxicity to adjacent neurons [1, 3, 18]. In addition, the peptide also inhibits uptake of cystine resulting in depletion of intracellular glutathione which may render cells more vulnerable to oxidative stress [3].

Oxidative stress is a most important factor of cell damage in spinal cord injury [17]. This is confirmed by the result that pretreatment with the new anti-oxidant compound H-290/51 [19] significantly attenuated edema formation, the microvascular permeability changes and cell injury in our model of spinal cord injury [5, 14, 19]. The mechanisms underlying anti-oxidants to afford neuroprotection are not well known. This investigation is undertaken to study the involvement of the substance P degrading enzyme, SP endopeptidase (SPE), in spinal cord injury using a sensitive radioimmunoassay technique. Furthermore, in order to understand the relationship between substance P metabolism and oxidative stress, the influence of the new antioxidant compound H-290/51 was examined on SPE activity following spinal cord injury.

Materials and Methods

Animals

The experiments were carried in 20 Sprague-Dawely rats (Alab, Stockholm) housed at controlled temperature ($21 \pm 1 °C$) with a 12 h light and 12 h dark schedule. The rats received food and tap water *ad libitum*.

Spinal Cord Injury

Under equithesin anaesthesia (3 ml/kg, i.p.) a segment laminectomy was carried out at T10-11 level as described previously [9–14]. Briefly, a longitudinal incision (about 2 mm deep and 5 mm long) was made in the right dorsal horn and the wound was covered with cotton soaked in 0.9% saline. The experiments were approved by the Ethical Committee of Uppsala University.

The SPE activity was assessed in extracts of the injured segments, T10-11, and of the immediate cranial, T9, and caudal, T12, segments as well as of segments located far away from the injury site, T4 and C5 (n = 5). In separate groups of rats (n = 10) the antioxidant H290/51 (Astra, Hässle, Mölndal, Sweden) was given orally (50 mg/kg). SCI was made in 5 animals 30 min after drug administration [5, 14]. Control animals treated with H 290/51 (n = 5) were sacrificed after 5.5 h. SPE activity was also examined in normal untreated control animals (n = 5).

Recovery of Substance P Converting Ezyme (SPE)

The spinal cord samples were homogenised in 1 ml 50 mM Na-phosphate buffer, at pH 7.4, with a motor-driven teflon pestle. The resulting homogenate was centrifuged ($10.000 \times g$, 10 min) and the supernatant was used for SPE-activity measurement.

Substance P Endopeptidase Assay

The conversion of SP to its N-terminal fragment was followed by a radioimmunoassay specific for the product, SP_{1-7}. Five µl (1:10 dilution) of the enzyme-containing supernatant were preincubated for 15 min at 37° in a volume of 50 µl, 50 mM Na-phosphate buffer, pH 7.4 in the presence of phosphoramidon 20 µM, amastatin 20 µM and captopril 10 µM. Following addition of 37 pmoles synthetic SP, the incubation was continued for another 5 or 15 min. The reaction was terminated by boiling the samples for 3 min following addition of 60 µl MeOH / 0.1 M HCl 1:1 and analysed by radioimmunoassay, as described earlier [8].

Chemicals

Substance P was purchased from Bachem Feinchemikalien AG (Bubendorf, Switzerland). Substance P_{1-7} and $Tyr-SP_{1-7}$ were prepared by Dr. G. Lindeberg, Dept. of Immunology, University of Uppsala, Sweden and Dr. J. M. Stewart, Dept. of Biochemistry, University of Colorado, Denver, CO, USA, respectively. The protease inhibitors phosphoramidon and amastatin were purchased from Sigma (St. Louis, MO, USA), captopril was supplied by Calbiochem Corp. (La Jolla, CA, USA). All other chemicals and solvents were of analytical-reagent grade from commercial sources. SP_{1-7} was iodinated by the chloramine T-method [6, 8].

Influence of the Anti-Oxidant H-290/51

In separate groups of rats (n = 20) a new inhibitor of lipid peroxidation H 290/51 (Astra Hässle AB, Mölndal, Sweden), was given orally (50 mg/kg). This dose effectively inhibits lipid peroxidation in the CNS by more than 95% within 30 min. The effect will last for up to about 6 h after drug administration [5, 14].

Statistical Analysis

The data were analysed using ANOVA followed by the Dunnett test. A p-value less than 0.05 was considered to be significant.

Results

SPE in the Normal Spinal Cord

The normal SPE activity of the spinal cord varied from segment to segment. Accordingly, there was a significant difference in SPE activity in the T9, T10-11, T12 segments as compared to the C5 and T4 segments (Table 1).

SPE Following Trauma to the Cord

Infliction of trauma by making an incision into the right dorsal horn of the T10-11 segment resulted in marked up-regulation of the SPE activity in the segments rostral to the lesion. On the other hand, the injured and adjacent caudal segments exhibited a marked downregulation of the SPE activity (Table 1).

Table 1. *Substance P Endopeptidase in Spinal Cord Injury and its Modification by the Anti-Oxidant Compound H-290/51*. The drug was given orally (50 mg/kg) 30 min before spinal cord injury. Spinal cord injury was produced by making an incision into the right dorsal horn of the T10-11 segment under equithesin anaesthesia. The rats were allowed to survive 5 h after injury

Type of experiment	Converted substance P (1-7) fmol/µg protein/min (spinal cord) (n = 5)				
	C5	T4	T9	T10-11[a]	T12
Control	63.53 ± 2.78	56.52 ± 3.34	69.21 ± 0.66	107.83 ± 8.58	116.84 ± 6.38
H-290/51 + control	76.43 ± 7.04	59.31 ± 6.77	109.49 ± 4.46[c]	75.45 ± 3.75[c]	70.46 ± 3.31[b]
Spinal cord injury[a]	98.57 ± 2.42[b]	84.08 ± 5.17[b]	79.38 ± 13.53	75.02 ± 4.35[c]	76.94 ± 7.72[b]
H-290/51 + spinal cord injury	76.55 ± 6.04[d]	72.55 ± 2.93[b]	109.86 ± 7.65[c, d]	72.59 ± 4.13[c]	56.40 ± 0.98[c, d]

Values are mean ± SD.
[a] Site of lesion; [b] P < 0.05; [c] P < 0.01, compared to control; [d] P < 0.05, compared to spinal cord injury (Student's unpaired t-test).

SPE in Normal Rats after Treatment with H-290/51

Pretreatment with the new anti-oxidant compound H 290/51 which is neuroprotective against edema and cell changes in this model led to alterations of the SPE activity in the spinal cord in normal animals. A significant increase of the SPE activity was seen in the T9 segment, whereas the T10-11 and T12 segments showed a profound decrease (Table 1).

SPE Activity in Trauma in Rats with H-290/51

The enzyme activity was not significantly altered by the trauma in the drug treated rats. Compared to the untreated injured rats, pretreatment resulted in a significant downregulation of the SPE activity in the C5 and T12 segments (Table 1).

Discussion

Our results demonstrate for the first time that focal spinal cord injury causes widespread alterations in SPE activity. SPE has recently been characterised as metallodependent endopeptidase capable of releasing the N-terminal fragment SP_{1-7} and SP_{1-8} of substance P (SP), an undecapeptide with a putative function as transmitter in sensory nerve fibres [6, 8]. The enzyme appears to be highly specific for SP and is suggested to regulate the level of the peptide in the central nervous system (CNS). The present observation is in line with our previous report on marked alterations of the SP content of the cord in a similar trauma model [12]. The perifocal spinal cord segments with an altered metabolism of substance P showed profound edema and cell changes [6, 12]. Taken together, the results indicate strongly an involvement of the peptide in spinal cord pathology *in vivo*, which has not been reported earlier.

The mechanism of the substance P induced pathology of the spinal cord is as yet unclear. The activity of SPE and the level of its substrate are affected during chronic pain conditions [8]. It appears, however, that a decrease in substance P endopeptidases in some segments after trauma prolongs metabolism of the peptide [3, 4]. The peptide can induce release of glutamate via NK1 receptor activation, resulting cell changes may be attributable to glutamate toxicity [2, 18]. For further confirmation, blockade of NK1 receptors by selective pharmacological agents is needed which requires additional investigations.

The other most important finding of this study is that pretreatment with the antioxidant compound H-290/51 in normal rats led to significant changes of the SPE content of the cord in many regions. This may suggest that pretreatment with the anti-oxidant influences metabolism of substance P via modifying endopeptidase activity [1]. This is in line with the idea that substance P and the endopeptidase activity is associated with cellular oxidative stress [2].

The new compound H 290/51 is an inhibitor of lipid peroxidation [16, 19]. Accordingly, lipid peroxidation is inhibited by more than 95% in the dosage used for the present investigation. This is also supported by the finding that superoxide anion production at a maximal rate of cytochrome (III) C reduction in phorbol ester stimulated neutrophils with H 290/51 had no effect on O_2^- formation. It appears therefore that H 290/51 reduces secondarily radical formation produced by lipid peroxidation rather than acting as a scavenger of oxygen radicals [5]. Pretreatment with H-290/51 was reducing edema and cell changes of the traumatised cord and attenuated significantly the microvascular permeability increase [5, 14]. These effects suggest the agent to be neuroprotective in spinal cord injuries. The present study has further shown that pretreatment with

H-290/51 in normal rats causes alterations of the SPE activity, which was not affected by trauma, indicating that SPE is somehow involved in pathomechanisms of cell injury.

A decrease in a SPE-like enzyme is found in senile dementia of the Alzheimer type in human post-mortem brain. The activity was well correlated in the cerebral cortex with substance P [18]. Senile dementia of the Alzheimer type is associated with marked cell damage and neuronal loss [18]. It is possible that the reduced enzyme activity and the thereby prolonged half-life of substance P is associated with cell damage via glutamate toxicity. Our results with the anti-oxidant treatment showed an elevation of SPE in the T9 segment after spinal cord injury associated with a reduction in cell changes and edema formation, which is supporting the above hypothesis. We did not observe similar correlations in others segments, however. The cause of this discrepancy is not clear. Further studies using other pharmacological agents on measurement of SPE activity are needed to clarify this point.

In conclusion, our results show that a focal cord trauma induces widespread alterations in spinal cord SPE activity. The alteration of the enzyme activity can be influenced by the anti-oxidant H 290/51, indicating that SPE is somehow involved in traumatic cell injury, which has not been reported earlier.

Acknowledgements

This study is supported by grants from Swedish Medical Research Council nrs. 2710, 9459, 9710, Astra Hässle, Mölndal, Sweden; Göran Gustafsson Foundation, Sweden; Alexander von Humboldt Foundation, Bonn, Germany; The University Grants Commission, New Delhi, India. The technical assistance of Ingamarie Olsson, Kärstin Flink, Gunilla Tibling, Inga Hjörte and Ulla Johansson is highly appreciated.

References

1. Brouillet E, Hyman BT, Jenkins BG, Henshaw DR, Schulz JB, Sodhi P, Rosen BR, Beal MF (1994) Systemic or local administration of azide produces striatal lesions by an energy impairment-induced excitotoxic mechanism. Exp Neurol 129: 175–182
2. Calvet JH, Jarreau PH, Levame M, D'Ortho MP, Lorino H, Harf A, Macquin-Mavier I (1994) Acute and chronic respiratory effects of sulfur mustard intoxication in guinea pig. J Appl Physiol 76: 681–688
3. Johnson CL, Johnson CG (1993) Substance P regulation of glutamate and cystine transport in human astrocytoma cells. Receptors Channels 1: 53–59
4. Mauborgne A, Bourgoin S, Benoliel JJ, Hamon M, Cesselin F (1991) Is substance P released from slices of the rat spinal cord inactivated by peptidase(s) distinct from both 'enkephalinase' and 'angiotensin converting enzyme'? Neurosci Lett 123: 221–225
5. Mustafa A, Sharma HS, Olsson Y, Gordh T, Thóren P, Sjöquist P-O, Roos P, Adem A, Nyberg F (1995) Vascular permeability to growth hormone in the rat central nervous system after focal spinal cord injury. Influence of a new anti-oxidant H 290/51 and age. Neurosci Res 23: 185–194
6. Nyberg F, Sharma HS, Wiesenfeld-Hallin Z (1995) Neuropeptides in the spinal cord. Prog Brain Res 104: 1–430
7. Olsson Y, Sharma HS, Nyberg F, Westman J (1995) The opioid receptor antagonist naloxone influences the pathophysiology of spinal cord injury. In: Nyberg F, Sharma HS, Wiesenfeld-Hallin Z (eds) Prog Brain Res 104: 381–399
8. Persson S, Post C, Holmdahl R, Nyberg F (1992) Decreased neuropeptide-converting enzyme activities in cerebrospinal fluid during acute but not chronic phases of collagen-induced arthritis in rats. Brain Res 581: 273–282
9. Sharma HS, Olsson Y, Nyberg F (1995) Influence of dynorphin-A antibodies on the formation of edema and cell changes in spinal cord trauma. Prog Brain Res 104: 401–416
10. Sharma HS, Nyberg F, Thörnwall M, Olsson Y (1993) Met-Enkephalin-Arg6-Phe7 in spinal cord and brain following traumatic injury of the spinal cord: influence of p-chlorophenylalanine. An experimental study in the rat using radioimmunoassay technique. Neuropharmacology 32: 711–717
11. Sharma HS, Nyberg F, Olsson Y (1992) Dynorphin A content in the rat brain and spinal cord after a localized trauma to the spinal cord and its modification with p-chlorophenylalanine. An experimental study using radioimmunoassay technique. Neurosci Res 14: 195–203
12. Sharma HS, Nyberg F, Olsson Y, Dey PK (1990) Alteration in substance P in brain and spinal cord following spinal cord injury. An experimental study in the rat. Neuroscience 38: 205–212
13. Sharma HS, Olsson Y, Nyberg F, Dey PK (1993) Prostaglandins modulate alterations of microvascular permeability, blood flow, edema and serotonin levels following spinal cord injury. An experimental study in the rat. Neuroscience 57: 443–449
14. Sharma HS, Olsson Y, Thóren P, Sjöquist P-O (1995) H 290/51, a new inhibitor of lipid peroxidation reduces edema and microvascular permeability changes following trauma to the rat spinal cord. J Neurotrauma 12: 453
15. Sharma HS (1987) Effect of captopril (a converting enzyme inhibitor) on blood-brain barrier permeability and cerebral blood flow in normotensive rats. Neuropharmacology 26: 85–92
16. Svensson L, Börjesson I, Kull B, Sjöquist P-O (1993) Automated procedure for measuring TBARS for in vitro comparison of the effect of antioxidants on tissues. Scand J Clin Lab Invest 53: 83–85
17. Tator CH, Fehlings MG (1991) Review of the secondary injury theory of acute spinal cord trauma with emphasis on vascular mechanisms. J Neurosurg 75: 15–26
18. Waters SM, David TP (1995) Alterations of substance P metabolism and neuropeptidases in Alzheimer's disease. J Gerontol A Biol Sci Med Sci 50: B315–319
19. Weterlund C, Östlund-Lindqvist A-M, Sainsbury M, Shertzer HG, Sjöquist P-O (1996) Characterization of novel indenoindoles. Part I. Structure-activity relationships in different model systems of lipid peroxidation. Biochem Pharmacol 51: 1397–1402
20. Winkler T, Sharma HS, Stålberg E, Olsson Y, Nyberg F (1994) Opioid receptors influence spinal cord electrical activity and edema formation following spinal cord injury. Experimental observations using naloxone in the rat. Neurosci Res 21: 91–101

Correspondence: Hari Shanker Sharma, Ph.D., Laboratory of Neuroanatomy, Department of Anatomy, Box 571, Biomedical Centre, Uppsala University, S-75123 Uppsala, Sweden.

Acta Neurochir (1997) [Suppl] 70: 216–219
© Springer-Verlag 1997

Benzodiazepine Receptors Influence Spinal Cord Evoked Potentials and Edema Following Trauma to the Rat Spinal Cord

T. Winkler[1], **H. S. Sharma**[2], **E. Stålberg**[1], and **J. Westman**[2]

[1] Department of Clinical Neurophysiology, University Hospital, and [2] Laboratory of Neuroanatomy, Department of Anatomy, Biomedical Centre, Uppsala University, Uppsala, Sweden

Summary

The possibility that diazepam will influence spinal cord evoked potentials (SCEP), edema formation and cell changes following spinal cord injury (SCI) was examined in a rat model. The SCI was produced in equithesin anaesthetised animals by making a longitudinal incision (about 2 mm deep and 5 mm long) in the right dorsal horn of the T10-11 segments. The SCEP were recorded from the epidural space of the T9 segment after stimulation of the right tibial and sural nerves. The SCEP consisted of a small positive peak followed by a broad and high negative peak. Infliction of trauma to the rats resulted in an immediate and pronounced decrease of the maximal negative peak (MNP) amplitude. The spinal cord edema and cell changes were markedly pronounced 5 h after injury. Pretreatment with diazepam attenuated the early SCEP changes induced by the trauma and reduced the later development of edema and cell injury. These results suggest that benzodiazepine receptors are involved in trauma induced alterations in SCEP changes, edema formation and cell injury, not reported earlier.

Keywords: Spinal cord evoked potentials; edema; spinal cord injury; epidural space; morphology.

Introduction

Spinal cord conduction is altered following spinal cord injury as a result of altered bioelectricity of the spinal cord [3, 8]. Previous work from our laboratory revealed involvement of various neurochemicals present in the spinal cord dorsal horn in modulating spinal cord evoked potentials [13, 16, 22]. Thus inhibition of serotonin and prostaglandin biosynthesis prior to spinal cord injury influences SCEP and reduces edema development in our rat model [16, 22]. Likewise blockade of opioid receptors using very high dose of naloxone also attenuated SCEP disturbances and edema formation following spinal cord trauma [23]. Recently, biochemical evidence for presence of benzodiazepine receptors in the central nervous system

(CNS) was suggested, however, the physiological function of such receptors is not yet understood [2, 5, 10]. There are two subtypes of benzodiazepine receptors located in the CNS based on the binding of zolpidam (Type I) and diazepam (Type II) [5, 10]. However, binding of zolpidam is not detectable in spinal cord indicating that the spinal cord possess mainly type II benzodiazepine receptors [12]. About 80% of benzodiazepine binding sites in the spinal cord are of type II and the binding is potentiated by GABA indicating that this receptor is a part of the $GABA_A$-Cl^- and benzodiazepine receptor complex [18, 20]. In the dorsal horn of the spinal cord, neurotransmission is modulated by many neurochemicals involved in inhibitory synaptic mechanisms such as opiates, 5-HT, glycine and GABA receptors [1, 4, 6, 7, 11, 18]. Benzodiazepine receptors are present in superficial laminae of the dorsal horn on neurons involved in processing of nociceptive information probably by exerting an inhibitory influence on other neurochemical transmission [2, 5, 7, 9]. Activation of benzodiazepine receptors co-localised on the $GABA_A$-Cl^- receptor complex [9] modulates nociception and influences other neurochemical transmitters in the spinal cord [12, 18, 20]. However, the role of benzodiazepine receptors in modulating spinal cord conduction is still unknown.

Benzodiazepine receptors influence nociceptive input and modulate inhibitory neurochemical transmission [10, 18]. Thus, a possibility exists that stimulation of benzodiazepine receptors with diazepam, a benzodiazepine receptor agonist, will influence SCEP changes following a focal trauma to the rat spinal cord. Since diazepam is an anti-stress drug, it seems quite likely that pretreatment with this drug will attenuate traumatic stress response resulting in a less severe cell reaction and consequently edema formation following injury. In the present investigation we examined the influence of diazepam on spinal cord trauma induced SCEP alterations, edema formation and cell changes in our rat model.

Material and Methods

Experiments were carried out on 15 Sprague-Dawley male rats (350 and 400 g, Alab, Stockholm) housed at a controlled room temperature (22 ± 1°C), with a 12 h light and 12 h dark schedule. Food and water were given *ad libitum* before experiments. Under equithesin anaesthesia (3 ml/kg i.p.) spinal cord injury was inflicted by making a longitudinal incision (2 mm deep and 5 mm long extending to Rexed's laminae VII) with a sterile scalpel blade in the right dorsal horn of the T10-11 segments [14, 16]. With this type of lesion, tracts within the white matter are mainly unaffected by the trauma [16]. The study was approved by the Ethical Committee of Uppsala University. Recording electrodes were made from a 10 cm long copper wire (denuded outer diameter 0.1 mm), inserted into the lumen of a 7 cm polythene tubing (PE 10). The denuded 3 cm end of the wire was taken out through a hole made in the wall of the tubing (5 mm below the tip) and wound 12–15 turns around the tubing (covering 2.5 to 3 mm of the tubing). Openings were sealed with araldite. The electrical resistance of these unipolar electrodes was less than 0.11 Ohm [16, 22, 23]. The recording electrode was inserted from the laminectomized region and advanced rostrally in the epidural space to T9. SCEP was recorded after supramaximal stimulation (5–10 mA) of the right tibial and sural nerves at a frequency of 6 Hz, and with a stimulus duration of 0.1 msec. Two hundred responses were collected and averaged by an EMG equipment (Dantec Keypoint, filter 3 Hz–5 kHz, sweep duration 20 msec). SCEP recordings were made 30 min before (–30), 2 min before (–2), immediately after (0), and 2, 4, 10, 30, and 60 min after injury [16]. Maximal negative amplitude (MNP) of the SCEP amplitude were measured and used in statistical calculations [22, 23]. Five hours after injury, the injured spinal cord segments (T10-11) were removed and weighed immediately to obtain the wet weight of the sample. The samples were then placed in an oven at 90°C for 48 h to obtain the dry weight. The water content of the spinal cord was calculated from the difference between the dry and wet weights of the sample. An increase in water content was used as a measure of edema [14, 16]. Light microscopy of toluidine blue stained sections was used to evaluate the gross pathology of the spinal cord in untreated and diazepam treated rats 5 h after injury according to the standard protocol [15]. Diazepam (ampoule, Smith Kline & French, U.K.) was injected subcutaneously (4 mg/kg) once 30 min before injury [17] and SCEP changes and water content were measured (n = 6). In the calculations, MNP amplitudes in each group measured 30 min before injury were set to 100%. Comparisons were then made for each parameter between 2 min and each recording time, and for each recording time between groups [16]. ANOVA followed by Fisher and Dunnett test was used in statistical calculations. P values less than 0.05 were considered significant.

Results

SCEP Changes in Spinal Cord Injury

The SCEP was markedly altered after spinal cord injury. In one animal MNP decreased to zero immediately (0 min) after injury and a positive injury potential

was seen. The depression of MNP showed some recovery in later recordings. Mean MNP showed a pronounced post- injury decrease (about 60%) which persisted throughout the recording period.

Effect of Diazepam

Pretreatment with diazepam markedly attenuated post injury SCEP changes. Thus the MNP did not show any significant diminution after injury in diazepam treated rats compared to the untreated group. However, the increase in SCEP latency was not influenced by diazepam treatment. The SCEP latency continued to increase after injury in both drug-treated and untreated groups.

Spinal Cord Edema

Edema formation after 5 h injury as seen by measurement of the water content was significantly attenuated

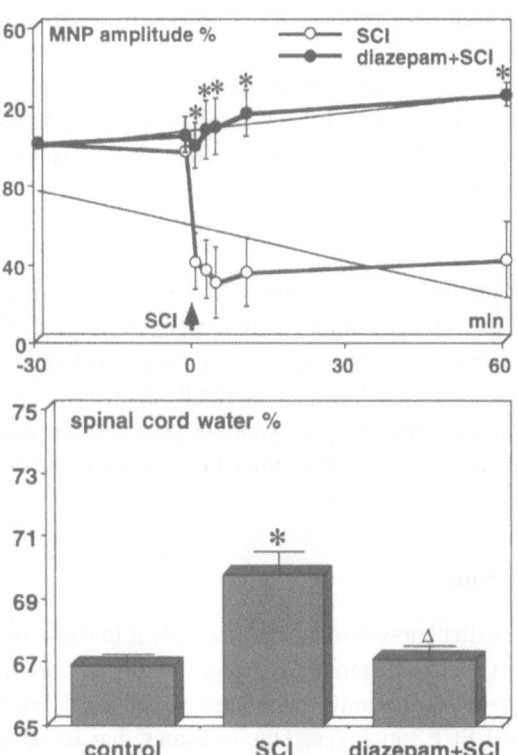

Fig. 1. Mean negative amplitudes (MNP) after spinal cord injury (SCI, arrow) in untreated (open circle) and diazepam pretreated (filled circle) animals. Straight thin lines are mathematical curve fit showing trend of MNP in untreated (downwards) and diazepam treated (upwards) rats after SCI. Upper: * p < 0.05, compared from SCI (ANOVA followed by Dunnet's test). Influence of diazepam on water content of the spinal cord segments (T10-11) at 5 h is shown below. Lower: * p < 0.05, compared from control group. Δ p < 0.05, compared from SCI

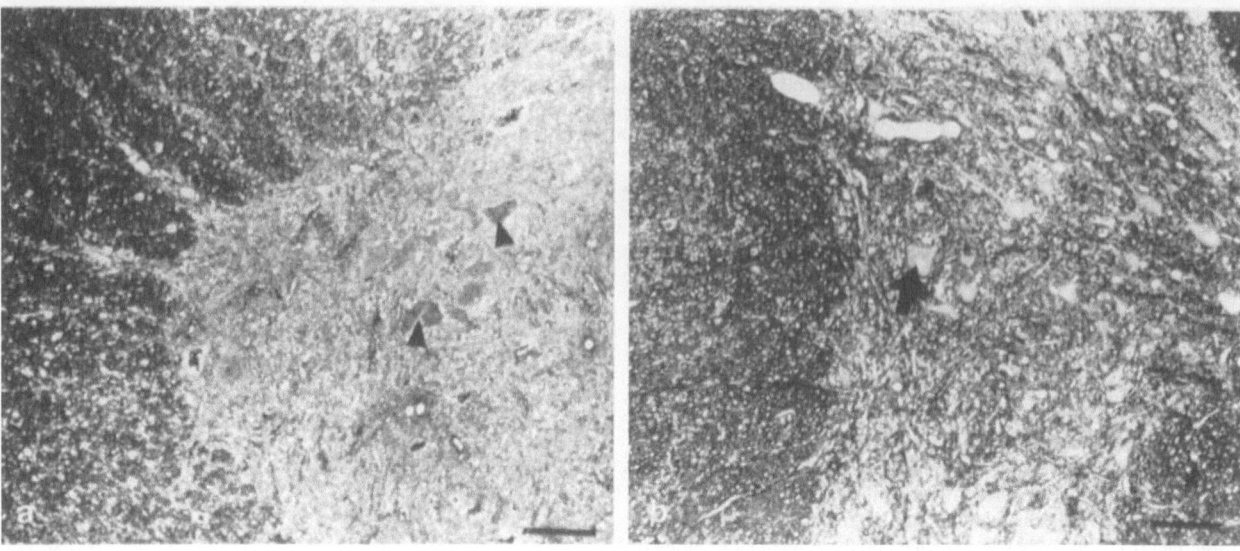

Fig. 2. Cell changes in the ventral horn of the T9 segment of one untreated (a) and one diazepam treated injured rat (b). Untreated traumatised rat showed many damaged and distorted neurons (arrow), whereas diazepam treated animal exhibited markedly less cell changes (bar = 80 μm)

in rats treated with diazepam compared to untreated traumatised rats. Thus the water content of the traumatised but untreated rats was elevated by 4% from the control values. On the other hand the water content of the spinal cord injured rats receiving diazepam before injury was only 1% higher than in the control group.

Spinal Cord Pathology

Morphological examination of 5 h spinal cord injured rats showed marked distortion of nerve cells, edema and general sponginess of the cord (Fig. 2a). Pretreatment with diazepam markedly attenuated these nerve cell changes (Fig. 2b) and the general expansion of the cord was less pronounced compared to the untreated traumatized rats.

Discussion

The salient new findings of this study is that stimulation of benzodiazepine receptors with its agonist diazepam significantly attenuates spinal cord injury induced SCEP changes. This indicates that benzodiazepine receptors participate in the spinal cord conduction, not reported earlier. The probable mechanisms by which benzodiazepine receptors influence SCEP is not further analyzed in this study. A possibility exists that diazepam can inhibit the "spinal shock" caused by trauma [18] due to its anti-stress effects in the CNS [17]. Spinal shock is a major contributor of SCEP disturbances in wide variety of spinal cord disturbanc-

es following trauma, ischemia or surgical manipulation [3, 6, 8, 13]. Thus a reduction in spinal shock will reduce SCEP abnormalities following injury. In addition, inhibitory influence of many neurochemicals [18], potentiation of the effects of inhibitory neurotransmitters such as GABA and glycine [20, 21] and reduction of traumatic stress [11, 17] by diazepam could play other important roles.

There are evidences that intrathecal or intravenously administered diazepam attenuates the responses in anterolateral quadrant neurons in the dorsal horn evoked by A- and C-fibre stimulation of the sural nerve in spinal rats [2, 7]. A-δ fibre evoked responses, but not C-fibre responses were depressed in convergent neurons of the dorsal horn following intravenous administration of misazolam, another benzodiazepine agonist [2, 9–11]. These observations suggest that benzodiazepines influence neuronal activity in the dorsal horn of the spinal cord following peripheral noxious or nonnoxious stimuli. It may be that benzodiazepine receptors also influence neuronal activity following spinal cord injury in the dorsal horn.

Our observations are in line with the idea that benzodiazepines are known inhibitors of mono- and polysynaptic reflexes via an interaction with the GABA$_A$-Cl$^-$ receptor complex [9, 11, 12, 20]. The primary action of diazepam on convergent neurons during ischemia or injury may be due to its binding with benzodiazepine receptors [5,10]. However, an interaction of diazepam with other receptor systems is also possible. There are recent evidences suggesting that stimulation of benzodiazepine receptors influence 5-HT receptor system [17]. Diazepam pretreatment will inhibit 5-HT release in the CNS probably via mediating central serotonergic transmission or stress response [17, 18].

That diazepam pretreatment will attenuate stress response is further evidenced by the fact that pretreatment with this drug attenuates serotonin release following heat stress and immobilisation [15, 17] and results in a reduction of the breakdown of the blood-brain barrier caused by stress [17]. This indicates that the antistress effect of the drug plays an important role in mediating stress induced disturbances of microvascular permeability.

In conclusion, our results show that pretreatment with diazepam reduces traumatic stress and attenuates spinal shock. These factors are important in preventing trauma induced changes in SCEP, edema formation and cell changes. Our results thus indicate an involvement of benzodiazepine receptors in the pathophysiology of traumatic injuries of the spinal cord and offer new possibilities of diazepam therapy in clinical usage where spinal cord handling is mandatory.

Acknowledgements

This investigation was supported by grants from the Swedish Medical Research Council project nos. 135 and 2710, the Göran Gustafsson Foundation, Sweden and the University Grants Commission, New Delhi, India. The skilful technical assistance of Ingamarie Olsson, Kärstin Flink, Gunilla Tibling, Inga Hjörte and Ulla Johansson is highly appreciated.

References

1. Balentine JD (1988) Spinal cord trauma: in search of the meaning of granular axoplasm and vesicular-myelin. J Neuropathol Exp Neurol 47: 77–92
2. Cartmell SM, Mitchell D (1994) Diazepam attenuates hyperexcitability and mechanical hypersensitivity of dorsal horn convergent neurons during reperfusion of the rat's tail following ischemia. Brain Res 659: 82–90
3. Ducker TB, Brown RH (1989) Neurophysiology and standards of spinal cord monitoring. Elsevier, Amsterdam
4. Faden AI, Salzman S (1992) Pharmacological strategies in CNS trauma. Trends Pharmacol Sci 13: 29–35
5. Faull RLM, Villiger JW (1986) Benzodiazepine receptors in the human spinal cord: a detailed anatomical and pharmacological study. Neuroscience 17: 791–802
6. Fehlings MG, Tator CH, Linden RD (1989) The relationships among the severity of spinal cord injury, motor and somatosensory evoked potentials and spinal cord blood flow. Electroenceph Clin Neurophysiol 74: 241–259
7. Goodchild CS, Serrao JM (1987) Intrathecal midazolam in the rat: evidence for spinally-mediated analgesia. Br J Anaesth 59: 1563–1570
8. Homma S, Tamaki T (1984) Fundamentals and clinical applications of spinal cord monitoring. Saikon, Tokyo
9. McLean BI, McDonald RL (1988) Benzodiazepines but not b-carbolines, limit high frequency repetitive firing of action potentials of spinal cord neurons in cell culture. J Pharmacol Exp Ther 344: 789–795
10. Maguire PA, Davies MF, Villar HO, Loew GH (1992) Evidence for more than two central benzodiazepine receptors in the rat spinal cord. Eur J Pharmacol 214: 85–88
11. Nagi SH, Tseng DTC, Wang SC (1983) Effect of diazepam and other CNS depressants on spinal reflexes in cats: a study of the site of action. J Pharmacol Exp Ther 153: 344–351
12. Niddam R, Dubois A, Scatton B, Arbilla S, Langer SZ (1987) Autoradiographic localization of [^{3}H]zolpidem binding sites in the rat CNS: comparison with the distribution of [^{3}H] flunitrazepam binding sites. J Neurochem 49: 890–896
13. Salzman SK (1990) Neural monitoring. The prevention of intraoperative injury. Humana Press, New Jersey
14. Sharma HS, Olsson Y, Dey PK (1990) Early accumulation of serotonin in rat spinal cord subjected to traumatic injury. Relation to edema and blood flow changes. Neuroscience 36: 725–730
15. Sharma HS, Cervós-Navarro J (1990) Nimodipine improves cerebral blood flow and reduces brain edema, cellular damage and blood-brain barrier permeability following heat stress in young rats. In: Krieglstein J, Oberpichler H (eds) Pharmacology of cerebral ischemia 1990. CRC, Boca Raton, pp 303–310
16. Sharma HS, Winkler T, Stålberg E, Olsson Y, Dey PK (1991) Evaluation of traumatic spinal cord edema using evoked potentials recorded from the spinal epidural space. An experimental study in the rat. J Neurol Sci 102: 150–162
17. Sharma HS, Dey PK (1986) Influence of long-term immobilization stress on regional blood-brain barrier permeability, cerebral blood flow and 5-HT level in conscious normotensive young rats. J Neurol Sci 72: 61–76
18. Stratten WP, Barnes CD (1971) Diazepam and presynaptic inhibition. Neuropharmacology 10: 685–696
19. Tator CH, Fehlings MG (1991) Review of the secondary injury theory of acute spinal cord trauma with emphasis on vascular mechanism. J Neurosurg 75: 15–26
20. Vicini S (1991) Pharmacological significance of the structural heterogeneity of the GABA$_A$ receptor-chloride ion channel complex. Neuropsychopharmacology 4: 9–21
21. Willis WD (1980) Spinal cord potentials. In: Windle WF (ed) Spinal cord and its reaction to traumatic injury. Marcel Dekker, New York, pp 159–187
22. Winkler T, Sharma HS, Stålberg E, Olsson Y (1993) Indomethacin, an inhibitor of prostaglandin synthesis, attenuates alteration in spinal cord evoked potentials and edema after trauma to the spinal cord. An experimental study in the rat. Neuroscience 52: 1057–1067
23. Winkler T, Sharma HS, Stålberg E, Olsson Y, Nyberg F (1994) Opioid receptors influence spinal cord electrical activity and edema formation following spinal cord injury. Experimental observations using naloxone in the rat. Neurosci Res 21: 91–101

Correspondence: Hari Shanker Sharma, Ph.D., Laboratory of Neuroanatomy, Department of Anatomy, Box 571, Biomedical Centre, Uppsala University, S-75123 Uppsala, Sweden.

Acta Neurochir (1997) [Suppl] 70: 220–221
© Springer-Verlag 1997

Induction of Matrix Metalloproteinases Following Brain Injury in Rats

M. Shibayama[1], **H. Kuchiwaki**[1], **S. Inao**[1], **K. Ichimi**[1], **J. Yoshida**[1], and **M. Hamaguchi**[2]

Departments of [1] Neurosurgery and [2] Molecular Pathogenesis, Nagoya University School of Medicine, Nagoya, Japan

Summary

Matrix metalloproteinases (MMPs) are important in various pathophysiological processes related with the tissue remodeling. We planned the experiments to determine whether MMPs participate in disruption and repair of the tissue following brain injury. We have studied induction of MMP-9, a 92 kilodalton (kDa) gelatinase, in traumatic brain tissue, which may be produced by brain residual cells. We speculate that MMP-9 plays a role in post-traumatic brain edema formation.

Keywords: Brain injury; metalloproteinase; extracellular matrix.

Introduction

Severe brain injury is followed by brain edema and modification of the tissue, although underlying mechanisms are not entirely clear yet. Matrix metalloproteinase (MMP) is a proteinase, degrading various components of the extracellular matrix [1]. Recently, it has been shown that MMP is involved in numerous pathophysiological processes, such as development, tumor cell invasion, or tissue remodeling [1]. Therefore, we suppose that MMP participates in brain edema formation and tissue repair after traumatic brain injury. In this study, we have examined MMP-9 in the injured brain.

Materials and Methods

Twenty-eight male rats were used for the experiments. After anesthesia, a craniectomy was made and a cortical stab wound stereotactically induced in the right brain hemisphere with a knife. At 3, 6, 12, 24, 48 hours, and 4 and 7 days after the operation, the rats were sacrificed by cardiac perfusion with saline for removal of the brain. The injured and corresponding contralateral brain was trimmed and weighed.

Then serum-free conditioned medium was added at a final concentration of 100 mg/ml, and the specimen was stored at 4°C for 48 hours. Supernatants were sampled and stored at –80°C until use. We have also obtained serum-free conditioned medium of a cultured human glioma cell line, U251-SP, which was incubated at 37°C for 48 hours with 15 ng/ml phorbol-12-myristate-13-acetate. We have performed then zymography and immunoblotting to determine the characteristics of MMP in the sample. We have also examined the time course of the activity by zymography, which was estimated by using an image analyzer. For statistical assessment, analysis of variance (ANOVA) was carried out by Fisher's protected least significant difference (PLSD) test. Statistical significance was assumed at $p < 0.05$. We have also studied the immunohistochemical localization of the enzyme in the brain sections (10 μm in thickness) using antibodies against MMP-9.

Results

We have determined the MMP-9 activity by gelatin zymography. Activity with 92 kilodalton (kDa) was found in the injured brain samples, as compared to the contralateral side and non-operated-control brain. We have also noticed activity with 72 kDa which, however, was also found in the control brain at almost the same intensity.

Further, we have studied the characteristics of the 92 kDa activity. For that purpose, the samples were added with p-aminophenylmercuric acetate (APMA), an organomercuric compound. APMA cleaves MMP-propeptide resulting in an active form of MMP [5]. Addition of APMA led to the appearance of molecular weight bands below 92 or 72 kDa, respectively. Incubation with 1,10-phenanthroline, a metal chelating agent, eliminated the activity of MMP. These results indicate that the gelatinolytic bands are caused by MMP. Moreover, by immunoblotting, the 92 kDa activity of the glioma cell line U251SP was identified as MMP-9. Because the 92 kDa activity in the brain was comparable to that of the glioma conditioned medium, we conclude that the injured brain samples contained MMP-9. Further, the 72 kDa activity was assumed to represent MMP-2.

In addition, we have studied the time course of MMP-9 by zymography. For that purpose, the gelati-

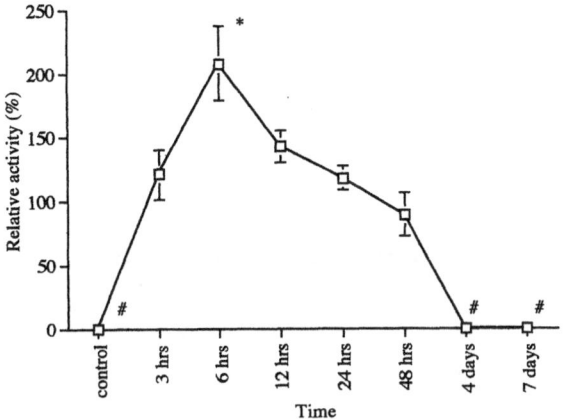

Fig. 1. MMP-9 was induced and detectable between 3 hours and 48 hours after the injury using gelatin zymography. As seen, the activity reached a maximum at 6 hrs. The increase in activity was statistically significant (ANOVA; $p < 0.001$). The value at 6 hrs (*) is significantly higher than that of any other time point (Fisher's PLSD; $p < 0.05$), n = 3 at each time point. At other time points (#) MMP-9 was not detectable by the image analyzer

nolytic activities were assessed by an image-analyzer, and statistically evaluated (Fig. 1). MMP-9 was undetectable in the control brain. It appeared at 3 hours after injury, and was reaching a maximum at 6 hours. It was decreasing then until 48 hours. By 4 days, the activity had disappeared. The changes in activity were statistically significant. On the other hand, the enzyme activity in the contralateral brain was not changing at all.

In order to examine MMP-3 activity, casein zymography was performed. It was confirmed thereby, using immunoblotting that glioma conditioned medium contains MMP-3. We have also noticed activity at 45 kDa in the brain samples, but were unable this to further characterize.

Finally, we have determined localization of MMP-9 by immunohistochemical staining. We found that the intra- and extracellular activities were restricted to the area around the wound. Histology was indicating that the MMP-9 positive cells were glia and neurons according to size and shape. Emigrating neutrophils had no activity.

Discussion

Brain injury promotes vasogenic edema early after trauma reaching a maximum at 24 hours [4]. In this context it is known that MMP-9 degrades type 4 collagen and laminin [2], which are localized in the basal membrane surrounding endothelium MMP-9 was found to increase vascular permeability in various cerebral disorders [3]. In our study, we have observed an increase of MMP-9 early after a cerebral stab wound. We suppose therefore that resident cells in the brain parenchyma produced MMP-9, which might participate in post-traumatic brain edema formation.

On the other hand, MMP-3 was not identified in the injured brain parenchyma. Nevertheless, we presume that proteases, like MMPs or serine proteases, may play a role during post-traumatic tissue remodeling.

In conclusion, we have provided evidence on the induction of MMP-9 in injured brain tissue. We postulate that MMP-9 participates in the formation of post-traumatic vasogenic brain edema.

References

1. Ennis BW, Martisian LM (1994) Matrix degrading metalloproteinase. J Neurooncol 18: 105–109
2. Morodomi T, Ogata Y, Sasaguri Y, Morimatsu M, Nagase H (1992) Purification and characterization of matrix metalloproteinase 9 from U937 monocytic leukaemia and HT1080 fibrosarcoma cells. Biochem J 285: 603–611
3. Rosenberg GA, Estrada EY, Dencoff JE, Stetler-Stevenson WG (1995) Tumor necrosis factor-α-induced gelatinase B causes delayed opening of the blood-brain-barrier: an expanded therapeutic window. Brain Res 703: 151–155
4. Schneider GH, Hennig S, Lanksch WR, Unterberg A (1994) Dynamics of post-traumatic brain swelling following a cryogenic injury in rats. Acta Neurochir (Wien) [Suppl] 60: 437–439
5. Stetler-Stevenson WG, Krutzsch HC, Wacher MP, Margulies IMK, Liotta LA (1989) The activation of human type IV collagenase proenzyme. J Biol Chem 265: 1353–1356

Correspondence: Mikine Shibayama, M.D., Department of Neurosurgery, Nagoya University School of Medicine, Turumai-cho 65, Showa-ku, Nagoya 466, Japan.

Acta Neurochir (1997) [Suppl] 70: 222–224
© Springer-Verlag 1997

Expression of Annexin and Annexin-mRNA in Rat Brain Under Influence of Steroid Drugs

P. H. Voermans[1], K. G. Go[1], G. J. ter Horst[2], M. H. J. Ruiters[3], E. Solito[4], and L. Parente[5]

[1] Department of Neurosurgery, [2] Biological Psychiatry, [3] Biomedical Technology Center, University Hospital Groningen, The Netherlands, [4] Institut Cochin de Génétique Moléculaire, Paris, France, and [5] Istituto di Farmacología e Farmacognosía, Palermo, Italy

Summary

Brain tissue of rats pretreated with methylprednisolone or with the 21-aminosteroid U74389F, and that of untreated control rats, was assessed for the expression of Annexin-1 (Anx-1) and the transcription of its mRNA. For this purpose Anx-1 cDNA was amplified and simultaneously a T7-RNA-polymerase promotor was incorporated into the cDNA using Polymerase Chain Reaction (PCR). Then digoxigenin-11-UTP was incorporated into the transcribed cRNA with T7-RNA-polymerase. With this probe *in situ* hybridization was carried out in sections of the brain. The probe was visualized by an immunoassay using an anti-digoxigenin antibody conjugate. Anx-1 protein was assessed by means of immunohistochemistry using a polyclonal antibody. The various brain areas of the control animals showed an appreciable amount of Anx-1 at mRNA or protein level; on the other hand, the animals which had been pretreated with either steroid, showed a more intense Anx-1 mRNA signal than the controls in many areas. In the pretreated animals Anx-1 immunostaining was unchanged in cortex, basal ganglia, amygdala and septum, but more intense in hippocampus, hypothalamus and thalamus. In ependyma, choroid plexus, meninges, and vascular walls there was no Anx-1 mRNA transcription detectable. An opposite profile was shown by the Anx-1 immunoreactivity, the protein was present in control animals as well as the steroid-pretreated animals, suggesting that here the protein was either from systemic origin, or has diffused from adjacent structures. The results indicate that Anx-1 mRNA transcription is upregulated by either steroid, and that in the untreated animals there is a resting level of Anx-1 mRNA transcription, presumably reflecting physiological influences on Anx-1 expression.

Keywords: Annexin-1; lipocortin; steroids; *in situ* hybridization; PCR.

Introduction

Annexins (or lipocortins) are proteins, which are produced in various tissues, and which are capable of inhibiting the enzyme phospholipase A_2 (Solito *et al.* 1991; Parente and Solito 1994). Therefore, they are assumed to mediate the anti-inflammatory actions of glucocorticosteroids since phospholipase A_2 releases arachidonic acid from phospholipids, and arachidonic acid is the precursor of eicosanoids, many of which are involved as mediators of inflammation. In the brain, arachidonic acid has been shown to be released after ischemia and other insults, and to be capable of inducing brain edema (Chan *et al.* 1983). In a previous study we have demonstrated that in the steroid-untreated brain annexins only occur sporadically, whereas steroid treatment induced widespread annexin-immunoreactivity in various cerebral structures (Go *et al.* 1994).

Material and Methods

A group of untreated (control) rats, a group of rats pretreated with methylprednisolone (2 mg/kg), and a group of rats pretreated with the 21-aminosteroid U74389F (10 mg/kg) 24 and 2 hrs previously, were killed by perfusion fixation under anesthesia. Brain sections were made which were assessed for Annexin-1 (Anx-1) by immunohistochemistry using a polyclonal antibody, and for Anx-1 mRNA by *in situ* hybridization (CISH) with a digoxigenin-conjugated cRNA.

The probe for *in situ* hybridization was prepared by the Polymerase Chain Reaction (PCR), using 10 ng of Anx-1 human cDNA as a template (justified by the 87% homology with the murine sequence (Kovacic *et al.* 1991). The PCR primers had the following sequences:

antisense PV5   5'-ATGGCAATGGTATCAGAATTCCTC-3'
antisense T7-PV3 5'-ATTAATACGACTCACTATAGGG-PV3-3'
(Young *et al.* 1993)

The PCR mixture consisted of 10 µl PCR buffer (pH 9.0), 1 nmol start and stop primers, 10 µl dNTP mixture H_2O to final volume of 100 µl. The PCR mixture was preheated at 94°C for 5 min with the addition of 2.5 U Taq DNA polymerase. The PCR profile was 1 min 94°C, 1 min 60°C, and 1 min 72°C for 30 cycles.

Transcription of Digoxigenin-conjugated cRNA was performed using a reaction mixture: 1 µl PCR-product + 2 µl transcription buffer + 2 µl NTP-mixture + 63 U T7-RNA-polymerase. Incubation at 37°C (2 hrs) and arrest of reaction by 0.2 M EDTA pH 8.0, was

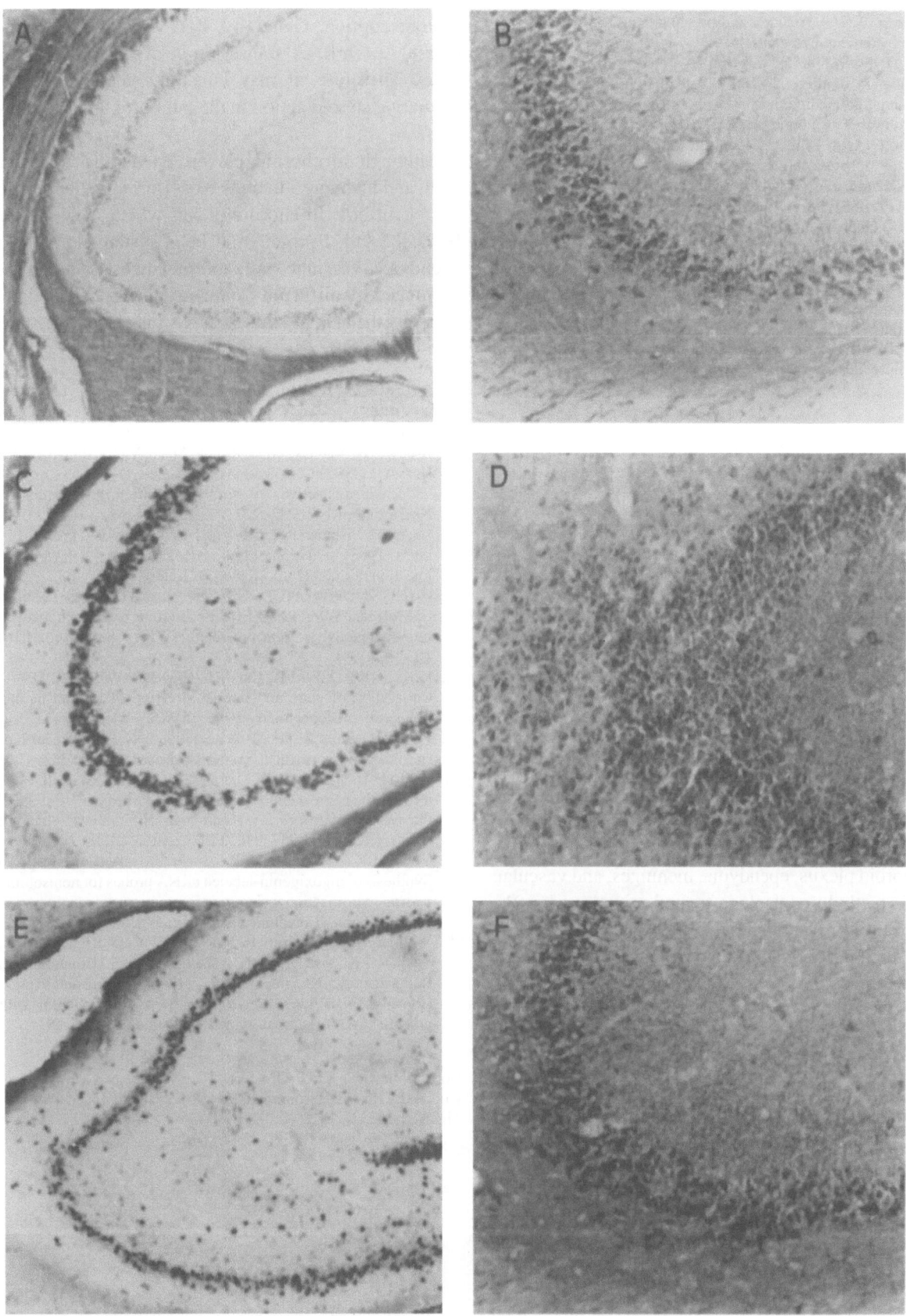

Fig. 1. Photomicrographs demonstrating Anx-1 mRNA by ISH using antisense digoxigenin-labeled cRNA (A, C and E), and immuno-reactive Anx-1 (B, D and F) in the hippocampal CA3 area of untreated controls (A and B), of methylprednisolone-pretreated (C and D), and of 21-aminosteroid-pretreated rats (E and F)

followed by RNA extraction and precipitation. The product was verified by the required controls.

In situ hybridization for Anx-1 mRNA detection was conducted by incubation of the slides in 100 µl of hybridization mixture (containing 1 µg/ml digoxigenin-labeled cRNA probe), overnight at 65°C, followed by immunological detection of the digoxigenin-labeled cRNA: the slides were incubated with anti-digoxigenin alkaline phosphatase conjugated antibody (1: 500), and presence of the phosphatase was visualized by means of a solution containing 45 µl of 90 mM Nitro Blue Tetrazolium salt + 35 µl 120 mM 5-bromo-4-chloro-3-indolylphosphate toluidinium salt in dimethylformamide (Brouwer *et al.* 1992; Wallner *et al.* 1986).

Immunocytochemical detection of Anx-1 was performed on free floating 40 µm thick sections incubated with polyclonal rabbit antibody raised against the amino terminus of Anx-1 (1:40) for 18 hrs, the secondary antibody (goat anti-rabbit 1:800) for 4 hrs, rabbit peroxidase-antiperoxidase (1:500) for 2 hrs, and finally the reaction product was visualized with nickel-diaminobenzidine.

Results

ISH demonstrated in the control animals transcription of Anx-1 mRNA in: cerebral cortex layers 2–6, olfactory bulb, nuclei of amygdala, hippocampus (CA$_1$, CA$_2$, CA$_3$, dentate gyrus), septum, striatum, and scattered cells in hypothalamus and thalamus. In methylprednisolone-treated animals there was transcription of Anx-1 mRNA in the same areas as in the controls, but far more intense. In 21-aminosteroid-treated animals the transcription of Anx-1 mRNA was similar to that in methylprednisolone-treated animals, and also far more intense than in controls (see Fig. 1).

As shown by immunocytochemistry the expression of Anx-1 in control animals was located in: the cerebral cortex (layers 2 and 5), basal ganglia, amygdala, hippocampus, hypothalamus, thalamus, furthermore in the choroid plexus, ependyma, meninges, and vascular wall. In methylprednisolone-treated animals and in 21-aminosteroid-treated animals there was increased immunostaining only in the hippocampus, hypothalamus, and thalamus.

Discussion

Presence of Anx-1 mRNA and Anx-1 immunostaining in control animals probably reflect resting levels of transcription. Generally, both steroid classes increase Anx-mRNA transcription in the same structures. Therefore, it may constitute the mechanism mediating steroid action in the inhibition of phospholipase A$_2$.

Although in choroid plexus, ependyma, vascular wall, and meninges, there is Anx-1 protein, there is no Anx-1 mRNA. In choroid plexus which is devoid of BBB, the Anx-1 protein may be of systemic origin. In ependyma, vascular wall, and meninges, it may have originated by diffusion from surrounding cells. Alternatively, the lack of Anx-1 mRNA may be due to rapid turn-over.

References

1. Brouwer N, Van Dyken H, Ruiters MHT, Van Willigen JD, ter Horst GJ (1992) Localization of dopamine D$_2$ receptor mRNA with non-radioactive *in situ* hybridization histochemistry. Neurosci Lett 142: 223–227
2. Chan PH, Fishman RA, Caronna J, Schmidley JW, Prioleau G, Lee J (1983) Induction of brain edema following intracerebral injection of arachidonic acid. Ann Neurol 13: 625–632
3. Go KG, Zuiderveen F, De Ley L, ter Haar JG, Parente L, Solito E, Molenaar WM (1994) Effect of steroids on brain lipocortin immunoreactivity. Acta Neurochir (Wien) [Suppl] 60: 101–103
4. Kovacic RT, Tizard R, Cate RL, Frey AZ, Wallner B (1991) Correlation of gene and protein structure of rat and human lipocortin 1. Biochemistry 30: 9015–9021
5. Parente L, Solito E (1994) Association between glucocorticosteroids and lipocortin 1. Trends Pharmacol Sci 15: 362
6. Solito E, Raugei G, Melli M, Parente L (1991) Dexamethasone induces the expression of the mRNA of lipocortin 1 and 2 and the release of lipocortin 1 and 5 in differentiated, but not undifferentiated U-937 cells. FEBS Lett 291: 238–244
7. Young ID, Stewart RJ, Ailles L, MacKie A, Gore J (1993) Synthesis of digoxigenin-labeled cRNA probes for nonisotopic *in situ* hybridization using reverse transcription polymerase chain reaction. Biotechnic Histochem 68: 153–158
8. Wallner BP, Mattalino RJ, Hesion C, Cate RL, Tizard R, Sinclair LK, Foeller C, Pingchang Chow E, Browning JL, Ramachandran KL, Pepinsky RB (1986) Cloning and expression of human lipocortin, a phopholipase A$_2$ inhibitor with potential anti-inflammatory activity. Nature 320: 77–81

Correspondence: K. G. Go, M.D., Department of Neurosurgery, University Hospital Groningen, Hanzeplein 1, Groningen 9700 RB, The Netherlands.

Acta Neurochir (1997) [Suppl] 70: 225–227
© Springer-Verlag 1997

Role of Protein Kinase C in Acidosis Induced Glial Swelling – Current Understanding

R. C. C. Chang[1], **N. Plesnila**[1], **F. Ringel**[1], **C. Grönlinger**[1], **F. Staub**[2], and **A. Baethmann**[1]

[1] Institute for Surgical Research, Klinikum Grosshadern, University of Munich, Germany, and [2] Department of Neurosurgery, University of Cologne, Federal Republic of Germany

Summary

A major factor in secondary brain injury following cerebral trauma is accumulation of lactic acid resulting in glial swelling. Further, evidence obtained in this context demonstrates activation of protein kinase C (PKC) under these circumstances. Glial swelling from acidosis is attributable to activation of the Na^+/H^+-exchanger, mediating influx of Na^+-ions in exchange for the extrusion of H^+ ions. The antiporter is activated following phosphorylation by PKC. The current study was made to elucidate the role of PKC activation in acidosis-induced glial swelling. For that purpose, suspended C6 glioma cells were used to examine changes of the cell volume and intracellular pH (pH_i). Acidosis was induced by administration of isotonic lactic acid. Stimulation of PKC by the phorbol-ester PMA was significantly enhancing glial swelling from severe acidosis (pH 6.2), whereas the decrease of pH_i was somewhat attenuated. On the other side, inhibition of PKC by staurosporine did not affect cell swelling nor the decrease of pH_i from acidosis. The results indicate that activation of PKC in cerebral trauma or ischemia may enhance glial swelling from lactacidosis.

Keywords: Brain injury; lactic acidosis; protein kinase C; glial swelling.

Introduction

Cerebral trauma or ischemia has been shown to induce a massive increase of intracellular Ca^{2+}-ions and of free fatty acids [1,11]. These processes together with the release of the excitotoxic amino acid glutamate may profoundly affect second messenger systems of neuronal- and glial cells. A major second messenger system, protein kinase C (PKC), has been observed to become activated in experimental brain trauma [8, 12–13]. Under physiological conditions, stimulation of PKC is associated with translocation of the enzyme molecule from the cytosol into the cell membrane. Translocation of the enzyme into the cell membrane has also been demonstrated in brain injury or ischemia, respectively [8, 12–13]. The many biochemical and physiological functions of PKC notwithstanding clear evidence concerning the significance of its activation in traumatic or ischemic brain injury is not yet available, particularly whether this is a beneficial or detrimental response for the brain under these circumstances.

As in the case of PKC activation, accumulation of lactic acid is almost always found in cerebral trauma or ischemia. In cerebral ischemia it has been reported that glial cells may become more acidotic than the extracellular environment [5]. Previous studies of this laboratory have demonstrated that lactacidosis is a potent factor to initiate and sustain glial swelling in a dose-dependent manner [2]. The acidosis-induced swelling is mediated by activation of the Na^+/H^+-exchanger (NHE), which extrudes intracellular H^+-ions in exchange for Na^+-ions in a one-to-one ratio [6]. An involvement of the exchanger has been shown experimentally, e.g. in studies on the special inhibitor amiloride or omission of Na^+-ions from the medium which both were inhibiting the acidosis-induced cell swelling [4]. Energy for the Na^+/H^+ exchange process is provided by the down-hill movement of Na^+-ions across the cell membrane. The exchanger is activated by an increase of the intracellular H^+-ion concentration above the normal level, or decrease of pH_i, respectively. Enhancement of the activity of the exchanger is accomplished following phosphorylation by protein kinases, for example, PKC. Sequence analysis has indicated that phosphorylation by PKC mainly occurs at the C-terminus of the exchanger as activating step. Not all NHE isoforms, however, are activated by PKC, neither are the mechanisms of stimulation of the different NHE isoforms identical. In mammalian cells including those of brain tissue, NHE-1 is believed to be the most abundant "house-keeping" isoform. Nevertheless, mRNA of NHE-2 is also found in brain tissue. PKC activates NHE-1 by increasing the affinity of H^+-ions to the exchanger, while NHE-2 is stimulated by increasing its maximum velocity [6].

In brain trauma or ischemia, the massive increase of intracellular Ca^{2+}-ions and of free fatty acids can be considered to stimulate PKC, which in turn phosphorylates NHE. Since the NHE is an important factor of regulation of the intracellular pH, thus, of the cell volume, this study was carried out to elucidate the role of PKC in the acidosis-induced glial swelling.

Material and Methods

Details of the experimental protocol have been previously described [2]. In brief, C6 glioma cells were cultured in Dulbecco's minimum essential medium (DMEM, Seromed, Germany) supplemented with 10% fetal calf serum (Gibco-BRL, Germany) and 1% (100 U / 0.1 mg) Penicillin/Streptomycin (Seromed, Germany). For the experiment, the cells were harvested by trypsinization, suspended and incubated in a plexiglass chamber. The suspension medium was equilibrated with O_2, N_2, CO_2. Temperature and pH of the medium were tightly controlled.

The cell volume was measured by flow cytometry utilizing an advanced Coulter method. The cell sizing system (Metricell®) was calibrated with plastic beads of known size. The intracellular pH (pH_i) was measured by flow cytometry utilizing the pH-dependent fluorescence indicator, BCECF-AM, the membrane permeable ester form (Molecular Probes, U.S.A.). Cells were incubated with BCECF-AM for 20 minutes at 37°C. Thereafter, pH_i was calibrated by incubating cell aliquots at 8 different pH levels in medium with a high K^+-concentration containing nigericin. The BCECF fluorescence was excited at 488 nm wavelength by a mercury arc lamp, while the fluorescence emission was recorded at 520 nm (F_2, pH-dependent) and 630 nm (F_1, pH-independent) and expressed as F_2/F_1 ratio. By utilizing assessment of the fluorescence emission ratio problems, such as leakage of fluorochromes or bleaching were minimized.

In order to elucidate the role of PKC the activator phorbol 12-myristate 13-acetate (PMA) and the inhibitor staurosporine were employed. Cells were incubated with either PMA or staurosporine for 30 minutes at 37°C at a different dose but normal pH. Acidosis was induced by adminstration of lactic acid lowering the medium pH from 7.4 to 6.8, or to 6.2, representing "mild" or "severe" acidosis, respectively. After 60 minutes, the suspension medium was neutralized to pH 7.4 by administration of 1N NaOH.

Results and Discussion

The intracellular pH (pH_i) of glial cells under physiological conditions was between 7.13 ± 0.02 and 7.19 ± 0.03 (n = 13). pH_i fell to 6.74 ± 0.02 (n = 6) in mild acidosis (medium pH: 6.8), or to 6.31 ± 0.02 (n = 7) in severe acidosis (medium pH: 6.2). The cell volume under control conditions did not change significantly

during 40 minutes. Upon induction of acidosis, glial cell swelling reached a maximum of $113 \pm 2\%$ (n = 7), or $122 \pm 2\%$ (n = 7) in mild or severe acidosis, respectively. Following neutralization of the medium pH, the cell volume of glial cells recovered, albeit imcompletely within 30 minutes.

Activation of PKC by PMA (100 nM or 500 nM) led to cellular alkalinization at normal medium pH. pH_i was increased by about 0.08 units. Hence, these experiments provide for first findings on the pH_i response of glial cell elements to activation of PKC under normal conditions using bicarbonate buffer. Further, activation of PKC by PMA appeared to inhibit or at least attenuate the fall of pH_i in acidosis. In severe acidosis, this effect required a higher PMA dose (500 nM). However, attenuation of the fall of pH_i by PMA notwithstanding, the acidosis-induced glial swelling (mild acidosis) reached the same maximum as without activation of PKC. The corresponding findings in severe acidosis were markedly different, however. Stimulation of PKC by 500 nM PMA resulted in a 10% enhancement of the glial swelling from severe acidosis as compared to the acidosis- induced swelling without PKC-activation.

At normal pH_i, inhibition of PKC by staurosporine did not significantly influence pH_i, whereas the agent led to shrinking of the glial cells by 3% or 10% at 0.4 or 4 µM, respectively. Shrinking of glial cells was apparently not a sequelae of apoptosis, as respective changes, for example membrane budding or DNA condensation was not observed. The extent of glial swelling from acidosis was not different in the experiments with

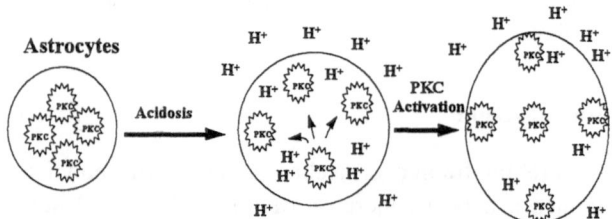

Acidosis-Induced Swelling   PKC Mediated Acidosis-Induced Swelling

Fig. 1. Significance of activation of protein kinase C in acidosis-induced glial swelling. Accordingly, brain tissue acidosis as evolving in cerebral ischemia or trauma causes swelling of glial cells in a dose-dependent manner. Acidosis may transiently translocate (i.e. activate) PKC from the cytosol into the cell membrane. Also other cytotoxic factors, for example glutamate, may activate PKC via metabotropic glutamate receptors. PKC upon activation may in turn phosphorylate the Na^+/H^+-exchanger, leading to enhancement of its activity. As the acidosis-induced glial swelling is mainly attributable to activation of the Na^+/H^+-exchanger, enhancement of its activity, thus, may augment the extent of cell swelling in acidosis

administration of staurosporine, whereas the recovery of the cell volume following pH neutralization was accelerated. pH_i was neither affected by inhibition of PKC with staurosporine in any phase of the experiment.

Taken together, the results demonstrate that activation of PKC by PMA results in both cellular alkalinization at normal pH and enhancement of glial swelling from severe acidosis. These effects most likely were mediated by activation of the Na^+/H^+-exchanger, as the observed changes of the intracellular pH and the cell volume can be attributed to this mechanism. Conversely, it has been demonstrated that inhibition of PKC by H-7 has a therapeutic effect on brain edema in an animal model of cerebral ischemia [3].

It is well known that acidosis is an important factor in ischemic and traumatic brain injury. In a recent report [7] it was confirmed again that tissue acidosis develops already within minutes after onset of ischemia. In this time span also other cytotoxic factors may come into play, for example glutamate which stimulates PKC via binding to its AMPA- and NMDA-receptor, resulting in influx of Ca^{2+}-ions, or to the metabotropic glutamate receptors. The metabotropic glutamate receptor is a $mGlu_5$ gene product of glial cells [10] coupled to the $Ins(1,4,5)P_3$-Ca^{2+} signal transduction system. In addition, acidosis per se may induce an increase of $[Ca^{2+}]_i$ [9], which in turn could stimulate PKC. Our results demonstrate that once PKC is stimulated, it can markedly enhance glial swelling from acidosis (Fig. 1). Although the stimulation of PKC by PMA was partly inhibiting the fall of pH_i from acidosis, its activation in ischemically and traumatically injured brain may be considered as a detrimental factor in view of the enhancement of the acidosis-induced cell swelling. Activation of PKC in brain tissue may be deleterious also in other pathophysiological conditions, such as status epilepticus due to the development of tissue acidosis.

Whereas activation of PKC enhances glial swelling from acidosis, inhibition of PKC is not necessarily protecting glial cells against swelling, as currently demonstrated in the experiments using the serine/threonine protein kinase inhibitor staurosporine, which did not affect cell swelling from acidosis. This may indicate either that PKC only is a facultative regulator of the Na^+/H^+-exchanger, implying that inhibition of PKC does not affect activity of the exchanger, or that other transport mechanisms not controlled by PKC are also involved in the acidosis-induced swelling process. The

present findings are promising, nevertheless, to further explore the physiological and pathological significance of PKC activation in ischemic and traumatic brain injury.

Acknowledgement

The authors appreciate the excellent technical advice of Dr. J. Peters in pH- and cell volume measurement, and the technical assistance of Ingrid Kölbl. The project is supported by a grant (Sta 406 2/1) from German Research Council (DFG). R.C.C. Chang has been awarded a fellowship from the German Academic Exchange Service.

References

1. Baethmann A, Maier-Hauff K, Kempski O, Unterberg A, Wahl M, Schürer L (1988) Mediators of brain edema and secondary brain damage. Crit Care Med 16: 972–978
2. Chang RCC, Plesnila N, Staub F, Peters J, Haberstok J, Baethmann A (1995) Glial cell volume and pH-response to acidosis – underlying mechanisms. J Cereb Blood Flow Metab 15 [Suppl 1]: 570
3. Joó F, Tósaki A, Olah Z, Koltai M (1989) Inhibition by H-7 of the protein kinase C prevents formation of brain edema in Sprague-Dawley CFY rats. Brain Res 490: 141–143
4. Kempski O, Staub F, Jansen M, Schödel F, Baethmann A (1988) Glial swelling during extracellular acidosis in vitro. Stroke 19: 385–392
5. Kraig RP, Chesler M (1990) Astrocytic acidosis in hyperglycemic and complete ischemia. J Cereb Blood Flow Metab 10: 104–114
6. Levine SA, Montrosse MH, Tse CM, Donowitz M (1993) Kinetics and regulation of three cloned mammalian Na^+/H^+-exchangers stably expressed in a fibroblast cell line. J Biol Chem 268: 25527–25535
7. Li PA, Kristian T, Shamloo M, Siesjö BK (1996) Effects of pre-ischemic hyperglycemia on brain damage incurred by rats subjected to 2.5 or 5 minutes of forebrain ischemia. Stroke 27: 1592–1602
8. Padmaperuma B, Mark R, Dhillon HS, Mattson MP, Prasad MR (1996) Alterations in brain protein kinase C after experimental brain injury. Brain Res 714: 19–26
9. OuYang YB, Mellergard P, Kristian T, Kristianova V, Siesjö BK (1994) Influence of acid-base changes on the intracellular calcium concentration of neurons in primary culture. Exp Brain Res 101: 265–271
10. Porter JT, McCarthy KD (1995) GFAP-positive hippocampal astrocytes in situ respond to glutamatergic neuroligands with increases in $[Ca^{2+}]_i$. Glia 13: 101–112
11. Siesjö BK (1993) Basic mechanisms of traumatic brain damage. Ann Emerg Med 22: 959–969
12. Sun FY, Faden AI (1994) N-methyl-D-aspartate receptors mediate post-traumatic increases of protein kinase C in rat brain. Brain Res 661: 63–69
13. Yang K, Taft WC, Dixon CE, Todaro CA, Yu RK, Hayes RL (1993) Alterations of protein kinase C in rat hippocampus following traumatic brain injury. J Neurotrauma 10: 287–295

Correspondence: A. Baethmann, M.D., Institute for Surgical Research, Klinikum Grosshadern, University of Munich, Marchioninistrasse 15, D-81366 Munich, Federal Republic of Germany.

Acta Neurochir (1997) [Suppl] 70: 228–230
© Springer-Verlag 1997

Dependence of Basal Cerebral Blood Flow and Cerebral Vascular Resistance in Spontaneously Hypertensive Rats Upon Vasoconstrictor Prostanoids

M. Osęka and E. Koźniewska

Department of Clinical and Applied Physiology, School of Medicine, Warsaw, Poland

Summary

The effects of indomethacin (inhibitor of cyclooxygenase), imidazole (inhibitor of thromboxane A_2 synthase) and SQ 29548 (antagonist of TxA_2/PGH_2 receptors) on basal CBF and CVR were studied in normocapnic and normoxic SHR and WKY rats. CBF was measured by the intracarotid ^{133}Xe technique. CVR was calculated as ratio of mean arterial blood pressure and CBF. Resting CBF did not differ between SHR and WKY. MABP and CVR were significantly higher ($p < 0.01$) in SHR than in WKY. Indomethacin (6 mg/kg, i.v.) produced a significant long-lasting decrease of CBF and increase of CVR in both strains, although these effects were more pronounced ($p < 0.01$) in WKY. Imidazole (20 mg/kg, i.v.) had no effect on measured variables in either strain. SQ 29548 (1 mg/kg, i.v.) produced a significant increase of CBF in SHR ($p < 0.001$) but not in WKY. CVR decreased in SHR parallel to the increase of CBF but remained unchanged in WKY. Our results demonstrate that, in contrast to WKY, basal CBF and CVR in SHR depend upon vasoconstricting prostanoids which act on TxA_2/PGH_2 receptors but are distinct from thromboxane A_2.

Keywords: Cerebral blood flow; cerebral vascular resistance; thromboxane A_2/endoperoxide receptors; spontaneously hypertensive rats.

Introduction

Basal cerebral blood flow (CBF) in normotensive subjects, both in animals and man, depends on vasodilator prostanoids [9, 10]. Consequently, inhibition of the activity of cyclooxygenase with indomethacin results in a long-lasting reduction of CBF and increase of cerebral vascular resistance (CVR) without affecting cerebral metabolism. These effects are attributed to the decreased production of prostacyclin (PGI_2) in cerebral blood vessels, since PGI_2 represents the main cyclooxygenase-dependent product of the metabolism of arachidonic acid in blood vessels under physiological conditions which dilates blood vessels.

Experimental evidence based on results obtained with isolated peripheral blood vessels *in vitro* or cere-

bral blood vessels *in vivo* suggests that in essential hypertension (spontaneoulsy hypertensive rats) there is an increased vascular production of vasoconstrictor prostanoids or increased sensitivity of vascular thromboxane-endoperoxide receptors [1, 5] which may be responsible for the increase of vascular resistance associated with hypertension.

Aim of the present study was to examine the role of endogenous vasoconstrictor prostanoids in the maintenance of CBF and CVR in adult spontaneously hypertensive rats.

Material and Methods

Animal Models

The experiments were performed using male spontaneously hypertensive rats (SHR) and aged-matched Wistar-Kyoto rats (WKY) of 240–320 g b.w. The animals were anaesthetized with chloral hydrate (36 mg 100 g^{-1} body weight, i.p.), paralyzed with d-tubocurarin (0.05 mg 100 g^{-1} body weight, i.v.) and mechanically ventilated (Rodent Harvard Ventilator) through a tracheal tube with oxygen enriched air ($FiO_2 = 0.3$). Body temperature was maintained around 37°C with a heating pad. Both femoral arteries were cannulated for continuous measurement of mean arterial blood pressure (MABP) and for collecting of arterial blood samples for gasometric analysis (PaO_2, $PaCO_2$ and pH), the femoral vein was cannulated for drug administration and supplementation of anaesthesia.

Methods

CBF was measured using the intracarotid ^{133}Xe injection technique [3]. CBF was calculated from the initial slope (15 s) of the semilogarithmically displayed clearance curve and expressed in ml 100 $g^{-1}min^{-1}$. CVR was calculated as ratio of MABP to CBF and expressed in mmHg ml^{-1} 100 g min. Arterial blood pH and partial pressure of blood gases (PaO_2 and $PaCO_2$) were determined during each CBF measurement (AVL gas check 995-Hb, AVL).

Experimental Protocol

Three groups of experiments were performed in each strain of rats. In group 1 (WKY n = 8, SHR n = 8) the inhibitor of prostaglandin synthase, indomethacin (INDO, Sigma) dissolved in 4% glucose solution in 0.4% sodium carbonicum and buffered at pH = 7.4 with 0.05 M HCl, was injected in a dose of 0.6 mg /100 g body weight (0.1 ml/100 g, i.v.). In group 2 (WKY n = 6, SHR n = 7) the thromboxane A_2 (Tx A_2) synthesis inhibitor, imidazole (IMI, Sigma) was administered in a dose of 2 mg/100 g body weight (1 ml/100 g, i.v.). In group 3 (WKY n = 7, SHR n = 7) an antagonist of thromboxane/endoperoxide receptors, SQ 29548 (RBI) dissolved in 0.9% NaCl solution was given in a dose of 0.1 mg/100 g body weight (0.1 ml / 100 g, i.v.). CBF was measured and CVR was calculated at rest and every 15 min for 1 hr (group 1 and 2) or for 2 hrs (group 3) following administration of drugs. The effect of i.v. administration of 0.3 ml of 0.9% NaCl (vehicle of SQ 29548 and IMI) and 0.3 ml of buffered vehicle of INDO on CBF and MABP were studied in separate groups of four rats. Since neither saline nor the vehicle had an effect in any group, it was not administered to the rest of the animals.

Statistical Analysis

All data are presented as mean ± SD. Statistical differences were evaluated by analysis of variances (ANOVA) for repeated or independent measurements. Individual comparisons were analyzed using the Newman-Keuls and simple comparison tests. In the case of significant differences between control values, delta analysis was used. p values < 0.05 were considered statistically significant.

Results

Control CBF was not different in SHR (55 ± 5 ml/ 100 g/min) and WKY (59 ± 4 ml/100 g/min). There were, however, significant differences in MABP and in CVR between WKY and SHR. MABP in SHR (163 ± 6 mmHg) was higher (p < 0.001) than in WKY (92 ± 9 mmHg). CVR was also significantly higher (p < 0.001) in SHR (2.9 ± 0.2 mmHg min/ml/100 g) when compared with WKY (1.7 ± 0.1 mmHg min/ml/100 g). Both groups of rats were normoxic and normocapnic under control conditions (WKY: pH = 7.44 ± 0.02, $PaCO_2$ =34 ± 1 mmHg, PaO_2 = 118 ± 3 mmHg; SHR: pH = 7.43 ± 0.03, $PaCO_2$ = 35 ± 2 mmHg, PaO_2 = 120 ± 9 mmHg) and throughout the experiment.

INDO produced a significant long-lasting decrease of CBF (Fig. 1) and increase of CVR both in WKY and in SHR. Both effects were much more pronounced in WKY than in SHR (p < 0.01), MABP was not affected in either strain.

IMI did not affect CBF, MABP and CVR in either strain, whereas SQ 29548 albeit without an effect on CBF and CVR in WKY resulted in a substantial and long-lasting increase of CBF and decrease of CVR in SHR (Fig. 2). CBF in SHR increased progressively attaining a maximum (144% of control on average, p < 0.001) at 105 min after administration of the drug. At the same time CVR in SHR attained its minimum (72% of control on average, p < 0.001) and was not different from CVR in WKY. SQ 29548 did not affect MABP, neither in WKY nor in SHR.

Discussion

The main finding of our study is that vasoconstricting prostanoids, distinct from TxA_2, contribute to the maintenance of the basal tone of cerebral blood vessels in SHR, whereas in WKY the basal tone of cerebral blood vessels depends on vasodilating prostaglandins. This conclusion is based on the observation that administration of indomethacin resulted in a significantly greater decrease of CBF and increase of CVR in WKY than in SHR, whereas inhibition of TxA_2 synthesis did not affect CBF and CVR in either strain, and that the specific antagonist of prostanoid receptors which mediate vasoconstriction resulted in an increase of CBF and decrease of CVR only in SHR rats. Moreover, administration of the antagonist of thromboxane/endoperoxide receptors resulted in a decrease of CVR in SHR to a "normotensive" level.

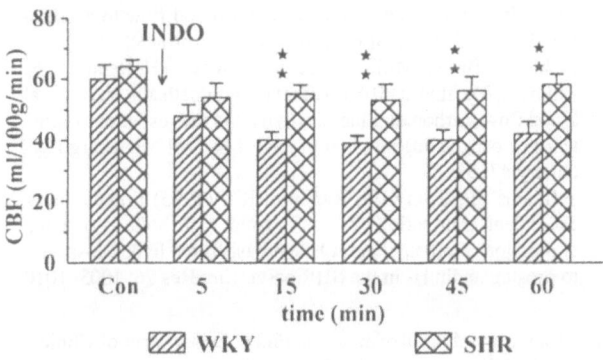

Fig. 1. Effect of intravenous administration of indomethacin on cerebral blood flow in WKY and in SHR. ** p < 0.01

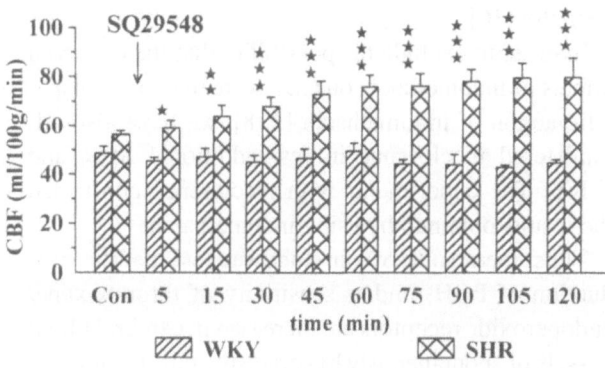

Fig. 2. Effect of intravenous administration of SQ 29548 on cerebral blood flow in WKY and in SHR. * p < 0.05, ** p < 0.01, *** p < 0.001

The fact that inhibition of the production of prostanoids resulted a smaller effect in SHR suggests that cerebral blood vessels in SHR produce less vasodilating PGI_2 or more vasoconstricting prostanoids in comparison with WKY. According to data published by others production of PGI_2 in SHR (isolated peripheral blood vessels) is not decreased [4, 7] in comparison with WKY. An increased production of the vasoconstrictor prostaglandin PGH_2 has been suggested for the cerebral circulation in SHR by Mayhan [5], who showed that the impaired vasodilatation of pial arterioles in SHR to acetylcholine and ADP was restored to normal by SQ 29548. It has been also demonstrated that in isolated SHR but not WKY PGH_2 is released in aortas following stimulation with acetylcholine [1]. Moreover Ge et al. [1] demonstrated that in addition to the release of vasoconstricting PGH_2, SHR aortas show a hypersensitivity of thromboxane/endoperoxide receptors. Such a hypersensitivity could also result in a vasoconstricting effect of PGI_2 as it has been demonstrated that PGI_2 in higher concentrations causes vasoconstriction mediated by thromboxane/endoperoxide receptors [4, 11]. Alternatively, a similar effect is conceivable if the receptors have a higher sensitivity and the concentration of the agonist is not increased above normal. Although it can not be excluded in our studies that due to a hypersensitivity of thromboxane/endoperoxide receptors, PGI_2 could result in vasoconstriction instead of vasodilation, such an explanation seems to be very speculative.

In contrast to our results, Mayhan [5] was not able to demonstrate that the basal tone of pial arterioles in SHR, which are resistance vessels, depends upon a stimulation of thromboxane/endoperoxide receptors. A possible explanation of this apparent discrepancy is that the SHR in our experiments were younger than those used by Mayhan, and that they did not show an impaired CBF response to endothelium-dependent vasodilators [6].

In order to exclude the possibility that the observed effects of indomethacin on CBF were due to a nonspecific action of indomethacin [2, 8], we have also administered meclofenac in few additional SHR and WKY. The experiments with meclofenac confirmed the results obtained by using indomethacin.

Thus, the results of our study suggest that the production of PGH_2 and/or sensitivity of thromboxane/ endoperoxide receptors are increased in cerebral blood vessels of spontaneously hypertensive rats in comparison with normotensive rats.

In conclusion, vasoconstricting prostanoids contribute to the maintenance of basal CBF and CVR in spontaneously hypertensive rats in contrast to normotensive rats. These prostanoids are distinct from TxA_2 but activate thromboxane A_2/endoperoxide receptors. The most probable candidate for such a prostanoid is the endoperoxide PGH_2.

Acknowledgment

This study was supported by the Medical School of Warsaw Grant H51.

References

1. Ge T, Hughes H, Junquero DC, Wu KK, Vanhoutte PM, Boulanger CM (1995) Endothelium-dependent contractions are associated with both augmented expression of prostaglandin H synthase-1 and hypersensitivity to prostaglandin H_2 in the SHR aorta. Circ Res 76: 1003–1010
2. Kontor HS, Hampton M (1978) Indomethacin in submicromolar concentration inhibits cyclic AMP dependent protein kinase. Nature 276: 841–842
3. Kozniewska E, Oseka M, Stys T (1992) Effect of endothelium-derived nitric oxide on cerebral circulation during normoxia and hypoxia in the rat. J Cereb Blood Flow Metab 12: 311–317
4. Lüscher TF, Romero JC, Vanhoutte PM (1986) Bioassay of endothelium-derived vasoactive substances in the aorta of normotensive and spontaneously hypertensive rats. J Hypertens 4 [Suppl 6]: 81–83
5. Mayhan WG (1992) Role of prostaglandin H_2-thromboxane A_2 in responses of cerebral arterioles during chronic hypertension. Am J Physiol 262: H539–H543
6. Oseka M, Kozniewska E (1995) Interaction of nitric oxide and prostanoids in the maintenance of cerebral blood flow in adult normotensive and spontaneously hypertensive rats. J Cereb Blood Flow Metab 15 [Suppl 1]: S 47
7. Pace-Asiak CR, Carrara MC (1979) Age-dependent increase in formation of prostaglandin I_2 by intact and homogenized aortae from developing spontaneously hypertensive rat. Biochim Biophys Acta 574: 177–181
8. Parfenova H, Hsu P, Leffler CW (1995) Dilator prostanoid-induced cyclic AMP formation and release by cerebral smooth muscle cells: inhibition by indomethacin. J Pharmacol Exp Therap 272: 44–52
9. Pickard JD (1981) Role of prostaglandins and arachidonic acid derivatives in the coupling of cerebral blood flow to cerebral metabolism. J Cereb Blood Flow Metab 1: 361–384
10. Pickles H, Brown MM, Thomas M, Hewazy AH, Redmond S, Zilkha E, Marshall J (1984) Effect of indomethacin on cerebral blood flow, carbon dioxide reactivity and the response to epostenol (prostacyclin) infusion in man. J Neurol Neurosurg Psychiatry 47: 51–55
11. Williams SP, Dom GW, Rapoport RM (1995) Endothelium-dependent contractions are associated with both augmented expression of prostaglandin H synthase-1 and hypersensitivity to prostaglandin H_2 in the SHR aorta. Circ Res 76: 1003–1010

Correspondence: Ewa Kozniewska, Ph.D., Department of Clinical and Applied Physiology, School of Medicine, Krakowskie Przedmiecie 26/28, 00-927 Warsaw, Poland.

Acta Neurochir (1997) [Suppl] 70: 231–233
© Springer-Verlag 1997

The Mechanism of Reversible Osmotic Opening of the Blood-Brain Barrier: Role of Intracellular Calcium Ion in Capillary Endothelial Cells

T. Nagashima[1], **K. Ikeda**[1], **S. Wu**[1], **T. Kondo**[1], **M. Yamaguchi**[2], and **N. Tamaki**[1]

[1] Department of Neurosurgery and [2] Institute of Health Science, Kobe University School of Medicine, Kobe, Japan

Summary

Despite clinical and experimental interest in the osmotic opening of the blood-brain barrier (BBB), the mechanism underlying the phenomenon remain undetermined. The aim of this study is to investigate the mechanism of intracellular Ca^{2+} change in brain microvascular endothelial cells subjected to hyperosmotic stress.

Cultured rat brain capillary endothelial cells were obtained by two-step enzymatic purification. Intracellular Ca^{2+} was measured by a confocal laser scanning microscope. After exposing the endothelial cells to 1.4 M mannitol for 30 seconds, the change of intracellular Ca^{2+} concentration was monitored. Intracellular Ca^{2+} concentration increased rapidly and reached its peak value within 10 seconds after the application of mannitol. The Ca^{2+} concentration returned to the basal level within 200 seconds. A calcium channel blocker nifedipine (100 µM, 10 µM) did not block the increase. A specific blocker (KB-R7943) of Na^+/Ca^{2+} exchange did not affect the rapid elevation of intracellular Ca^{2+}. However, it blocked the return phase almost completely. The results indicated that the Na^+/Ca^{2+} exchanger pumped out the increased intracellular Ca^{2+} during the return phase.

Reversible osmotic disruption and reconstruction of the BBB is not due to simple mechanical shrinkage of the endothelial cells but is due to the intracellular Ca^{2+}-activated complex mechanism. The manipulation of the reconstruction phase, which depends on Na^+/Ca^{2+} exchanger, may have clinical implications.

Keywords: Blood-brain barrier; endothelium; calcium ion; laser scanning confocal microscopy.

Introduction

The osmotic opening of the blood-brain barrier (BBB) has been proved successful in consistently and innocuously opening the BBB [7, 10, 12, 13]. Despite clinical and experimental interest in a reversible opening of the BBB by a hyperosmotic solution, the mechanisms underlying this phenomenon remain undetermined. It has been repeatedly argued that the opening of tight junctions, an essential ultrastructural component of the BBB, is the dominant mode of leakage under hyperosmolar conditions [3, 13]. Rapoport and

Robinson hypothesized that a hyperosmotic solution opens the BBB by shrinking endothelial cells [13]. We reported the transient increase of intracellular Ca^{2+} concentration by the application of hyperosmotic solution and pointed out that the phenomenon is intracellular Ca^{2+}-mediated complex process [7]. The unique properties of brain endothelial cells are reflected in the expression of specific cell surface molecules that participate in the transport process across the BBB. As calcium ion is an important second messenger, the significant increase of intracellular calcium concentration may influence the intracellular signal transduction and cause BBB disruption. The aim of this study was to investigate the mechanism of intracellular calcium ion change during hyperosmotic disruption and reconstruction of the BBB.

Materials and Methods

1. Rat brain capillary endothelial cells were isolated from 10 male Sprague-Dawley rat brains [2]. The cerebral cortexes were digested by a two-step enzymatic treatment: dispase and collagenase/dispase. Then the endothelial cells were purified by centrifugation over a pre-established 50% Percoll gradient. Next the cells were seeded onto collagen-coated plastic plates and grown in a medium consisting of Dulbecco MEM (Gibco, Grand Island, NY, USA), 13% bovine calf serum, and 50 mg/ml endothelial growth factor (Beckton Dickinson Lab Ware, Bedford, MA, USA). Identification as endothelium was determined by the presence of factor VIII-related antigen and the capability of prostacycline production.

2. Intracellular Ca^{2+} was measured by a confocal laser scanning microscope using Indo-1/AM as a intracellular Ca^{2+} indicator. After the endothelial cells were labeled by Indo-1/AM for 30 minutes, they were exposed to 1.4 M mannitol (25%) in PBS for 30 seconds. The change of intracellular Ca^{2+} concentration was monitored for 30 minutes by the confocal laser scanning microscope and then expressed as an averaged value of 10–12 cells that were monitored simultaneously.

3. To study the source of increased intracellular Ca^{2+}, the cells were incubated in Ca^{2+} free extracellular PBS after the hyper-

osmotic treatment. A calcium channel blocker (nifedipine 100 μM, 10 μM) or a specific blocker of Na^+/Ca^{2+} exchange (10 μM, KB-R7943, Kanebo Ltd, Osaka, Japan) was added to the PBS (+) to examine the mechanism of Ca^{2+} change.

Results

1. Intracellular Ca^{2+} concentration increased rapidly and reached its peak value within 10 seconds after the application of 1.4 M mannitol (Fig. 1). Peak Ca^{2+} concentration was about 250 nM.

2. The increased intracellular Ca^{2+} concentration returned to basal level within 200 seconds after the end of 1.4 M mannitol application. The cells, which were monitored simultaneously, showed a very homogeneous pattern of intracellular Ca^{2+} change (Fig. 1).

3. The intracellular Ca^{2+} concentration did not increase when the cells were incubated in Ca^{2+}-free extracellular PBS. This indicated that the elevated intracellular Ca^{2+} came from extracellular Ca^{2+}.

4. The calcium channel blocker, nifedipine, did not block the increase of intracellular Ca^{2+}.

5. The Na^+/Ca^{2+} exchange blocker did not affect the rapid elevation of intracellular Ca^{2+} concentration; however, it almost completely blocked the return phase (Fig. 2). This result indicates that the Na^+/Ca^{2+} exchanger pumped out the increased intracellular Ca^{2+}.

Discussion

Intracarotid infusion of hyperosmotic solution is the most thoroughly evaluated and consistently documented method to induce reversible disruption of the BBB. The hyperosmotic disruption of the BBB was initially applied to chemotherapy of malignant brain tumors [8]. Then the application was extended to deliver monoclonal antibodies into the brain. Doran *et al.* recently reported that BBB disruption with mannitol can facilitate the delivery of functional viral vectors to the central nervous system [4]. Hyperosmotic BBB disruption will no doubt be applied to other clinical fields as well. On the other hand, after continued clinical experience in chemotherapy, Neuwelt [9] reported an increased incidence of focal and generalized seizures during the procedures. Considering the risks and multiple factors underlying brain tumor chemotherapy or gene therapy, further clinical applications of osmotic disruption of the BBB remain controversial.

The phenomenon of reversible opening of the BBB consists of two different processes, the disrupting process and the reconstructing process. The underlying mechanisms of these two processes are considered to

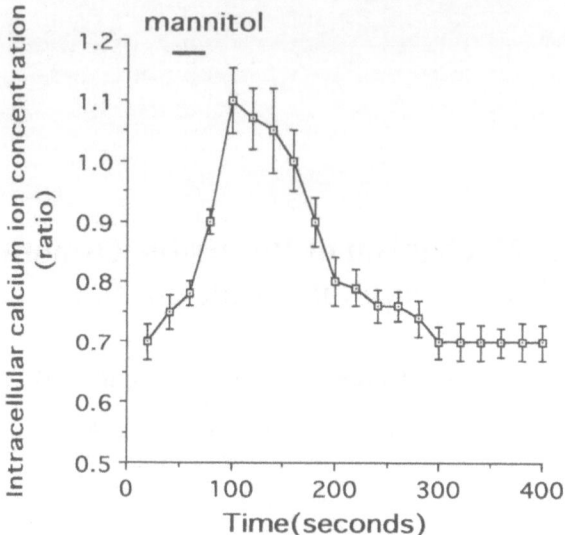

Fig. 1. The change of intracellular calcium ion of cultured brain microvascular endothelial cells caused by the application of 1.4 M mannitol. Twelve cells were monitored simultaneously. The ordinate presents intracellular calcium ion concentration expressed by the calculated ratio of calcium chelated Indo-1 to free Indo-1

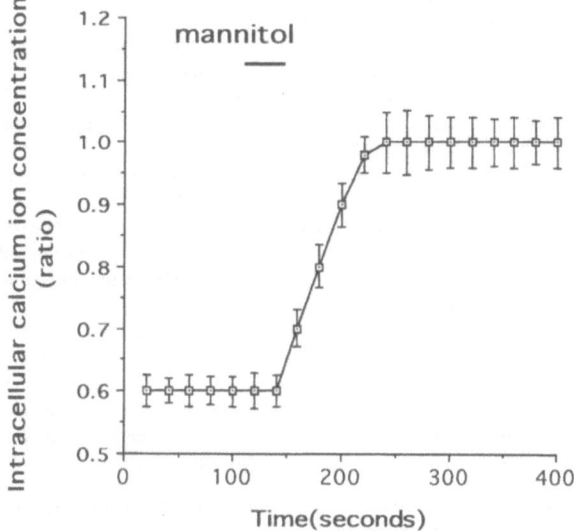

Fig. 2. The change of intracellular calcium ion of cultured brain microvascular endothelial cells caused by the application of 1.4 M mannitol. The blocker of Na^+/Ca^{2+} exchanger (10 μM, KB-R7943) was added to the extracellular PBS (+). Ten cells were monitored simultaneously. The ordinate presents intracellular calcium ion concentration expressed by the calculated ratio of calcium chelated Indo-1 to free Indo-1

be different. Using electron microscopy, Brightman *et al.* demonstrated that tight junctions open to a peroxidase tracer after intracarotid infusion of 3 M urea [3]. It has been suggested that intracarotid hyperosmotic infusion leads to osmotically mediated-shrinkage of endothelial cells, which then mechanically disrupts the endothelial cell layer [6, 12, 13]. In the present study, we demonstrated that the the hyperosmotic treatment induced the rapid alteration of Ca^{2+} concentration in cultured brain capillary endothelial cells. Calcium ion is an important second messenger of intracellular signal transduction. Therefore, the rapid increase of intracellular calcium ion induced by the hyperosmotic condition may cause drastic changes in cellular functions, such as BBB integrity. Calcium ion entry into endothelial cells may occur via four different mechanisms: (1) a receptor-mediated channel, (2) a Ca^{2+} leak channel dependent on the elecrochemical gradient, (3) a stretch-activated nonselective cation channel, and (4) internal Na^+-dependent Ca^{2+} entry (Na^+/Ca^{2+} exchanger) [1]. As our results show that increased intracellular Ca^{2+} comes from an extracellular pool, an L-type calcium channel and Na^+/Ca^{2+} exchanger do not seem to affect the process of the BBB disruption. Popp *et al.* suggested that the opening of stretch-activated cation channels in the antiluminal membrane of brain capillary by osmotic change of the interstitial fluid brings about an influx of Na^+ and Ca^{2+} into the endothelial cells [10]. The intracellular Ca^{2+} causing the BBB disruption may be induced via stretch-activated nonselective cation channels.

In spite of its physiological importances, the mechanism of reconstruction after hyperosmotic disruption of the BBB has not been elucidated. The results of the present study demonstrate that the reconstruction process depends on an Na^+/Ca^{2+} exchange of endothelial cells. The return of intracellular Ca^{2+} to basal level precedes the reconstruction of the disrupted BBB. The reversible osmotic disruption and reconstruction of BBB are not due to simple mechanical shrinkage of endothelial cells but are due to an intracellular calcium-activated complex process. Manipulation of the reconstruction phase, which depends on an Na^+/Ca^{2+} exchange, has clinical implications.

Further studies of the molecular mechanisms are necessary to understand osmotic disruption and reconstruction of the BBB.

References

1. Adams DJ, Barakeh J, Lakey R, Breemen CV (1989) Ion channels and regulation of intracellular calcium in vascular endothelial cells. FASEB J 3: 2389–2400
2. Bowman PD, Betz AL, Ar D, Wolinsky JS, Penney JB, Shivers RR, Goldstein GW (1981) Primary culture of capillary endothelium from rat brain. In vitro 17: 353–362
3. Brightman MW, Hori M, Rapoport SI, Reese TS, Westergard E (1973) Osmotic opening of tight junctions in cerebral endothelium. J Comp Neurol 152: 317–326
4. Doran SE, Ren XD, Betz AL, Pagel MA, Neuwelt EA, Rossler BJ, Davidson BL (1995) Gene expression from recombinant viral vectors in the central nervous system after blood-brain barrier disruption. Neurosurgery 36: 965–970
5. Dorovini-Zis K, Bowman PD, Betz AL, Goldstein GW (1984) Hyperosmotic arabinose solutions open the tight junctions between brain capillary endothelial cells in tissue culture. Brain Res 302: 383–386
6. Greenwood J, Luthert PJ, Pratt OE, Lantos PL (1988). Hyperosmolar opening of the blood brain barrier in the energy-depleted rat brain. Part 1. Permeability studies. J Cereb Blood Flow Metab 8: 9–15
7. Nagashima T, Wu S, Mizoguchi A, Tamaki N (1994) A possible role of calcium ion in osmotic opening of blood-brain barrier. J Auton Nerv Syst 49: 145–149
8. Neuwelt EA, Barnett PA, Glasberg RG (1983) Successful treatment of primary central nervous system lymphomas with chemotherapy after osmotic blood-brain barrier opening. Neurosurgery 12: 662–671
9. Neuwelt EA (1988) Blood-brain barrier disruption in the treatment of brain tumors. In: Neuwelt EA (ed) Implications of the blood-brain barrier and its manipulation, Vol 2. Plenum, New York, pp 107–261
10. Popp R, Hoyer J, Meyer J, Galla HJ, Gogelein H (1992) Stretch activated non-selective cation channels in the antiluminal membrane of porcine cerebral capillaries. J Physiol 454: 435–449
11. Rapoport SI (1970) Effect of concentrated solutions on blood brain barrier Am J Physiol 219: 270–274
12. Rapoport SI, Hori M, Klatzo I (1972) Testing of hypothesis for osmotic opening of the blood-brain barrier. Am J Physiol 223: 323–331
13. Rapoport SI, Robinson PJ (1986) Tight junctional modification as the basis of osmotic opening of blood-brain barrier. Ann NY Acad Sci 481: 250–266
14. Williams PC, Henner WD, Roman GS, Dahlborg SA, Brummett RE, Tableman M, Danna BW, Neuwelt WA (1995) Toxicity and efficacy of carbopaltin and etoposide in conjunction with disruption of the blood-brain barrier in the treatment of intracranial neoplasms. Neurosurgery 37: 17–27

Correspondence: Tatsuya Nagashima, M.D., Department of Neurosurgery, Kobe University School of Medicine, Kobe, Japan.

Acta Neurochir (1997) [Suppl] 70: 234–236
© Springer-Verlag 1997

Blood-Brain Barrier Disruption, Edema Formation, and Apoptotic Neuronal Death Following Cold Injury

K. Murakami, T. Kondo, and **P. H. Chan**

CNS Injury and Edema Research Center, Departments of Neurological Surgery and Neurology, School of Medicine, University of California, San Francisco, CA, U.S.A.

Summary

The temporal pattern of brain edema and apoptosis following cold injury was investigated. Extravasation of Evans blue from the disrupted blood-brain barrier (BBB) maximized immediately after injury and returned to the control level at 24 h. However, water content increased up to 24 h and was maintained at a higher level than the control at 72 h. Apoptotic cells as detected by *in situ* end labeling were observed in the entire lesion at 24 h. At 72 h after injury, these apoptotic cells were observed in the margin of the lesion, but not in the core. These results suggest that apoptosis contributes to neuronal damage following cold injury and may result from the development of vasogenic edema.

Keywords: Apoptotic neuronal death; blood-brain barrier; brain edema; cold injury.

Introduction

Apoptotic neuronal death has been known to be involved in brain injury following a variety of brain insults, including cerebral ischemia, trauma, and kainic acid-induced epileptic seizures. Apoptosis is characterized morphologically by cell shrinkage, nuclei condensation, and apoptotic bodies, and biochemically by the internucleosomal DNA fragmentation. Recently, the *in situ* terminal deoxynucleotidyl transferase-mediated uridine 5'-triphosphate-biotin nick end labeling (TUNEL) method and morphological observation have been commonly used to detect neuronal apoptosis in various forms of brain injury.

Vasogenic brain edema, which is characterized by increased permeability of the BBB, results after numerous brain insults [5] and causes secondary injury [13]. However, the role of vasogenic edema on neuronal apoptosis is unknown and has not been investigated.

The present experiment was designed to clarify the relationship of BBB disruption, edema formation, and neuronal injury, neuronal apoptosis in particular, following cold injury.

Materials and Methods

CD-1 mice (male, 3 months old) were subjected to cold injury according to the method of Chan *et al.* [3]. BBB disruption was evaluated by quantification of extravasated Evans blue in the injured hemisphere. Evans blue was injected intravenously 0.5 h prior to sacrifice. Evans blue content was calculated from the absorbance of Evans blue in brain samples at 610 nm and expressed as µg/hemisphere [2].

Water content in the injured hemisphere was calculated from the wet weight measured immediately after removal of the brain and the dry weight measured after drying at 105°C for 24 h. Water content is expressed as $\%H_2O$ calculated as (wet weight – dry weight) / wet weight × 100% [2].

Lesion volume was quantified using an image analysis system. Coronal sections were collected at intervals of 500 µm by a cryostat and stained with cresyl violet. Lesion volume was calculated by multiplying the unstained area and distance.

The *in situ* TUNEL staining method was used to investigate the distribution of apoptotic neurons after cold injury. Two regions in the cold lesion (core and margin) were used to access the anatomic distribution of TUNEL-positive cells. The TUNEL-positive cells were counted by a blinded investigator.

Results were expressed as mean ± standard deviation. The statistical significance of differences between groups was evaluated by analysis of variance, followed by Fisher's protected least significant difference test for multiple comparisons. Significance between groups was assigned at a level of less than 5% probability ($p < 0.05$).

Results

The mean values of Evans blue content at each time point are shown in Fig. 1A. Immediately after cold injury, extravasation of Evans blue through the disrupted BBB was significantly elevated from a control valne of 0.09 ± 0.02 (n = 6) to 1.38 ± 0.34 µg/hemisphere (n = 6) (p < 0.01, versus control). Although Evans blue content in the injured hemisphere was decreased to 0.29 ± 0.03 μg/hemisphere at 4 h (n = 6), it was significantly higher than the control value (p < 0.01, versus control). Thereafter it nearly returned to the control value at 24 and 72 h after cold injury and was 0.11 ± 0.01 (n = 6) and 0.13 ± 0.01 μg/hemisphere (n = 4), respectively.

The temporal change of cerebral water content is shown in Fig. 1B. Following cold injury, water content in the injured hemisphere was elevated from a control value of $77.99 \pm 0.39\%$ to $78.62 \pm 0.24\%$ at 30 min after cold injury. At 4 h, water content slightly increased to $78.71 \pm 0.10\%$. Thereafter water content reached the maximum of $79.49 \pm 0.57\%$ at 24 h. At 72 h, however, water content decreased to $78.92 \pm 0.56\%$ but was maintained at a higher level than the control (p < 0.01, versus control).

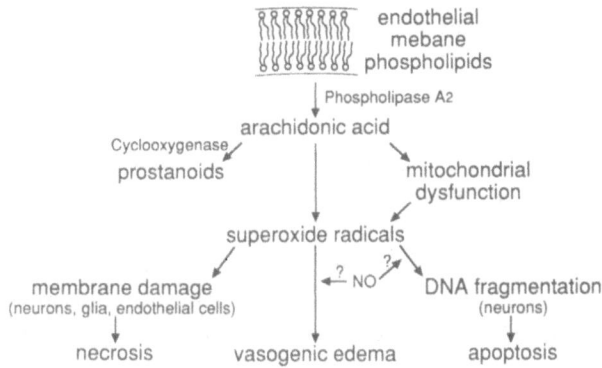

Fig. 2. A possible biochemical mechanism of the formation of neuronal apoptosis after cold injury

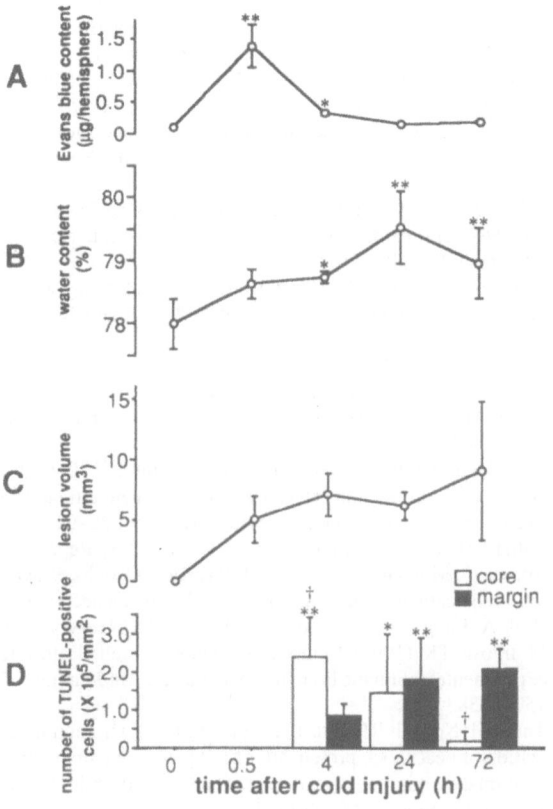

Fig. 1. Temporal profile of Evans blue content (A), water content (B), volume of lesion (C), and number of TUNEL-positive cells (D) following cold injury. Evans blue content increased immediately after cold injury, reached the maximum at 0.5 h, and decreased to the control level at 24 h. Water content increased gradually and maximized at 24 h. It remained higher than the control value at 72 h. Volume of the lesion was increased continuously up to 72 h. The distribution of TUNEL-positive cells changed as time progressed. In the margin, the number of TUNEL-positive cells increased up to 72 h, whereas in the core of the lesion these cells reached the maximum at 4 h and then decreased. * p < 0.05, ** p < 0.01, versus 0 h, † p < 0.05, versus margin

Fig. 1C shows lesion volume at various time points after cold injury. From 0.5 to 4 h after cold injury, lesion volume was gradually increased and was 4.8 ± 1.8 mm^2 (n = 4), $5.6 + 1.3$ mm^2 (n = 4), and 6.3 ± 1.5 mm^2 (n = 4) at 0.5, 1, 4 h, respectively. At 24 h, lesion volume was slightly decreased to 5.7 ± 1.2 mm^2 (n = 5) from 4 h. Lesion volume reached the maximum of 7.9 ± 4.8 mm^2 (n = 4) at 72 h after cold injury.

Fig. 1D shows the numbers of TUNEL-positive cells in each region at 0.5, 4, 24, 72 h after cold injury. At 0.5 h after cold injury, TUNEL-positive cells were not observed in either the center or periphery of the cold lesion. TUNEL-positive cells were scattered in the center of the lesion at 4 h [core; $(2.37 \pm 1.03) \times 10^5$ / mm^2, margin; $(0.83 \pm 0.29) \times 10^5$ / mm^2]. At 24 h apoptotic neurons were diffusely distributed over the entire cold lesion [core; $(1.42 + 1.54) \times 10^5$ / mm^2, margin; $(1.78 \pm 1.07) \times 10^5$ / mm^2]. At 72 h, the number of these cells was maximized in the margin [$(2.05 \pm 0.52) \times 10^5$ / mm^2), but decreased further in the core of the cold lesion $(0.15 \pm 0.26) \times 10^5$ / mm^2]. These TUNEL-positive cells were not detected in the area remote from the cold injury region.

Discussion

Recent investigations have shown that neuronal apoptosis contributes to neuronal injury after a variety of brain injuries [9–12]. It has been demonstrated that mild fluid percussion, which produces the BBB disruption with minimal hemorrhage, induces heat shock protein expression as evidence of neuronal stress and/ or injury [13]. In the present study, it was determined whether neuronal apoptosis is induced following cold injury-induced brain edema. Our results showed the temporal pattern of BBB disruption, brain edema, and distribution of apoptotic cells. Extravasation of Evans blue as a tracer of BBB disruption was restricted in the acute phase of cold injury, and returned to the control level by 24 h after injury, whereas brain edema maximized at 24 h and continued at 72 h after injury. The lesion volume quantified with image analysis, which is a mixture of both edematous and damaged brain tissue, reached its peak at 72 h. As measure for apoptosis, TUNEL-stained cells spread over the lesion in a time-dependent manner and the distribution of these cells expanded concurrently with the expansion of the lesion. At 72 h after injury, these cells were still detected in the margin of the lesion. We believe that this is the first report regarding the occurrence of neuronal apoptosis in a cold traumatized brain following the development of vasogenic edema. These data may also suggest that the apoptotic process contributes to the pathogenesis of neuronal death not only at the acute phase, but also in a delayed fashion, and that may result from the expansion of brain edema induced by cold injury.

The mechanisms underlying the neuronal apoptosis induced by vasogenic brain edema are not clear at present. We have previously demonstrated membrane phospholipid degradation and the release of arachidonic acid following cold injury [2]. Arachidonic acid, once released from the membrane, forms superoxide radicals and prostanoids [1]. Both arachidonic acid and free radicals are potent mitochondrial respiratory inhibitors, and increased superoxide radicals are likely to form in the mitochondria compartments due to mitochondrial dysfunction [7, 8]. It is known that oxygen free radicals, superoxide radicals in particular, participate in neuronal apoptosis in cerebral ischemia and in cultured neuronal cells that are subjected to nerve growth factor withdrawal [6, 9]. We have also demonstrated that neuronal apoptosis induced by hypoxia and reoxygenation was ameliorated in cultured cortical neurons overexpressing human copper, zinc-superoxide dismutase transgene [4]. These data, when put together, suggest that superoxide radicals are an important mediator in promoting neuronal apoptosis following cold injury-induced vasogenic edema (Fig. 2).

Acknowledgments

This work is supported by NIH grants NS14543, NS25372, AG08938, and N01NS5-2334. We thank Cheryl Christensen for editorial assistance.

References

1. Chan PH, Chen SF, Yu AC (1988) Induction of intracellular superoxide radical formation by arachidonic acid and by polyunsaturated fatty acids in primary astrocytic cultures. J Neurochem 50: 1185–1193
2. Chan PH, Longar S, Fishman RA (1983) Phospholipid degradation and edema development in cold-injured rat brain. Brain Res 277: 329–337
3. Chan PH, Yang GY, Chen SF, Carlson E, Epstein CJ (1991) Cold-induced brain edema and infarction are reduced in transgenic mice overexpressing CuZn-superoxide dismutase. Ann Neurol 29: 482–486
4. Copin J-C, Reola LF, Chan TYY, Li Y, Epstein CJ, Chan PH (1996) Oxygen deprivation but not a combination of oxygen, glucose, and serum deprivation induces DNA degradation in mouse cortical neurons *in vitro*: attenuation by transgenic overexpressing of CuZn-superoxide dismutase. J Neurotrauma 13: 233–244
5. Fishman RA (1975) Brain edema. N Engl J Med 293: 706–711
6. Greenlund LJ, Deckwerth TL, Johnson EM Jr (1995) Superoxide dismutase delays neuronal apoptosis: a role for reactive oxygen species in programmed neuronal death. Neuron 14: 303–315
7. Hillered L, Chan PH (1988) Role of arachidonic acid and other free fatty acids in mitochondrial dysfunction in brain ischemia. J Neurosci Res 20: 451–456
8. Hillered L, Chan PH (1989) Brain mitochondrial swelling induced by arachidonic acid and other long chain free fatty acids. J Neurosci Res 24: 247–250
9. Li Y, Chopp M, Jiang N, Yao F, Zaloga C (1995) Temporal profile of *in situ* DNA fragmentation after transient middle cerebral artery occlusion in the rat. J Cereb Blood Flow Metab 15: 389–397
10. MacManus JP, Buchan AM, Hill IE, Rasquinha I, Preston E (1993) Global ischemia can cause DNA fragmentation indicative of apoptosis in rat brain. Neurosci Lett 164: 89–92
11. Pollard H, Charriaut-Marlangue C, Cantagrel S, Represa A, Robain O, Moreau J, Ben-Ari Y (1994) Kainate-induced apoptotic cell death in hippocampal neurons. Neuroscience 63: 7–18
12. Rink A, Fung KM, Trojanowski JQ, Lee VM, Neugebauer E, McIntosh TK (1995) Evidence of apoptotic cell death after experimental traumatic brain injury in the rat. Am J Pathol 147: 1575–1583
13. Tanno H, Nockels RP, Pitts LH, Noble LJ (1993) Immunolocalization of heat shock protein after fluid percussive brain injury and relationship to breakdown of the blood-brain barrier. J Cereb Blood Flow Metab 13: 116–124

Correspondence: Pak H. Chan, Ph.D., CNS Injury and Edema Research Center, Departments of Neurological Surgery and Neurology, University of California, Box 0651, San Francisco, CA 94143-0651, U.S.A.

Acta Neurochir (1997) [Suppl] 70: 237–239
© Springer-Verlag 1997

Blood-Brain Barrier Disruption, HSP70 Expression and Apoptosis Due to 3-Nitropropionic Acid, a Mitochondrial Toxin

S. Sato[1], G. T. Gobbel[1], Y. Li[1], T. Kondo[1], K. Murakami[1], M. Sato[1], K. Hasegawa[2], J.-Ch. Copin[1], J. Honkaniemi[3], F. R. Sharp[3], and **P. H. Chan[1]**

Departments of [1] Neurological Surgery and [2] Anesthesia, University of California, School of Medicine, San Francisco, CA, and [3] Department of Neurology, Veterans Affairs Medical Center, San Francisco, CA, U.S.A.

Summary

3-Nitropropionic acid (3-NP), a mitochondrial toxin, induces apoptosis in the striatum. We wanted to determine if there was a relationship between mitochondrial dysfunction, disruption of the blood-brain barrier (BBB), and apoptosis. BBB disruption following intrastriatal injection of 3-NP was assessed by Evans blue leakage, brain water content, and by the expression of the 70 kDa heat shock protein (HSP70) and mRNA. Apoptosis was assessed by *in situ* terminal deoxynucleotidyl transferase-mediated uridine 5'- triphosphate-biotin nick end labeling (TUNEL) and gel electrophoresis to detect internucleosomal DNA fragmentation. Microscopic evidence of Evans blue leakage due to 3-NP was present only 3 hr after injection. Both internucleosomal DNA fragmentation and TUNEL-labeling did not appear until 24 hr after injection. HSP70 (protein and mRNA) was also elevated by 24 hr. There was a quantitative increase in Evans blue leakage and brain water content due to 3-NP by 3 days after injection. Our results suggest that BBB disruption is an early event followed by increased HSP70 expression and apoptosis. We speculate that 3-NP damages endothelial cells, leading to vasogenic edema and apoptosis.

Keywords: Apoptosis; blood-brain barrier; HSP70 expression; 3-nitropropionic acid.

Introduction

3-Nitropropionic acid (3-NP) is an irreversible inhibitor of a mitochondrial complex II enzyme, succinate dehydrogenase, and it induces apoptosis in the striatum. Apoptosis is a form of death resulting from the stimulation of genomic activity to carry out a suicide-like process. It is unclear whether apoptosis due to 3-NP is a direct effect of the toxin or secondary to other actions of 3-NP, such as endothelial damage leading to either ischemia or blood-brain barrier (BBB) disruption and vasogenic edema. To clarify the relationship between mitochondrial dysfunction, BBB disruption, and apoptosis, we measured leakage of Evans blue and brain water content following 3-NP injection. In addition, we measured the expression of the 70 kDa form of heat shock protein (HSP70) and its mRNA following intracerebral injection of 3-NP to induce apoptosis. HSP70 is a marker of cell injury that can be induced in response to BBB disruption [10, 12] and ischemia.

Materials and Methods

Male Sprague-Dawley rats weighing 190–210 gm were anesthetized, and 1 µl of a solution containing 500 nmoles of 3-NP or saline (control) was stereotaxically injected into the striatum unilaterally [1]. The brains were removed at 3, 6, and 24 hr and 3 days after the injection.

BBB disruption was detected by examining the brain microscopically after intravenous injection of Evans blue. A quantitative measure of BBB disruption was calculated from the absorbance of Evans blue in the supernatant of centrifuged brain homogenate and expressed as µg/hemisphere [2, 13]. Water content was calculated from wet and dry weights of the brain. Differences in water contents and Evans blue concentrations between the time points were evaluated using analysis of variance. For histologic evaluation, brains were sectioned and stained with cresyl violet for Nissl substance. To detect neuronal apoptosis, brain sections were stained by the *in situ* terminal deoxynucleotidyl transferase-mediated uridine 5'-triphosphate-biotin nick end labeling (TUNEL) method using a modification of the technique previously described by Gavrieli *et al.* [3]. Sections stained by the TUNEL method were 20 µm rostral to sections stained with cresyl violet. The expression of hsp70 mRNA was examined using *in situ* hybridization [5, 6] in sections 100 µm rostral to the sections stained by the TUNEL method. HSP70 was detected immunohistochemically using a mouse monoclonal antibody (Amersham, Arlington, IL, U.S.A.) [6].

Results

The first evidence of injury was the microscopic and macroscopic appearance of Evans blue leakage in animals treated with 3-NP. By 24 hr, DNA from rats treated with 3-NP showed evidence of internucleosomal fragmentation as evidenced by a ladder pattern due to cleavage into segments that are multiples of approximately 200 base pairs in length (Fig. 1, left). No ladder pattern was visible in DNA from saline-treated animals. At 24 hr following the injection of 3-NP, TUNEL-positive cells were observed in the striatum (Fig. 1, right). Histologically, there were large striatal lesions after 3-NP injection (Fig. 2A) that were accompanied by HSP70 staining in the border of the lesion (Fig. 2C). The number of cells that expressed hsp70 mRNA (Fig. 2D) appeared to be greater than the number that expressed HSP70 (Fig. 2B) and less than the number of TUNEL-positive cells. Evans blue content in the hemisphere injected with 3-NP increased from a value of 0.47 at 3 hr to 0.91 at 12 hr and to 1.05 µg/hemisphere at 3 days. Evans blue content in the hemisphere injected with saline increased from a value of 0.54 at 3 hr to 0.95 at 12 hr and decreased to 0.72 µg/hemisphere at 3 days. Water content was higher in the hemisphere injected with 3-NP. Water content in the hemisphere injected with 3-NP gradually increased from a value of 79.8% at 3 hr to 81.7% at 24 hr and decreased to 79.9% at 3 days. The water content of the hemisphere injected with saline was 79.6% at 3 hr and stayed at a similar level until 24 hr, before decreasing to 78.2% at 3 days.

Discussion

Our results support the idea that 3-NP induces apoptosis in the striatum. First, gel electrophoresis of DNA isolated from the striatum showed a laddering pattern typical of apoptosis. Second, cells in the striatum were stained by the TUNEL method, which is a staining technique to detect DNA breaks like those that occur due to apoptosis.

The apoptosis that occurred at 24 hr after 3-NP injection was accompanied by expression of hsp70 mRNA throughout the lesion and HSP70 protein within the border of the lesion. The reason that expression of hsp70 mRNA was more extensive than that of HSP70 may be related to the severity of the insult produced by 3-NP at the site of the injection; the high dose of 3-NP close to the site of injection may have produced an insult too severe and too rapid to allow translation of mRNA into protein.

HSP70 is commonly expressed in cells in response to stress [10, 12]. In the brain, increased HSP70 expression is seen following ischemia and is localized to

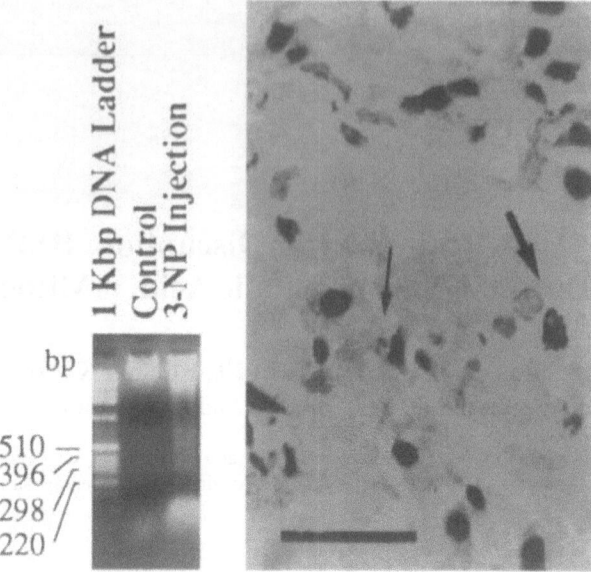

Fig. 1. Left: Electrophoresis of DNA isolated from the striatum of 3-NP-treated and saline-treated rats. DNA laddering, a biochemical marker of apoptosis, was also present in the lesioned brain of 3-NP-treated rats, but not in control animals. A standard with DNA lengths that are multiples of 123 base pairs is shown for comparison in the left lane. Right: At 24 hr after 3-NP injection, TUNEL-positive cells were observed in the lesion. Nuclear fragmentation, a characteristic of apoptosis, was visible in some of the TUNEL-positive cells (arrow). The scale bar is 10 µm

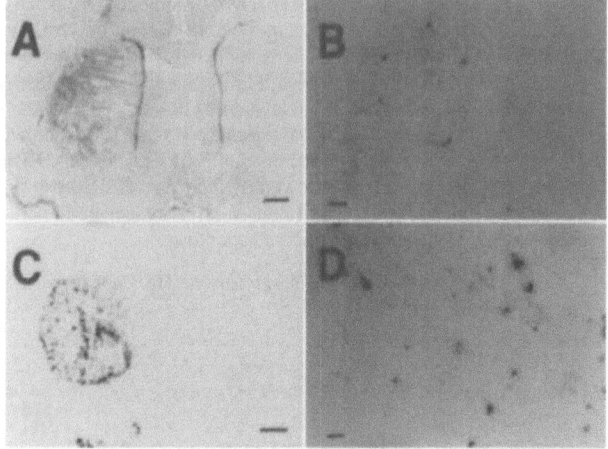

Fig. 2. (A) A coronal section stained with cresyl violet shows evidence of selective degeneration and selective striatal lesions within the striatum. (B) HSP70 immunostaining was predominantly within the border of the striatum. No staining was seen in the right, uninfected striatum. (C) Autoradiographs developed following *in situ* hybridization for hsp70 revealed expression throughout the striatum. (D) Microscopic localization of hsp70 mRNA revealed a patchy cellular distribution. All sections were collected 24 hr after 3-NP injection. Scale bars in (A) and (B) are 1 mm; scale bars in (C) and (D) are 10 µm

regions of BBB disruption following traumatic injury [6, 7, 10, 12]. Considering that Evans blue leakage was seen as early as 3 hr after 3-NP injection, whereas HSP70 expression was not detected until 24 hr, the HSP70 expression seen after 3-NP injection may also be due to BBB disruption. The regional distribution of HSP70 expression may also be related to the susceptibility of that brain region to BBB disruption [8, 9]. The BBB disruption is presumably due to an effect of 3-NP on the ability of the endothelial mitochondria to carry out cell metabolism and generate adenosine triphosphate from glucose – endothelial cells die when depleted of energy sources [4] – and exogenous energy sources, such as glycerol, can protect endothelial cells against BBB disruption [11]. Because endothelial cell injury could also disrupt cerebral blood flow, we cannot rule out the possibility that ischemia secondary to cell death may have contributed to HSP70 expression.

Quantitative measures of BBB disruption and vasogenic edema, namely Evans blue leakage and brain water content, were not increased in 3-NP-treated animals as compared to controls until 3 days after injection. Thus, although BBB disruption preceded apoptosis, apoptosis preceded the development of significant vasogenic edema. In addition, although BBB disruption following injection of 3-NP may contribute to the development of apoptosis, vasogenic edema and the associated tissue swelling probably does not. It may be that substances within the blood that leak into the brain following BBB disruption are the cause of the subsequent apoptosis. Further work is needed to establish the effect of 3-NP on brain endothelial cells and the role of BBB disruption in apoptosis.

Acknowledgments

The authors would like to thank S. Chen, B. Calagui and L. Reola for their technical assistance and C. Christensen for editorial assistance. This study was supported by National Institutes of Health grants NS 14543, NS 25372, AG 08938, and CA 13525.

References

1. Beal MF, Brouillet E, Jenkins BG, Ferrante RJ, Kowall NW, Miller JM, Storey E, Srivastava R, Rosen BR, Hyman BT (1993) Neurochemical and histologic characterization of striatal excitotoxic lesions produced by the mitochondrial toxin 3-nitropropionic acid. J Neurosci 13: 4181–4192
2. Chan PH, Yang GY, Chen SF, Carlson E, Epstein CJ (1991) Cold- induced brain edema and infarction are reduced in transgenic mice overexpressing CuZn-superoxide dismutase. Ann Neurol 29: 482–486
3. Gavrieli Y, Sherman Y, Ben-Sasson SA (1992) Identification of programmed cell death in situ via specific labeling of nuclear DNA fragmentation. J Cell Biol 119: 493–501
4. Gobbel GT, Chan TY, Gregory GA, Chan PH (1994) Response of cerebral endothelial cells to hypoxia: modification by fructose-1,6-bisphosphate but not glutamate receptor antagonists. Brain Res 653: 23–30
5. Honkaniemi J, Sagar SM, Pyykonen I, Hicks KJ, Sharp FR (1995) Focal brain injury induces multiple immediate early genes encoding zinc finger transcription factors. Mol Brain Res 28: 157–163
6. Kinouchi H, Sharp FR, Chan PH, Koistinaho J, Sagar SM, Yoshimoto T (1994) Induction of c-fos, junB, c-jun, and hsp70 mRNA in cortex, thalamus, basal ganglia, and hippocampus following middle cerebral artery occlusion. J Cereb Blood Flow Metab 14: 808–817
7. Nowak TS Jr (1985) Synthesis of a stress protein following transient ischemia in the gerbil. J Neurochem 45: 1635–1641
8. Sato S, Suga S, Yunoki K, Mihara B (1994) Effect of barrier opening on brain edema in human brain tumors. Acta Neurochir (Wien) [Suppl] 60: 116–118
9. Sato S, Toya S, Ohtani M, Suga S, Harada S (1990) Effect of blood-brain barrier disruption on the permeability of peritumoral edema. Adv Neurol 52: 555
10. Sharp FR, Lowenstein D, Simon R, Hisanaga K (1991) Heat shock protein Hsp72 induction in cortical and striatal astrocytes and neurons following infarction. J Cereb Blood Flow Metab 11: 621–627
11. Suga S, Sato S, Ishihara N, Togashi O, Yunoki K, Kobari M (1990) Effect of glycerol on ischemic edema. Adv Neurol 52: 185–194
12. Tanno H, Nockels RP, Pitts LH, Noble LJ (1993) Immunolocalization of heat shock protein after fluid percussive brain injury and relationship to breakdown of the blood-brain barrier. J Cereb Blood Flow Metab 13: 116–124
13. Yang G, Chan PH, Chen J, Carlson E, Chen SF, Weinstein P, Epstein CJ, Kamii H (1994) Human copper-zinc superoxide dismutase transgenic mice are highly resistant to reperfusion injury after focal cerebral ischemia. Stroke 25: 165–170

Correspondence: Pak H. Chan, Ph.D., Departments of Neurological Surgery and Neurology, University of California, Box 0651, San Francisco, CA 94143, U.S.A.

Acta Neurochir (1997) [Suppl] 70: 240–242
© Springer-Verlag 1997

Blood-Brain Barrier Breakdown Occurs Early After Traumatic Brain Injury and is not Related to White Blood Cell Adherence

R. Härtl, M. Medary, M. Ruge, K. E. Arfors, and **J. Ghajar**

The Aitken Neuroscience Institute and Cornell University Medical College, New York, NY, U.S.A.

Summary

The time course of blood-brain barrier (BBB) breakdown after traumatic brain injury (TBI) has important implications for therapy. This study was conducted in order to test post-traumatic BBB dysfunction in a model of fluid-percussion induced TBI in rabbits at 1 and 6 hours after TBI and relate it to white blood cell (WBC) activation. Ten anesthetized rabbits had chronic cranial windows implanted three weeks prior to experimentation. Fluid-percussion injury (3.5 atm.) was induced and animals were followed for 1 or 6 h. Intravital fluorescence videomicroscopy was used to assess BBB permeability and WBC adhesion to pial venules. Na^+-fluorescein was infused continuously over 30 min at either 30 min (Group I, n = 5) or 5.5 h (Group II, n = 5) after TBI. Microvascular permeability in individual postcapillary venules was assessed qualitatively at 1 and 30 min after start of infusion. TBI led to a transient mean arterial blood pressure (MAP) surge after trauma and a progressive increase in the number of sticking WBCs per mm^2 vessel wall. Na^+-fluorescein extravasation was observed in 4 out of 5 Group I animals and in none of Group II. BBB breakdown was not associated with WBC sticking. We conclude that after fluid-percussion injury the BBB is damaged at 1 h post-trauma and that its function is restored 6 h later. Increased WBC sticking at 6 h is not associated with BBB breakdown. Whether WBCs may cause vascular permeability changes at a later point needs further investigation.

Keywords: Traumatic brain injury; leukocytes; white blood cells; blood-brain barrier; intravital videomicroscopy.

Introduction

The time course of blood-brain barrier (BBB) breakdown after traumatic brain injury (TBI) has not been fully understood. While some authors describe early BBB disruption occurring within the first few hours after TBI, others have reported delayed BBB breakdown with initially intact cerebrovasculature. The present experiments were conducted in order to shed light on the time course of posttraumatic BBB dysfunction in a model of fluid-percussion induced TBI and its relationship to early inflammatory changes and white blood cell (WBC) activation.

Material and Methods

Permission was granted by the local Institutional Ethics Committee. New Zealand rabbits were employed in this study. In order to avoid artifacts associated with the surgical procedure (skin incision, trephination, dura reflection and exposure of the brain surface) the modified version of a chronic cranial window described previously by Levasseur *et al.* was implanted 2–4 weeks prior to the final experiments [5].

Brain injury: For the final experiments anesthesia was induced by repetitive i.m. administration of xylazine/ketamine. Experimental brain injury was produced using a modified fluid-percussion injury device. A drill hole (diameter 4 mm) over the left hemisphere anterior to the cranial window was prepared and the dura was left intact. To produce an insult, the piston was impounded by a 3.4 kg metal weight from a specific fall height. This resulted in a 3.5 atm. barotraumatic injury delivered to the brain over 20–25 msec.

Intravital videomicroscopy: A custom-designed Leitz microscope for intravital videomicroscopy equipped with a 50 W mercury light source (Opti Quip 1200), Ploem-Pak illuminator filter block (Leitz, Wetzlar, FRG) for epi-illumination, 5× to 32× objectives and a MTI VE1000 SIT camera with external control board was used for assessment of microcirculatory parameters. Images were recorded on a SONY U-Matic VCR, VO 9600, and were for off-line evaluation displayed on a 20 inch Sony videomonitor. An image analysis software program (NIH image version 1.55) on a Macintosh Quadra 700 computer was used to measure vessel diameters.

WBC behavior: WBCs in postcapillary pia venules were visualized by injection of Rhodamine 6 G (0.3 ml/kg of a 0.05% R6G, Sigma) i.v. for *in vivo* labelling. Selective observation of rhodamine 6G-stained WBCs was possible using epi-illumination with a Leitz N2 filter block (excitation 530–560 nm, emission > 580 nm). Results are given as number of WBCs sticking > 30 sec per mm^2 vessel wall.

Blood-brain barrier integrity: Blood-brain barrier integrity was assessed qualitatively by i.v. infusion of Na^+-fluorescein 30 min before termination of the experiments. The initial dose of Na^+-fluorescein was 1 ml/kg body weight of a 2% solution followed by continuous intravenous infusion at a rate of 1 ml/kg b.w. to maintain stable plasma concentration. Microvascular permeability in individual postcapillary venules was evaluated qualitatively by checking for leaky sites per region of interest 30 min after start of infusion [7, 14].

Experimental protocol: Animals equipped with chronic cranial windows were assigned to one of two experimental groups: After a baseline period of one hour animals underwent fluid-percussion brain injury and were followed for either 1 h (Group I) or 6 h (Group II) and sacrified by i.v. injection of euthanasia solution. Na+-fluorescein was infused continuously over 30 min at either 30 min (Group I, n = 5) or 5.5 h (Group II, n = 5) after TBI.

Results

No difference was found in injury severity (3.5 atm.) and mean arterial blood pressure (MAP) between groups. MAP after trauma increased transiently from 79 ± 8 (SD) to a maximum of 93 ± 16 mmHg at 15 min postinjury and from 81 ± 11 to 95 ± 17 mmHg at 15 min in Group I and in Group II, respectively. Thereafter, MAP returned to values not significantly different from baseline.

TBI led to extravasation of Na+-fluorescein in 4 of 5 experiments in Group I. In none of the experiments of Group II, however, did we observe breakdown of the BBB. The relationship between numbers of WBCs sticking to the vessel wall of postcapillary venules and BBB disruption is given in Table 1. No association was found between WBC sticking and increased leakiness of pia vessels after trauma; BBB disruption at 1 h was not paralleled by WBC sticking in corresponding vessels and increased WBC activation at 6 h after TBI was not associated with BBB damage.

Discussion

The time course of BBB breakdown has been discussed controversially in the past. A better understanding of the dynamics of posttraumatic alterations in vascular permeability is far from being of purely academic interest. BBB breakdown gives rise to the development of vasogenic brain edema and intracranial hypertension. On the other hand, a disrupted BBB may offer the possibility to deliver neuroprotective drugs to the brain.

The integrity of the BBB after fluid-percussion injury has been investigated before. Our findings are in accordance with Tanno *et al.* who reported that in rats undergoing fluidpercussion injury BBB leakage was most pronounced within the first hour after TBI [12, 13]. Fukuda *et al.* recently reported transient extravasation of horseradish peroxidase after lateral fluid percussion injury in rats and found that the injured BBB was restored in most regions by 30 min after TBI [2]. Others also reported that the BBB sealed after fluidpercussion injury and speculated that the initial breakdown was related to the hypertensive surge typically associated with this type of injury [15]. Enters and coworkers, however, found that pretreatment of animals with hexamethonium, a drug that prevents the MAP increase, did not prevent TBI-induced disruption of the BBB [1]. Van den Brink *et al.* compared the role of acute post-traumatic hypertension in BBB breakdown in two different models of TBI in rats [15]. They found that after impact acceleration injury, a model characterized by relative absence of a pressure rise, the BBB was compromised to a much lesser degree than after fluid-percussion injury, which was typically followed by a severe blood pressure surge. The increase in MAP observed in our experiments was relatively mild compared to previous results with a maximum of 14 mmHg in both groups at 15 min post-trauma.

We find that in fluid-percussion brain injury the BBB is damaged at 1 h post-trauma, while its function is restored by 6 h. Over the past years interest has shifted towards WBCs as possible mediators of secondary brain damage after brain injury [3].

Our results indicate that 1) BBB breakdown at 1 h after Trauma is not related to increased WBC sticking and 2) that WBC sticking in pia venules at 6 h after TBI is *not* associated with increased vessel permeability. This latter finding was unexpected because studies in the past have reported a positive correlation between

Table 1. *Relationship Between WBC Sticking in Postcapillary Pia Venules and BBB Disruption*

Group/experiment number	I-1	I-2	I-3	I-4	I-5	II-1	II-2	II-3	II-4	II-5
Na+-fluorescein extravasation	yes	yes	yes	yes	no	no	no	no	no	no
WBC sticking per mm²										
vessel wall at baseline	3	18	0	23	8	5	17	7	0	20
1 h after TBI	17	24	11	35	23	–	–	–	–	–
6 h after TBI	–	–	–	–	–	0	111	136	64	50

brain edema and WBC accumulation in brain tissue after experimental cerebral ischemia [6]. Moreover, from intravital videomicroscopy studies it is known that WBC sticking in peripheral organs is associated with increased vascular permeability [4]. Recently, Soares et al. reported that in rats undergoing lateral fluid-percussion injury recruitment of WBCs was only observed in regions of concomitant BBB damage [11]. Data from Baethmann and co-workers, on the other hand, indicated that *depletion* of WBCs after cryogenic lesion was associated with more pronounced edema formation, suggesting that WBCs may actually confer neroprotection [10].

Some points deserve mentioning: The degree of WBC sticking observed in the present experiments at 6 h after TBI (mean: 72 ± 48 WBCs/mm^2 endothelium) was less than reported by others in peripheral organs. Experimental ischemia/reperfusion in striated muscle appears to trigger an earlier WBC response with 400–1500 sticking WBCs/mm^2 endothelium after only 2 h [8, 9]. It is therefore possible that WBC-mediated BBB disruption after TBI might occur at a later timepoint when more WBCs are activated. Also, one may speculate that morphological characteristics of the BBB, such as the existence of tight junctions, confers resistance to WBC toxicity. Finally, based on our findings and the data by Soares et al. WBCs may not induce BBB damage at all, but rather act as passive responders to tissue injury and depend on an allready compromised microvasculature to migrate into brain parenchyma.

Taken together, our data provide *in vivo* evidence for transient opening of the BBB very early after TBI. WBC activation at 6 h after TBI is not associated with increased vascular permeability. Whether activated WBCs injure the cerebral vasculature at a later point will be investigated further.

Acknowledgements

This study was supported by the Annie Laurie Aitken Charitable Trust as part of their commitment to the advancement of brain injury research.

References

1. Enters EK, Pascua JR, McDowell KP, et al (1992) Blockade of acute hypertensive response does not prevent changes in behavior or in CSF acetylcholine (ACH) content following traumatic brain injury (TBI). Brain Res 576: 271–276
2. Fukuda K, Tanno H, Okimura Y, et al (1995) The blood-brain barrier disruption to circulating proteins in the early period after fluid percussion brain injury in rats. J Neurotrauma 12: 315–324
3. Härtl R, Schürer L, Schmid-Schönbein, et al (1996) Antileukocyte interventions in experimental cerebral ischemia. J Cereb Blood Flow Metab: in press
4. Kubes P, Suzuki M, Granger DN (1990) Modulation of PAF-induced leukocyte adherence and increased microvascular permeability. Am J Physiol 259: G859–864
5. Levasseur JE, Wei EP, Raper AJ, et al (1975) Detailed description of a cranial window technique for acute and chronic experiments. Stroke 6: 308–317
6. Matsuo Y, Onodera H, Shiga Y, et al (1994) Correlation between myeloperoxidasequantified neutrophil accumulation and ischemic brain injury in the rat. Effects of neutrophil depletion. Stroke 25: 1469–1475
7. Mayhan WG, Heistad DD (1985) Permeability of blood-brain barrier to various sized molecules. Am J Physiol 248: H712–718
8. Menger MD, Steiner D, Messmer K (1992) Microvascular ischemia-reperfusion injury in striated muscle: significance of "no reflow". Am J Physiol 263: H1892–1900
9. Nolte D, Hecht R, Schmid P, et al (1994) Role of Mac-1 and ICAM-1 in ischemiareperfusion injuy in a microcirculation model of BALB/C mice. Am J Physiol 267: H1320–H1328
10. Schürer L, Prugner U, Kempski O, et al (1990) Effects of antineutrophil serum (ANS) on posttraumatic brain oedema in rats. Acta Neurochir (Wien) [Suppl] 51: 49–51
11. Soares HD, Hicks RR, Smith D, et al (1995) Inflammatory leukocytic recruitment and diffuse neuronal degeneration are separate pathological processes resulting from traumatic brain injury. J Neurosci 15: 8223–8233
12. Tanno H, Nockels RP, Pitts LH, et al (1992) Breakdown of the blood-brain barrier after fluid percussion brain injury in the rat. Part 2: Effect of hypoxia on permeability to plasma proteins. J Neurotrauma 9: 335–347
13. Tanno H, Nockels RP, Pitts LH, et al (1992) Breakdown of the blood-brain barrier after fluid percussive brain injury in the rat. Part 1: Distribution and time course of protein extravasation. J Neurotrauma 9: 21–32
14. Unterberg A, Wahl M, Baethmann A (1988) Effects of free radicals on permeability and vasomotor response of cerebral vessels. Acta Neuropathol 76: 238–244
15. van den Brink WA, Santos BO, Marmarou A, et al (1994) Quantitative analysis of blood-brain, barrier damage in two models of experimental head injury in the rat. Acta Neurochir (Wien) [Suppl] 60: 456–458

Correspondence: Roger Härtl, M.D., Aitken Neuroscience Institute, 523 E 72nd Street, New York, NY 10021, U.S.A.

Acta Neurochir (1997) [Suppl] 70: 243–246
© Springer-Verlag 1997

Acute Blood-Brain Barrier Changes in Experimental Closed Head Injury as Measured by MRI and Gd-DTPA

P. Barzó[1], **A. Marmarou**[1], **P. Fatouros**[2], **F. Corwin**[2], and **J. G. Dunbar**[1]

[1] Division of Neurosurgery and [2] Department of Radiology, Medical College of Virginia, Richmond, VA, U.S.A

Summary

The objective of this study was to determine the early time course of blood-brain barrier (BBB) changes in diffuse closed head injury (CHI) and to what extent BBB is affected by secondary insult.

The BBB disruption was quantified using T_1-weighted MRI following administration of Gd-DTPA. The maximal signal intensity (SI) enhancement was used to calculate BBB disruption. A new CHI model was used to induce injury. Adult SD rats were separated into four groups: Group I: Sham (n = 4), II: Hypoxia and Hypotension (HH, n = 4), III: Trauma alone (n = 23), and IV: Trauma coupled with HH (THH, n = 14). Following trauma, a 30 minute insult of hypoxia (PaO_2 = 40 mmHg) and hypotension (MABP = 30 mmHg) were imposed.

In trauma animals, SI increased dramatically immediately following impact. By 15 minutes, permeability decreased exponentially and by 30 minutes was equal to that of control. In THH animals, SI enhancement was lower after the trauma, consistent with reduced blood pressure and blood flow. However, the SI increased dramatically upon reperfusion and was equal to that of control after 60 minutes.

In conclusion we may consider, that CHI is associated with a rapid and transient BBB opening which begins at the time of the trauma and lasts not more than 30 minutes. It has been also shown that addition of hypoxia and hypotension prolongs the time of BBB breakdown.

Keywords: Traumatic brain injury; blood-brain barrier; magnetic resonance imaging; gadolinium-DTPA; brain watrer determination.

Introduction

Traumatic brain edema has long been considered a result of blood-brain barrier (BBB) compromise and exudation of fluid to the extracellular space. The vascular origin of this fluid led to the classification of the edema type as "vasogenic" in contrast to the ischemic form of edema which is bound intracellularly and termed "cytotoxic" [1]. If indeed the edema component is of the so called vasogenic type, then it is reasonable to posit that the blood brain barrier in diffuse injury must remain compromised for a considerable period as the effects of the swelling process are most pronounced 3 to 4 days post injury when intracranial hypertension is problematic. If however, the BBB opening is short-lived, then it is reasonable to conclude that the ensuing swelling process is not exclusively a "vasogenic" form but must involve cellular swelling as well, particularly when the injury is coupled with hypoxia and hypotension which may exacerbate the swelling process.

To help resolve these issues, our goal was to describe both the duration of opening and extent of permeability change of the blood brain barrier in an experimental model of diffuse CHI produced by impact acceleration [2] and injury coupled with secondary insult. Magnetic resonance imaging with Gd-DTP provides a means for the noninvasive detection of BBB injury [3]. Gd-DTPA does not normally cross the BBB, but has been shown to cross if the BBB is damaged.

Therefore, the objective of this study were threefold: first, to develop a new method for *in vivo* quantification of BBB permeability; secondly, use this method to follow the time course of early BBB changes following diffuse CHI and thirdly to examine the effect of hypoxia and hypotension upon BBB permeability.

Materials and Methods

Adult male Sprague-Dawley rats weighing 340 to 375 grams were divided into four groups (n = ICP/CBF bench study and the MRI study): I. Control (n = 4 and 4), II. Hypotension plus hypoxia (n = 4 and 4), III. Trauma alone (n = 4 and 23), and IV. Trauma plus hypoxia coupled with hypotension (THH) (n = 4 and 14). In fifteen animals of Group III (trauma alone) GD-DTPA was injected 15 (Group IIIb, n = 5), 30 (Group IIIc, n = 5) and 60 minutes (Group IIId, n = 5) after the trauma, whereas in six animals of Group IV (trauma and secondary insult) Gd-DTPA was injected only 60 minutes postinjury (IVb). Rats were initially anesthetized with halothane, then intubated and ventilated with a gas mixture of N_2O (70%), O_2 (30%), and halothane. Body temperature was maintained at $37 \pm 0.5°C$. In the HH and the THH groups, hypotension was induced by withdrawing arterial blood during the first five minutes following trauma until a MABP of 30–40 mmHg was sustained for 30 minutes. After hypotension, all withdrawn blood was returned. Hypoxia was maintained at approximately 40 mmHg for 30 minutes. A new impact acceleration head injury model was used to produce trauma [2].

Experiments were performed using a 2.35 T, 40 cm bore magnet (Biospec, Bruker Instruments, Billerica, MA) equipped with a 12 cm inner diameter actively shielded gradient insert. T1- and T2-weighted images were acquired from the same coronal slice (3 mm thickness), placed at a standardized anatomical plane chosen to be 7.5 mm from the tip to the forebrain, employing conventional single and multiecho spin echo sequences, respectfully. T1-weighted images (TR/TE 700/22) were sequentially acquired using an image matrix of 128×128 (1.5 minutes per image). T2-weighted images (TR/TE 3000/160) were acquired for elucidation of structures within the brain. The average T1-weighted signal intensities for six regions of interest (ROI's) within the brain (bilateral cerebral cortex, caudate nucleus, the corpus callosum and the whole brain) and one within the muscle, were determined for each image in both the control and post trauma runs. Five T1-weighted and one T2-weighted control images were collected prior to the trauma. Following the acquisition of control images Gd-DTPA was injected at a dose of 0.2 mmol/kg and the animals were subjected to the insult. The animals were then repositioned in the magnet and data acquisition was carried out at 1.5 minutes intervals from 4 to 73 minutes post injury. The percentage change in signal intensity (SI) of the previously described regions was calculated as follows: SI (%) = (SI_t − SI_0) / $SI_0 \times 100$ where SI_t is the intensity t minutes after trauma, and SI_0 the intensity before trauma.

Microgravimetric analysis was performed on the same slices for which MRI was performed. Specific gravity and water content were obtained by using a calibrated gravimetric column of kerosene and bromobenzene.

Results

Dynamic progression of blood-brain-barrier damage: The signal intensity enhancement changes in the brain for the four groups (Group I–IV) is shown in Fig. 1. To illustrate more clearly the BBB disruption, the duration (as long as SI increased) and the severity (maximum SI) of the BBB opening was calculated and plotted.

Group I (control): SI gradually increased in the brain during the first 13 minutes after Gd-DTPA injection and achieved a maximum value of $2 \pm 1\%$ between 13 and 75 minutes (Fig. 1).

Group II (HH, hypoxia and hypotension): The Gd-DTPA injection did not alter the SI during the time of hypotension and hypoxia. At 30 minutes, however a rapid enhancement ($6 \pm 1\%$, $p < 0.001$) was observed, which paralleled the recovery of the blood pressure (Fig. 1).

Group IIIa (trauma alone, trauma and Gd-DTPA inj. in the same time): Four minutes after the head injury and Gd-DTPA injection, significant bilateral

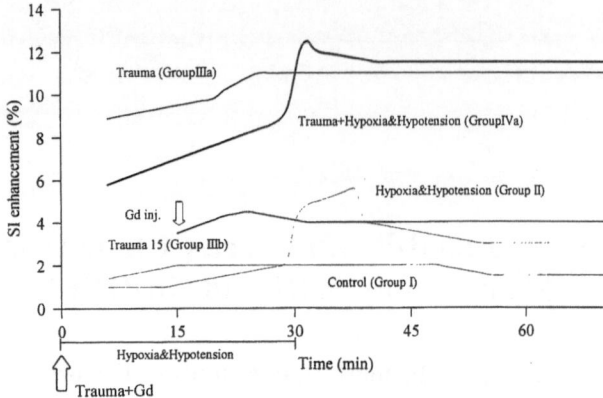

Fig. 1. Time course of signal intensity (SI) changes in T_1-weighted images – trauma alone and trauma with secondary insult groups: Values showed means. Control: Gd-DTPA injection, no trauma (Group I); hypoxia and hypotension (Group II): hypoxia and hypotension; trauma (Group IIIa): trauma and Gd-DTPA inj. in the same time; trauma-15 (Group IIIb): Gd-DTPA inj. at 15 min post injury; trauma-30 (Group IIIc): Gd-DTPA inj. at 30 min post injury; trauma + hypoxia and hypotension (Group IVa): trauma and Gd-DTPA inj. in the same time)

increases in SI ($9 \pm 4\%$, $p < 0.01$) were visible on the MR images. During the next 20 minutes, SI increased only slightly and reached its maximum value of $11.5 \pm 6\%$ at 26 minutes after trauma (Fig. 1).

Group IIIb (trauma alone, Gd-DTPA inj. 15 min after trauma): Following the Gd-DTPA, a slight but significant increase in SI was visible corresponding to the whole brain (Fig. 1).

Group IIIc-d (trauma alone, Gd-DTPA 30 or 60 min after trauma): In the five-five animals no significant increase in SI was observed.

Group IVa (trauma and secondary insult, trauma and Gd-DTPA at the same time): A significant intensity enhancement was observed on the first images ($6 \pm 3\%$, $p < 0.01$); however, it was less pronounced as compared to the trauma alone animals. Although the further time course study of MR signals showed gradually increased SI during hypotension and hypoxia, the most definitive change occurred at the time of recovery (30 minutes post injury). The SI increased 4%, and reached its maximum value ($12 \pm 3\%$) within 3 minutes (Fig. 1). The cerebral cortex and the corpus callosum showed the highest enhancement of $13 \pm 4\%$ and $15 \pm 6\%$.

Group IVb (trauma and secondary insult, Gd-DTPA 60 min after trauma): In the six animals no significant increase was observed indicating that the BBB was closed.

Water content of the cerebrum and cerebellum at 90 minutes post injury is summarised in Fig. 2.

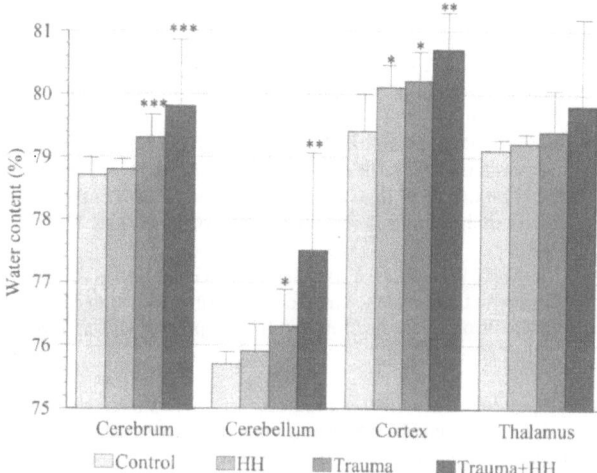

Fig. 2. Water content (WC) 90 minutes after trauma: The estimated WC of the total brain was significantly increased in both Group III and IV. Cortex and cerebellum of Group III and IV revealed the highest WCs whereas the WC in the thalamus did not change significantly in any of Group II, III or IV. This water increase was consistent with traumatic opening of the blood-brain barrier

Discussion

Our observations indicate, that MRI due to its non-invasive character is an excellent technique to follow (time resolution 1–1.5 min) the evolution of trauma-induced BBB damage from as early as few minutes up to hours or even longer after the trauma. Only two other studies have followed the early BBB changes quantitatively with similar method. Rhine *et al.* using hyperosmotic shock for demonstrating BBB disruption, found that Gd-DTPA enhances SI in the tissues outside the barrier by 17–33%, without affecting the intensity in the normal brain tissue [3]. However, these results are in accordance with our findings, it should be noted that the hyperosmotic barrier opening is not an equivalent to the insult due to head injury. We think that this is one of the reasons why we could not observe such a high increase (24%) in the SI even in our THH group animals (12%). Moreover, this difference suggests that the BBB breakdown observed in the trauma or in the THH group was only partial. This supports the principal finding of this study, namely, that the BBB opening is transient and rapidly re-establishes itself.

The evidence of the transient opening can be seen from the time course of the intensity changes (Fig. 1). The BBB for the trauma alone group opens within a few minutes after injury, approaches gradually a plateau at 26 minutes post trauma and remains constant thereafter. Since the elevated SI did not change during

the next 60 minutes, we also presume that the Gd-DTPA is trapped in the brain. Since at 15 minutes post injury Gd-DTPA injection revealed only slight permeability disturbances, we may also assume that the BBB breakdown is most severe during the first 15 minutes following brain injury. This rapid closure of the barrier provides further support to our hypotheses that the vasogenic component of edema may be overemphasized and that the predominant form of edema may be cellular in nature [4].

The fact that the BBB is closed at 30 minutes after the injury in the trauma alone (Group IIIc) and 60 minutes even in the THH Group (Group IVb, Fig. 1) supports our contention of the transient pattern of BBB opening in diffuse injury and with secondary insult. Although many studies have been published on the BBB disruption due to traumatic brain injury, only very few investigations followed the early changes [5, 6]. Our results are consistent with previous reports on the integrity of the BBB and the role of a permeability deficit in the formation of cerebral edema using other models of head injury [5]. These studies analyzed permeability defect of short duration and showed that the peak of the BBB leakage was seen between 0 and 30 minutes.

Based on these observations we conclude that during the transient breakdown of the BBB, Gd-DTPA may enter both extracellular space and cellular compartments. Following the rapid closure of the barrier and sealing of the axons [7], Gd-DTPA is trapped intra- and extracellularly and it is reasonable to assume that with barrier closure, subsequent edema development must be of cellular nature.

The mild and transient hypertension, followed by a period of sustained hypotension seen in this CHI model is in contrast to the documented prolonged surge of arterial pressure following fluid percussion model. Whereas in both models the barrier is compromised, in CHI other pathological events, rather than severe hypertension are also responsible for the BBB disruption. However the difference in SI enhancement between the trauma alone and the THH group (Fig. 1) during the first 30 minutes postinjury reflect the importance of blood pressure and blood flow in the initial BBB breakdown.

In conclusion, diffuse CHI is associated with a rapid and transient BBB onening which begins at the time of the trauma and approaches closure at about 25–30 minutes. Post traumatic secondary insult prolongs the breakdown of the BBB. MRI due to its noninvasive character is an excellent technique to follow (time resolution 1–1.5 min) the evolution of trauma-induced BBB damage from as early as few minutes up to hours or even longer after the trauma.

References

1. Reulen HJ, Graham R, Spatz M, Klatzo (1997) Role of pressure gradients and bulk flow in dynamics of vasogenic brain edema. J Neurosurg 46: 24–36
2. Foda MAA, Marmarou A (1994) A new model of diffuse brain injury in rats. Part II: Morphological characterization. J Neurosurg 80: 301–313
3. Rhine WD, Benaron DA, Enzmann DR, Chung C, Gonzales-Mendez R, Sayre JR, Stevenson DK (1993) Gd-DTPA MR detection of blood-brain barrier opening in rats after hyperosmotic shock. J Comp Assist Tomogr 17: 563–566
4. Marmarou A (1994) Traumatic brain edema: an overview. Acta Neurochir (Wien) [Supp] 60: 421–424
5. Povlishock JT, Becker DP, Miller JD, Jenkins LW, Dietrich WD (1979) The morphologic substrates of concussion. Acta Neuropath 47: 1–11
6. Bullock R, Statham P, Patterson J, Wyper D, Hadley D, Teasdale E (1990) The time course of vasogenic oedema after focal human head injury – evidence from SPECT mapping of blood brain barrier defects. Acta Neurochir (Wien) 51: 286–288
7. Maxwell WL, Watt C, Graham DI, Gennarelli TA (1993) Ultrastructural evidence of axonal shearing as a result of lateral acceleration of the head in hon-human primates. Acta Neuropathol 86: 136–144

Correspondence: Anthony Marmarou, M.D., Division of Neurosurgery, P.O. Box 508, MCV Station, Sanger Hll, Room 8004a, 1101 E Marshal St., Richmond, VA 23298, U.S.A.

Acta Neurochir (1997) [Suppl] 70: 247–249
© Springer-Verlag 1997

Transport of Human β-Amyloid Peptide Through the Rat Blood-Brain Barrier After Global Cerebral Ischemia

R. Pluta[1,3], A. Misicka[2,4], S. Januszewski[1], M. Barcikowska[1], and A. W. Lipkowski[2]

[1] Department of Neuropathology and [2] Neuropeptide Laboratory, Medical Research Centre, Polish Academy of Sciences,
[3] Department of Medical Sciences, Academy of Physical Education, and [4] Department of Chemistry, Warsaw University,
Warsaw, Poland

Summary

In an attempt to produce an animal model of the Alzheimer's disease (AD), β-amyloid-(1-42)-peptide (βA1-42) was injected into the femoral vein in rats after single and repeated cardiac arrest (CA). After survival of 3.5 months, the brains immunoreactivity was evaluated using light microscopic immunocytochemistry of monoclonal β-amyloid peptide (βA) antibody 4G8 (mAb 4G8). Rats receiving βA1-42 after CA demonstrated multifocal and widespread extravasation of βA1-42 in extra- and intracellular space. The permeability to βA1-42 was significantly higher in rats after repeated cerebral ischemia. As in AD, there were irregular diffuse amyloid plaque-like deposits and neuronal loss with reactive gliosis. Our data in ischemic rats with βA1-42 represent a novel animal model of Alzheimer's pathology.

Keywords: Alzheimer's disease; blood-brain barrier; β-amyloid; cerebral ischemia.

Introduction

The extracellular accumulation of βA in the brain parenchyma and vasculature of patients with AD is a neuropathological hallmark of the disease [7]. The origin of βA in brain plaques and vessels of AD victims is not known and the effect of βA *in vivo* remains unresolved. Soluble βA has been detected in normal biological fluids [8] and in the media of cultured cells [2]. Recently, clinical studies reported the increased level of soluble βA in the plasma of AD cases [3]. Therefore, we decided to test the hypothesis that repeated injections of human βA1-42 [4] in conjunction with repeated opening of the blood-brain barrier (BBB) induced by CA [5] would facilitate the development of a rat model in which to study the consequences of βA deposition in brain.

Material and Methods

Wistar rats under ether anesthesia, were subjected to a single 10 min global cerebral ischemia or to three repeated ischemic episodes (first 10 min global cerebral ischemia, followed by two episodes each of 3.5 min global cerebral ischemia at 1 month intervals). A special metal hook-like device was inserted into the mediastinum through the third right intercostal space for occluding the cardiac vessel bundle. The effect of this procedure was CA with total cessation of systemic circulation [5]. Heart activity and brain circulation were restored by external heart massage and artificial ventilation [5]. All rats received synthetic, human βA1-42 [4] given as three injections, each of 1 mg, per week into the femoral vein for 3 months (a total of 36 injections). The peptide infusion begun 15 min after the first ischemic insult. Controls were sham-operated rats with or without βA1-42 injections and rats with single and repeated ischemia only. Two weeks after last βA1-42 injection the rats were perfused transcardially with phosphate-buffered saline followed by 2% paraformaldehyde containing 1% glutaraldehyde [5]. At least three rats were included in each group. For βA visualization we used human-specific mAb 4G8 [6]. Recent studies showed that cerebral ischemia induced in rats β-amyloid deposits in brain parenchyma, but these deposits showed no immunoreactivity with human-specific mAb 4G8 [6]. For this reason we used a synthetic βA1-42 homologous to a major form of human soluble βA, which was found to react with mAb 4G8 in rats [4].

Results

Following ischemia and injection of βA1-42, brain microvessels of various kinds and sizes showed remarkable extravasation of βA1-42, spreading multifocally predominantly in the hippocampus and cerebral cortex. Neuronal, glial and ependymal cell bodies were observed filled with βA1-42. The βA1-42 immunoreactivity was found in both morphologically unchanged and markedly damaged neurons. Blood vessels were frequently surrounded by a number of

Table 1. *Extravasation of βA1-42 Following Global Cerebral Ischemia*

Deposits of βA1-42 in brain	Single ischemia	Repeated ischemia
Extracellular space	+	+ + +
Intracellular space		
Neurons	+ +	+ + +
Glia	+	+ +
Pericytes	+	+ + +
Ependymal cells	+	+ + +
Intraventricular space	+ + +	+ + +

Deposits: + single; ++ few; +++ multiple.

pericytes filled with βA1-42 reaction product. The size of βA1-42 deposition ranged from numerous small immunopositive dots to irregular diffuse plaques. The latter were often observed without any visible connection with blood vessels. The leakage of βA1-42 increased significantly with frequency of ischemic episodes (Table 1).

Discussion

The link of βA with AD has been well established [7]. The deposition of soluble βA into amyloid plaques is believed to be a primary event in the neuropathology of the disease. It is not yet known what causes the abundance of plaques in AD brain. Our studies suggest that soluble βA from the circulation in conjunction with alterations in the BBB permeability could lead to an increase in plaque formation. The present study implies that, the BBB in normal conditions seems to possess the ability to control the cerebrovascular sequestration and penetration of βA into the brain parenchyma. Halting or reducing plaque formation, either by preventing the deposition of βA, or by reducing the amount of βA transported from the circulation by open BBB could potentially lead to therapy for the disease.

Direct evidence that soluble human βA1-42 floods from vascular bed into the brain parenchyma in environmental condition is provided here for the first time. Injection of βA1-42 was stopped 2 weeks before the end of experiments. This results suggest either the protein within brain could not be efficiently removed/metabolized or that it was continuously supplied from the circulation in response to ischemic opening of BBB. As in AD, we observed irregular diffuse amyloid plaque-like deposits and neuronal loss with reac-

tive gliosis. This finding demonstrates that an amyloid deposit with the morphological appearance of a human amyloid diffuse plaque can be artificially produced in an animal model. Factors such as chronic, silent and repeated ischemia with frequent opening of BBB, may be critical for the development of AD symptoms.

Unlike AD, βA1-42 deposition in our rat model was not associated with accumulation of fibrillar amyloid. Since tioflavine S labeling was not detected in any region of the ischemic/βA1-42 rat brains examined, the compact fibrillar structure of βA1-42 was probably not formed. On the other hand fibrillar βA1-42 could be formed but in amount to small to be recognized by tioflavine S. Rats may have a higher capacity to metabolize and remove βA1-42 from the brain. This was not confirmed in our study. Finally, the possibility that 3.5 months of survival may be insufficient to produce detectable amounts of fibrillar βA1-42 cannot be excluded. Deposition of βA in the brain is a slow process that in humans takes decades to develop. In our rat model may be the time factor plays a central role in the maturation of βA1-42 deposits as in transgenic mice [1]. Longer study intervals may clarify this issue.

Acknowledgement

Supported by grant from the CSR 6 P207 051 05.

References

1. Games D, Adams D, Alessandrini R, Barbour R, Berthelette P, Blackwell C, Carr T, Clemens J, Donaldson T, Gillespie F, Guido T, Hagopian S, Johnson-Wood K, Khan K, Lee M, Leibowitz P, Lieberburg I, Little S, Masliah E, McConlogue L, Montoya-Zavala M, Mucke L, Paganini L, Penniman E, Power M, Schenk D, Seubert P, Snyder B, Soriano F, Tan H, Vitale J, Wadsworth S, Wolozin B, Zhao J (1995) Alzheimer-type neuropathology in transgenic mice overexpressing V717F β-amyloid precursor protein. Nature 373: 523–527
2. Haass C, Schlossmacher MG, Hung AY, Vigo-Pelfrey C, Mellon A, Ostaszewski BL, Lieberburg L, Koo EH, Schenk D, Teplow DB, Selkoe DJ (1992) Amyloid beta-peptide is produced by cultured cells during normal metabolism. Nature 359: 322–325
3. Jensen M, Song XH, Suzuki N, Lannfelt L, Younkin SG (1995) The A NL Alzheimer mutation (Swedish) increases plasma amyloid β-protein concentration. J Neurochem [Suppl] 65: S136
4. Misicka A, Lipkowski AW, Barcikowska M, Pluta R (1995) Synthesis and formulation for biological study of the β-amyloid (1-42) polypeptide. In: Maia HLS (ed) Peptides 1994. ESCOM, Leiden, pp 377–378
5. Pluta R, Lossinsky AS, Mossakowski MJ, Faso L, Wisniewski HM (1991) Reassessment of a new model of complete cerebral ischemia in rats. Method of induction of clinical death, patho-

physiology and cerebrovascular pathology. Acta Neuropathol 83: 1–11

6. Pluta R, Kida E, Lossinsky AS, Golabek AA, Mossakowski MJ, Wisniewski HM (1994) Complete cerebral ischemia with short-term survival in rats induced by cardiac arrest. I. Extracellular accumulation of Alzheimer's β-amyloid protein precursor in the brain. Brain Res 649: 323–328

7. Selkoe DJ (1994) Alzheimer's disease: a central role for amyloid. J Neuropathol Exp Neurol 53: 438–447

8. Seubert P, Vigo-Pelfrey C, Esch F, Lee M, Dovey H, Davis D, Sinha S, Schlossmacher M, Whaley J, Swindlehurst C, McCormack R, Wolfert R, Selkoe DJ (1992) Isolation and quantification of soluble Alzheimer's β-peptide from biological fluids. Nature 359: 325–327

Correspondence: Ryszard Pluta, M.D., Ph.D., Department of Neuropathology, Medical Research Centre, Polish Academy of Sciences, Dworkowa 3 Str., 00-784 Warsaw, Poland.

Acta Neurochir (1997) [Suppl] 70: 250–253
© Springer-Verlag 1997

Enhanced Brain Opioid Receptor Activity Precedes Blood-Brain Barrier Disruption

P. Ting[1], P. A. Cushenberry[1], T. C. Friedman[2], and Y. P. Loh[2]

[1] Department of Pediatrics, Howard University, Washington, D.C., and [2] Cellular Neurobiology Section, National Institute of Child Health, NIH, Bethesda, MD, U.S.A.

Summary

We studied the effects of transient postischemic increased opioid receptors (OPR) binding (μ, ∂, k) on blood-brain barrier (BBB), brain water content and brain mitochondrial oxidative enzymes system. Cats were exposed to temporary middle cerebral artery occlusion (MCAO). The significant increased OPR bindings observed 10 min after the release of MCAO (ischemic rCBF= 7 ± 1 to 11 ± 2 ml/100 g/min) preceded the early and late BBB disruptions, brain edema and postischemic impaired mitochondrial oxidative enzymes functions. Further, the study suggests indirectly that the latter process was irreversible and hence associated with subsequent ischemic cerebral infarction. In addition, the results revealed a possible viable therapeutic window in the early postischemic recirculation period, before the onset of impaired mitochondrial oxidative function.

Keywords: Cerebral ischemia; blood-brain barrier; opioid receptors/peptides; 2,3,5-triphenyltetrazolium chloride.

Introduction

Enhanced endogenous opioid system activity has been suggested to mediate ischemic neurological dysfunction and neuronal damage, however, the mechanisms are not clear [5, 9, 10, 13, 16]. We recently reported that following temporary focal cerebral ischemia in cats, there was a transient significant increase in brain opioid receptors (μ, ∂, k) [17]. The present study was conducted to evaluate the effects of enhanced brain opioid activity on subsequent microcirculatory and neuronal homeostasis, specifically on bloodbrain barrier, brain water content and brain mitochondrial oxidative enzymes system.

Materials and Methods

Adult male mongrel cats with body weight between 2.5 and 3.5 kg were fasted overnight before an experiment. A cat was

intubated and placed on a respirator following initial anesthesia induction with Ketamin 20 mg/kg 1M, and then, maintained on alpha-chloralose 60 mg/kg i.v. Rectal temperature was kept between 37–38 degrees Celsius by adjusting the thermostat control of a heating pad. Femoral artery and vein were cannulated for direct continuous recording of arterial blood pressure, pH, pCO_2, pO_2 and i.v. infusion of fluid and drugs. The cat's head was then fixed on a stereotaxic apparatus for transorbital exposure of a left middle cerebral artery (MCA), and for stereotaxic insertion of recording platinum microelectrodes, one each in ipsilateral cortex and caudate coordinates supplied by the MCA (Synder's Atlas). A miniature stainless steel screw was affixed to the skull and used as the reference electrode. The regional cerebral blood flow (rCBF) was measured by standard hydrogen clearance technique described elsewhere [2, 8] The rCBF is calculated using the formula $F = \lambda$ $0.693 / T) \times 100$, where F = flow in ml/100 g/min, λ = brain blood partition coefficient (for H_2, $\lambda = 1$), $0.693 = \log_e 2$, and T is the effective half time in minutes for desaturation. Blood-brain barrier (BBB) opening to albumin was evaluated by 2% Evans blue (EB) dye tracer (2 ml/kg i.v.). The EB was injected (1) just prior to MCA occlusion for cats sacrificed at the end of one hour (h) of occlusion (MCAO); (2) immediately upon release of MCAO for cats sacrificed at 10, 60, and 180 minutes of recirculation (R) (Early BBB opening); (3) after 3 h R for cats sacrificed at 6 h R (late BBB opening) and (4) one hour post surgery in sham operated controls which were sacrificed 5–6 h later. Passage of the tracer into the brain tissue was assessed macroscopically in the brain sections, in the vicinity of the recording electrode tips. For brain water content evaluation, the specific gravity (SG) method [14] was used on regional brain tissue samples close to the recording electrode tips. Brain opioid receptor subtypes (μ, ∂, k°) were determined by radioligand binding technique [6, 18]. Brain opioid peptides were measured by radioimmunoassay technique as described elsewhere [7]. Briefly, brain tissue samples of 50–70 mg (w/w) were obtained from regions close to the microelectrode tips and frozen immediately on dry ice and stored at −70°C. Different receptor subtypes were studied by sequential displacement of the "overall" binding of the unselective opioid antagonist, $< 10^{-9}$ M [^{3}H]-diprenorphine (DPN), with highly selective ligand for various subsites: 10^{-7} M [D-Ala^2, MePhe^4, Gly(ol)^5]-enkephalin (DAGO = μ agonist), 10^{-6} M ICI 174,864 (ICI = delta antagonist), 10^{-5} U-50488H (U-50 = kappa agonist) and 10^{-5} Naloxone (NAL) to define non-specific binding. The receptor concentration was expressed as fmol/mg protein in the sample. For opioid peptides measurements, approximately 10 mg (w/w) brain samples were homogenized in a solution containing 1N HCl, 5% formic acid, 1% trifluoroacetic acid (TFA), 1% NaCl, 1 mM phenylmethane sulfonylfluoride, 1 mM iodoacetamide, 50 μM pepstatin A, 30 K1U aprotinin and 1 mM EDTA. The homogenate was passed through an octadecyl silylsilica cartridge. The eluent was lyophilized and reconstituted in radioimmunoassay (RIA) buffer provided, and the peptides measured by the commercially available RIA kits. For evaluation of brain mitochondrial oxidative enzymes system, fresh brain sections were stained with 2% 2,3,5-triphenyl-tetrazolium chloride (TTC) as described elsewhere [3, 4]. The stain acts as a proton acceptor for mitochondrial oxidative cellular metabolism, and it is reduced to a redformazan product in normal brain (TTC–). However, when there is impaired oxidative metabolism, the dye is not reduced and the brain remains pale (TTC+).

Following an hour of stabilization from surgery, rCBF was determined before, during and after the release of 1 h MCAO. Arterial BP and rectal temperature were recorded continuously until the animal was sacrificed with an overdose of i.v. pentobarbital. The brain was rapidly removed and a coronal section was made through the H_2 electrode entrance marks, the anterior 5 mm block was used for SG, and the posterior 5 mm section was frozen immediately for opioid receptors/peptides assays or for TTC staining.

Statistical analysis. T-Test and ANOVA were used with the aid of PC JMP program. Statistical significance was established at $P \leq 0.05$. Data were expressed as mean ± SE.

Results

There were 9 sham operated control without and 44 cats with temporary MCAO. The arterial BP and blood pH, and gases remained fairly stable without significant changes throughout the experiment, and likewise the rCBF in control group showed insignificant changes. However, in cats subjected to MCAO, the rCBF dropped from preischemic value of 78 ± 10 and 79 ± 20 to between 7 ± 1 and 11 ± 2 ml/100 g/min ($p < 0.01$) during ischemia, and upon recirculation, a significant hyperemia was noted ($p < 0.05$; Table 1). Early BBB opening with diffuse areas of EB extravasations were seen in upper lateral caudate and ectosylvian cortex ipsilateral to MCAO in 58% of cats (N = 19) sacrificed at 1 and 3 h of recirculation, but in none of the 10 cats euthanized at 10 min after the release of MCAO. The late BBB disruption was observed in 50% of cats (N = 6) sacrificed at six hours of recirculation. However, BBB was intact in all control

Table 1. *Regional Cerebral Blood Flow (ml/100 g/min) of Cats with (Ischemic) and without (Control) Temporary MCAO*

Group	Site	Baseline	MCAO		Recirculation		
			15	45	10	30	60 minutes
Controls (7)	caudate	78 ± 10	69 ± 13	78 ± 16	75 ± 16	69 ± 17	68 ± 21
	cortex	79 ± 20	79 ± 13	80 + 20	80 ± 23	88 ± 31	84 + 25
Ischemic (44)	caudate	39 ± 4	7 ± 1[a]	9 ± 2[a]	98 ± 11[a]	77 ± 12	78 ± 14
	cortex	57 ± 5	11 ± 24[a]	8 ± 1[a]	106 ± 22[a]	96 ± 26	70 ± 11

[a] $p < 0.05$ vs baseline.

Table 2. *Specific Gravity profile (Mean ± SE) of Controls and Cats Exposed to Temporary MCAO*

Site	Baseline	1 h MCAO	Recirculation (minutes)			
			10	60	180	360
Caudate	1.0439 ± 0.0006	1.0424 ± 0.0002	1.0426 + 0.0003	1.0399 ± 0.0007[a]	1.0387 ± 0.0012[a]	1.0361 ± 0.0025[a]
Cortex	1.0443 ± 0.0004	1.0422 ± 0.0007	1.0421 ± 0.0004	1.0422 ± 0.0008	1.0385 ± 0.0012[a]	1.0357 ± 0.0014[a]

[a] $p < 0.01$ vs baseline of controls.

Table 3. *Brain Cortical Opioid Peptides Concentrations (Mean ± SE) of Cats with and without MCAO*

Group	Opioid peptides fm/mg protein)		
	β-END	Leu-ENK	Dyn A1-13
Control	0.51 ± 0.06	7.75 ± 1.96	2.54 ± 0.76
1 h MCAO	0.60 ± 0.06	6.56 ± 2.32	3.98 ± 0.90
10 min R	0.56 ± 0.06	10.16 ± 2.11	2.60 ± 0.82

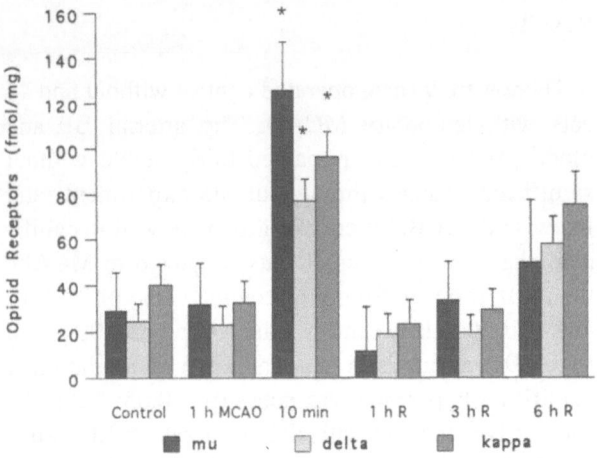

Fig. 1. Ipsilateral cortex. Ipsilateral brain opioid receptors (μ, ∂, k) concentrations (fm/mg protein) of controls (N = 7) and temporarily MCA occluded cats (N = 29). * p < 0.01 vs. control values

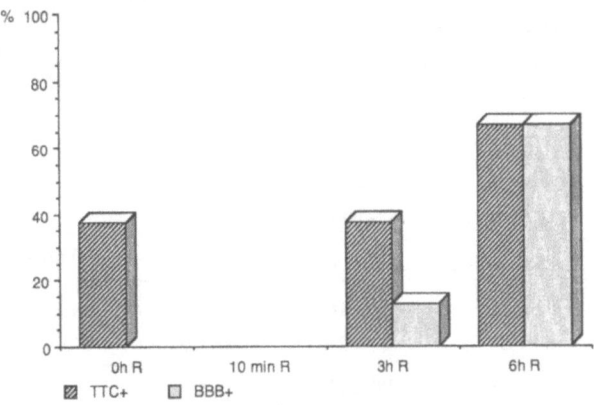

Fig. 2. Percentage of positive sites after MCAR. Ipsilateral caudate and cortex depicting TTC + stain (% of total sites) and BBB disruption (% of TTC + sites) in 21 cats subjected to temporary MCAO

cats (N = 9) and those sacrificed at the end of 1 h MCAO (N = 8). The ipsilateral SG values were significantly lower than controls at 1 h (caudate), 3 h (caudate and cortex) and 6 h (caudate and cortex) of recirculation (p < 0.01, Table 2). The opioid peptides, β-endorphin (β-END), leucine-enkephalin (Leu-ENK), and dynorphin A1-13 (Dyn A1-13) concentrations (fm/mg protein) in ipsilateral cortex were not significantly changed during and at 10 min after release of MCAO when compared with the controls (Table 3). However, brain opioid receptors concentrations (μ = 125.5 ± 21.5; ∂ = 77.1 ± 9.4; k = 96.1 ± 11.4 fm/mg protein) were significantly higher (p < 0.01) in ipsilateral cortex at 10 min R than controls (μ = 28.8 ± 17; ∂ = 24.5 ± 7.5; k = 40.1 ± 9 fm/mg protein) (Fig. 1). In ipsilateral caudate, only μ subtype OPR level (μ =

269.7 ± 41.3) was significantly increased at 10 min R when compared to controls (μ = 116 ± 32.7) (p < 0.01). Twenty-one cat's brains were stained with 2% TTC, and all non-ischemic contralateral brain sections were TTC negative. However, the incidence of positive TTC stain in ipsilateral caudate and cortex was 38% at 1 h MCAO (N = 4), none at 10 min R (N = 6), 43% at 180 min R (N = 5) and 60% at 360 min R (N = 6) (Fig. 2). All cats with TTC+ sites at 360 min R also depicted late BBB disruption.

Discussion

The present study revealed that the transient significant increased brain opioid receptors binding (μ, ∂, k) observed shortly upon release of MCAO preceded the early BBB disruption, brain edema, late BBB disruption and the late mitochondrial oxidative enzymes dysfunction. The early transient BBB disruption has been shown to be causally related to progression of postischemic brain edema, late BBB disruption and cerebral infarction, whereas, the late BBB disruption was always associated with cerebral infarction [8, 15]. It is possible that the increased OPR binding mediates early BBB disruption because, treatment with a high dose of Naloxone significantly reduced the postischemic BBB disruption and improved neurological outcome in newborn lambs [16]. In addition, a recent report revealed that NAL (high dose) significantly reduced the hypertensive BBB disruption and edema [12]. However, mechanisms for the OPR-induced BBB disruption are not known. Brain opioids concentrations in ipsilateral cortex were not significantly different from control cats both during ischemia and at 10 min of recirculation in the present study. Thus, endogenous opioids appear, not to be involved prior to the onset of early postischemic neuropathophysiology in the present study. However, more measurements at subsequent time intervals are needed to clarify this important issue. Two recent studies [1, 11] revealed a significant increase in brain OPR binding following temporary cerebral ischemia, one revealed a transient increase during the recirculation period prior to the onset of histological evidence of neuronal necrosis; the other study showed a significant increase in brain k-binding prior to the onset of ischemic neuronal lesions. TTC stain has been used as a histochemical marker for mitochondrial oxidative enzymes function. But, the enzymes dysfunctional status may be reversible, and therefore, may not indicate a permanent ischemic neuronal damage [4]. Our results revealed that the impaired TTC strain observed during MCAO recovered at 10 min R, and was associated with an intact BBB. However, this was followed by a recurrence of, and a progressive increase in the incidence of impaired mitochondrial oxidative system at 3 and 6 h of recirculation. This late deterioration in mitochondrial enzymes function always coincided with the onset of the late BBB disruption. Since earlier report [15] on the same animal model of focal cerebral ischemia indicated, that the early BBB opening was causally related to, and that the late BBB was always associated with cerebral infarction, we believe, that the positive TTC stain associated with both early and late BBB disruptions is an irreversible process, culminating with subsequent neuronal death.

In conclusion, the study suggests that enhanced brain OPR binding may be responsible for the early postischemic BBB disrutpion, progression of brain edema, late BBB disruptio and the irreversible mitochondrial oxidative enzymes function. The study also depicted a possible therapeutic window in the early postischemic recirculation period, prior to the onset of impaired mitochondrial enzymes function.

Acknowledgement

The study was funded by NIH, NIGMSS06-GM 08244-06. The authors thank Ms. Joanne H. Adelberg and the Howard University Veterinary Services for their excellent technical support.

References

1. Araki T, Murakami F, Kanai Y, Kato H, Kogure K (1993) Naloxone receptor binding in gerbil striatum and hippocampus following transient cerebral ischemia. Neurochem Int 23: 319–325
2. Aukland K, Bruce BF, Berliner RW (1964) Measurement of local blood flow with hydrogen gas. Cir Res 14: 164–187
3. Bederson JB, Pitts LH, Germano SM, Nishimura MC, et al (1986) Evaluation of 2,3,5-triphenyltetrazoilum chloride as a stain for detection and quantification of experimental cerebral infarction in rats. Stroke 17: 1304–1308
4. Cole DJ, Drummond JC, Ghazal EA, Shapiro HM (1989) A reversible component of cerebral injury as identified by the histochemical stain 2,3,5-triphenyltetrazolium chloride. Acta Neuropathol 80: 152–155
5. Faden AI (1986) Neuropeptides and central nervous system injury. Arch Neurol 32: 501–504
6. Fedynyshyn JP, Lee GK, et al (1989) Characterization of high affinity opioid binding sites in rat periaquecductal gray P2 membrane. Eur J Pharmacol 159: 83–88
7. Friedman TC, Chen HC, Loh YP (1993) Generation of 1-37 and 1-38 forms of adrenocorticortropin by mono-and dipeptidyl serine carboxypeptidase activities in bovine pituitary secretory vesicles. Endocinology 133: 2951–2961
8. Kuroiwa TT, Ting P, Martinez H, Klatzo I (1985) The biphasic opening of the blood-brain barrier to proteins following temporary middle cerebral artery occlusion. Acta Neuropathol 68: 122–129
9. Olinger CP, Adams HP Jr, Brott TG, et al (1990) High-dose intravenous naloxone for the treatment of acute ischemic stroke. Stroke 21: 721–725
10. Rozza A, La Torre G, Scavini C, Lanza E, et al (1992) K-opioid receptor changes in experimental models of cerebral ischaemia and atherosclerosis in the rabbit. Phamarcol Res 26: 409–415
11. Scavini C, Rozza A, Bo P, Lanza E, et al (1990) K-opioid receptor changes and neurophysiological alterations during cerebral ischemia in rabbits. Stroke 21: 943–947
12. Sharma HS, Westman J, Cervós-Navarro J, Nyberg F (1996) Role of neurochemicals in brain edema and cell changes following hyperthermic brain injury in the rat. TheTenth International Brain Edema Symposium, Abstract 8
13. Takahashi H, Kirsch JR, Hashimoto K, London ED, et al (1995) PPBP (4-Phenyl-1-(4-P-phenylbutyl) Piperidinel), a potent α-receptor ligand, decreases brain injury after transient focal ischemia in cats. Stroke 26: 1676–1682
14. Tengvar C, Hultstrom D, Olsson Y (1983) An improved Percoll density gradient for measurements of experimental brain edema. Acta Neuropathol 61: 201–206
15. Ting P, Masaoka H, Kuroiwa T, Wagner H, et al (1986) Influence of blood-brain barrier opening to proteins on development of postischemic brain injury. Neurol Res 8: 146–151
16. Ting P, Pan Y (1994) The effects of naloxone on the post-asphyxic cerebral pathophysiology of newborn lambs. Neurol Res 16: 359–364
17. Ting P, Xu S, Krumins S (1994) Endogenous opioid system activity following temporary focal cerebral ischemia. Acta Neurochir (Wien) [Suppl] 60: 253–256
18. Wood MS, Traynor JR (1989) 3(H) diprenorphine binding to k-sites in guinea-pig and rat brain: evidence for apparent heterogeneity. J Neurochem 53: 173–178

Correspondence: Pauline Ting, M.D., Howard Universtiy Hospital, 2041 Georgia Ave N.W., Washington, D.C. 20060, U.S.A.

Acta Neurochir (1997) [Suppl] 70: 254–256
© Springer-Verlag 1997

The Effects of Methylmethacrylate's Hyperthermic Polymerization on Cerebral Vascular Permeability

D. F. Jimenez[1], C. M. Barone[2], T. Tigno[3], X-F. Yang[2], and A. Clapper[1]

[1] Division of Neurosurgery and [2] Division of Plastic Surgery, University of Missouri Health Sciences Center, Columbia, MO, U.S.A., and [3] Division of Neurosurgery, AFP Medical Center, Queen City, Phillipines

Summary

This study was undertaken to analyze the effects of significant hyperthermia ($> 100°C$) associated with the polymerization of polymethlymethacrylate (PMM) on the permeability of the cerebral vasculature in rats. The method used to visualize the pial vasculature included the open pial window technique and epifluorescence microscopy. Results indicated that there is a significant increase in cerebral vascular permeability following *in situ* polymerization of PMM over the craniectomy site.

Keywords: Polymethylmethacrylate; hyperthermia; cerebral vascular permeability; fluorescence isothiocyanate (FITC) albumin; cranioplasty.

Introduction

Historically, a large variety of materials have been used to repair and close calvarial defects. Polymethylmethacrylate (PMM) has been the allograft most widely used by neurosurgeons for decades. During polymerization of the acrylic, there is a significant exothermic reaction which takes place prior to hardening and settling of the material. Due to the need to obtain a perfect match between the cranioplasty and the cranial defect, the semisolid mixture must be allowed to harden *in situ*; this requires close contact between the polymerizing agent in the underlying dura and brain. Concern over the effect of the extreme exothermic reaction (up to $100°C$) on the underlying brain, led to the analysis presented herein.

Methods

Ten Sprague-Dawley female rats (225–250 gm) were induced under anesthesia with intraperitoneal Nembutal (at a concentration of 50 mg/kg) and underwent placement of intravenous and intra-arterial (common carotid artery) lines followed by tracheostomy. The animals were placed in a three point rigid fixation frame and allowed to breath spontaneously. Bilateral, 10×10 mm frontoparietal craniotomies were performed with a 30,000 rpm drill. A plastic reservoir was secured in place with Coe tray surrounding the craniotomies. The group was divided into two subgroups: fast and slow set PMM. There were 8 control animals in a separate group.

Two types of PMM monomers were studied and included the slow setting (Codman cranioplastic™) and fast setting (Codman aneuroplastic™). Each monomer was mixed and allowed to polymerize and harden on the exposed dura. A miniature temperature probe was inserted into the acrylic close to the dural interface and the temperature elevation was measured during the hardening process. Once the reaction was completed, the acrylic was removed and the dura opened in a cruciate fashion. The reservoir was filled with pH balanced, $37°C$, artificial CSF and allowed to fill and irrigate the reservoir at a rate of 2 cc per minute. Fluorescein isothiocyanate (FITC) was injected intravenously and the animal placed under epifluorescence microscope with the appropriate optical filter. The pial vasculature was visualized for 2.0 hours. Increases in cerebral permeability and disruption of the blood brain barrier were defined as leakage of the FITC coupled albumin into the interstitium from the intravascular space. Analysis of the albumin-FITC leakage was done with NIH Image 1.6 software. Eight animals were included in the control group. These animals were treated in the same way except for the lack of PMM polymerization. The data was analyzed by using a two factor ANOVA analysis.

Results

Thermocouple analysis of the heat generated by the polymerizing mixture revealed a significant increase in temperature from the baseline. The slow set PMM group reached a peak temperature of $92°C$ at 17 minutes and lasted for 25 seconds (Fig. 1). The fast set PMM group reached a peak temperature of $112°C$ at 5 minutes and lasted for 31 seconds (Fig. 2). The percent of albumin leakage from the intra to the extravascular compartment was considered to be the percent change in cerebral vascular permeability. The increase in permeability was found to be significant

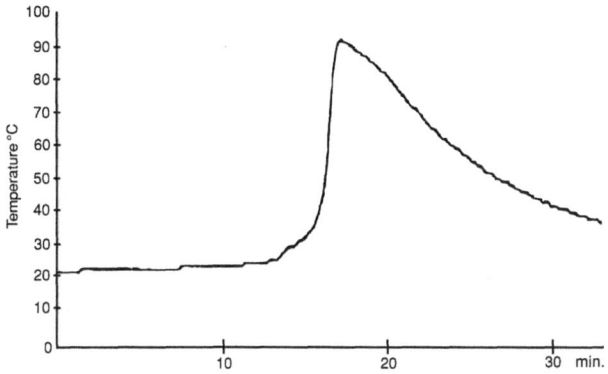

Fig. 1. Temperature curve for slow set PMM

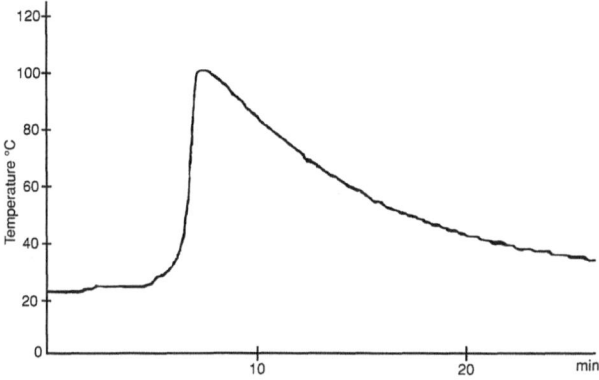

Fig. 1. Temperature curve for fast set PMM

(p = 0.0052) for both experimental groups over control, but not significant between the fast and slow set groups (Table 1).

Discussion

The acrylic polymethylmethacrylate (PMM) is manufactured and packaged in two forms: a powder polymer which contains the activator benzoyl peroxide and the initiator dimethylparatoludene. The liquid form in a monomer which contains the polymerization inhibitor hydroquinone. This inhibitor prevents spontaneous and slow polymerization into a solid form. Once the

polymer and mononer are mixed, the activator plus the initiator lead to polymerization and hardening by generating free radicals. Chain lengthening of the PMM occurs by consequent free radical addition. Growth of these chains is terminated by the reaction of two free radicals yielding a stable product unavailable for further addition.

In the process, an exothermic reaction occurs which releases energy at a rate of 1300 calories per 100 grams of mononer (5.4×10^5 J/kg) [3]. Several factors are known to affect the rate and extent of heat production: mixing temperature, pressure to which mixture is subjected, humidity, relative mounts of liquid and powder, the mass of the mixture, and thermodynamic properties of PMM such as heat capacity and thermal [2] conductivity. Perhaps the most important factor determining the maximal temperature generated is the amount (mass) used. Because of the total heat content is fixed by the weight of the reacting monomer, maximum temperature increases with increasing mass. This is clinically relevant when closing large calvarial defects with PMM.

The effects of termal injury on bone secondary to PMM polymerization has been well studied and documented in the orthopaedic literature. Bone necrosis surrounding the implant has been well documented [6]. At temperatures of 70°C, osteon cellular loss, disruption of the orderly lamellar bone matrix, depressed blood perfusion and loss of remolding activity have been demonstrated [1, 4, 5]. Fifty six degrees centigrade is considered the temperature at which proteins begin to demature in living systems. Irreversible enzymatic disturbances occur at 50°C for 30 second exposure. Concern over the known effects of thermal injury on body tissues, led to the present study of cerebral vascular permeability and blood brain barrier (BBB) integrity. Our results indicate that there is a signficant increase in leakage of labelled albumin into the interstitial space from the intravascular compartment. The negative effects of thermal injury on the vascular integrity in the peripheral systemic circulation has been well documented in the burn literature. The leakage noted in

Table 1. *Percent of Albumin Leakage from the Intra- to the Extravascular Compartment Following PMM Polymerization*

	0 Minutes	15 Minutes	60 Minutes	120 Minutes
Control	1.2 ± 0.5	–2.1 ± 1.1	–2.3 ± 1.3	–5.3 ± 1.5
Slow PMM	3.5 ± 1.0	31.2 ± 2.1	38.3 ± 1.4	48.6 ± 4.0
Fast PMM	6.3 ± 2.1	32.1 ± 1.9	44.5 ± 5.1	59.3 ± 2.8

PMM polymethylmethacrylate.

the experimental animals took place immediately following polymerization. Along with BBB disruption, adherence of labelled leukocytes to the vessel wall was also found to increase significantly over control animals. The significance of this finding is currently being studied. This is the first study to demonstrate the effects of high temperature PMM polymerization on the underlying brain. The clinical implications need to be further studied.

References

1. Berman AT, Reid JS, Yanicko DR Jr, Sih GC, Zimmerman MR (1983) Thermally induced bone necrosis in rabbits. Relation to implant failure in humans. Clin Orthop 186: 284–291

2. Jeferiss CD, Lee AJC, Ling RSM (1975) Thermal aspects of self-curing polymethylmethacrylate. J Bone Joint Surg Br 57B (4): 511–518
3. Nelson CG, Krishnan EC, Neff JR (1986) Consideration of physical parameters to predict thermal necrosis in acrylic cement implants at the site of giant cell tumors of bone. Med Phys 13 (4): 462–468
4. Schultz RJ, Johnston AD, Krishnamurthy S (1987) Thermal effects of polymerization of methylmethacrylate on small tubular bones. Int Orthop (SICOT) 11: 277–282
5. Stürup J, Nimb L, Kramhøft M, Jensen J (1994) Effects of polymerization heat and monomers from acrylic cement on canine bone. Acta Orthop Scand 65 (1): 20–23
6. Toksvig-Larsen S, Johnsson R, Ströqvist B (1995) Heat generation and heat protection in methylmethacrylate cementation of vertebral bodies. Eur Spine J 4: 15–17

Correspondence: David F. Jimenez, M.D., F.A.C.S., One Hospital Drive, N521, Columbia, MO 65212, U.S.A.

Acta Neurochir (1997) [Suppl] 70: 257–259
© Springer-Verlag 1997

Intraischemic Hypothermia During Pretreatment with Sublethal Ischemia Reduces the Induction of Ischemic Tolerance in the Gerbil Hippocampus

K. Wada, T. Miyazawa, H. Kato, N. Nomura, A. Yano, K. Shima, and **H. Chigasaki**

Department of Neurosurgery, National Defense Medical College, Saitama, Japan

Summary

We examined whether mild brain hypothermia during pretreatment with sublethal 2-min ischemia affected the tolerance to subsequent lethal 5-min ischemia.

The neuronal densities in the hippocampal CA1 sector of gerbils preconditioned at mild brain hypothermia (32% of normal) were significantly lower than those in gerbils preconditioned at brain normothermia (70% of normal). 72-kDa heat-shock protein immunoreactivity in the CA1 sector preconditioned at mild hypothermia was reduced.

These results suggest that mild brain hypothermia during pretreatment with sublethal ischemia reduces the tolerance to subsequent lethal ischemia.

Keywords: Transient global ischemia; ischemic tolerance; intraischemic hypothermia; delayed neuronal death; gerbil.

Introduction

Pretreatment with sublethal ischemia has been shown to induce tolerance to subsequent lethal ischemic injury in hippocampal neurons [5, 6], although the influence of brain temperature during pretreatment on the induction of tolerance has not been demonstrated. We examined whether mild brain hypothermia during pretreatment with sublethal ischemia affected the tolerance to subsequent lethal ischemic insults.

Method

Male Mongolian gerbils, weighing 60 to 80, were subjected to 2 min of forebrain ischemia at mild brain hypothermia; 32°C (n = 8) or normothermia; 36.5°C (n = 8) under anesthesia with 1% halothane.

The animals were then subjected to a second 5-min ischemia under 1% halothane anesthesia with 2 days interval following the first ischemic insult.

The onset of ischemia in both the sublethal and lethal insults were confirmed by the electroencephalogram (EEG) isoelectricity; animals with incomplete EEG suppression during either procedure were excluded.

Seven days after surviving the second insult, the brains were embedded in paraffin, cut into 5-μm sections, and stained with cresyl violet. The neuronal density of each hippocampal CA1 subfield, i.e., the number of intact pyramidal cells per 1 mm of linear length of the CA1, was determined according to the method of Kirino *et al.* [4]. Statistical comparisons were made using the Kruskal-Wallis and the two-tailed Mann-Whitney U test.

Two days following 2-min ischemia, immunostaining of gerbil brain tissue with a mouse monoclonal antibody against 72-kDa heat-shock protein (HSP-72) was performed to examine the expression of the stress response following the 2-min period of first ischemia in brain subjected to normo- or hypothermia. Each group consisted of five animals.

Result

The results of the histologic examination of CA1 neurons are summarized in Table 1. The sham-operated group (group A) showed no evidence of neuronal death and had an average neuronal density of 327.9 ± 28.9 (mean ± SD). The gerbils in the normothermic ischemic control group (group B) and the hypothermic ischemic control group (group C) showed extensive neuronal damage in the CA1 sector, with CA1 neuronal densities of 28.5 ± 14.7/mm (8.7% of normal) and 28.2 ± 12.6/mm (8.6% of normal), respectively. There was no significant difference between these two groups. Animals in the normothermic induced-tolerance group (group E), in contrast, showed significant preservation of CA1 cells, with a neuronal density of 228.5 ± 20.2/mm (69.7% of normal). On the other hand, a significant reduction in the neuroprotective effect was observed in animals in the hypothermic induced tolerance group (group D), with a neuronal density of 104.9 ± 57.4/mm (32.0% of normal) ($P < 0.01$).

Table 1. *Neuronal Density in CA1 Sector* (mean ± SD)

	Animals used	First ischemia	Brain temperature during primary ischemia	Second ischemia	Neuronal density of CA1 (/mm)
Group A	5	–	normothermia	–	327.9 ± 28.9
Group B	5	–	normothermia	+	28.5 ± 14.7
Group C	5	–	hypothermia	+	28.2 ± 12.6
Group D	8	+	hypothermia	+	104.9 ± 57.4[a]
Group E	8	+	normothermia	+	228.5 ± 20.2[a]

Statistically significant difference: [a] P < 0.01.
– Sham operation was performed.
+ Ischemia was induced.

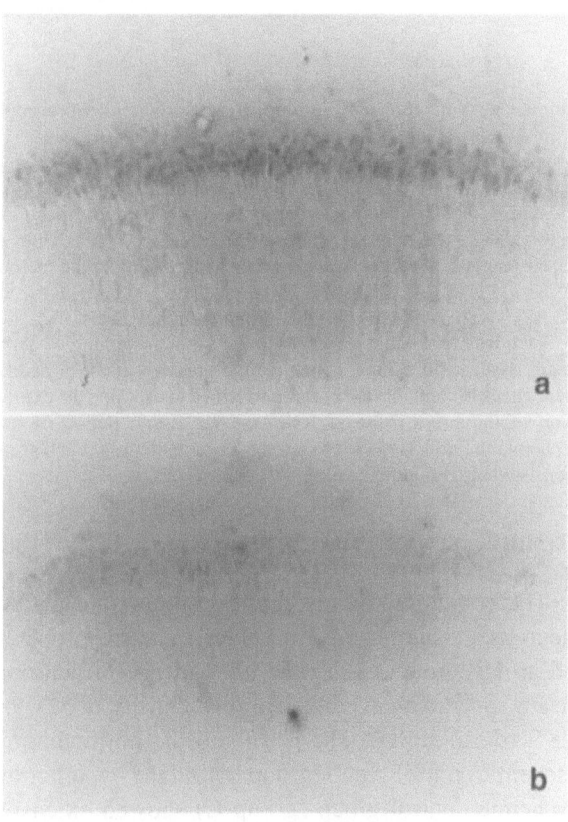

Fig. 1. Immunostaining with a monoclonal antibody against HSP-72 following the 2-min period of nonlethal ischemia. Strongly positive staining is visible in the normothermic pretreatment group (a), whereas only faint staining is visible in the hypothermic pretreatment group (b)

Immunohistochemical staining for HSP-72 in CA1 pyramidal neurons revealed moderate expression in four and weak expression in one gerbil in the normothermic pretreatment group (Fig. 1a), but only weak staining in all five of the gerbils in the hypothermic pretreatment group (Fig. 1b). There was a significant difference between these two groups (P < 0.05).

Discussion

The results of this study suggest that mild brain hypothermia during preceding sublethal ischemia reduces the induction of ischemic tolerance. Moreover, we have demonstrated that mild hypothermia likewise reduces HSP-72 synthesis in the gerbil brain after transient sublethal forebrain ischemia. HSP-72 is selectively expressed in neurons subjected to sublethal stress, and lethal ischemic damage can be ameliorated by preceding hyperthermia [1, 2, 7], brief ischemia [5, 8], or oxidative stress [9], all of which can induce HSP-72 synthesis. HSP-72 may exert a protective effect by maintaining the structure of normal or partially denatured proteins [3]. Therefore, one possibile mechanism for the reduction in ischemic tolerance is the reduction of HSP-72 synthesis [5].

Acknowledgment

The authors would like to thank Ms. O. J. Natsume, Ms. T. Hayashi, Ms. Y. Ichiki, Dr. A. Shimizu, Mr. M. Takahashi, and Mr. K. Murata for their technical assistance.

References

1. Barbe MF, Tytell M, Gower DJ, Welch WJ (1988) Hyperthermia protects against light damage in the rat retina. Science 241: 1817–1820
2. Chopp M, Chen H, Ho KL, Dereski MO, Brown E, Hetzel FW, Welch KMA (1989) Transient hyperthermia protects against subsequent forebrain ischemic cell damage in the rat. Neurology 39: 1396–1398
3. Gething MJ, Sambrook J (1992) Protein folding in the cell. Nature 355: 33–45
4. Kirino T (1982) Delayed neuronal death in the gerbil hippocampus following ischemia. Brain Res 239: 57–69
5. Kirino T, Tsujita Y, Tamura A (1991) Induced tolerance to ischemia in gerbil hippocampal neurons. J Cereb Blood Flow Metab 11: 299–307
6. Kitagawa K, Matsumoto M, Tagaya M, Hata R, Ueda H, Niinobe M, Handa N, Fukunaga R, Kimura K, Mikoshiba K, Kamada T (1990) Ischemic tolerance phenomenon found in the brain. Brain Res 528: 21–24

7. Kitagawa K, Matsumoto M, Tagaya M, Kuwabara K, Hata R, Handa N, Fukunaga R, Kimura K, Kameda T (1991) Hyperthermia-induced neuronal protection against ischemic injury in gerbils. J Cereb Blood Flow Metab 11: 449–452

8. Li Y, Chopp M, Zhang ZG, Zhang RL, Garcia JH (1993) Neuronal survival is associated with 72-kDa heat shock protein expression after transient middle cerebral artery occlusion in the rat. J Neurol Sci 120: 187–194

9. Ohtsuki T, Matsumoto M, Kuwabara K, Kitagawa K, Sukuki K, Taniguchi N, Kamada T (1992) Influence of oxidative stress on induced tolerance to ischemia in gerbil hippocampal neurons. Brain Res 599: 246–252

Correspondence: Kojiro Wada, M.D., Department of Neurosurgery, National Defense Medical College, 3-2 Namiki, Tokorozawa, Saitama 359, Japan.

Acta Neurochir (1997) [Suppl] 70: 260–261
© Springer-Verlag 1997

The Relationship Between Brain Temperature and Neutrophil Accumulation After Traumatic Brain Injury in Rats

M. J. Whalen, T. M. Carlos, R. S. B. Clark, D. W. Marion, M. S. T. DeKosky, S. Heineman, J. K. Schiding, F. Memarzadeh, C. E. Dixon, and P. M. Kochanek

The Safar Center for Resuscitation Research, and the Brain Trauma Research Center, University of Pittsburgh, Pittsburgh, PA, U.S.A.

Summary

Mild hypothermia reduces secondary damage after traumatic brain injury (TBI) in rodent models; however, the mechanisms involved in this beneficial effect remain unclear. We previously reported that TBI induces the upregulation of adhesion molecules and infiltration of neutrophils (PMN) in brain. Since PMN accumulation may be associated with the development of hyperemia and blood-brain barrier injury, we hypothesized that hypothermia would reduce acute inflammation after TBI in rats. To test this hypothesis, rats were anesthetized and subjected to TBI by controlled cortical impact to left parietal cortex. Brain temperature was controlled at 32°C, 37°C, or 39°C (n = 8 per group) for 4 h after TBI, then rats were sacrificed and brain were harvested. Immunohistochemistries were performed on brain sections using antibodies that recognize the adhesion molecules E-selectin and intercellular adhesion molecule-1 (ICAM-1), and PMN. PMN were also quantified using a myeloperoxidase (MPO) assay. PMN accumulation in injured brain was decreased in rats maintained at 32°C vs 39°C (4-fold by immunohistochemistry and 8-fold by MPO, $p < 0.05$). E-selectin was induced after TBI, but not attenuated by hypothermia. ICAM-1 was not up-regulated at this early time after TBI. Based on these preliminary data, we conclude that mild hypothermia reduces PMN accumulation in injured brain during the initial 4 h after TBI, without decreasing adhesion molecule expression.

Keywords: Neutrophil accumulation; traumatic brain injury (TBI); hypothermia; intercellular adhesion molecule-1 (ICAM-1); hyperthermia; polymorphonuclear leukocyte (PMN).

Introduction

Mild hypothermia reduces secondary damage after TBI in rats, even when applied after the injury [4, 5, 7, 9, 10]. Recent studies suggest that the beneficial effects of hypothermia applied after TBI may not be mediated by reduced excitotoxicity or energy demands [10], although there are conflicting data on this issue [7]. Mechanisms of benefit remain to be determined. We previously reported that TBI induces an acute inflam-matory response (endothelial adhesion molecule up-regulation and PMN accumulation) in rat brain [2, 3, 14]. Since PMN accumulation may be associated with hyperemia and blood-brain barrier injury [14], we hypothesized that hypothermia would reduce acute inflammation after TBI.

Methods

All studies were approved by the University of Pittsburgh Animal Care and Use Committee. Sprague-Dawley rats were anesthetized with 1% isoflurane in nitrous oxide and oxygen, intubated, and subjected to TBI by controlled cortical impact (CCI) to the left parietal cortex. CCI parameters were a 2.5 mm depth of penetration and a 4 m/s impact velocity.

Brain temperature was controlled at 32°C, 37°C, or 39°C (n = 8 per group) for 4 h after TBI, then rats were decapitated after saline perfusion and brains were harvested. Each brain was coronally sectioned through the lesion.

Immunohistochemistries were performed on brain sections using monoclonal antibodies (MoAb) including TM-8 (anti-rat ICAM-1, mouse IgG$_1$, provided by Dr. Heidi Horner, Athena Neurosciences, South San Francisco, CA); anti-rabbit E-selectin (mouse IgG$_1$, MoAb 14G2, provided by Dr. Barry Wolitsky, Hoffman-LaRoche, Nutley, NJ); and RP-3 (anti-rat neutrophil, mouse IgM, hybridoma provided by Dr. Warren Lo, Ohio State University) [12]. PMN were also quantified using a myeloperoxidase (MPO) assay [3].

Results

PMN accumulation in injured brain was markedly decreased in rats maintained at 32°C vs 39°C (4-fold by immunohistochemistry, 8-fold by MPO assay, both $p < 0.05$). E-selectin was induced after TBI ($p < 0.05$ injured vs non-injured cortex), but was not significantly attenuated by hypothermia. ICAM-1

Table 1. *Effect of Brain Temperature on Markers of Acute Inflammation at 4 h After TBI in Rats*

Inflammatory marker[a]	32°C	37°C	39°C
PMN (cortex, immunohistochemistry)	2–3[b]	4+	6–7+
PMN (MPO)	0.02[b]	0.04	0.19
E-selectin (cortex)	0–1 +	1+	1+
ICAM-1 (cortex)	0–1+	0–1+	0–1+

[a] Estimates of positive cells per high-power field for immunohistochemistries. The MPO data are expressed as units of MPO activity per gram of brain. For immunohistochemistries, the number of PMN and vessels reactive with the corresponding MoAb were counted in 48–75 $100 \times$ fields within cortical regions.
[b] $p < 0.05$, 32°C vs 39°C.

was not up-regulated at this early time after TBI (Table 1).

Discussion

Classic studies have demonstrated pronounced effects of hypothermia on acute inflammation outside of the central nervous system (CNS) [1, 13]. Even mild hypothermia reduces PMN influx into inflammatory foci outside of the CNS [1, 13]. Despite recent work suggesting both a beneficial effect of mild hypothermia on secondary damage after TBI [4, 5, 9, 10] and marked augmentation of damage to posttraumatic cerebral microcirculation by mild hyperthermia [6], the effect of brain temperature on the acute inflammatory response in injured brain has received limited study. Rosomoff *et al.* [11] suggested a dramatic effect of hypothermia on acute inflammation in injured brain over 30 years ago; however, these studies were not pursued further.

In this preliminary report, compared to hyperthermia, hypothermia reduced early PMN accumulation after TBI in rats, without a significant decrease in cerebrovascular adhesion molecule expression. The failure of hypothermia to attenuate the expression of E-selectin on cerebrovascular endothelium suggests that hypothermia may confer some of its anti-inflammatory effects by producing qualitative changes on neutrophils (such as avidity changes) or via a reduction in chemotaxin production following TBI.

These studies compliment the work of Goss *et al.* [8] who reported a marked reduction of IL-1 mRNA and protein by mild hypothermia in injured rat brain.

The direct relationship between brain temperature and PMN accumulation after TBI suggests that beneficial effects of hypothermia may be mediated, in part, by effects on the acute inflammatory response.

Acknowledgments

This work was supported by grant 2P50 NS30318-04A21 from the NINDS. Dr. Kochanek is supported in part by an Established Investigator Grant from the Society of Critical Care Medicine.

References

1. Biggar WD, Bohn DJ, Kent G, Barker C, Hamilton G (1984) Neutrophil migration *in vitro* and *in vivo* during hypothermia. Infect Immun 46: 857–859
2. Carlos TM, Clark RSB, Franicola-Higgins D, Schiding JK, Kochanek PM (1995) Expression of endothelial adhesion molecules after traumatic brain injury in rats. J Neurotrauma 12: 458
3. Clark RSB, Schiding J, Kaczorowski SL, Marion DW, Kochanek PM (1994) Neutrophil accumulation after traumatic brain injury in rats: comparison of weight drop and controlled cortical impact models. J Neurotrauma 11: 499–506
4. Clifton GL, Allen S, Barrodale P, Plenger P, Berry J, Koch S, Fletcher J, Hayes RL, Choi SC (1993) A phase II study of moderate hypothermia in severe brain injury. J Neurotrauma 10: 263–271
5. Dietrich WD, Alonso O, Busto R, Globus MY, Ginsberg MD (1994) Post-traumatic brain hypothermia reduces histopathological damage following concussive brain injury in the rat. Acta Neuropathol (Berl) 87: 250–258
6. Dietrich WD, Busto R, Halley M, Valdes I (1990) The importance of brain temperature in alterations of the blood-brain barrier following cerebral ischemia. J Neuropathol Exp Neurol 49: 486–497
7. Globus MY, Alonso O, Dietrich WD, Busto R, Ginsberg MD (1995) Glutamate release and free radical production following brain injury: effects of posttraumatic hypothermia. J Neurochem 65 (4): 1704–1711
8. Goss JR, Styren SD, Miller PD, Kochanek PM, Palmer AM, Marion DW, DeKosky ST (1995) Hypothermia attenuates the normal increase in interleukin 1 beta RNA and nerve growth factor following traumatic brain injury in the rat. J Neurotrauma 12 (2): 159–167
9. Marion DW, Obrist WD, Carlier PM, Penrod LE, Darby JM (1993) The use of moderate therapeutic hypothermia for patients with severe head injuries: a preliminary report. J Neurosurg 79: 354–362
10. Palmer AM, Marion DW, Botscheller ML, Redd EE (1993) Therapeutic hypothermia is cytoprotective without attenuating the traumatic brain injury-induced elevations in interstitial concentrations of aspartate and glutamate. J Neurotrauma 10 (4): 363–372
11. Rosomoff HL, Clasen RA, Hartstock R, Bebin J (1965) Brain reaction to experimental injury after hypothermia. Arch Neurol 13: 337–345
12. Sekiya S, Gotoh S, Yamashita T, Watanabi T, Saitoh S, Sendo F (1989) Selective depletion of rat neutrophils by *in vivo* administration of a monoclonal antibody. J Leuk Biol 46: 96–102
13. Thomas G, Sousa PS (1986) Early inflammatory response to carrageenan in the pleural cavity and paw of rats with altered body temperature. J Pharm Pharmacol 38: 936–938
14. Uhl MW, Biagas KV, Grundl PD, Barmada MA, Schiding JK, Nemoto EM, Kochanek PM (1994) Effects of neutropenia on edema, histology, and cerebral blood flow after traumatic brain injury in rats. J Neurotrauma 11 (3): 303–315

Correspondence: Patrick M. Kochanek, M.D., Safar Center for Resuscitation Research, 3434 Fifth Avenue, Pittsburgh, PA 15260, U.S.A.

Acta Neurochir (1997) [Suppl] 70: 262–264
© Springer-Verlag 1997

Effect of Mild and Moderate Hypothermia on the Acidosis-Induced Swelling of Glial Cells

N. Plesnila[1], F. Ringel[1], R. C. C. Chang[1], J. Peters[1], F. Staub[2], and **A. Baethmann[1]**

[1] Institute for Surgical Research, Klinikum Grosshadern, Ludwig-Maximilians University, Munich, and
[2] Department of Neurosurgery, University of Cologne, Federal Republic of Germany

Summary

The effect of mild (32°C) and moderate (27°C) hypothermia was analyzed on the cell volume and intracellular pH (pH_i) of C6 glioma cells at normal pH and during lactacidosis at pH 6.2 *in vitro*. The cells were suspended in an incubation chamber under continuous control of pH, PO_2 and temperature. Cell swelling was quantified by an advanced Coulter-system. pH_i was measured by flow cytometry using the fluorescent dye bis-carboxyethyl carboxyfluorescein (BCECF). Following a control period at 37°C, the ambient temperature was decreased to 32°C for 30 min, and subsequently to 27°C for another 30 min. Hypothermia alone led to an immediate and significant cell volume increase of $107.3 \pm 0.4\%$ (mean ± SEM) of control after 30 min at 32°C, and further swelling to $110.5 \pm 0.9\%$ after 30 min at 27°C. Yet, hypothermia (27°C) afforded partial protection against the acidosis-induced cell swelling at pH 6.2, which was reaching to $120.4 \pm 0.9\%$ in the normothermic control group after 60 min, while only to $111.3 \pm 0.9\%$ at 27°C. Hypothermia, however, was associated with a more pronounced decrease of the pH_i during acidosis (6.3 ± 0.04) as compared to that of the normothermic control falling then to 6.5 ± 0.03. The results demonstrate that mild and moderate hypothermia induce glial cell swelling, but simultaneously inhibit cell swelling from acidosis. The protection against cell swelling, however, has its price as indicated by the enhancement of the intracellular acidification.

Keywords: Hypothermia; glial cell swelling; acidosis; flow-cytometry; C6 glioma cell; bis-carboxyethyl carboxyfluorescein (BCECF).

Introduction

Head injury and cerebral ischemia are associated with tissue hypoxia resulting in a sustained activation of anaerobic glycolysis with accumulation of lactic acid. The evolving lactacidosis is an important factor for the development of secondary brain damage following the primary insult [9]. Lactic acid may leak from the core of the necrosis into the perifocal still viable tissue leading there to cytotoxic brain edema and further tissue damage. The "acidosis-induced" cell swelling is most likely mediated by activation of membrane transporters, e.g. the Na^+/H^+-antiporter or the Na^+/HCO_3^--cotransporter [8]. Since many transport processes are known to be temperature dependent, the objective of the current experiments was to investigate whether mild or moderate hypothermia inhibits the acidosis-induced cell swelling and intracellular acidification following administration of lactic acid to suspended glial cells *in vitro*.

Materials and Methods

C6 glioma cells were cultured as monolayers under standard conditions (humidified room air, 5% CO_2, 37°C, pH 7.4, DMEM + 10% FCS + 100 IU/ml Penicillin + 50 µg/ml Streptomycin). The cells were harvested upon reaching confluence (0.05% trypsin / 0.02% EGTA in PBS) and suspended in serum-free DMEM with 25 mM bicarbonate at a density of $1–2 \times 10^6$ cells/ml. The cells were transferred then to a temperature-controlled incubation chamber furnished with a membrane oxygenator to supply the cell suspension with a mixture of CO_2, O_2 and N_2. Temperature, pH and PO_2 were continuously monitored and if necessary adjusted. A magnetic stirrer prevented cell sedimentation [7]. Cell volume and intracellular pH (pH_i) were determined by flow cytometry. The cell volume measurement is based on an advanced Coulter system with hydrodynamic focusing [4]. Calibration was made using latex beads of known size. The sensitivity of the system allows detection of cell volume changes of $\leq 1–2\%$. $1–2 \times 10^4$ cells were used for a single measurement. The PH_i was also assessed by flowcytometry utilizing the fluorescent dye BCECF. The method has been described in details elsewere [11].

After a control period at 37°C the temperature of the cell suspension in the chamber was lowered to 32°C for 30 min, and subsequently to 27°C for the same period of time. Cell volume and pH_i were repeatedly assessed at least every 5 min. In further experiments the temperature was lowered to 27°C in combination with induction of acidosis by addition of isotonic lactic acid (350 mM) for 60 min. The pCO_2 in the chamber was increased to 80–100 mmHg to compensate for the loss of CO_2 and to prevent a secondary recovery of the pH_e in the medium. The medium pH was subsequently restored to 7.4 by addition of isotonic NaOH for another observation period of 30 min.

Table 1. *Volume Response (Mean ± SEM) of Glial Cells to Hypothermia at Normal pH and During Lactacidosis of pH 6.2*

pH	Temperature [°C]	Cell volume after 30 min [% baseline]	Cell volume after 60 min [% baseline]
7.4	37	100.03 ± 0.16	100.61 ± 0.42
7.4	32	107.09 ± 0.41	–
7.4	27	–	110.53 ± 0.92
6.2	37	118.46 ± 1.17	120.35 ± 0.97
6.2	27	110.11 ± 0.88	111.17 ± 0.88

Results

During the control phase of 30 min at 37°C the volume and pH_i of C6 glioma cells remained constant (n = 5). With induction of mild hypothermia (32°C), however, rapid and significant cell swelling was observed to 107.3 ± 0.4% (mean ± SEM) of control (p < 0.016, n = 4). Upon lowering the temperature subsequently to 27°C, cell volume was further increased to 110.5 ± 0.93% (Table 1), although pH_i remained unchanged at both levels of hypothermia.

As reported earlier, lactacidosis of pH 6.2 induced in normothermia led to significant cell volume increase of 114.4 ± 0.8% at 15 min reaching a maximum of 120.4 ± 0.9% at 60 min. Upon normalization of the medium pH (pH_e) to 7.4 cell volume recovered to near baseline level. When, however, acidosis was induced in moderate hypothermia (27°C), glial swelling response was significantly inhibited. Following addition of lactic acid the cell volume increase was only 108.3 ± 0.68% of control at 15 min, while 111.3 ± 0.89% at 60 min, corresponding to inhibition of the acidosis-induced cell swelling by more than 40%. Neutralization of the medium to pH 7.4 resulted in complete recovery of the cell volume in both groups.

Induction of acidosis (pH 6.2) in the medium was associated with a significant decrease of pH_i in both, normo- and hypothermically suspended glial cells. In

Table 2. *PH_i (Mean + SEM) of Glial Cells Exposed to Lactacidosis at pH 6.2 During Normothermia (37°C) and Hypothermia (27°C) in Comparison with Cell Suspension at pH 7.4*

pH	Temperature [°C]	pH_i after 10 min
7.4	37	7.22 ± 0.03
6.2	37	6.50 ± 0.02
7.4	27	7.18 ± 0.03
6.2	27	6.31 ± 0.02

the normothermic group at 37°C, pH_i fell immediately to 6.5 ± 0.03 after induction of acidosis and remained at this level until the end of the observation period at 60 min. Addition of lactic acid during hypothermia at 27°C resulted in moderate, yet significant (p < 0.007) additional decrease of PH_i to 6.3 ± 0.04 (n = 6). Following neutralization of the medium, however, PH_i was found in both groups to recover to the baseline level obtained prior to acidosis (7.2 ± 0.03).

Discussion

For many years hypothermia is known to afford tissue protection against ischemia, e.g. in organ transplantation or open heart surgery [12]. Recently, the procedure is attracting renewed attention for the treatment of cerebral ischemia or traumatic brain injury [2, 6]. Various reports have been published on beneficial effects of mild or moderate hypothermia on brain edema based on animal studies [5] and on clinical observations [2]. However, there is only scarce information about the mechanisms how hypothermia is brain protective and how it inhibits brain edema on the cellular level [1, 3].

The present results clearly demonstrate that hypothermia is markedly attenuating acidosis-induced swelling of glial cells *in vitro,* notwithstanding that the procedure itself was eliciting a dose-dependent swelling response of glial cells suspended at normal pH. It should be mentioned in this context that the experimental parameters, which might be influenced by temperature as the actual pH or gas concentrations in the medium were carefully monitored including correction of the results for the temperature change, if necessary. Since measurement of cell volume by a conventional Coulter system is temperature dependent, a custom designed flowcytometer with electrical temperature compensation was used for the study [4].

Some contents are adequate concerning the influence of hypothermia on cell volume control. The transmembrane Na^+ concentration gradient is fueling a variety of passive transport processes across the cell membrane, including those involved in cell volume regulation. That Na^+-gradient is actively maintained by the Na^+/K^+-ATPase, which is dependend on the cellular energy metabolism. Accordingly, hypothermia might inhibit the active Na^+-transport afforded by the ATPase, leading to an accumulation of Na^+-ions in the cells together with water for osmotic reasons, thus leading to cell swelling.

During extracellular lactacidosis hypothermia (27°C) reduces the acidosis-induced cell swelling observed under normothermic conditions, but increases the intracellular acidification. In essence, the acidosis-induced cell swelling is brought about by activation of the Na^+/H^+-antiporter in an attempt to defend pH_i. Thereby, H^+-ions are exchanged against Na^+-ions in the medium leading to a subsequent influx of water, i.e. cell swelling [10]. The reduction of the acidosis-induced cell swelling with enhancement of intracellular acidification by hypothermia may be attributed to inhibition of the Na^+/H^+-antiporter, either directly or by flattening of the transmembrane Na^+-concentration gradient (see above).

Taken together the present findings demonstrate intriguing effects of hypothermia on the glial cell volume under normal conditions and after exposure to lactic acid. Both, induction of swelling at normal pH and inhibition of swelling from acidosis by hypothermia may be reconciled by assuming that lowering of the ambient temperature is differentially affecting membrane transporters involved in cell volume regulation, particularly the Na^+/K^+-ATPase and Na^+/H^+-antiporter. Further data, however, are required, especially to identify the therapeutically useful level of hypothermia, which provides protection against cell swelling without enhancing adverse effects, e.g. intracellular acidosis.

References

1. Arai H, Uto A, Ogawa Y, Sato K (1993) Effect of low temperature on glutamate-induced intracellular calcium accumulation and cell death in cultured hippocampal neurons. Neurosci Lett 163 (2): 132–134
2. Clifton GL (1995) Systemic hypothermia in treatment of severe brain injury: a review and update. J Neurotrauma 12 (5): 923–927
3. Huang R, Shuaib A, Hertz L (1993) Glutamate uptake and glutamate content in primary cultures of mouse astrocytes during anoxia, substrate deprivation and simulated ischemia under normothermic and hypothermic conditions. Brain Res 618 (2): 346–351
4. Kachel V (1976) Basic principles of electrical sizing of cells and particles and their realization in the new instrument "Metricell". J Histochem Cytochem 24: 211–230
5. Karibe H, Zarow GJ, Graham SH, Weinstein PR (1994) Mild intraischemic hypothermia reduces postischemic hyperperfusion, delayed postischemic hypoperfusion, blood-brain barrier disruption, brain edema, and neuronal damage volume after temporary focal cerebral ischemia in rats. J Cereb Blood Flow Metab 14: 620–627
6. Karibe H, Zarow G1, Weinstein PR (1995) Delayed induction of mild hypothermia to reduce infarct volume after temporary middle cerebral artery occlusion in rats. J Neurosurg 83: 93–98
7. Kempski O, Chaussy L, Gross U, Zimmer M, Baethmann A (1983) Volume regulation and metabolism of suspended C6 glioma cells: an *in vitro* model to study cytotoxic brain edema. Brain Res 279: 217–228
8. Mellergard PE, Ouyang YB, Siesjö BK (1992) The regulation of intracellular pH in cultured astrocytes and neuroblastoma cells, and its dependence on extracellular pH in a HCO3-free solution. Can J Physiol Pharmacol 70 [Suppl]: S293–300
9. Siesjö BK, Katsura K, Mellergard P, Ekholm A, Lundgren J, Smith ML (1993) Acidosis-related brain damage. Prog Brain Res 96: 23–48
10. Staub F, Plesnila N, Chang R, Peters J, Baethmann A (1995) Effect of lactacidosis on volume and intracellular pH of astrocytes. J Neurotrauma 12 (3): 378
11. Staub F, Winkler A, Peters J, Kempski O, Kachel V, Baethmann A (1994) Swelling, acidosis, and irreversible damage of glial cells from exposure to arachidonic acid *in vitro*. J Cereb Blood Flow Metab 14: 1030–1039
12. Tharion J, Johnson DC, Celermajer JM, Hawker RM, Cartmill TB, Overton JH (1982) Profound hypothermia with circulatory arrest: nine years' clinical experience. J Thorac Cardiovasc Surg 84 (1): 66–72

Correspondence: Nikolaus Plesnila, M.D., Institute for Surgical Research, Klinikum Grosshadern, Marchioninistr. 15, D-81366 Munich, Federal Republic of Germany.

Acta Neurochir (1997) [Suppl] 70: 265–266
© Springer-Verlag 1997

Cerebral Vascular Response to Hypertonic Fluid Resuscitation in Thermal Injury

M. Barone[1], **D. F. Jimenez**[2], **V. H. Huxley**[3], and **X.-F. Yang**[1]

[1] Division of Plastic Surgery, [2] Division of Neurosurgery, and [3] Department of Physiologie, University of Missouri, Columbia, MO, U.S.A.

Summary

The purpose of this project was to study the effects of various resuscitation fluid protocols in a systemically thermally injured rat sustaining 70% body surface area third degree burn using the pial window model in rats. The results show that there was a significant albumin leak in the cerebral vessels in both the experimental group which underwent no resuscitation fluid, as well as the experimental group that was resuscitated with Lactated Ringer's solution using the Parkland formula. When this was compared with the control group, as well as to the experimental group which received hypertonic hyperosmotic saline (HMS) boluses every hour, there was little if any leakage seen.

Keywords: Thermal injury; resuscitation; hypertonic hyperosmotic saline; lactated Ringer's solution; fluorescence isothiocyanate (FITC) albumin.

Introduction

Burn injury is characterized by increased microvascular permeability, which causes massive fluid volume requirements during resuscitation. This has clearly been shown in the peripheral vessels [5, 12] not in the cerebral circulation. Since burn injury remains one of the leading causes of childhood death in the United States (1 million children are injured and 3,000 children die each year as a result of burn trauma, according to the Children's Burn Awareness Program, Chicago, IL) and since generalized encephalopathy is the most common neurological complication of burns in children occurring with a 14% incidence [1, 3, 6, 7, 11], research on the effects of thermal injury on the cerebral blood brain barrier is essential. The use of hypertonic saline has been successfully used for initial resuscitation of hemorrhagic shock [8] and has also been effectively used to treat resuscitation of major burns [9]. Our previous work using a pial window model has shown that systemic thermal injury causes a disruption of the blood brain barrier [2, 4]. The purpose of this project is to study the effects of various resuscitation fluid protocols i.e., the Parkland formula versus 7.5% hypertonic saline solution.

Methods

Adult Sprague-Dawley rats weighing 250 grams were anesthetized intraperitoneally with 50 mg/kg of Pentobarbital. A tracheostomy was performed and the animals were allowed to breathe spontaneously. Polyethylene catheters were placed in the right jugular vein for the infusion of fluorochrome fluorescence isothiocyanate (FITC) albumin. All animals were given a bolus injection of FITC albumin [3 mg FITC/100 g wt in 0.5 ml Lactated Ringer's solution (LR)], then a constant infusion of FITC-albumin (0.5 mg FITC/100 g wt) dissolved in (2 ml LR/100 g wt/hr × 6 hrs). Another catheter was inserted into the femoral artery and attached to the arterial pressure monitoring system. Mean arterial pressure and heart rates were monitored throughout the experiment and at all times the core body temperature was maintained at 37°C using a rectal probe and heating pad. The animals were placed in rigid 3-point fixation frame and sagittal incision was made on the scalp and a plastic reservoir with an inflow and outflow tubing was secured to the skull and a biparietal craniotomy was performed and the dura reflected. The reservoir was filled with modified Elliot's solution and the pH adjusted to 7.4 and the temperature adjusted to 37°C. Solution was constantly infused with a gas mixture of 5% CO_2 and 95% N_2. Microcirculation was visualized with epifluorescent microscopy attached to a closed circuit TV monitor and video recorder. The camera location and specific vessels and adjacent parenchyma was kept constant and the data stored. A fluorescent microscope photometer was used to evaluate the fluorescent intensity of the FITC albumin within the vessels in the perivascular interstitium.

An index of albumin leakage was determined from the ratio of perivascular to intravascular florescence. The experimental group then underwent immersion into water of 100°C for six seconds. This produced a 70% body surface area third degree burn[3] and the control group was immersed in water of 37°C for six seconds. Therefore, the following groups were tested: Group A = control group, no thermal injury; Group B = thermal injury and no resuscitation fluid; Group C = thermal injury + LR (4 cc/kg/%burn, Parkland formula); Group D = thermal injury + 7.5% hyperosmotic hypertonic saline bolus given at 4 cc/kg after thermal injury, once every hour. FITC albumin was administered intravenously at a constant infusion rate.

Recordings were made every 15 minutes with exposure of filtered ultra violet light of 480 nm for a 10 second duration. The experiments were continued for six hours after thermal injury.

Results

Group A which was the control group (N = 6) had a mean percent albumin leakage of $1 \pm 6\%$ (mean $\pm$ SEM) at six hours. Group B which was the experimental group which received no resuscitation fluid (N = 6) had a mean percent albumin leak of $104 \pm 4\%$. Group C which was the experimental group which received the Lactated Ringer's using the Parkland formula had (N = 6) with a mean percent albumin leak at six hours of $91 \pm 21\%$. Group D which was the experimental group which underwent resuscitation using hyperosmotic hypertonic saline (N = 6) had a mean percent albumin leak of $3 \pm 2\%$ at six hours.

Conclusion

Thermal injury leads to an increased permeability of cerebral vessels. Treatment with Lactated Ringer's did not improve the leakage. Treatment with hypertonic hyperosomotic saline post thermal injury seemed to essentially eliminate the albumin leakage in the cerebral vessels, comparable to control levels. Therefore, hyperosomotic saline may be a beneficial addition to burn resuscitation protocols.

Acknowledgement

This work was supported by the Alumni Faculty Award, NIH #RR07053, Research Board Grant, Children's Miracle Telethon Grant, and Edna M. Jeffries Trust Fund.

References

1. Antoon AY, Volpe JJ, Crawford JD (1972) Burn encephalopathy in children. Pediatrics 50: 609–616
2. Barone CM, Jimenez DF, Huxley VH, *et al* (1997) Morphologic analysis of the cerebral microcirculation after thermal injury and the response to fluid resuscitation. Brain Edema X. Acta Neurochir (Wien) [Suppl] 70: 267–268
3. Emery JL, Campbell-Reid DA (1962) Cerebral oedema and spastic hemiplegia following minor burnsin young children. Br J Surg 50: 53–56
4. Jimenez DF, Barone CM, Huxley VH. *In vivo* visualization of cerebral microcirculation in systemic thermal injury: a new animal model. Int J Microcirc (Submitted)
5. Matsuda T, Tanaka H, Williams S, *et al* (1991) Reduced fluid volume requirement for resuscitation of third-degree burns with high-dose vitamin C. J Burn Care Rehabil 12: 525–532
6. McManus WF, Hunt JL, Pruitt BA Jr (1974) Postburn convulsive disorders in children. J Trauma 14: 396–401
7. Mohnot D, Snead OC 3rd, Benton JW Jr (1982) Burn encephalopathy in children. Ann Neurol 12: 42–47
8. Nakayama S, Kramer GC, Carlsen RC, *et al* (1985) Infusion of very hypertonic saline to bled rats: membrane potentials and fluid shifts. J Surg Res 38: 180–186
9. Onarheim H, Missavage AK, Kramer GC, *et al* (1990) Effectiveness of hypertonic saline-dextran 70 for initial fluid resuscitation of major burns. J Trauma 30 (5): 597–603
10. Saez JC, Ward PH, Gunther B, *et al* (1984) Superoxide radical involvement in the pathogenesis of burn shock. Circ Shock 12: 229–239
11. Shahar E, Keidan I, Brand N, *et al* (1991) Uncommon neurologic complications of burns in infants: a parkinsonian extrapyramidal disorder and massive cerebral infarction. J Burn Care Rehabil 12: 54–57
12. Tanaka H, Wada T, Simazaki S, *et al* (1991) Effects of cimetidine on fluid requirement during resuscitation of third-degree burns. J Burn Care Rehabil 12: 425–429

Correspondence: C. M. Barone, M.D., Division of Plastic Surgery, M349, University of Missouri, One Hospital Drive, Columbia, MO 65212, U.S.A.

Acta Neurochir (1997) [Suppl] 70: 267–268
© Springer-Verlag 1997

Morphologic Analysis of the Cerebral Microcirculation After Thermal Injury and the Response to Fluid Resuscitation

M. Barone[1], **F. Jimenez**[2], **V. H. Huxley**[3], and **X.-F. Yang**[1]

[1] Division of Plastic Surgery, [2] Division of Neurosurgery, and [3] Department of Physiologie, University of Missouri, Columbia, MO, U.S.A.

Summary

Using the pial window model, we have previously demonstrated that there is a disruption of the blood brain barrier with distal thermal injury [1–3]. Our laboratory has shown that treatment with Lactated Ringer's Solution did not improve labeled albumin leakage. However, treatment with hypertonic hyperosmotic saline (HHS) solution post thermal injury seemed to essentially eliminate the albumin leakage in cerebral vessels. Using adult Sprague-Dawley rats and epifluorescent microscopy, the cerebral vessel size and diameter were measured, as well as the number of leukocytes rolling or adherent to the endothelium. The results show that there was significant progressive arterial dilatation over six hours in the thermally injured animals treated with HHS. There was also a significant increase in leukocyte number if the animals were thermally injured and had no resuscitation fluid or if the animals were thermally injured and underwent resuscitation fluid with Lactated Ringer's compared to either the control group or the group that was treated with HHS after thermal injury.

Keywords: Thermal injury; cerebral microcirculation; resuscitation; hypertonic hyperosmotic saline; lactated Ringer's solution.

Introduction

Our pial window model has shown that there is a disruption of the blood brain barrier with distal thermal injury [1–3]. Review of the literature has failed to produce any studies examining the changes which occur in cerebral vessels after thermal body injury. Our laboratory has shown that treatment with Lactated Ringer's (LR) solution did not improve labeled albumin leakage, however, treatment with solution post thermal injury seemed to essentially eliminate the albumin leakage in cerebral vessels. The purpose of this study was to evaluate leukocyte endothelial adherence characteristics and dynamic changes in cerebral microvessels after thermal injury. In addition, the effects of various resuscitation fluid protocols on the cerebral microcirculatory changes was investigated.

Materials and Methods

Adult Sprague-Dawley rats (250 grams) were anesthetized intraperitoneally with 50 mg/kg of Pentobarbital. A tracheostomy was performed and the animals were allowed to breathe spontaneously. Polyethylene catheters were placed in the femoral vein for infusion of acridine red and another catheter was inserted into the femoral artery and attached to an arterial pressure monitor. The animal was placed in a rigid 3-point fixation frame, a sagittal incision was made on the scalp, and a plastic reservoir with an inflow and outflow tubing was secured to the skull. A biparietal craniotomy was performed and the dura reflected. The reservoir was filled with modified Elliot's solution which was constantly infused with a gas mixture of 5% CO_2 plus 95% N_2. Microcirculation was visualized with epifluorescent microscopy attached to a closed circuit TV. Camera location was kept constant and the data stored. The experimental group underwent immersion into water of 100°C for six seconds. This produced a 70% body surface area third degree burn. The control group, or the nonthermally injured group, was immersed in water of 37°C for six seconds. Baseline arteriolar and venular diameters were measured. Repeat measurements were done every 15 minutes for six hours. At the end of six hours, acridine red was injected to visualize leukocytes (0.1 ml/100 gms weight at 1 mg/ml concentration) and observed for 20 times magnification. Fifty micron segments of vein were video recorded for thirty seconds and the number of leukocytes rolling or adherent to the endothelium were counted and the experimental group compared to the control group. At the end of this time period. The animals were sacrificed. The following groups were examined with a control or nonthermally injured animals versus the experimental or thermally injured animals in each group: Group A (no resuscitation fluid) control N = 6, experimental N = 6. Group B (LR at 4 cc/kg / %burn, Parkland formula) control N = 6, experimental N = 6. Group C (7.5% HHS bolus post injury at 4 cc/kg Q 1 hour) control N = 6, experimental N = 6.

Results

There was a significant increase in leukocyte number in Group A [+ 15.7 ± 2.0% (m ± S.E.M.)] and in Group B (+13.7 ± 2.1%) when the experimental was compared to the control group. However, Group C had a significant decrease (−0.2 ± 1.0%) There was no significant percent change in mean arteriolar diameter over the six hour period in Group A or Group B. However, there was a significant progressive arteriolar dilatation over six hours in the thermally injured animals treated with HHS with percent mean arteriolar change in Group C: control (+6.3 ± 6.7%) versus experimental (+58.1 ± 7.9%) with a p value of less than 0.001.

Discussion

Thermal injury leads to an increased number of leukocytes along the vessel wall. Treatment with LR did not improve this. However, treatment with HHS seemed to essentially eliminate the number of rolling and adherent leukocytes with a progressive significant arteriolar dilatation over six hours. These findings provide important mechanistic information that may have explained the beneficial effects of hypertonic saline in the treatment of thermally injured patients. Hypertonic saline has been used to treat hemorrhagic shock [4] and it has also been effectively used to treat major burns

[5]. The progressive arteriolar dilatation seen in the HHS treated animals seemed to suggest an improvement in the intravascular volume.

Acknowledgement

This work was supported by NIH #RR07053, Alumni Faculty Award, Children's Miracle Network Telethon Grant, Research Board Grant, and the Edna M. Jeffries Trust Fund.

References

1. Barone CM, Jimenez DF, Huxley VH, *et al* (1994) The effect of thermal injury on cerebral permeability. 39th annual meeting of the Plastic Surgery Research Council (Abstract)
2. Barone CM, Jimenez DF, Huxley VH (1997) Cerebral vascular response to hypertonic fluid resuscitation in thermal injury. Brain Edema X. Acta Neurochir (Wien) [Suppl] 70: 265–266
3. Jimenez DF, Barone CM, Huxley VH. *In vivo* visualization of cerebral microcirculation in systemic thermal injury: a new animal model. Int J Microcirc (Submitted)
4. Nakayama SI, Kramer GC, Carlsen RC, *et al* (1985) Infusion of very hypertonic saline to blood rats: membrane potentials in fluid shifts. J Surg Res 38: 180–186
5. Onarheim H, Missavage AK, Kramer GC, *et al* (1990) Effectiveness of hypertonic saline dextran for initial fluid resuscitation of major burns. J Trauma 30 (5): 597–603

Correspondence: C. M. Barone, M.D., Division of Plastic Surgery, M349, University of Missouri, One Hospital Drive, Columbia, MO 65212, U.S.A.

Acta Neurochir (1997) [Suppl] 70: 269–274
© Springer-Verlag 1997

Role of Neurochemicals in Brain Edema and Cell Changes Following Hyperthermic Brain Injury in the Rat

H. S. Sharma[1,2], **J. Westman**[1], **J. Cervós-Navarro**[3], and **F. Nyberg**[2]

[1] Laboratory of Neuroanatomy, [2] Department of Anatomy and Department of Pharmaceutical Biosciences, Biomedical Centre, Uppsala University, Uppsala, Sweden, and [3] Institute of Neuropathology, Free University Berlin, Berlin, Federal Republic of Germany

Summary

The involvement of three potent neurochemical mediators of the edema formation such as serotonin, prostaglandins and opioids in the pathophysiology of hyperthermic brain injury was examined in a rat model using a pharmacological approach. Hyperthermic brain injury was induced in conscious young rats by exposing them to heat stress at 38°C for 4 h. In these rats the blood-brain barrier (BBB) permeability, brain edema, cerebral blood flow (CBF), heat shock protein 72 kD (HSP) response and cell changes were examined. Pretreatment with ketanserin (a serotonin-2 receptor antagonist), indomethacin (prostaglandin synthesis inhibitor) and naloxone (opioid receptor antagonist) in separate groups of rats reduced hyperthermia and HSP response following heat stress and significantly attenuated changes in the BBB permeability, brain edema, CBF and cell reaction. These results suggest that the pathophysiology of hyperthermic brain injury is a complex mechanisms and several neurochemicals are involved in the brain pathology caused by heat stress.

Keywords: Hyperthermic brain injury; neurochemicals; heat shock protein response.

Introduction

Heat stress (HS) and associated hyperthermia is a serious clinical condition in which profound brain damage occurs if the body temperature exceeds beyond 41°C [4, 11, 15, 16]. The mechanisms underlying brain damage in HS is not well known. Experiments carried out in our laboratory in the last 10 years suggest that increased microvascular permeability following hyperthermic brain injuries may play a crucial role [11–13, 15]. An increased extravasation of serum protein will lead to vasogenic edema which is primarily responsible for secondary brain damage in hyperthermic brain injuries [1, 2, 17]. Recently, various neurochemical mediators such as serotonin, prostaglandins, histamine, neuropeptides and bradykinin have been suggested to influence BBB and brain edema in vari-

ous pathological conditions [1, 2, 17]. Interestingly, these neurochemicals are also involved in the physiological mechanisms of thermoregulation [5, 18]. Thus it seems quite likely that altered metabolism of neurochemicals in the plasma and brain following hyperthermia may lead to breakdown of the BBB permeability, alterations in the blood flow and vasogenic edema [1, 2, 17]. These factors either alone or in combination may influence the neuronal function and induce adverse cell reaction in the brain following hyperthermic brain insults.

This study was performed in order to investigate the involvement of serotonin, prostaglandins and neuropeptides in the secondary mechanisms of hyperthermic brain damage in a rat model using pharmacological approach.

Materials and Methods

Animals

Experiments were carried out on male Wistar rats (80–90 g, 8–9 weeks old) housed in a controlled ambient temperature (21 ± 1°C) with 12 h light and 12 h dark schedule. The rat food and tap water were supplied ad libitum.

Exposure to Heat Stress

Rats were exposed to heat for 4 h in a biological oxygen demand (B.O.D.) incubator maintained at 38°C (relative humidity 45–50%, wind velocity 20–25 cm/sec). Normal rats kept at room temperature served as controls [7, 18].

Stress Symptoms

The occurrence of hyperthermia, salivation and behavioural prostration were examined at every 1 h hour interval during 4 h heat exposure. Gastric ulceration in the mucosa of the stomach wall was examined at autopsy [18].

Blood-Brain Barrier Permeability

The blood-brain barrier (BBB) permeability was examined using Evans blue (2% of 0.3 ml solution, pH 7.4) and radiolabelled iodine, ^{131}I-sodium (10 μCi/rat) as protein tracers as described earlier [6, 8]. The extravasation of iodine in brain was expressed as ratio over blood radioactivity. The Evans blue dye entered into the brain was measured colorometrically [18].

Cerebral Blood Flow

The cerebral blood flow (CBF) was measured in separate groups of rats using carbonised microspheres (15 ± 0.6 μm) labelled with [125]Iodine as described earlier [6, 18].

Brain Edema

In separate groups of rats, the brain edema was measured using the brain water content determined from the differences in the dry and wet weight of the samples [12, 13].

Immunohistochemistry of Heat Shock Protein (HSP 72 kD)

For morphological examination, separate groups of rats were anaesthetised with equithesis and perfused with 4% paraformaldehyde in 0.1 M phosphate buffer (pH 7.4) at room temperature. The immunohistochemistry of heat shock proteins (72 kD) using constitutive isoform of HSP antiserum (Amersham, Germany) was done on 60 μm free floating vibratome sections using standard protocol [10]. In some selective immunostained sections, ultrastructural investigation at electron microscopy was done to identify the HSP labelling into the intracellular compartments [10].

Light and Electron Microscopy

For routine morphological investigations, few tissue pieces were embedded in paraffin and 3 μm thick sections were cut and stained for routine Nissl, glial fibrillary acidic protein (GFAP) and myelin basic protein (MBP) immunostaining [12, 13]. For electron microscopy, tissue pieces were embedded in epon, postfixed in osmium and processed for routine electron microscopy, counterstained with lead acetate and uranyl sulphate and examined in a Philips or Hitachi Transmission Electron microscope. Ultratsructural investigation of the BBB was examined using lanthanum (2.5% of Lanthanum chloride) as an electron dense small molecular tracer (18 A°) added into the fixative solution [9, 12, 13].

Drug Treatments

In separate groups of rats influence of ketanserin (a serotonin-2 receptor antagonist, Janssen Pharmaceuticals, Beerse, Belgium), indomethacin (a prostaglandin synthesis inhibitor, Sigma Chemical Co., USA) or naloxone (an opioid receptor antagonist, Sigma Chemical Co., USA) was examined in rats subjected to 4 h heat stress. All these drugs were injected in a dose of 10 mg/kg intraperitoneally 30 min before the onset of heat stress after which the BBB permeability, CBF, edema and cell changes were examined.

Statistical Analysis

The unpaired Student's t-test was used to evaluate statistical significance of the data obtained. For multiple group comparison, ANOVA followed by Dunnet test was used. A p-value less than 0.05 was considered significant.

Results

Stress Symptoms

Subjection of untreated animals to a 4 h HS resulted in profound hyperthermia (41.86 ± 0.23°C), salivation and behavioural prostration. Post mortem examination showed many microhaemorrhages in the mucosal wall of the stomach. Pretreatment with ketanserin (39.76 ± 0.34, p < 0.05), indomethacin (39.54 ± 0.23, p < 0.05) or naloxone (40.24 ± 0.34, p < 0.05) significantly reduced the hyperthermic response however the behavioural symptoms were only mildly reduced. The occurrence of gastric haemorrhages were considerable attenuated.

BBB Permeability and CBF

The BBB permeability to Evans blue (from 0.24 ± 0.04 to 1.56 ± 0.23 mg%, p < 0.001) and ^{131}I-sodium (from 0.28 ± 0.06 to 1.84 ± 0.28%, p < 0.001) was increased significantly in these heat stressed animals compared to control values. Pretreatment with ketanserin, indomethacin or naloxone significantly reduced the increased permeability of the BBB to Evans blue (0.32 ± 0.04, 0.35 ± 0.06 and 0.42 ± 0.08% respectively, p < 0.05) and radiolabelled iodine (0.38 ± 0.06, 0.44 ± 0.08 and 0,46 ± 0.10% respectively, p < 0.05) following heat stress. The CBF in heat stressed animals was reduced significantly (from 1.01 ± 0.06 to 0.74 ± 0.08 ml/g/min, p < 0.01) from the control group. Pretreatment with ketanserin, indomethacin or naloxone significantly restored (0.96 ± 0.05, 0.88 ± 0.04 and 0.91 ± 0.06 ml/g/min respectively, p < 0.05) the CBF values near normal level in heat stressed rats.

Brain Edema

The brain water content was elevated (81.57 ± 0.36%, p < 0.001) in heat stressed animals from control value (77.24 ± 0.23%). This increase in the brain water content was significantly thwarted by pretreatment with ketanserin, indomethacin or naloxone (78.23 ± 0.18, 78.56 ± 0.32 and 78.89 ± 0.34% respectively, p < 0.05).

Light Microscopy

Light microscopy showed many distorted neurons and gliosis in several brain regions of heat stressed rats (Fig. 1). Thus degeneration of Nissl substance in the neuronal cytoplasm and upregulation of glial fibrillary acidic protein (GFAP) immunoreactivity, a marker of astrocytes, was very common finding (Fig. 1). Pretreatment with ketanserin, indomethacin and naloxone markedly attenuated these nerve cell and glial cell changes. A representative example of nerve cell dam-

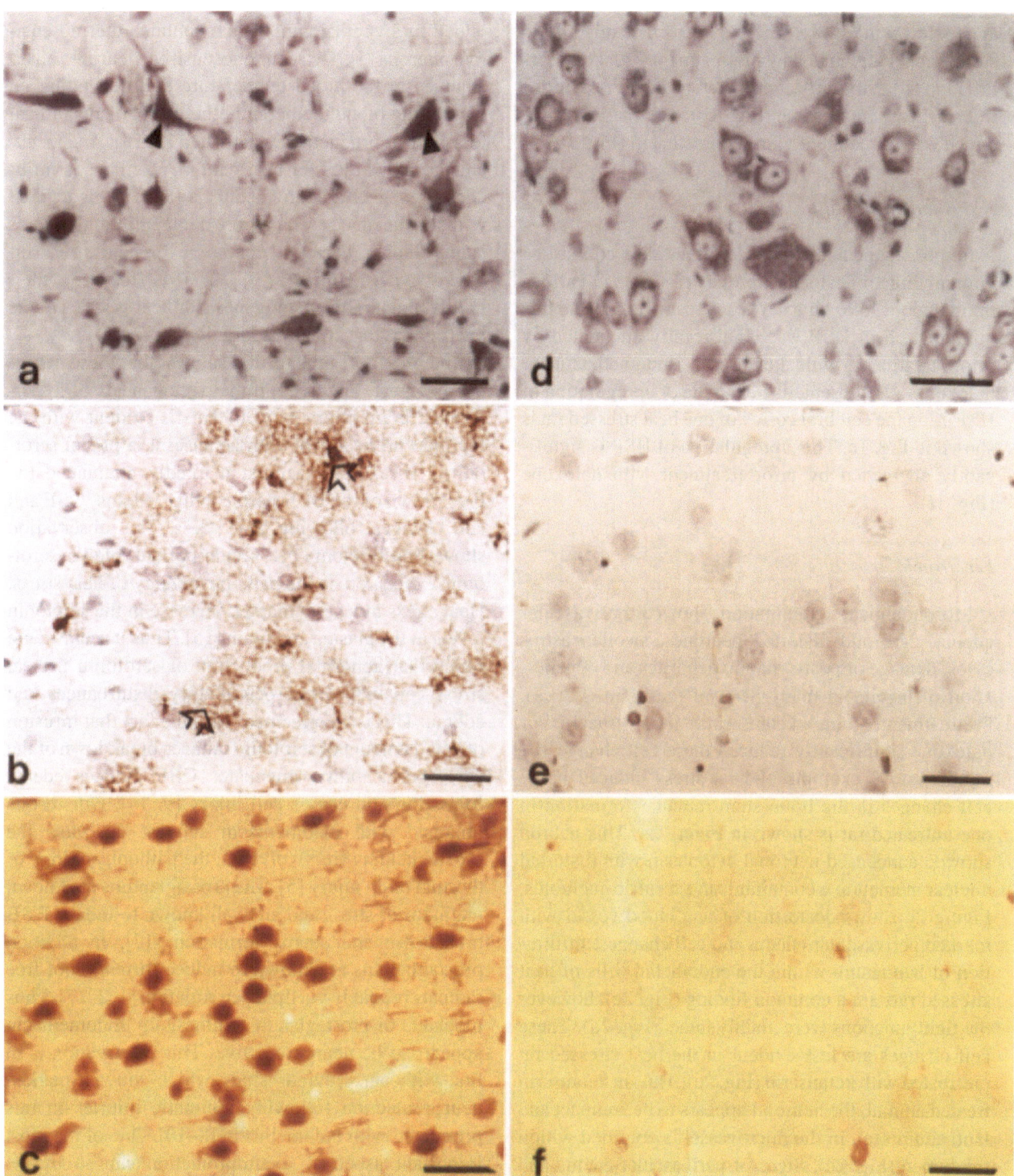

Fig. 1. 4 h heat stress 58°C. Left: untreated, right: treated. Shows distortion of nerve cells (arrow head) (a) and upregulation of glial fibrillary acididc protein (GFAP) immunoreactivity in the astrocytes (arrow) (b) in the brain stem reticular formation following heat stress in one heat stressed rat. Upregulation of constitutive isoform of heat shock protein (HSP) immunoreactivity (72 kD) in the cerebral cortex is shown in one heat stressed rat (c). These cell changes were markedly reduced by pretreatment with ketanserin (d), indomethacin (e) and naloxone (f) pretreatment (bar = 50 μm)

age is shown in Fig. 1a. These nerve cell changes were significantly attenuated by pretreatment with ketanserin (Fig. 1d). Similarly, upregulation of GFAP in untreated heat stressed rat (Fig. 1b) was markedly reduced by pretreatment with indomethacin (Fig. 1d).

HSP Immunostaining

Immunocytochemical observations showed marked upregulation of heat shock protein response in various brain regions following 4 h heat stress (Fig.1c) and this upregulation of HSP was significantly attenuated by prior treatment with ketanserin, indomethacin or naloxone. A representative example of upregulation of HSP 72 in the cerebral cortex of one heat stressed rat is shown in Fig. 1c. This upregulation of HSP is significantly attenuated by prior treatment with naloxone (Fig. 1f).

Electron Microscopy

Morphological examination showed perivascular edema, dark and distorted neurones, swollen astrocytes, damage of post-synaptic dendrites and degeneration of myelin in many parts of the brain (Fig. 2). Pretreatment with ketanserin, indomethacin or naloxone significantly reduced these cell changes. A representative example of heat stress induced nerve cell changes in the brain stem reticular formation in one untreated rat is shown in Figure 2a. This neuron showed condensed neuronal cytoplasm with distorted nuclear memebrane containing an eccentric nucluolus. Figure 2b shows dostortion of one blood vessel with marked perivascular edema and cell changes. Infiltration of lanthanum within the endothelial cells of heat stressed rats are a common finding (Fig. 2c), however the tight junctions were mainly intact (Fig. 2d). These cell changes are less evident in the heat stressed rat pretreated with ketanserin (Fig. 2e). Thus in ketanserin treated animal, the neuropil appears to be compact and lanthanum seen in the microvessel is confined within the lumen (Fig. 2e). Signs of perivascular edema and membrane damage is largely absent.

Discussion

Heat stress is associated with a marked increase in the body temperature [4, 16]. An increase in body temperature may result either by fever [5, 18], radiotherapy [16] or exercise in hot environment [5, 7, 18]. Under normal condition, the body temperature is main-

tained by hypothalamus which contains thermosensitive neurons [5]. These thermosensitive neurons senses changes in the blood temperature and depending on circulating blood temperature the mechanisms of heat loss or heat production is activated [5, 18]. The mechanisms of heat loss or heat gain mechanisms is influenced by several neurochemicals [5]. This is evident with the fact that serotonin, prostaglandins and opioids can influence bacterial endotoxin or heat stress induced hyperthermia [5, 7, 16, 18]. However, their involvement in the pathogenesis of heat injuries to the central nervous system is largely ignored.

The present results further suggest that these neurochemicals are involved in the pathogenesis of hyperthermic brain injury as well. This is evident with the fact that pretreatment with ketanserin, a potent serotonin-2 receptor antagonist markedly attenuated the breakdown of the BBB permeability, edema, CBF and cell changes following heat stress. This observation shows that serotonin plays an important role via serotonin-2 receptors in the pathophysiology of heat stress. Heat stress induces a marked increase in the serotonin levels in the plasma and brain [15]. Thus it seems quite likely that abnormal production of serotonin in heat stress can induce microcirculatory disturbances and edema. This is in agreement with the fact that infusion of small amount of serotonin induces breakdown of the BBB permeability, attenuates CBF induces edema formation and causes cell injury [9, 14]. Our results obtained with indomethacin suggest that also the prostaglandins are involved in the pathophysiology of thermal brain injury [5]. The prostaglandins are known mediator of stress and are well known to induce BBB breakdown and edema formation [17]. In addition prostaglandins are known to induce formation of free radicals probably via lipid peroxidation [1, 2, 17]. Thus blockade of prostaglandin synthesis by indomethacin appears to be neuroprotective. This observation is in line with our previous study which showed marked neuroprotection following traumatic injuries in rats pretreated with indomethacin [8–10]. One of the most important aspect of neuroprotection caused by indomethacin is its ability to reduce breakdown of the BBB permeability [8, 11].

The other most important findings of this investigation is that blockade of opioid receptors by naloxone also significantly reduced the BBB leakage, edema formation, disturbances in the CBF and cell changes. This observation suggest that opioid peptides are involved in the pathological mechanisms of heat stress induced brain injury. Previously it has been shown that

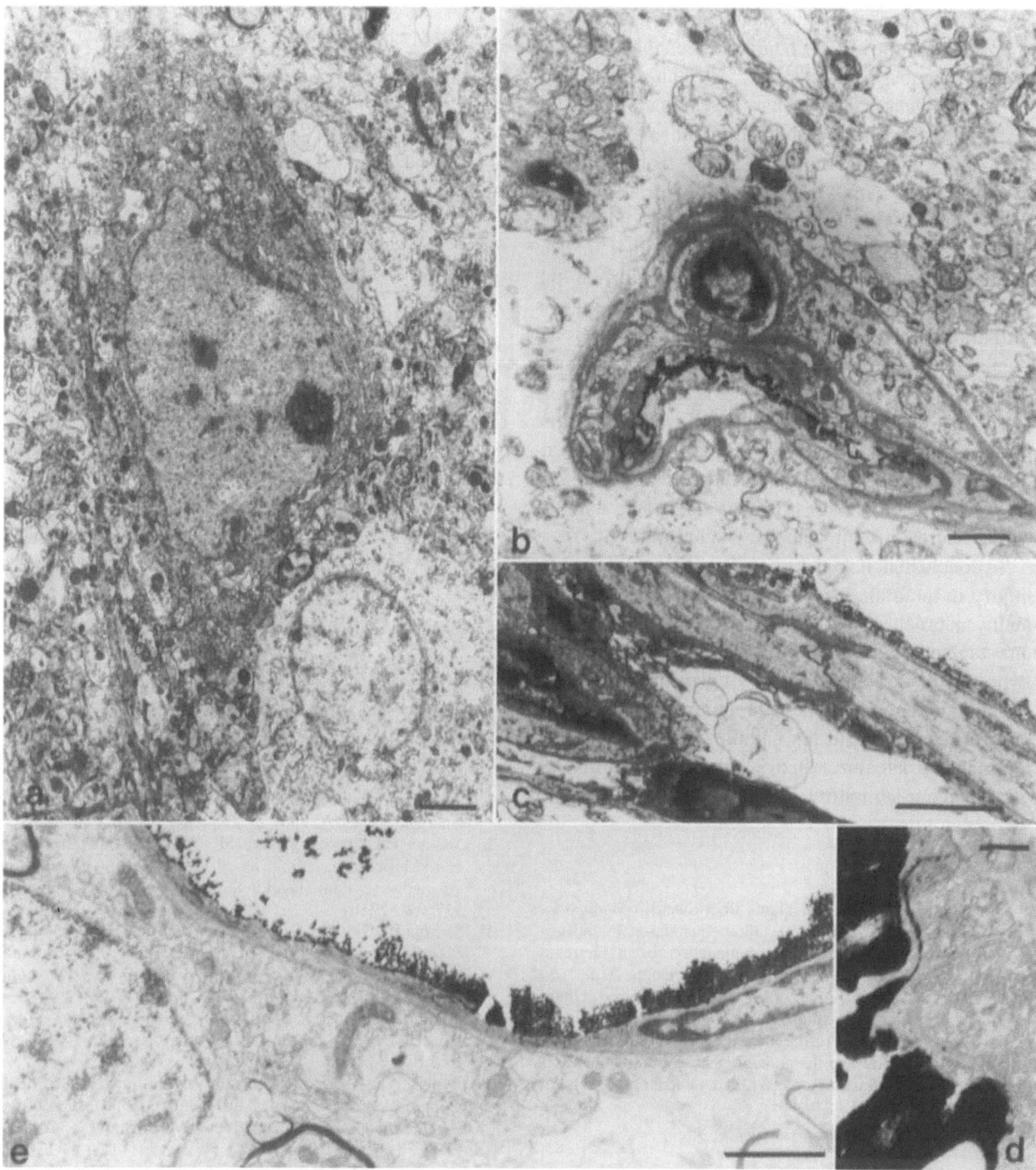

Fig. 2. Low power electron micrograph from the brain stem reticular formation of a heat stressed rat showing one dark and distorted neuron with an eccentric nucleolus (a). Disruption of one blood vessel, memebrane, vacuolation, edema and synaptic damage is quite frequent in this heat stressed rat (b). Lanthanum infliltration into the endothelial cell and in vesicular profiles within the endothelium can be clearly seen (c), whereas, the tight junction remained intact (d). These cell changes and vascular reaction were less apparent in the ketanserin pretreated and heat stressed rat (e) (bar = 1 μm)

opioids receptor antagonist naloxone can induce neuroprotection following ischemia or mechanical injuries to the brain and spinal cord [1, 17]. Thus, our results obtained in heat stress further suggest that opioids are also involved in the underlying mechanisms of thermal brain injury. Recent observations show that opioids are involved in the pathophysiology of fever [5, 18]. Thus blockade of opioid receptors by naloxone attenuated bacterial endotoxin induced hyperthermia [5]. The mechanisms of naloxone-induced reduction in the body temperature following endotoxin challenge is still unclear. However, it appears that naloxone has the capacity to reduce stress response caused by bacterial endotoxin [18]. Our results further show that naloxone prevented the HSP response caused by hyperthermia which suggest that blockade of opioid receptors contribute to the reduction of stress response. Obviously a reduction in cellular stress response is related with the lesser degree of brain pathology in heat stress.

In conclusion, it appears that heat stress induced cell injury in the brain is a complex phenomena in which many neurochemicals are involved. Since serotonin, prostaglandins and opioids have multiple receptor subtypes in the CNS, additional studies using specific receptor antagonist to these compounds are needed to get further insight in the pathology of hyperthermic brain injury, a feature which is currently under investigation in our laboratory.

Acknowledgements

This study is supported by grants from Swedish Medical Research Council nrs. 2710, 9459, Göran Gustafsson Foundation, Sweden; Alexander von Humboldt Foundation, Bonn, Germany; The University Grants Commission, New Delhi, India. The technical assistance of Kärstin Flink, Ingamarie Olsson, Gunilla Tibling, Madeleine Järild, Inga Hjörte, Ulla Johansson; the secretarial assistance of Gun Britt Lind, Agneta Bergström, Gunnila Aberg, Aruna Misra; and the photographic and computer assistance of Frank Bittkowski and William Schannöng are highly appreciated.

References

1. Black KL (1995) Biochemical opening of the blood-brain barrier. Adv Drug Del Rev 15: 37–52
2. Greenwood J, Begely J, Segel M (1995) The new concept of a blood-brain barrier. Plenum, New York, pp 1–438
4. Malmud N, Haymaker MW, Custer CR (1946) Heat stroke. A clinicopathological study of 125 fatal cases. Milit Surg 99: 397–449
5. Milton AS (1993) Temperature regulation. Adv Pharmacol Sci. Birkhäuser, Basel, pp 1–450
6. Sharma HS (1987) Effect of captopril (a converting enzyme inhibitor) on blood-brain barrier permeability and cerebral blood flow in normotensive rats. Neuropharmacology 26: 85–92
7. Sharma HS, Westman J, Cervós-Navarro J, Nyberg F (1997) Pathophysiology of brain edema and cell changes in hyperthermic brain injury. In: Sharma HS, Westman J (eds) Brain function in hot environment. Prog Brain Res. Elsevier, Amsterdam
8. Sharma HS, Nyberg F, Westman J, Cervós-Navarro J, Dey PK (1996) Probable involvement of serotonin in the increased permeability of the blood-brain barrier by forced swimming. An experimental study using Evans blue and ^{131}I-sodium tracers in the rat. Behav Brain Res 72: 189–196
9. Sharma HS, Olsson Y, Dey PK (1995) Serotonin as a mediator of increased microvascular permeability of the brain and spinal cord. Experimental observations in anaesthetised rats and mice. In: Greenwood J, Begley D, Segal M, Lightman S (eds) New concepts of a blood-brain barrier. Plenum, New York, pp 7580
10. Sharma HS, Olsson Y, Westman J (1995) A serotonin synthesis inhibitor, p-chlorophenylalanine reduces the heat shock protein response following trauma to the spinal cord. An immunohistochemical and ultrastructural study in the rat. Neurosci Res 21: 241–249
11. Sharma HS, Westman J, Nyberg F, Cervós-Navarro J, Dey PK (1994) Role of serotonin and prostaglandins in brain edema induced by heat stress. An experimental study in the rat. Acta Neurochir (Wien) [Suppl] 60: 65–70
12. Sharma HS, Kretzschmar R, Cervós-Navarro J, Ermisch A, Rühle H-J, Dey PK (1992) Age-related pathophysiology of the blood-brain barrier in heat stress. Prog Brain Res 91: 189–196
13. Sharma HS, Cervós-Navarro J (1990) Brain oedema and cellular changes induced by acute heat stress in young rats. Acta Neurochir (Wien) [Suppl] 51: 383–386
14. Sharma HS, Olsson Y, Dey PK (1990) Blood-brain barrier permeability and cerebral blood flow following elevation of circulating serotonin level in the anaesthetized rats. Brain Res 517: 215–223
15. Sharma HS, Dey PK (1987) Influence of long-term acute heat exposure on regional blood-brain barrier permeability, cerebral blood flow and 5-HT level in conscious normotensive young rats. Brain Res 424: 153–162
16. Sminia P, Van der Zee J, Wondergem J, Haveman J (1994) Effect of hyperthermia on the central nervous system: a review. Int J Hyperthermia 10: 1–30
17. Wahl M, Unterberg A, Baethmann A, Schilling L (1988) Mediators of blood-brain barrier dysfunction and formation of vasogenic edema. J Cereb Blood Flow Metab 8: 621–634
18. Zeisberger E, Schönbaum E, Lomax P (1994) Thermal balance in health and disease, recent basic research and clinical progress. Adv Pharmacol Sci. Birkhäuser, Basel, pp 1–457

Correspondence: Hari Shanker Sharma, Ph.D., Laboratory of Neuroanatomy, Department of Anatomy, Box 571, Biomedical Centre, Uppsala University, S-75123 Uppsala, Sweden.

Acta Neurochir (1997) [Suppl] 70: 275–278
© Springer-Verlag 1997

Acute Heat Stress Induces Edema and Nitric Oxide Synthase Upregulation and Down-Regulates mRNA Levels of the NMDAR1, NMDAR2A and NMDAR2B Subunits in the Rat Hippocampus

P. Le Grevès[1], H. S. Sharma[1, 2], J. Westman[2], P. Alm[3], and F. Nyberg[1]

[1] Department of Pharmaceutical Biosciences and [2] Laboratory of Neuroanatomy, Department of Anatomy, Biomedical Centre, Uppsala University, Uppsala, and [3] Department of Pathology, University Hospital Lund, University of Lund, Lund, Sweden

Summary

The influence of heat stress on constitutive isoform of neuronal nitric oxide synthase (cNOS) and NMDA receptor gene expression in hippocampus was examined in a rat model. Subjection of animals to 4 h heat stress at 38°C resulted in a marked upregulation of cNOS in the hippocampus accompanied with a marked general expansion and edematous cell changes. On the other hand NMDA receptor messenger RNA encoding NMDAR1, NMDAR2A and NMDAR2B subunits showed a marked downregulation in the hippocampus of heat stressed rats compared to the controls. Our results show that upregulation of cNOS is instrumental in heat stress associated edema and cell injury. Furthermore, an increased production of NO as evident with upregulation of cNOS appears to be a key factor in the downregulation of NMDA receptor gene expression in heat stress.

Keywords: Heat stress, nitric oxide, NMDA receptor gene expression, hyperthermia.

Introduction

Heat stress (HS) and associated hyperthermia is quite frequent during fever, exposure to high ambient temperature and following radiotherapy for tumours [22]. It is known from previous reports that longterm elevation of body temperature (exceeding 41°C) is associated with abnormal cell reaction in the brain [15, 18, 20–22]. The mechanisms of brain damage following hyperthermic insults is not known in all its details. However, experimental studies carried in our laboratory in the past several years suggest that a global increase in the blood-brain barrier (BBB) permeability may play an important role in vasogenic edema formation and cell changes in the brain [15, 18–21].

Recent observations show that NO production is associated with inhibition of selective NMDA receptor activation and exogenously applied NO blocks

NMDA and kianate induce increase in the intracellular calcium [1, 10, 14, 23, 24]. Since NO is involved in signal transduction via NMDA receptors, it is possible that hyperthermia can influence NMDA receptor regulation. Therefore, in this investigation we examined the expression of mRNAs encoding the NMDA receptor NMDAR1, NMDAR2A and NMDAR2B subunits in the hippocampus of normal and heat stressed rats using Northern blot analysis. In addition, NOS histochemistry and edema in the hippocampus were also examined.

Materials and Methods

Animals

Experiments were carried out on 20 male Wistar rats (100–150 g body weight) housed at controlled ambient temperature 21°C with 12 h light and 12 h dark schedule. The rat feed and tap water were supplied ad libitum before the experiments.

Exposure to Heat Stress

Rats were exposed to heat stress at 38°C for 4 h as described earlier [20, 21]. Normal animals kept at room temperature served as controls. This experimental condition is approved by the Ethical committee of Uppsala University.

NOS Immunohistochemistry

For immunostaining, immediately after heat stress animals were anaesthetised with equithesin and the chest was rapidly exposed and the intravascular blood was washed out by perfusing 0.1 M phosphate buffer saline through heart at 90 torr followed by perfusion with 4% paraformaldehyde containing 1.5% glutaraldehyde in 0.1 M phosphate buffer, pH 7.4 at room temperature. After perfusion, the brains were removed and tissue pieces containing hippocampus were dissected out. Immunohistochemistry of NOS was examined on vibratome sections (60 μm thick) obtained from hippocampus of normal and heat stressed rats using antibodies directed against constitutive isoform of neuronal nitric oxide synthase (cNOS) according to the standard protocol [16, 17].

Edema and Cell Changes

Edema in the hippocampus was examined by measuring water content. The cell changes were examined by light microscopy on paraffin embedded 3 μm thick sections stained with haemotoxylin and eosin, as described earlier [18–20].

NMDA Receptor Gene Expression

Immediately after heat exposure, the animals were anaesthetised with Equithesin (3 ml/kg, i.p.) and decapitated. Hippocampus was dissected out on ice and frozen on dry ice and stored at –70°C until further analysed. Total RNA was extracted using the single step acid guanidium thiocyanate-phenol-chloroform method [6] and electrophoresed on agarose MOPS-formaldehyde gels. The RNA was transferred to nylon filters and hybridised against cDNA probes for the NMDA receptor subunits, NMDAR1, NMDAR2A and NMDAR2B. After stringent washing the filters were subjected to autoradiography and the hybridisation signals were measured by use of an image-analysing system. The signals for NMDAR1, NMDAR2A and NMDAR2B mRNA were normalised to the ethidium bromide fluorescence signal of 28S ribosomal RNA [8]. The values were mathematically transformed so that the mRNA levels for the control group were set to 1.0 arbitrary unit [9].

Statistical Analysis

The data were analysed using Student's unpaired t-test. A p-value less than 0.05 were considered to be significant.

Results

NOS Immunohistochemistry

Subjection of rats to a 4 h HS resulted in a marked hyperthermia ($41.89 \pm 0.34°C$). There was a marked increase in cNOS immunostaining in the hippocampus of heat stressed rats. This increase in cNOS immuno-

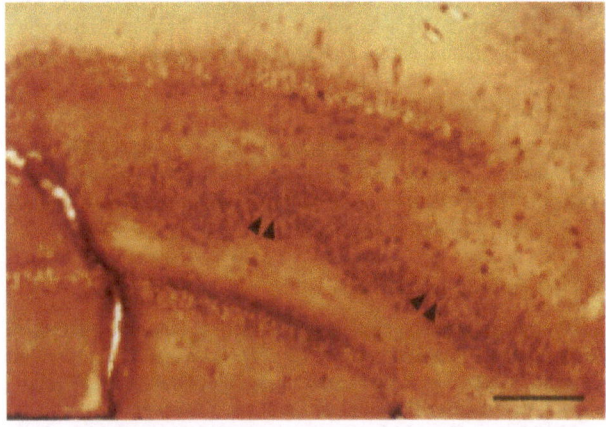

Fig 1. cNOS immunostaining, hippocampus. 4 h heat stress, 38°C. Immunohistochemical staining of constitutive isoform of neuronal nitric oxide synthase (cNOS) in the hippocampus of a heat stressed rat. Marked upregulation of cNOS (arrowheads) in neurons located in the CA-4 and CA-3 regions are clearly visible (bar = 250 μm)

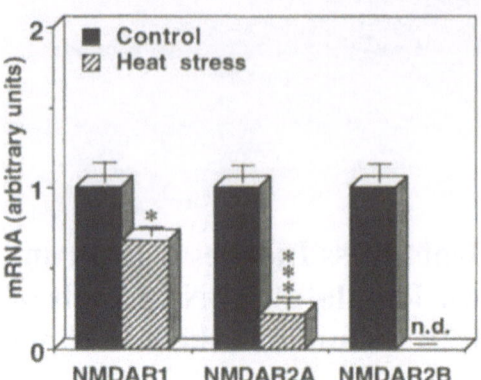

Fig. 2. Heat stress induced downregulation of NMDAR1, NMDAR2A and NMDAR2B mRNA levels in the hippocampus compared to control. * p < 0.05, *** p < 0.001 (Student's unpaired t-test), *n.d.* not detectable

staining was most marked in the CA-3 and CA-4 subfields of the hippocampus (Fig. 1). Normal rats showed only few cNOS immunostained neurons present in the dentate gyrus.

Edema and Cell Changes

Measurement of water content in heat stressed animals indicated a marked increase in the hippocampus ($81.58 \pm 0.35\%$, p < 0.01) compared to control group ($79.23 \pm 0.56\%$). Examination of gross morphology showed marked general expansion of hippocampus and edematous cell changes were quite frequent. The most pronounced distortion and degeneration of neurons were seen in the CA-3 and CA-4 regions compared to other regions of the hippocampus.

NMDA Receptor Gene Expression

Northern blot studies showed transcripts of expected sizes for the three NMDA receptor subunits (NMDAR1; 4.4 kD, NMDAR2A; 12 kD and NMDAR2B; 15 kD). HS resulted in a slight reduction in the NMDAR1 mRNA levels whereas NMDAR2A and NMDAR2B mRNAs showed profound downregulation compared to the levels detected in the control group (Fig. 2).

Discussion

The most important new finding of this study is a downregulation of NMDA receptor gene expression in the hippocampus following heat stress. This indicates that hyperthermia affects the transmission of excitatory amino acids at the receptor level in this area of the brain. An altered regulation of NMDA receptor gene expression could be due to compensatory factors in order to enhance neuronal plasticity associated with cell protection [14, 23, 24]. An increased release of glutamate is associated with a downregulation of NMDA receptor gene expression [3, 7, 10, 14]. Likewise an increased production of NO in the hippocampus following heat stress as indicated by an upregulation of cNOS could be associated with a compensatory downregulation of the NMDA receptor gene expression. This is apparent with the fact that abnormal production of excess glutamate or NOS will induce cell damage or death via activation of excitatory amino acid receptors [4, 5]. It is well documented that the subunit composition of the NMDA receptor can modify its properties and function [11, 12]. The NMDAR2A and NMDAR2B are modulatory subunits and marked downregulation of their mRNAs compared to the NMDAR1 mRNA in heat stress further support this role in the regulation of the receptor specificity. However, whether the decreased expression of NMDA receptor subunits on heat stress is due to a direct effect of NO on the transcriptional level is not known.

In present study, heat stress induced a marked upregulation of cNOS in the hippocampus. Thus, it seems quite likely that hyperthermia is associated with increased production of NO [2, 4, 16, 17]. NOS is the main enzyme responsible for conversion of L-arginine to NO [2, 14]. Thus an upregulation of NOS is compatible with increased production of NO in the nervous system [2, 4, 14, 24] and may induce cell injury as seen in ischemia, spinal cord trauma or peripheral nerve lesion [7, 13, 14, 16, 17]. It is interesting to note that a marked increase in NOS immunostaining appears in the CA-3 and CA-4 regions of the hippocampus. These subfields of the hippocampus are the most susceptible regions exhibiting cell injury and edema [18–20]. Previous observations from our laboratory show a profound increase in the BBB permeability and a reduction of the cerebral blood flow in the hippocampus of heat stressed rats [21]. Thus, ischemia and disruption of the BBB can induce vasogenic edema [15, 20]. Edema associated with disturbances in the microenvironment of the hippocampus such as alteration in the function of membrane ion channels or transporters and accumulation of intracellular calcium either alone or in combination will induce cell injury [16, 24].

Heat stressed induced upregulation of cNOS is prevented by drugs such as serotonin synthesis inhibitor, p-CPA or antioxidant compound H-290/51 [17]. Interestingly, these drugs also exhibited good neuroprotec- tion. Thus, a prevention of cNOS upregulation in heat stress is neuroprotective. However, it is not known whether these drugs also affect the downregulation of NMDA receptor gene expression in this model. It would be interesting to further testify this hypothesis by studying NMDA receptor gene expression using various neuroprotective drugs and selective NOS inhibitors in this model.

In conclusion, our data suggest that heat stress has the capacity to induce upregulation of NOS in the hippocampus indicating an increased production of NO. Abnormal production of NO appears to be injurious to the hippocampus and can cause downregulation of NMDA receptor gene expression.

Acknowledgements

This study is supported by grants from Swedish Medical Research Council nrs. 2710, 9710, 9459, Göran Gustafsson Foundation, Torsten and Ragner Söderberg Foundation, Sweden; Alexander von Humboldt Foundation, Bonn, Germany and The University Grants Commission, New Delhi, India. The technical assistance of Kärstin Flink, Ingamarie Olsson and Ulla Johansson is highly appreciated.

References

1. Baader SL, Schilling K (1996) Glutamate receptors mediate dynamic regulation of nitric oxide synthase expression in cerebellar granule cells. J Neurosci 16: 1440–1449
2. Bredt DS, Hwang PH, Snyder SH (1990) Localization of nitric oxide synthase indicating a neural role for nitric oxide. Nature 347: 768–770
3. Casabona G, L'Episcopo MR, Di Iorio P, Ciccarelli R, De Bernardis E, Shinozaki H, Nicoletti F, Caciagli F (1994) Interaction between metabotropic receptors and purinergic transmission in rat hippocampal slices. Brain Res 645: 13–18
4. Chiueh CC, Gilbert DL, Colton CA (1994) The neurobiology of NO˙ and ˙OH. Ann NY Acad Sci 738: 1–471
5. Choi DW (1993) Nitric oxide: foe or friend to the injured brain. Proc Natl Acad Sci USA 90: 9741–9743
6. Chomczynski P, Sacchi N (1987) Single-step method of RNA isolation by acid guanidinium thiocyanatephenol-chloroform extraction. Ann Biochem 162: 156–159
7. Dawson TM, Snyder SH (1994) Gases as biological messengers: nitric oxide and carbon monooxide in the brain. J Neurosci 14: 5147–5159
8. Duhl DM, Gillespie DD, Sulser F (1992) Ethidium bromide fluorescence of 28S ribosomal RNA can be used to normalize samples in Northern or dot blots when analyzing small drug-induced changes in specific mRNA. J Neurosci Methods 42: 211–218
9. Le Grevès P, Hoogendoorn K, Synnergren B, Meyerson B, Nyberg F (1996) The relationship between the NMDA receptor NR1 subunit mRNA and [³H]MK-801 binding in the embryonic and early postnatal rat CNS. Neurosci Res Comm 19
10. Manzoni OS, Bockaert J (1993) Nitric oxide synthase activity endogenously modulates NMDA receptors. J Neurochem 61: 368–370
11. Meguro H, Mori H, Araki K, Kushiya E, Kutsuwada T, Yamazaki M, Kumanishi T, Arakawa M, Sakimura K, Mishina M (1992)

Functional characterization of a heteromeric NMDA receptor channel expressed from cloned cDNAs. Nature 357: 70–74

12. Monyer H, Sprengel R, Schoepfer R, Herb A, Higuchi M, Lomeli H, Burnashev N, Sakmann B, Seeburg PH (1992) Heteromeric NMDA receptors: molecular and functional distinction of subtypes. Science 256: 1217–1221

13. Regodor J, Montesdeoca J, Ramirez-Gonzalez J A, Hernandez-Urquia CM, Divac I (1993) Bilateral induction of NADPH-diaphorase activity in neocortical and hippocampal neurons by unilateral injury. Brain Res 631: 171–174

14. Schuman EM, Madison DV (1994) Nitric oxide and synaptic function. Ann Rev Neurosci 17: 153–158

15. Sharma HS, Westman J, Cervós-Navarro J, Nyberg F (1996) Pathophysiology of brain edema and cell changes in hyperthermic brain injury. In: Sharma HS, Westman J (eds) Brain function in hot environment. Prog Brain Res. Elsevier, Amsterdam

16. Sharma HS, Westman J, Olsson Y, Alm P (1996) Involvement of nitric oxide in acute spinal cord injury: an immunocytochemical study using light and electron microscopy in the rat. Neurosci Res 24: 373–384

17. Sharma HS, Westman J, Cervós-Navarro J, Alm P (1996) Involvement of nitric oxide in hyperthermic brain injury. Neuropath App Neurobiol 22 [Suppl 1]: 14–15

18. Sharma HS, Westman J, Nyberg F, Cervós-Navarro J, Dey PK (1994) Role of serotonin and prostaglandins in brain edema induced by heat stress. An experimental study in the rat. Acta Neurochir (Wien) [Suppl] 60: 65–70

19. Sharma HS, Kretzschmar R, Cervós-Navarro J, Ermisch A, Rühle H-J, Dey PK (1992) Age-related pathophysiology of the blood-brain barrier in heat stress. Prog Brain Res 91: 189–196

20. Sharma HS, Cervós-Navarro J (1990) Brain oedema and cellular changes induced by acute heat stress in young rats. Acta Neurochir (Wien) [Suppl] 51: 383–386

21. Sharma HS, Dey PK (1987) Influence of long-term acute heat exposure on regional blood-brain barrier permeability, cerebral blood flow and 5-HT level in conscious normotensive young rats. Brain Res 424: 153–162

22. Sminia P, Van der Zee J, Wondergem J, Haveman J (1994) Effect of hyperthermia on the central nervous system: a review. Int J Hyperthermia 10: 1–30

23. Tanaka T, Saito H, Matsuki N (1993) Endogenous nitric oxide inhibits NMDA- and kainate-responses by a feedback system in rat hippocampal neurons. Brain Res 631: 72–76

24. Whittle BJR (1995) Nitric oxide in physiology and pathology. Histochem J 27: 727–737

Correspondence: Hari Shanker Sharma, Ph.D., Laboratory of Neuroanatomy, Department of Anatomy, Post Box 571, Biomedical Centre, Uppsala University, S-75123 Uppsala, Sweden.

Acta Neurochir (1997) [Suppl] 70: 279–281
© Springer-Verlag 1997

Choroid Plexus Ion Transporter Expression and Cerebrospinal Fluid Secretion

R. F. Keep[1], **J. Xiang**[1], **L. J. Ulanski**[1], **F. C. Brosius**[2, 4], and **A. Lorris Betz**[1, 3]

Departments of [1] Surgery (Neurosurgery), [2] Internal Medicine, [3] Neurology and Pediatrics, University of Michigan, and [4] Veterans Affairs Hospital, Ann Arbor, MI, U.S.A.

Summary

The $Cl^-/HCO3^-$ exchanger (AE2 isoform) and the Na^+/K^+-ATPase at the choroid plexus are both thought to be involved in CSF secretion. However, both transport mechanisms are also postulated to have a role in CSF ion homeostasis raising questions as to which parameters control the expression of these transporters? Northern blots have been used to assess AE2 mRNA levels in rats subjected to alterations in blood pH or blood osmolality (a factor affecting CSF secretion). Six hours of alkalosis induced a 40% increase in AE2 mRNA ($p < 0.01$), suggesting that alterations in the expression of this transporter play a role in CSF pH homeostasis. In contrast, changes in osmolality did not affect AE2 mRNA. Western blots of Na^+/K^+-ATPase subunits were also examined to determine whether hypo and hyperkalemia affect protein levels of this transporter. There was a positive correlation between the plasma K^+ concentration and both $\alpha 1$- and $\beta 1$ subunit protein levels suggesting a role for this transporter in CSF K^+ homeostasis. As changes in plasma K^+ and pH affect choroid plexus ion transporters but do not appear to alter CSF production, these results suggest the presence of compensatory mechanisms. Understanding of such mechanisms may facilitate therapeutic control of CSF production.

Keywords: Cerebrospinal fluid; choroid plexus; ion transport.

Introduction

The choroid plexus possesses an array of ion transport mechanisms. These include $Cl^-/HCO3^-$ and Na^+/H^+ exchangers, Na^+/K^+-ATPase, and $Na^+/K^+/2Cl^-$ and K^+/Cl^- cotransporters, by inhibitor studies suggested to be involved in cerebrospinal fluid secretion [5, 7, 9]. However, a number of these transporters have been proposed to have multiple functions. For example, the exchange of $Cl^-/HCO3^-$ and Na^+/H^+ may also be involved in CSF pH homeostasis, whereas Na^+/K^+-ATPase may regulate both the CSF K^+ concentration and the Na^+-dependent transport of nutrients, such as amino acids. This raises questions as to the parameters that control expression of these transporters and whether changes in expression for ion- or nutrient regulation are uncoupled from CSF secretion.

In this study, we have examined whether blood pH or blood osmolality affect choroid plexus mRNA levels for the $Cl^-/HCO3^-$ exchanger (AE2 isoform) to investigate the importance of the exchanger in both CSF pH regulation and changes in CSF secretion that occur with osmotic stress [8]. We have also examined whether hypo- and hyperkalemia alter protein levels of the Na^+/K^+-ATPase subunits.

Methods

All experiments used adult male Sprague Dawley rats with surgery and sacrifice being performed under sodium pentobarbital anesthesia (50 mg/kg). For the AE2 experiments, four groups of rats were examined involving either acute (1 hour) or chronic (6 hour) acid-base or osmotic perturbations. For the acid-base experiments, nephrectomized rats received intraperitoneal injection of either HCl, NaCl or $NaHCO_3$ (235 mM; 2 ml/100 g). For the osmotic stress experiments the rats received intraperitoneal injection of either 1.5 M NaCl (2 ml/100 g at time 0 and 0.5 ml/100 g at 180 min), deionized water (10 ml/100 g at time 0,5 ml/100 g at 40 min and 1.5 ml/100 g at 210 min) or isotonic saline. For the Na^+/K^+-ATPase experiments, rats were made hypo- and hyperkalemic by feeding them either a potassium-deficient diet or one supplemented with 20% KCl for two weeks. To ensure a more uniform rise in plasma K^+ concentration, the rats fed the high K^+ diet were uninephrectomized.

At sacrifice, arterial blood samples were taken for determination of plasma osmolality and ions as well as blood gases. Rats then underwent intracardiac perfusion with physiological buffer to remove blood elements from the choroid plexuses prior to decapitation and excision of the choroid plexuses for either Western or Northern blotting.

Northern Blots

Total RNA was isolated from lateral and 4th ventricle choroid plexuses. AE2 mRNA expression was examined using Northern blots with a 32P-labeled cDNA probe. Results were quantified using a phosphorimager and normalized using a probe to cyclophilin, a housekeeping gene.

Western Blots

Lateral ventricle choroid plexuses were used for Western blots. After electrophoresis, samples were transferred to polyvinylidene difluoride membranes and immunoblotted with rabbit anti-rat Na^+/K^+-ATPase α and β subunit antibodies (Upstate Biotechnology Incorporated; Lake Placid, NY) followed by peroxidase-linked anti- rabbit IgG antibody (Amersham; Arlington Heights, IL). Membranes were developed with the ECL system (Amersham; Arlington Heights, IL) and the images transferred to x-ray film. The developed images were acquired via a CCD camera and band densities analyzed using a public domain program (NIH Image Version 1.55; NTIS, Springfield, VA).

Statistics

The relation between physiological parameters and choroid plexus AE2 mRNA or Na^+/K^+-ATPase protein was examined by linear regression analysis or analysis of variance with a Newman-Keuls post-hoc test.

Results

Cl^-/HCO_3^- Exchange

Although a wide range of changes of plasma osmolality was achieved in both the 1 hour (267 to 362 mOsmol/kg) and 6 hour (271 to 366 mOsmol/kg) osmotic stress experiments, there was no correlation between osmolality and AE2 mRNA expression in either type of experiment.

Similarly, the one hour experiments with acidosis and alkalosis also failed to alter AE2 mRNA expression. However, in the 6 hour experiments, alkalosis (pH: 7.47 ± 0.02; [HCO_3^-]: 37 ± 2 mM) increased

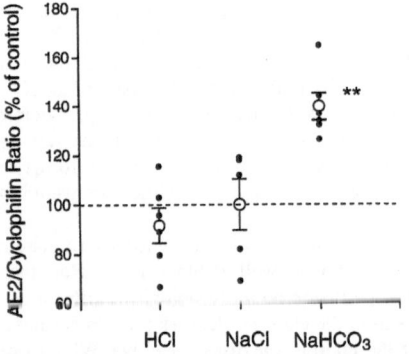

Fig. 1. Effect of 6 hours of acidosis (HCl injection) and alkalosis (NaHCO₃ injection) on choroid plexus AE2 mRNA. Data was nomalized to cyclophilin and is expressed as a percentage of average control (NaCl injection) levels. Closed circles represent individual data points, open circles are means ± S.E; **indicates significant difference from control at the p < 0.01 level

choroid plexus AE2 mRNA expression (Fig. 1; p < 0.01) to $140 \pm 6\%$ of that in controls (pH: 7.34 ± 0.01; [HCO_3^-]: 28 ± 1 mM). Six hours of acidosis (pH: 7.19 ± 0.02; [HCO_3^-]: 13 ± 1 mM) did not significantly alter expression ($92 \pm 7\%$ of control).

Na^+/K^+-ATPase

The hypo-, normo- and hyperkalemic groups in this study had plasma K^+ concentrations of 2.3 ± 0.1, 3.9 ± 0.1 and 7.2 ± 0.6 mM. Western blots failed to demonstrate the presence of the $\alpha2$ and $\alpha3$ subunits of Na^+/K^+-ATPase in the choroid plexuses of any group. Of the $\alpha1$, $\beta1$ and $\beta2$ subunits, which were present, both the $\alpha1$ and β_1 subunits showed a positive correlation with plasma [K^+] (p < 0.01 and p < 0.05 respectively). The $\alpha1$ and $\beta1$ levels were respectively 62 and 30% higher in the hyperkalemic group compared to the hypokalemic group. In contrast there was no correlation between plasma [K^+] and the $\beta2$ subunit.

Discussion

This study demonstrates changes in both the $\alpha1$ and $\beta1$ isoforms of Na^+/K^+-ATPase with alterations in plasma potassium concentration supporting a role for the choroid plexus Na^+/K^+-ATPase in CSF potassium homeostasis. Similarly, the mRNA for the AE2 isoform of the Cl^-/HCO_3^- anion exchanger was increased in response to alkalosis supporting a role of this transporter in CSF pH homeostasis. Husted and Reed [4] have demonstrated that the choroid plexus regulates CSF bicarbonate during changes in plasma pH or CSF bicarbonate concentration. In contrast, osmotic stress did not affect AE2 mRNA levels at the choroid plexus although Wald *et al.* [8] have demonstrated increasing CSF production with increasing osmolality indicating exchange of Cl^-/HCO_3^- to play a pivotal role in CSF secretion. Indeed, there appears to be a disparity between the changes reported here for ion transporters and those published for CSF secretion. Alkalinization increased AE2 mRNA levels but most studies have failed to find a change in CSF secretion. Although pH changes [4] and hyperkalemia increased choroid plexus Na^+/K^+-ATPase protein levels, CSF secretion was not affected [6].

There are a number of potential explanations for this apparent disparity. In this study, we did not measure charges in transport activity, since this parameter may not correlate with either protein or mRNA levels. Hyperosmotic activation of the AE2 anion exchange in transfected Xenopus oocytes is attributable to changes in intracellular pH mediated by Na/H exchange [3] but may not require changes in the amount of the AE2 protein. However, it should be noted that we have measured choroid plexus Na^+/K^+-ATPase activity (ouabain-sensitive 86Rb transport) in hypo- and hyperkalemia (Klarr, Stummer, Xiang, Betz and Keep; unpublished observations) where similar changes were found to those observed with Western Blots. Other potential explanations are that these transporters may not be rate limiting for CSF secretion unless they are markedly inhibited, or that compensatory pathways prevent changes in transport from affecting CSF secretion. In particular, non-selective cation [1] and chloride [2] channels present at the choroid plexus may prevent changes in HCO_3^- or K^+ transport from affecting net Cl^- and Na^+ transport and thus CSF secretion.

Understanding the exact relation between choroid plexus ion transport and CSF secretion is important for developing better methods for reducing CSF secretion. If compensatory pathways can prevent changes in ion transport from being reflected in changes in CSF secretion, it is possible that those pathways may reduce the effectiveness of inhibitors of CSF secretion such as acetazolamide. More consistent reductions in CSF secretion may occur if inhibitors are given in combination to prevent potential compensatory pathways.

Acknowledgements

This work was supported by grants from the National Institutes of Health (HL-18575 and NS-23870).

References

1. Christensen O (1987) Mediation of cell volume regulation by Ca^{2+} influx through stretch-activated channels. Nature 330: 66–68
2. Garner C, Brown PD (1992) Two types of chloride channel in the apical membrane of rat choroid plexus epithelial cells. Brain Res 591: 137–145
3. Humphreys BD, Jiang L, Chernova MN, Alper SL (1995) Hypertonic activation of AE2 anion exchanger in Xenopus oocytes via NHE–mediated intracellular alkalinization. Am J Physiol 268: C201–C209
4. Husted RF, Reed DJ (1977) Regulation of cerebrospinal fluid bicarbonate by the cat choroid plexus. J Physiol 267: 411–428
5. Johanson CE (1989) Potential for pharmacologic manipulation of the blood-cerebrospinal fluid barrier. In: Neuwelt EA (ed) Implications of the blood-brain barrier and its manipulation. Plenum, New York, pp 223–269
6. Keep RF, Cawkwell RD, Jones HC (1987) Choroid plexus structure and function in young rats on a high-potassium diet. Brain Res 413: 45–52
7. Pollay M, Hisey B, Reynolds E, Tomkins P, Stevens FA, Smith R (1985) Choroid plexus Na^+/K^+-activated adenosine triphosphatase and cerebrospinal fluid formation. Neurosurgery 17: 768–772
8. Wald A, Hochwald GM, Malhan C (1976) The effects of ventricular fluid osmolality on bulk flow of nascent fluid into the cerebral ventricles of cats. Exp Brain Res 25: 157–167
9. Zeuthen T (1991) Secondary active transport of water across ventricular cell membrane of choroid plexus epithelium of Necturus maculosus. J Physiol 444: 153–173

Correspondence: Richard F. Keep, Ph.D., Department of Surgery (Neurosurgery), University of Michigan, R5605 Kresge I, Ann Arbor, MI 48109-0532, U.S.A.

Acta Neurochir (1997) [Suppl] 70: 282–284
© Springer-Verlag 1997

Effect of Infection Brain Edema on NMDA Receptor Binding in Rat Brain *in vivo*

G. S. Cheng[1], J.-F. Chen[1], X. Chen[2], L.-H. Chen[3], Y.-G. Tao[2], and Y.-J. Yang[2, 4]

[1] Central Laboratory, [2] Department of Pediatrics, [3] Department of Neurosurgery, and [4] National Laboratory of Medical Genetics, Hunan Medical University, Changsha, Hunan, Peoples Republic of China

Summary

The purpose of this study was to determine the effect of infection brain edema (IBE) in the rat model induced by injecting pertussis bacilli (PB) into the left carotid artery. The specific binding of N-methyl-D-aspartate (NMDA) receptor with [³H] MK-801 was measured in the neuronal membrane of cerebral cortex. The Scatchard plots were performed. The B_{max} values were 0.623 ± 0.082 and 0.606 ± 0.087 pmol/mg protein in the group that received normal saline (NS) and PB respectively ($P < 0.05$). The K_d values were 43.1 ± 4.2 and 30.5 ± 3.0 nM in the groups NS and PB respectively.

The results indicated that the affinity of NMDA receptor was significantly higher in the group PB than group NS, whereas the total number of NMDA receptors had not changed in the IBE model. The increase of affinity of NMDA receptor can be blockaded by MK-801 pretreatment *in vivo*.

Keywords: Brain edema; infection; pertussis; NMDA receptor.

Introduction

Infection brain edema (IBE) is seen with a high morbidity and mortality in the pediatric population. The mechanisms of IBE is not well understood. The prevention and treatment of IBE is difficult. It is known that the concentrations of excitatory amino acid (EAA) in brain tissue and intracellular free calcium in neuron are significantly increased during brain edema induced by ischemia and injury [1, 3, 7, 13]. Nimodipine (an inhibitor of calcium channels) has protective role for ischemic or traumatic brain edema [2, 10]. It has been known that antagonists of NMDA receptor MK-801 and dextromethorphan have protective effect for ischemic brain edema [4, 5]. Wahlestedt [9] reported the anti-sense oligodeoxynucleotides of NMDA-R1 can reduce the area of ischemic infarction in rat brain. This suggested that the mechanism of ischemic brain edema maybe involve abnormal increase in EAA, overexcitation of NMDA receptor and an excessive increase of calcium influx. Our previous studies showed that histopathological features of IBE was a complex brain edema, i.e., vasogenic and cytotoxic brain edema in its early stage [11, 12]. This model of IBE is more similar to that of the sick children with IBE. The purpose of this study was to determine the effect of the IBE in the rat model using the method of [³H] MK-801 binding assay.

Materials and Methods

Male Sprague-Dawley rats weighing 200–280 g were divided into three groups: 1) Group control (NS, n = 11); 2) Group IBE (PB, n = 12); 3) MK-801 pretreatment group (MK-801, n=4). Rats were anesthetized with 25% urethane (125 mg/100 g body weight) intraperitoneal. The left common carotid artery, external carotid artery and its branch (superior thyroid artery and occipital artery), internal carotid artery and pterygopalatine artery were exposed. The pterygopalatine artery and the branch of external carotid artery were ligated, the external carotid artery was temporarily closed by a clip. Pertussis bacilli (contained bacilli in 10.8×10^9/ml, Beijing Institute for Biologic Products) 0.02 ml/100 g body weight was injected into left internal carotid artery by 1 ml syringe with needle size 4 via left common carotid over 30 s'. Normal saline 0.02 ml/100 g body weight was injected in the normal saline group (NS). Then the clip was removed from the external carotid artery, 2% Evans blue (3 ml/kg) was injected intravenously. MK-801 (Research Biochemical International, Natick MA01760-2447, USA) 0.5 mg/kg per day was injected by intraperitoneal route two days before injection of PB, in this group. Rats were killed by decapitation at 24 hrs after injection PB. The left hemisphere was rapidly removed and placed in a glass homogenizer with 9 times (w/v) Tris-acetate acid buffer (TAB, 0.05 M, pH 7.4) and homogenized in the ice water for 3 minutes. The homogenate was centrifuged for 10 min at $1000 \times g$, the supernatant was centrifuged at $43,000 \times g$ for 20 min. Abandoning the supernatant, the pellet was suspended in 1 ml ice-cold TAB. The protein concentration was measured with HITACHI 7170 full automatic biochemical analyzer and the protein concentration was regulated to final concentration of 1 mg/ml by ice-cold TAB. NMDA receptor binding assays were performed in 150 µl of this crude membrane suspension (0.15 mg protein), 100 µl MK-801 (final concentration 0.3 mM, non-specific binding) or 100 µl buffer alone (total binding); 10 µl [³H] MK-801 (final concentration 1, 2, 4, 8, 16, and 32 nM) and 50 µl TAB at 37°C for 30 min. The incubation was terminated by adding 10 ml ice-cold TAB and then rapidly filtrated through a glassfiber filter, followed by two 10 ml washes with cold TAB within 10 seconds. The radioactivity on the filters was determined by liquid scintillation counting in plastic vials with a 5 ml scintillation solution.

Results

[³H] MK-801 labeled a site of neuronal membranes in rat cerebral cortex with high affinity. The specific binding curves of groups NS, PB, and [³H] MK-801 are seen in Fig. 1. Scatchard plots of the specific binding curves of groups NS and PB are showed in Fig. 2. The site density (B_{max}) values were 0.623 ± 0.082 and 0.606 ± 0.087 pmol/mg protein in groups NS and PB respectively, there was no difference between the two groups ($p > 0.05$). The dissociation constant (K_d) values were 43.1 ± 4.2 nM and 30.5 ± 3.0 nM in the groups NS and PB respectively. The affinity was significantly higher in group PB than group NS ($p < 0.05$). The specific

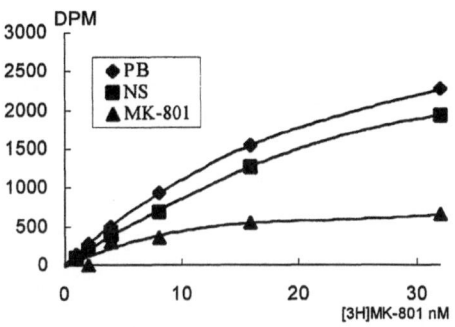

Fig. 1. Specific binding curves. The radioactivity of the filters appeared a saturated characteristic with increasing ³H-MK-801. ◆ PB: Pertussis bacilli group; ■ NS: normal saline control group; ▲ MK-801 pretreatment group

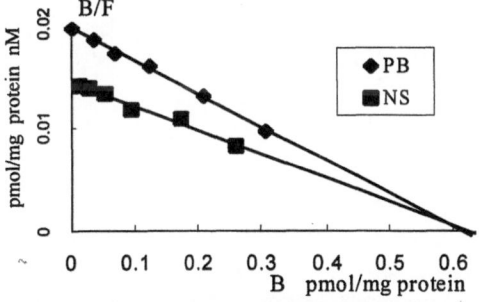

Fig. 2. Scatchard plots of specific binding curves of PB and NS control groups. The site density (B_{max}) values were 0.623 ± 0.082 and 0.606 ± 0.087 pmol/mg protein in groups NS and PB respectively. The dissociation constant (K_d) values were 43.1 ± 4.2 nM and 30.5 ± 3.0 nM in the groups NS and PB respectively. ◆ PB: Pertussis bacilli group; ■ NS: normal saline control group

binding was significantly lower in group MK-801 than in groups NS and PB ($p < 0.05$).

Discussion

NMDA receptor-ion channel complex located neuronal membrane is a receptor of EAA and as a channel of calcium ion [8]. Under neuropathological conditions, the EAA in brain tissue is significantly increased, NMDA receptor is excessively excited, overload of calcium ion enter neurons through NMDA gate channels. Elevation of intracellular calcium could activate lipase and protease and damage mitochondria (Faber 1981). On the other hand, depolarization of neuron induced by calcium also draws chloride into the neuron, and the electrochemical gradient is lowered. The increase in the chloride and cation entry draws water into cells and leads to cation swelling of the neuron. The quantity and activity of NMDA receptor may be important factors in brain edema. In this study, with brain edema the B_{max} of NMDA-channel complex was unchanged. The result showed that the mechanism of IBE was not affected by the expression of NMDA receptor genes. The Kd values were 43.1 ± 4.2 nM and 30.5 ± 3.0 nM in the groups NS and PB respectively, indicating that the affinity was significantly higher in the group PB than group NS. Thus the brain edema induced by PB was relative to the excitation of NMDA receptor. This is a mechanism similar to that of ischemic and traumatic edema. MK-801 is a non-competitive antagonist of NMDA receptor, its binding sites are located in the channels themselves. When MK-801 bound with its binding site, the calcium ion channels are blocked and the influx of calcium is inhibited [6]. In this study, pretreatment with MK-801 i.p. decreased [³H] MK-801 binding with NMDA receptor (Fig. 1). The result suggested that MK-801 attenuated the effect on PB-induced increase in affinity of NMDA receptor, and on IBE.

Acknowledgement

The project supported by the National Natural Science Foundation of China (Number 3940233).

References

1. Baethmann A, Maier-Hauff K, Schurer L, Lange M, Guggenbichler C, Vogt W (1989) Release of glutamate and of free fatty acids in vasogenic brain edema. J Neurosurg 70: 578–591
2. Benveniste J, Jorgensen MB, Diemer NH, Hansen AJ (1988) Calcium accumulation by glutamate receptor activation is involved in hippocampal cell damage after ischemia. Acta Neurol Scand 78: 529–536

3. Collins RC, Dobkin BH, Choi DW (1989) Selective vulnerability of brain: new insights into the pathophysiology of stroke. Ann Intern Med 110: 992–1000
4. George CP, Goldberg MP, Choi DW, Steinberg GK (1988) Dextromethorphan reduces neocortical ischemic neurons damage *in vivo*. Brain Res 440: 375–379
5. Gill R, Foster AC, Woodruff GN (1987) Systemic administration of MK-801 protects against ischemia induced hippocampal neurodegeneration in the gerbil. J Neurosci 7: 3343–3349
6. Lipton SA (1993) Prospects for clinically tolerated NMDA antagonists: open-channel blockers and alternative redox states of nitric oxide. TINS 16: 527–531
7. Liu D-C, Tang W-X, Zhang S-A, Yang Y-J (1989) Pyroantimonate method for localization of intracellular calcium ions. Bul Hunan Med Uni 14: 300–308
8. Mac Dermott AB, Mayer ML, Westbrook GL, Smith SJ, Barker JL (1986) NMDA-receptor activation increases cytoplasmic calcium concentration in cultured spinal cord neurons. Nature 321: 519–522
9. Wahlestedt C, Golanow E, Yamamoto S, Yee F, Ericson H, Yoo H, Inturrisi CE, Reis DJ (1993) Antisense oligodeoxynucleotides to NMDA-R1 receptor channel protect cortical neurons from excitotoxicity and reduce focal ischemic infarctions. Nature 363: 260–263
10. Xiu R-X, Yi S-Y, Wu S-L,Wang P-Y (1992) The changes of neurons Ca^{2+} channel and its influence on permeability of blood brain barrier and injury brain edema in rats. Chin J Neurosurg 8: 41–44
11. Xu Z-G, Yu P-L, Li Y-Y, Zong Q-S, Sheng A-X (1987) Brain edema model induced by pertussis bacilli. Bul Hunan Med Uni 12: 47–50
12. Yu P-L, Zhou P-F, Yang Y-J, Peng L-X, Feng B-C (1985) Edema model induced with typhoid endotoxin in rabbits. In: Inaba Y (eds) Brain edema. Springer, Berlin Heidelberg New York Tokyo, pp 113–116
13. Zhang T-X, Zhao W-G (1990) Experiment study of acute ischemic brain edema-neurotoxic role of excitatory aminoacids. Chin J Neurosurg 6: 14–17

Correspondence: Yu-Jia Yang, M.D., National Laboratory of Medical Genetics, Hunan Medical University, Changsha, Hunan 410008, Peoples Republic of China.

Acta Neurochir (1997) [Suppl] 70: 285–287
© Springer-Verlag 1997

The Rapid Flow of Cerebrospinal Fluid from Ventricles to Cisterns via Subarachnoid Velae in the Normal Rat

J. D. Fenstermacher[1, 2], **J.-F. Ghersi-Egea**[1], **W. Finnegan**[1], and **J.-L. Chen**[1]

[1] Department of Neurological Surgery, State University of New York, Stony Brook, NY, and [2] Department of Anesthesiology, Henry Ford Hospital, Detroit, MI, U.S.A.

Summary

[14]C-sucrose in 0.5 μl of buffered saline was infused over 30 sec into one lateral ventricle, and its subsequent distribution was determined in brain, meninges, cerebral blood vessels, and cerebrospinal fluid (CSF) by quantitative autoradiography. Within 3.5 min, infused radiotracer had moved into the third ventricle, the velum interpositum (an extension of the subarachnoid system that contains many blood vessels), the aqueduct, the mesencephalic and fourth ventricles, and the superior medullary velum (a part of the subarachnoid system that touches the mesencephalic and fourth ventricles). The CSF within both of these velae appears to empty into the quadrigeminal and ambient cisterns. Within 5 min radioactive sucrose was also found in the interpeduncular cistern. About 15% of the injected sucrose quickly left the ventricles and entered these large cisterns. In contrast to most CSF-brain interfaces, little sucrose moved from CSF into the medulla next to the lateral recesses and tissues such as the superior colliculus that lie adjacent to the large CSF cisterns. A thick, multilayered glia limitans visible on electron micrographs seemed to form a CSF-brain barrier at these interfaces. Some of the infused ^{14}C-sucrose persisted in the perivascular spaces and walls of arteries and arterioles for more than 3.5 hr. These findings suggest that CSF may function to deliver various agents and factors to pial and parenchymal arteries and arterioles.

Keywords: Cerebrospinal fluid; rapid subarachnoid flow; radioactive tracer study; animal model.

Introduction

A number of studies have shown that the choroid plexuses synthesize transport proteins such as transthyretin and secretes them into the CSF [4, 5]. In addition, protease inhibitors, e.g., cystatin C, and growth factors, e.g., insulin-like growth factors I and II, are apparently produced by the choroid plexus at various stages in development and into adulthood [1, 6]. If such regulatory materials are secreted with choroidal fluid, as seems to be the case, then they may be delivered to brain, cerebral blood vessels and meninges by way of the CSF. The present study was designed to examine the potential "delivery function" of the CSF system. Most of these findings have recently been published [2, 3].

Experimental Procedures

For these experiments, 0.5 μl of artificial CSF containing radiolabeled sucrose (a commonly used, metabolically inert extracellular space marker) was infused into one lateral ventricle of anesthetized adult rats over 30 sec and allowed to circulate from 3.5 min to 3.5 hr. Following decapitation, the severed heads were rapidly frozen and the brain with meninges, blood vessels, and CSF in place and still frozen was removed. This frozen specimen was then sectioned in a cryostat; subsequently tissue and CSF radioactivity were measured by quantitative autoradiography. Tissue samples for electron microscopy were prepared and viewed in the usual manner. The methods are given in more detail by Ghersi-Egea *et al.* [2, 3].

Results

Within 3.5 min of intraventricular injection, ^{14}C-sucrose was found in the third ventricle, the aqueduct, the mesencephalic ventricle, and the fourth ventricle. By 7.5 min, radioactivity was evident in the tissue around the injected (ipsilateral) lateral ventricle, ipsilateral Foramen of Monro, the dorsal and ventral parts of the third ventricle, and the lateral and third ventricle choroid plexuses. At this time some radioactivity had even reached the optic recess, which is an extension of the third ventricle immediately above the optic chiasma.

Starting beside the subfornical organ and projecting caudally alongside it and below the roof of the third ventricle are the two pouches of the velum interpositum (VI), an elongate, inward extension of the subarachnoid space. Before reaching the pineal recess and the posterior commisure, the two pouches fuse to form the body of the VI, which runs beneath the pineal recess. The ipsilateral pouch and body of the velum interpositum were lightly labeled by 3.5 minutes and heavily marked at 7.5 min. At the latter time, the contralateral pouch was also labeled. Because sucrose can be seen throughout the VI within minutes and the VI is 5–6 mm long, it must have been carried convectively by bulk flowing fluid, presumably CSF, and not by simple diffusion.

The body of the velum interpositum apparently opens into and terminates at the quadrigeminal and ambient cisterns. These two cisterns, which are continuous, partially wrap around the superior and inferior colliculi and the pineal gland and extend to the cerebellum, where they join the superior medullary velum. Radioactivity appeared in these two cisterns and the superior medullary velum within 5 minutes. The interpeduncular cistern is located at the base of the brain, surrounds the pituitary gland, mammillary body, and circle of Willis, and joins the ambient cistern along the side of the midbrain. Radiolabel appeared in the interpeduncular cistern after 5 min, and the amount there continued to increase up to 20 min. From this time up to and beyond 3.5 hr, the arteries and arterioles in these cisterns retained considerable ^{14}C-sucrose. The relatively rapid appearance of the radioactivity in different regions of these cisterns was consistent with a convective (bulk flow) delivery of sucrose.

In the rat the anterior or superior medullary velum (SMV) is an extension of the subarachnoid space that lies between the inferior colliculus and the cerebellum; this membranous pouch separates the mesencephalic ventricle (also known as the recess of the inferior colliculus) and the rostral part of the fourth ventricle from the anterior aspects of the cerebellum. At its distal end, the superior medullary velum opens into the caudal part of the quadrigeminal cistern. The front of radiolabelled material reached the mesencephalic ventricle and the rostral part of the fourth ventricle within 3.5 min and the proximal SMV within 5.0 min. By 7.5 min post-injection, the radioactivity had spread into the infoldings of the SMV along the surface of the cerebellum, probably by bulk fluid flow through the intravelar subarachnoid space.

At the level of the fourth ventricle, ^{14}C-sucrose was seen in the subependymal and underlying medullary tissue at 7.5 min. By 30 min most of the radioactivity had left the fourth ventricle. In contrast, a fairly large amount of ^{14}C-activity was evident in parts of the lateral recesses and a very sharp, very dark rim of it demarcated the border between the lateral recess and the lateral surfaces of the medulla. Ultrastructural observations showed there was a complex glia limitans on the outer edge of the medulla similar to that described above for the colliculi and cerebral peduncles.

No radioactivity was detected in the cortical subarachnoid space during the first 20 min. Some radiolabel was observed thereafter in the area of the rhinal fissure, probably reaching here via the extensions of the ambient cistern. The lack of ^{14}C-sucrose in the cortices may be reflective of CSF loss via basal structures such as the cranial nerves.

In some experiments a 5–10 μl sample of CSF was "cut" from the cisterna magna of the frozen brain-meninges-blood-vessel specimen before sectioning it for autoradiography; the amount of radioactivity in the lateral recesses, other cisterns, and the two velae could be directly read from the autoradiograms. The time-courses of ^{14}C-sucrose were then quantitatively determined for these CSF compartments. Radiolabel was present in the lateral recesses and cisterna magna at 3.5 min after lateral ventricle injection. The radioactivity gradually rose thereafter to reach a maximal value of 20% of the amount injected after 15–20 minutes but decreased continuously from then on as radiotracer began to wash out of the ventricles and periventricular tissue. Incidently, the lateral recesses are much larger structures than the cisterna magna in the rat, and most of the radioactivity within these two CSF compartments is in the lateral recesses.

As for the remaining subarachnoid compartments, the percentage of radioactivity in both the interpeduncular cistern and the velum interpositum increased slowly from 3.5 to 15 min and remained around 2% as long as 3.5 hr after injection. The radioactivity in the quadrigeminal and ambient cisterns and the superior medulary velum (SMV) also was appreciable at 3.5 min, with the highest concentration being in the SMV. The percentage of radioactivity in this set of structures quickly rose through the next 30 min, mainly as a result of increases within the two midbrain cisterns. The total percentage of radioactivity present in the interpeduncular, ambient, and quadrigeminal cisterns and the two velae was 10% of the injected amount at 10 min, 15% at 15 min, and 25% at 30 min. All of the radioactive sucrose in the two velae and the three cisterns at 15 min appeared to have come via the velum interpositum and superior medullary velum rather than by the lateral recesses and fourth ventricular foraminae that comprise the well-known route of CSF exit from ventricles to subarachnoid space.

At 30 min after administration, approximately 75% of the radioactivity was still in the CSF system and brain, and 25% was in the three cisterns and the two velae. About one-half of the latter percentage of radioactivity apparently came into the subarachnoid space via the lateral recesses and foraminae of Magendie and Luschka, which our analysis indicates is the major pathway of CSF flow into the subarachnoid space.

Discussion

Several technical procedures have enabled us to generate these observations. First, the severed head was immediately frozen at –50°C after decapitation; this action instantly freezes the cut stump of the head and neck and effectively traps blood in the cerebral microvessels and CSF within the ventricular and subarachnoid systems. Second, the tissue was maintained in a frozen state up to the moment of heat drying and fixing the sections; this was done by picking up the frozen tissue sections on chilled (–18°C) coverslips prior to drying. Third, CSF radioactivity was assessed by quantitative autoradiography (QAR), which has the potential to localize accurately radioactivity in brain and CSF at the 50 μm level. To make the QAR technique quantitative for these studies, injectate radioactivities were selected that yield tissue and CSF ^{14}C-concentrations at the times of sampling in the linear range of the optical density vs. radioactivity curve.

The movement of sucrose from the cisterns into the superior and inferior colliculi, cerebral peduncles, and other pericisternal structures appears to be greatly restricted, despite a relatively large amount of radioactivity in the adjacent cisternal CSF. This lack of cisternal CSF-to-tissue penetration contrasted with the diffuse spread of radioactivity into the midbrain around the aqueduct. Electron micrographs indicated that the subarachnoid surface of the superior colliculus contained a 6–8 μm thick, convoluted subpial "membrane," the glia limitans. The latter consisted of 7 to 15 layers of interleaved processes of protoplasmic astrocytes that separated the underlying parenchyma from the subpial space, pie mater, pial vasculature, and subarachnoidal CSF. In contrast, the glia limitans was simple and only 1–2 layers thick on the surface of the cortex. A multilayered glia limitans may, thus, be responsible for the apparently restricted entry of ^{14}C-sucrose from these cisterns into adjacent brain.

^{14}C-sucrose was expected to pass readily into the perivascular spaces of pial blood vessels but not to mark more strongly pial arteries than pial veins nor to remain in the perivascular spaces and/or walls of these vessels for 3.5 or more hours. The velum interpositum and superior medullary velum, VI and SMV, respectively, and the quadrigeminal, ambient, and intrapeduncular cisterns are filled with arachnoid membranes, arteries, arterioles, and veins. In less than 7.5 min, the arteries, arterioles, veins, and arachnoid trabeculae within the VI and SMV were radiolabeled; at 20 min, most of the dark figures on the autoradiograms were associated with pial arteries and arterioles within these velae and cisterns. Virtually all subarachnoidal radioactivity after 2 hr was in and around pial arteries and arterioles.

The rapid labeling of pial arteries and arterioles via CSF flow through the VI and SMV suggests a not previously described function for the CSF system. To be specific, various biological factors, regulators, and pathogens in third and fourth ventricular CSF could be rather quickly transmitted into the VI and SMV and various cisterns, and in turn be distributed to and affect pial blood vessels.

References

1. Bondy C, Werner H, Roberts Jr CT, LeRoith D (1992) Cellular pattern of type-I insulin-like growth factor receptor gene expression during maturation of the rat brain: comparison with insulin-like growth factors I and II. Neuroscience 46: 909–923
2. Ghersi-Egea J-F, Finnegan W, Chen J-L, Fenstermacher J: Rapid distribution of intraventricularly administered sucrose into cerebrospinal fluid cisterns via subarachnoid velae in rat. Neuroscience: in press
3. Ghersi-Egea J-F, Gorevic P, Ghiso J, Frangione B, Patlak C and Fenstermacher J (1996b) Fate of cerebrospinal fluid-borne amyloid β-peptide: rapid clearance into blood and appreciable accumulation by cerebral arteries. J Neurochem 67: 880–883
4. Schreiber G, Aldred AR, Jaworowski A, Nilson C, Achen MG, Segal MB (1990) Thyroxine transport from blood to brain via transthyretin synthesis in choroid plexus. Am J Physiol 258: R338–R345
5. Tu G-F, Cole T, Southwell BR, Schreiber G (1990) Expression of genes for transthyretin, cystatin C and A4 amyloid precursor protein in sheep choroid plexus during development. Develop Brain Res 55: 203–208
6. Tu G-F, Aldred AR, Southwell BR, Schreiber G (1992) Strong conservation of the expression of cystatin C gene in choroid plexus. Am J Physiol 263: R195–R200

Correspondence: J. D. Fenstermacher, Department of Anesthesiology, Henry Ford Hospital, 2799 West Grand Boulevard, Detroit, MI 48202, U.S.A.

Acta Neurochir (1997) [Suppl] 70: 288–290
© Springer-Verlag 1997

Quantitative Analysis of Brain Edema Resolution into the Cerebral Ventricles and Subarachnoid Space

E. Wrba[1], V. Nehring[1], R. C. C. Chang[2], A. Baethmann[2], H.-J. Reulen[1], and E. Uhl[1]

[1] Department of Neurosurgery and [2] Institute for Surgical Research, Grosshadern University Hospital, University of Munich, Federal Republic of Germany

Summary

Resolution of vasogenic brain edema was examined using a model of infusion of fluid into the brain of rabbits. For this purpose infusion of Texas Red-albumin (MW 67.000 D) and sodium fluorescein (MW 376 D) dissolved in artificial cerebrospinal fluid (mock CSF) was made into the white matter of the left frontal lobe of the brain. In order to quantify the portion of edema fluid which was cleared by the ventricular system, a ventriculo-cisternal perfusion was performed with mock CSF. A closed cranial window was implanted above the left parietal brain for superfusion of the cerebral cortex with mock CSF, in order to study resolution of the artificial edema fluid via the subarachnoid space. CSF-samples were collected in 30 minutes-intervals and analysed with a spectrophotometer. The clearance of edema fluid was examined under low (2–5 mmHg) and medium (9–12 mmHg) intracranial pressure (ICP). In the low-pressure group both edema fluid markers were found in the ventriculo-cisternal and subarachnoid perfusate at 60 min and 90 min, respectively, after start of infusion. In the group with moderately increased ICP the markers appeared at 90 min and 120 min, respectively. The amount of clearance of fluorescent dye via the subarachnoid space was the same in both groups and independent of the intracranial pressure.

Keywords: Vasogenic brain edema; infusion edema model; resolution of edema fluid.

Introduction

Resolution of vasogenic brain edema occurs mainly via bulk flow along a pressure gradient from the site of fluid entry [5]. Previous studies have shown that part of the edema fluid is reabsorbed into the cerebral ventricles or taken up by the vascular system [3, 6–8]. Very little is known, however, whether and to what extent clearance of edema fluid into the subarachnoid space is involved, and how the actual intracranial pressure (ICP) level influences reabsorption of the edema fluid into these compartments. The purpose of the present study was a quantitative analysis of clearance of the edema fluid into the ventricles and the subarachnoid space under different ICP-levels, utilising fluorescence indicators of different molecular size for labelling of the edema fluid.

Materials and Methods

New Zealand white rabbits (n = 19) were used as experimental animals. Anesthesia was induced with thiopental, and continued with alpha-chloralose (50 mg/kg). After tracheostomy the animals were ventilated under airway-pressure control. The body temperature was regulated by a heating pad. The arterial blood pressure was continuously recorded, blood gases every hour. For surgical preparation the animals were placed in a stereotactic holder. The skin overlying the skull was surgically opened in the midline. For administration of the mock edema fluid an infusion cannula was inserted into the white matter of the left frontal lobe. A second cannula was implanted into the right lateral ventricle serving as inflow line for the ventriculo-cisternal perfusion (3 ml/h). An outflow cannula was implanted into the cisterna magna after opening of the atlanto-occipital membrane. By adjustment of the height of the cisternal outflow tube, the intracranial pressure could be modified. For superfusion of the subarachnoid space a closed cranial window was implanted over the left parietal cortex as previously described in detail [2], and the brain cortex was permanently superfused with mock CSF (3 ml/h). Mock edema was induced by infusion of 1 mM sodium fluorescein (MW 376 D) and 0.9 mM Texas Red-albumin (MW 67,000) dissolved in artificial CSF. After termination of the surgical preparation, ventriculo-cisternal perfusion and superfusion of the subarachnoid space commenced at the same time. The cisternal outflow tube was adjusted to a given height depending on the ICP level which was desired (group 1: 2–5 mmHg; group 2: 9–12 mmHg). Infusion of the edema fluid into the white matter was started at time point 0 min at a rate of 100 μl/h, and was continued during 5 hours. CSF-samples were collected from the beginning of the edema infusion in 30 minutes intervals for 8 hours. Clearance of the edema fluid into the perfusate was measured by fluorescence spectrophotometry using two different filter sets (sodium fluorescein: exc.: 485 nm, em.: 515 nm; Texas Red-albumin: exe.: 590 nm, em.: 650 nm).

Table 1. *Clearance of Fluorescence Markers of Edema Fluid at Different ICP-Levels*

| Time after start of infusion | Group 1 (ICP = 2–5 mmHg; n = 9) | | | | Group 2 (ICP = 9–12 mmHg; n = 10) | | | |
| | Ventricular system | | Subarachnoid space | | Ventricular system | | Subarachnoid space | |
	NaFl	TeRe	NaFl	TeRe	NaFl	TeRe	NaFl	TeRe
60 min	3.0 ± 1.7	3.9 ± 1.7	0.5 ± 0.3	0.6 ± 0.4	0.5 ± 0.4	1.1 ± 0.7	0.0 ± 0.0	0.0 ± 0.0
120 min	7.6 ± 2.3	12.9 ± 3.7	2.1 ± 1.1	2.1 ± 0.9	2.6 ± 1.6	4.4 ± 2.1	1.2 ± 1.0	1.6 ± 1.4
180 min	9.3 ± 2.9	16.5 ± 4.6	2.2 ± 1.1	2.5 ± 1.1	4.3 ± 2.4	7.3 ± 3.2	1.9 ± 1.3	2.6 ± 1.8
240 min	9.3 ± 2.7	17.5 ± 4.4	2.6 ± 1.3	2.9 ± 1.3	5.7 ± 2.7	10.0 ± 3.6	2.6 ± 1.5	3.3 ± 1.8
300 min	9.3 ± 2.6	17.8 ± 4.1	2.7 ± 1.2	3.2 ± 1.2	7.0 ± 3.1	12.3 ± 4.1	2.5 ± 1.5	3.3 ± 1.8
360 min	10.5 ± 2.9	21.5 ± 4.5	3.0 ± 1.3	3.7 ± 1.3	8.6 ± 3.7	15.0 ± 4.9	2.6 ± 1.5	3.4 ± 1.8
420 min	10.9 ± 3.0	23.1 ± 4.8	3.3 ± 1.4	4.0 ± 1.4	9.2 ± 3.9	16.4 ± 5.3	2.6 ± 1.5	3.5 ± 1.8
480 min	11.1 ± 3.1	23.8 ± 5.0	3.5 ± 1.5	4.2 ± 1.5	9.5 ± 4.1	17.2 ± 5.6	2.6 ± 1.5	3.5 ± 1.8

The proportion of both fluorescent dyes reabsorbed via the ventricular system or the subarachnoid space, respectively, is given in % of the total amount of label infused up to the time of sampling (mean ± SEM). Enhanced figures are statistically significant ($p < 0.05$). *NaFl* Sodium fluorescein; *TeRe* Texas Red-albumin.

Results

ICP in the low-pressure group had a range of 1 to 3.8 mmHg (mean 1.7 ± 1.1), while from 8.4 to 13.4 mmHg (mean 10.8 ± 1.5) in the medium-pressure group, respectively. Both fluorescence labels started to appear in the cerebral ventricles at 60 min following onset of edema infusion in group 1 (low ICP), whereas at 90 min in group 2 (medium ICP), respectively. In the two groups a different clearance kinetic of both fluorescent dyes, with low or high molecular weight, could be found, demonstrating a more rapid increase of the ventricular marker concentration in group 1. The difference was found to be significant when studying Texas Red-albumin at 60 and 90 min ($p < 0.05$). Accordingly, Texas Red-albumin was reabsorbed via the ventricular system at a higher amount than sodium fluorescein. On the other hand, in the subarachnoid space no differences between the low- and the high molecular weight marker were observed. Both fluorescent dyes appeared at 90 min for the first time. The total amount of marker clearance and the time of their appearance in the subarachnoid space was independent from the intracranial pressure. In contrast, reabsorption of edema fluid via the ventricular system was found to depend on the intracranial pressure. The results are given in Table 1.

Discussion

The present findings demonstrate and confirm that vasogenic edema fluid is cleared via both the ventricles and the subarachnoid space. Edema reabsorption is mainly attributable to bulk flow of the fluid along a pressure gradient from the site of edema entry towards the ventricles [5], which also was found in this study. On the other hand, reabsorption of edema fluid into the subarachnoid space appeared to be independent of the intracranial pressure. Further, the proportion of clearance of the edema fluid into the subarachnoid space was definitely smaller as compared to the ventricular reabsorption. There was no differential clearance behavior of the low- and the high-molcular weight edema marker as concluded from the similar clearance kinetics of both labels. Obviously, the clearance does not depend on diffusion mechanisms, which is at variance with respective conclusions of Ohata *et al.* [4] using FITC-dextran of different molecular size as edema label.

In conclusion, the present findings show that edema fluid is reabsorbed both via the ventricular system and the subarachnoid space, although the latter route appears to be less significant. Moreover, while clearance into the ventricles is modified by the intracranial pressure, reabsorption via the subarachnoid space was found to be pressure independent.

Acknowledgements

This work was supported by the "BMBF-Verbund 'Neurotrauma' Munich", FKZ: 01 K0 94026.

References

1. Bauknight GC, Faraci FM, Heistad DD (1992) Endothelium-derived relaxing factor modulates noradrenergic constriction of cerebral arterioles in rabbits. Stroke 23: 1522–1526

2. Kawamura S, Schuerer L, Goetz A, Kempski O, Schmucker B, Baethmann A (1990) An improved closed cranial window technique for investigation of blood-brain barrier function and cerebral vasomotor control in the rat. Int J Microcirc: Clin Exp 9: 369–383

3. Marmarou A, Hochwald G, Nakamura T, Tanaka K, Weaver J, Dunbar J (1994) Brain edema resolution by CSF pathways and brain vasculature in cats. Am J Physiol 267: H514–H520

4. Ohata K, Marmarou A (1992) Clearance of brain edema and macromolecules through the cortical extracellular space. J Neurosurg 77: 387–396

5. Reulen HJ, Graham R, Spatz M, Klatzo I (1977) Role of pressure gradients and bulk flow in dynamics of vasogenic brain edema. J Neurosurg 46: 24–35

6. Reulen HJ, Tsuyumu M, Tack A, Fenske AR, Prioleau GR (1978) Clearance of edema fluid into cerebrospinal fluid. J Neurosurg 48: 754–764

7. Tsuyumu M, Reulen HJ, Prioleau GR (1981) Dynamics of formation and resolution of vasogenic brain edema I. Measurement of edema clearance into ventricular CSF. Acta Neurochir (Wien) 57: 1–13

8. Vorbrodt AW, Lossinsky AS, Wisniewski HM, Suzuki R, Yamaguchi T, Masaoka H, Klatzo I (1985) Ultrastructural observations on the transvascular route of protein removal in vasogenic brain edema. Acta Neuropathol 66: 265–273

Correspondence: Eberhard Uhl, M.D., Department of Neurosurgery, Grosshadern University Hospital, University of Munich, Marchioninistrasse 15, D-81366 Munich, Federal Republic of Germany.

Acta Neurochir (1997) [Suppl] 70: 291–292
© Springer-Verlag 1997

Responses of Cerebral Blood Flow Regulation to Activation of the Primary Somatosensory Cortex During Electrical Stimulation of the Forearm

K. Ichimi, H. Kuchiwaki, S. Inao, M. Shibayama, and **J. Yoshida**

Department of Neurosurgery, Nagoya University School of Medicine, Nagoya, Japan

Summary

We assessed the cerebral blood flow (CBF) response to electrical stimulation of the contralateral forearm over the primary somatosensory cortex (S-I) in anesthetized cats. CBF was monitored continuously using laser-Doppler flowmetry (LDF). In the first set of experiments, the effects of varying stimulus frequency and intensity were examined. During stimulation, CBF in S-I was increased significantly. At high stimulus intensity, response reached a near-plateau level. In the second set of experiments, the CBF response after introduction of an intracerebral mass was investigated using a mechanical microballoon model to simulate an intracerebral hematoma. A microballoon was inserted into the ventral posterolateral nucleus of the thalamus (VPL). Following gradual balloon inflation, there was a rapid reduction in CBF response. We conclude that CBF regulation to neuronal activation is affected by stimulation parameters, and is impaired by an intracerebral mass obstructing the afferent sensory pathway.

Keywords: Cerebral blood flow; activation; somatosensory stimulation; electrical stimulation.

Introduction

It is widely accepted that cerebral blood flow (CBF) is tightly coupled to brain function, although its regulation is still unclear. In this study, we investigated the CBF response in the primary somatosensory cortex (S-I) during stimulation of the forearm in cats utilizing laser-Doppler flowmetry (LDF). We also evaluated whether an experimental intracerebral mass altered the CBF response to somatosensory activation using a microballoon model to simulate an intracerebral hematoma.

Materials and Methods

Twelve adult cats of both sexes were used in the study. Anesthesia was induced with ketamine hydrochloride, then maintained with α-chloralose and urethane. The animals were tracheotomized, immobilized with pancuronium bromide, and mechanically ventilated with room air. The femoral artery and vein were cannulated for monitoring blood pressure (BP), blood gas sampling, and drug administration. The animals were secured in a stereotactic frame. After unilateral frontoparietal craniectomy, the dura mater was removed from S-I.

CBF was monitored continuously using LDF. A needle probe mounted on a stereotaxic manipulator was placed perpendicularly on the forearm area of S-I according to known somatotopic maps [1]. S-I was activated by electrical stimulation of the contralateral forearm with two needle electrodes introduced into the subcutaneous tissue. The corresponding receptive fields in the forearm were localized while maximizing the recorded CBF response by slightly changing the position of the electrodes. The animals were divided into two groups.

Study I (n = 6): The effects of varying stimulus intensity and frequency were examined to assess the optimal stimulation parameters.

Study II (n = 6): The effects of an intracerebral mass were investigated. A microballoon mounted on a micromanipulator was inserted stereotaxically into the ventral posterolateral nucleus of the thalamus (VPL). The balloon was inflated step by step with normal saline.

Results

The physiological variables for all animals were within normal range and were maintained stable throughout each experiment.

Electrical stimulation of the forearm induced a significant increase of CBF in the contralateral corresponding area of S-I. The CBF response was strictly confined to the forearm area of S-I.

Study I: When stimulus intensity was increased, there was a rapid increase in CBF response. At higher intensities the response exhibited a near-plateau trend. In contrast, BP was decreased as the intensity became higher. However, at higher intensities, BP was increased in some animals. When frequency was increased, there was a graded increase in CBF response. Further elevation of frequency exhibited a downward trend. Frequency changes had no apparent effect on BP response.

Study II: When the balloon was inflated gradually, there was a rapid reduction in CBF response to stimulation.

Discussion

Our results indicate that CBF over the S-I cortex is regulated by the degree of somatosensory stimulation.

When we increased stimulus intensity, there was a rapid increase in CBF response. At higher intensities the response reached its near-plateau level. BP was decreased with increased intensity. However, at higher intensities, BP was increased in some animals. This fluctuation in BP may confound data interpretation.

The effect of stimulus frequency on the CBF response is similar to that of other investigators. Ngai *et al.* [4] showed that maximum dilation of pial arteriolar diameter to sciatic nerve stimulation in rats was obtained at a frequency of 5 Hz, but with significant attenuation when frequency was increased beyond 10 Hz. Leniger-Follert *et al.* [3], who analyzed CBF responses in cats utilizing the local hydrogen clearance method, stated that the maximum CBF increase was obtained at 2–3 Hz. These minor discrepancies may be explained by differences between protocols, including species, the recording techniques, the anesthetic agents used, and the degree of anesthesia.

In the second set of experiments, we evaluated the effect of an experimental intracerebral mass on CBF response during somatosensory activation, using a mechanical microballoon model to simulate an intracerebral hematoma. CBF response to stimulation rapidly decreased as the balloon was inflated.

The VPL is a key station in the lateral system of ascending pain pathways. As the balloon is inflated, this key station is gradually impaired by mechanical distortion and destruction of the tissue, which causes decline in CBF response over S-I. However, temporal progression of ischemia should also be considered. Increased local tissue edema and pressure due to mass effect may play important roles in the ischemic damage [2].

References

1. Felleman DJ, Wall JT, Cusick CG, Kaas JH (1983) The representation of the body surface in S-I of cats. J Neurosci 3: 1648–1669
2. Kingman TA, Mendelow AD, Graham DI, Teasdale GM (1987) Experimental intracerebral mass: time-related effects on local cerebral blood flow. J Neurosurg 67: 732–738
3. Leniger-Follert E, Hossmann K-A (1979) Simultaneous measurements of microflow and evoked potentials in the somatomotor cortex of the cat brain during specific sensory activation. Pflügers Arch 380: 85–89
4. Ngai AC, Ko KR, Morii S, Winn HR (1988) Effect of sciatic nerve stimulation on pial arterioles in rats. Am J Physiol 254: H133–H139

Correspondence: Kazuyoshi Ichimi, M.D., Department of Neurosurgery, Nagoya University School of Medicine, 65 Tsurumai-cho, Showa-ku, Nagoya 466, Japan.

Acta Neurochir (1997) [Suppl] 70: 293–295
© Springer-Verlag 1997

A New Model of Spinal Cord Edema

H. Naruse[1], **K. Tanaka**[2], **A. Kim**[2], and **A. Hakuba**[2]

[1] Department of Neurosurgery, Tane Hospital, and [2] Department of Neurosurgery, Osaka City University Medical School, Osaka, Japan

Summary

Edema of the spinal cord has not been well understood. Brain edema produced by Marmarou's infusion method is essentially similar to vasogenic edema. This infusion method for producing edema was applied to a cat spinal cord. After laminectomy, a 30-gauge needle was inserted into the intumescentia cervicalis. A total amount of 10 µl of 2% Evans' blue or autoserum were infused using an infusion pump at a rate of 5 µl/hr. Macroscopally, Evans' blue was observed in the vicinity of infused site at the same level of the needle insertion and was seen spreading mainly longitudinally in the lateral column for a certain distance. The extracellular space was markedly distended in the in fused white mater and filled with electron-dense materials which were thought to be proteins in the electron microscopic study. The fine structural features were similar to the findings which were seen in Marmarou's infusion type of brain edema. Using this model, it seems to be feasible to produce reproducible spinal cord edema at any location in order to investigate not only the morphological aspect but also physiological aspect of the edema.

Keywords: Spinal cord edema; infusion method; animal model.

Introduction

There have been a few reports of experimental spinal cord edema. In the previous studies, major attention was focused on changes of cellular architecture of the spinal cord, because edema was produced by cold injury or trauma [1, 2, 7]. We have previously reported that edema fluid widely spread along the extracellular- and the perivascular space toward the CSF space in the brain edema using Marmarou's method [4–6].

In order to develop an experimental spinal cord edema, Marmarou's infusion method for producing edema was applied to a cat spinal cord. Evans' blue and autoserum were used as tracers, and the structural features were studied.

Materials and Methods

Production of Spinal Cord Edema

Adult mongrel cats were anesthetized with intraperitoneal injection of pentobarbital sodium (30 mg/kg), intubated and mechanically ventilated using halothane in a mixture of nitrous oxide and oxygen (1:1). A 1 ml-syringe connected to a 30-gauge needle with a stiff polyethylene tubing was mounted on a variable speed infusion pump. After laminectomy at levels of C3-7, the needle was inserted slowly into the intumescentia cervicalis at the position of 1/6th of the spinal cord width from its lateral border. A total amount of 10 µl of 2% Evans' blue or autoserum were infused using an infusion pump at a rate of 5 µl/hr.

Morphological Study

In the group of infusion of Evans' blue, the animals were sacrificed with an intravenous injection of saturated KCl immediately after infusion. The spinal cord was removed and fixed by immersion in alcohol, followed by paraffin embedding for cutting slices of 5 µm thickness. The slices were inspected macroscopically and microscopically with fluorescent microscope. In the group of infusion of autoserum, after infusion was terminated, the animals were perfused by the transcardiac route with 0.9% saline for no longer than 2 min, followed with 4% paraformaldehyde in 0.1 M phosphate buffer solution at a pressure of 100 mmHg for about 10 min at room temperature. Finally, with a mixture containing 4% paraformaldehyde and 0.5% glutaraldehyde in 0.1 M phosphate buffer solution for about 10 min. The spinal cord was removed and immersed in the same fixative overnight. Some of these slices were stained with hematoxylin and eosin (H & E) after paraffin embedding. Small pieces of tissues were cut and postfixed in 1% osmium tetroxide in phosphate buffer for 2 hours and embedded in Epon after dehydration. Thin sections were prepared and examined with a transmission electron microscope (H-300, Hitachi).

Results

Infusion of Evans' Blue

Macroscopic observations. Evans' blue was observed widely in the vicinity of infused site at the same level of needle insertion and was seen spreading longitudinally in the lateral column for a certain distance

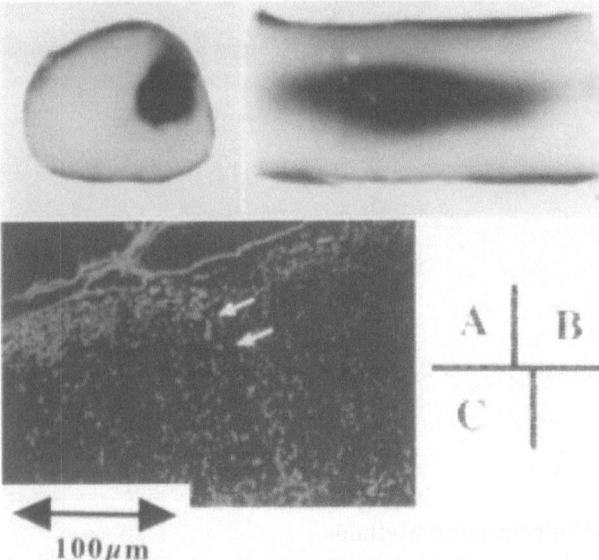

Fig. 1. (A) The coronal section of the lower cervical spinal cord: Evans' blue was observed widely in the vicinity of infused site at the same level of the needle insertion. However, there were no remarkable changes in the grey matter even in the infusion site. (B) The sagittal section of the cervical and upper thoracic spinal cord: Evans' blue was seen spreading longitudinally in the lateral column for a certain distance (ca. 20 mm). The extension of Evans' blue was obviously longer in longitudinal direction than in horizontal direction. The tracer was also observed over the surface of the spinal cord. (C) A photograph of fluorescent microscope of the infused white matter: Red staining which was observed along vessels led to the surface of the spinal cord (arrows)

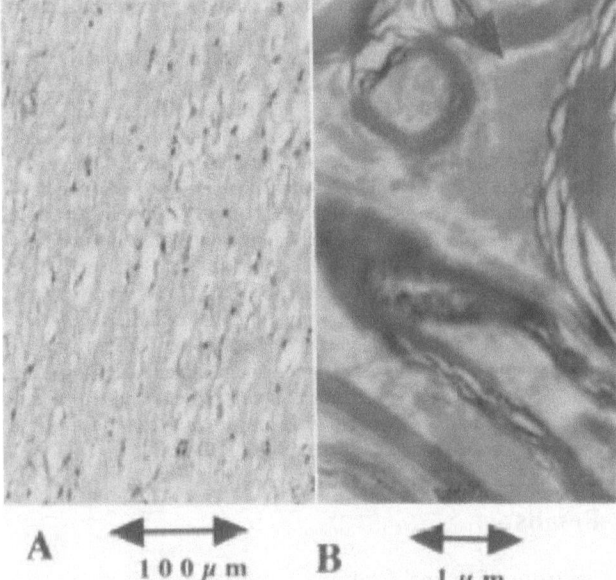

Fig. 2. (A) A photograph of the sagittal section of the infused white matter. The extracellular space was markedly distended in the infused white matter. (B) Appearance of the edematous white matter in the electron microscopic aspect: The extracellular space was markedly distended and filled with electron-dense materials (arrows). However, swelling of astrocytes was not observed

(ca. 20 mm) (Fig. 1A, B). The extension of Evans' blue was obviously longer in longitudinal direction than in horizontal direction. The tracer was also observed over the surface of the spinal cord.

Microscopic observations. Using fluorescent microscope, red staining indicative of presence of Evans' blue was observed in the infused white matter. The tracer was also observed in the subarachnoid space and was slightly noticed in the grey matter in the vicinity of the infused site. Red staining which was observed along vessels led to the surface of the spinal cord (Fig. 1C).

Infusion of Autoserum

Microscopic observations. Using hematoxylin and eosin, expansion of the extracellular space was seen in the infused site. However, there were no remarkable changes in the grey matter even in the infusion site (Fig. 2A).

Electron microscopic observations. The extracellular space was markedly distended and filled with electron-dense materials. However, swelling of astrocytes was not observed (Fig. 2B).

Discussion

We have previously reported structural and fine structural features of the brain edema produced by Marmarou's infusion method [5, 6]. In this type of edema, fine structural features such that marked expansion of the extracellularspace and the perivascular region which were filled with electron-dense materials, were essentially similar to the condition associated with vasogenic edema. There was no BBB breakdown even along the needle tract. Because of these characteristics, this type of edema is appropriate in research into the effect of edema per se.

The infusate was observed mainly in the infused lateral column and this did not reach the midline. The tracer was seen spreading longitudinally in the lateral column for a certain distance. The extension of Evans' blue was obviously longer in longitudinal direction than in horizontal direction. The tracer was also observed over the surface of the spinal cord. The extracellular space was markedly distended in the infused white mater. Electron-dens materials which were observed in the extracellular space in the electron microscopic study were thought to be proteins in autoserum.

The structural features of the infused areas of the spinal cord are similar to the findings which were seen in Marmarou's infusion type of brain edema [3, 5, 6]. The major route of the expansion of the edemafluid was seemed to be the extracellular space and spread mainly longitudinally. The area of edema might depend on an amount of infusate. Using this model, it is possible to change an amount of infusate and to produce edema at any areas in the spinal cord.

References

1. Balentine JD (1978) Pathology of experimental spinal cord trauma. I. The necrotic lesions as a function of vascular injury. Lab Invest 39: 236–253
2. Collins GH, West NR, Parmely JD, Samson FM, Ward DA (1986) The histopathology of freezing injury to the rat spinal cord. A light microscopic study. 1. Early degenerative change. J Neuropathol Exp Neurol 45: 721–741
3. Hirano A, Marmarou A, Nakamura T, Inoue A (1984) The fine structural study of brain response to intracerebral infusion of serum in the cat. In: Inaba Y, Klatzo I, Spatz M (eds) Brain edema. Springer, Berlin Heidelberg New York Tokyo, pp 32–39
4. Marmarou A, Tanaka K, Shulman K (1982) The brain response of infusion edema: dynamics of fluid resolution. In: Hartmann A, Brock M (eds) Treatment of cerebral edema. Springer, Berlin Heidelberg New York, pp 11–18
5. Naruse H, Tanaka K, Nishimura S, Fujimoto K (1990) A microstructural study of oedema resolution. In: Reulen H-J, Baethmann A (eds) Brain edema VIII. Acta Neurochir (Wien) [Suppl 51] 87–89
6. Tanaka K, Ohata K, Katsuyama J, Nishimura S, Marmarou A (1986) Effect of steroids on the resolution of edema. In: Miller JD, Teasdale GM, Rowan JO, et al (eds) Intracranial pressure VI. Springer, Berlin Heidelberg New York Tokyo, pp 611–614
7. Wang R, Ehara K, Tamaki N (1993) Spinal cord edema following freezing injury in the rat: relationship between tissue water-content and spinal cord blood flow. Surg Neurol 39: 348–354

Correspondence: K. Tanaka, M.D., Department of Neurosurgery, Osaka City University Medical School, 1-5-7, Asahi-machi, Abeno-ku, Osaka 545, Japan.

Acta Neurochir (1997) [Suppl] 70: 296–298
© Springer-Verlag 1997

Assessment of the CAMINO Intracranial Pressure Device in Clinical Practice

L. Schürer[1], **E. Münch**[2], **A. Piepgras**[1], **R. Weigel**[1], **L. Schilling**[1], and **P. Schmiedek**[1]

Departments of [1] Neurosurgery and [2] Anesthesiology, Klinikum Mannheim, University of Heidelberg, Federal Republic of Germany

Summary

The purpose of this study was to investigate reliability, handling characteristics and complication rate of the CAMINO-ICP-monitor-system in clinical routine. In a case controlled study 82 patients with intracranial pathology necessitating ICP-monitoring received either a ventricular or a parenchymal CAMINO-device. Clinical assessment of curve shape and apparent reliability of the measurement was documented. Probe postition and presence of hematoma was evaluated in all patients with a CT after probe insertion. Handling complications, i.e. dislocation were recorded. At the end of the measuring period the drift of the probe was checked ex vivo and a two point calibration was performed using a water column. During one year 82 patients received 95 probes (parench. 73, ventric. 22). The average measuring period was 91.3 ± 70.6 hrs. Catheter position was verified by CCT for 67 (70.5%) probes. 92.5% of the devices were placed correctly. Clinically 88.4% of the measurements were assessed plausible, in 8.2% the displayed ICP-values were judged to be too high, in 2.1% too low. Probe drift after explantation was −0.21 mmHg/24 hrs. The mean value of the recalibrated probes in the water column corresponding to 15.8 mmHg was 14.7 ± 1.9 mmHg. There was no correlation between neither drift nor funtion in the water column and the duration of the measurement. Technical complications exclusively related to the construction of the CAMINO-system like kinking of the cable, dislocation (probe pulled out) or dislocated fixation screw were too high (25.3%).

Keywords: Intracranial pressure; monitoring; CAMINO device; fiberoptic system.

Introduction

The fiberoptic intracranial pressure monitor (CAMINO) is extensively used in our interdisciplinary intensive care unit for monitoring patients with increased intracranial pressure (ICP). Experimental *ex vivo* and *in vivo* studies in animals and humans have shown that there is a close correlation between ventricular fluid pressure measured by the standard manometric method and brain tissue pressure using the fiberoptic device [1, 2, 4].

We adopted the CAMINO-intracranial pressure monitoring device in 1993. The nursing as well as the medical personal is now well familiar with the advantages and pitfalls of the system. The purpose of this study was to investigate reliability, handling characteristics and complication rate of the device in routine clinical practice 2 years after introduction of the CAMINO-system in our intensive care unit. Respective data in the literature is scarce [3, 5] and often difficult to assess due to small sample sizes.

Methods

During August 1995 and August 1996 in a case-controlled prospective investigation eighty-two patients with intracranial pathology necessitating intracranial pressure monitoring who were admitted to the interdisciplinary intensive care unit of Klinikum Mannheim were monitored. The patients were all equipped with a CAMINO-fiberoptic ICP-measuring device. The patients had sustained either a servere head injury or nontraumatic intracranial hemorrhage. Prehospital GCS ranged from 3 to 14 points. At least one CT scan was obtained in all patients. Thereafter, implantation of either a ventricular or parenchymal CAMINO-probe (as felt necessary) was performed via a precoronal burr hole in the operating theatre using standard techniques. Subjective assessment of curve shape, and apparent reliability of ICP (according to the clinical condition of the patient) was done by 2 neurosurgeons (L.S., R.W.) and one intensivist (E.M.) during the course of the measurement and documented in an open questionnaire. In all cases with a control CT after probe implantation, probe position and occurrence of hematoma related to probe insertion was documented. Handling complications, i.e. dislocation (probe pulled out), dislocation of the fixation screw and kinking of the fiberoptic cable was also recorded. In selected cases, where the reliability of the measurement was doubted, *in vivo* recalibration and reinsertion of probes was performed.

At the end of the measuring period the drift of the probe was checked *ex vivo* and a two-point calibration was performed with the help of a water column corresponding to 15.8 mmHg.

Results

During August 1995 and August 1996, 82 patients with intracranial pathology necessitating ICP-monitoring were equipped with 95 CAMINO-devices (parenchymal 73, ventricular 22). The mean age was 42 ± 20 (range 11–89), the prehospital GCS ranged between 3–14. The average measuring period was 91.3 ± 70.6 hrs (range 1–403 hrs). There was no statistical difference between the duration of the measuring period of parenchymal and ventricular devices. 13 patients received 2 devices (only parenchymal).

Probe Position in CT

Catheter position was verified by CT for 67 (70.5%) probes. Sixty- two (92.5%) devices were placed correctly (frontal lobe, white matter), 2 (3%) probes were located too close to the falx (< 1 cm). The tip of the catheter was not located in the brain parenchyma in three patients (4.5%). A summary of the clinical plausibility assessment of the fiberoptic devices is given in Table 1.

Recalibration

Nine parenchymal probes were recalibrated. Five of them were recalibrated because of "ICP estimated too high". The drift was +4, +2, +8, ±0, ±0 mmHg respec-

Table 1. *Clinical Assessment of Plausibility of Measurement*

	Type	n	%	Total %
ICP-values plausible	parenchymal	63	(86.3)	
	ventricular	21	(95.5)	88.4
ICP-values too high	parenchymal	6	(8.2)	
	ventricular	0	(0)	8.2
ICP-values too low	parenchymal	1	(1.4)	
	ventricular	1	(4.6)	2.1
ICP-values negative	parenchymal	3	(4.1)	
	ventricular	1	(4.6)	4.2

More than one answer possible.

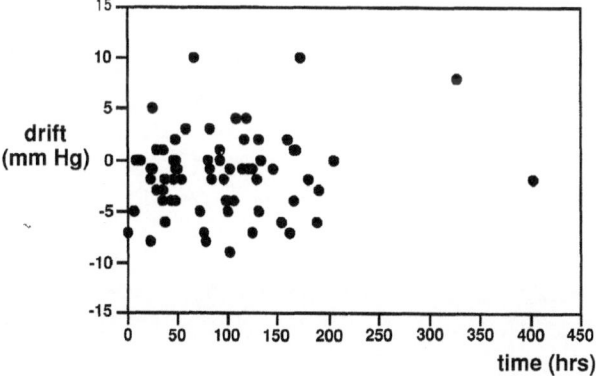

Fig. 1. Correlation between duration of implantation and drift after explantation. Mean drift was –0.21 mmHg/24 hrs

tively. Two probes were recalibrated because of "ICP estimated too low". The drift was +2 and +4 mmHg. Two probes were recalibrated because of dislocation. The drift was –1 and –7 mmHg respectively.

Drift and Two-Point Calibration

After explantation of the probes the drift of each catheter was documented (Fig. 1). There was no correlation between the measuring period and the drift. Mean drift was –0.21 mmHg/24 hrs. Thereafter each probe was recalibrated to zero and the function checked in a calibration vial corresponding to 15.8 mmHg. The mean value obtained was 14.7 ± 1.9 mmHg. A correlation between function of the probe in the calibration vial and the drift was lacking.

Complications

Most technical complications occurred during nursing or transport of the patient. In detail 12 probes were pulled out (12.6%), 3 screws dislocated (3.2%), in three cases the fiberoptic cable broke (3.2%) and in 6 cases no reason was found for defective probes (6.4%). We observed a total or 24 technical complications (25.4%). Complications related to insertion were hematoma in insertion canal (n = 4, 4.2%) and one case of bacterial meningitis (1.05%) after implantation of a CAMINO-ventricular catheter.

Discussion

During one year 95 CAMINO intracranial pressure probes were implanted in 82 patients with intracranial pathology in our interdisciplinary intensive care unit. Correct positioning of the catheter was performed in 92.5% the catheters controlled by CT. Implantation is easy and quick. During the clinical course the measurements were assessed plausibe in 88.4%. Nine catheters were recalibrated *in vivo* under sterile conditions either because the measurement was felt to be inaccurate according to the patients clinical condition (n = 7) or because the catheter was pulled out of the head into the protection hose accidentally (n = 2). The construction of the system (catheter sticks out perpendicularly) allows this recalibration manoeuvre, in selected cases (personal communication).

It is known from the literature that there is a good correlation between the ICP measured with the fiberoptic device and the manometrically measured ICP with a ventricular catheter [1, 4]. We were able to confirm the stability of the measurement in our study. After explantation the mean drift was −0.21 mmHg per 24 hrs, a value which is well acceptable and below the companies specification [2]. There was no correlation between the measuring period and the drift. The two-point calibration performed *ex vivo* also showed acceptable performance of the explanted catheters. Medical complications were hematoma in the insertion canal in 4 instances and one case of bacterial meningitis. All of the patients who developed hematoma after parenchymal CAMINO implantation were severely injured and had profound disturbance of their clotting system (low platelet count or elevated partial thromboplastine time).

The complication rate due to technical reasons was high (25.4%). Despite the fact that the nursing staff was used to the system for two years and well aware of the sensitivity of the rigid fiberoptic cable and the fragility of the insertion screw, probes were pulled out during nursing and screws broke during patient transport. It is important to note that the staff was not informed about the ongoing study, a fact which might serve as an explanation for our high technical complication rate as compared to the literature. It is especially remarkable that in a series of 209 CAMINO-probes published by Gambardella [3] not a single technical complication was reported. Yablon and co-workers [5] documented 55 probes and found a total rate of technical complications of 12.7%.

In conclusion we feel that the overall reliability of the fiberoptic ICP-monitoring system (CAMINO) appears to be acceptable. The screw and the rigid fiberoptic cable stick out of the head perpendicular, carrying a high risk of damage or dislocation. However, the perpendicular way of catheter insertion allows for explantation, recalibration and reinsertion of probes in selected cases where the displayed ICP-value is felt not to be plausible.

The screw fixation system and the fiberoptic cable stability have to be improved.

References

1. Cruchfield JS, Narayan RK, Robertson CS, Michael LH (1990) Evaluation of a fiberoptic intracranial pressure monitor. J Neurosurg 72: 482–487
2. Czosnyka M, Czosnyka Z, Pickard JD (1996) Laboratory testing of three intracranial pressure microtransducers: technical report. Neurosurgery 38: 219–224
3. Gambardella G, d'Avella D, Tomasello F (1992) Monitoring of brain tissue pressure with a fiberoptic device. Neurosurgery 31: 918–922
4. Ostrup RC, Luerssen TG, Marshall LF, Zornow MH (1987) Continous monitoring of intracranial pressure with a miniaturized fiberoptic device. J Neurosurg 67: 206–209
5. Yablon JS, Lantner HJ, McCormack TM, Nair S, Barker E, Black P (1993) Clinical experience with a fiberoptic intracranial pressure monitor. Clin Monit 9: 171–175

Correspondence: Ludwig Schürer, M.D., Ph.D., Neurochirurgische Klinik, Klinikum Mannheim, University of Heidelberg, Theodor-Kutzer-Ufer 1–3, D-68135 Mannheim, Federal Republic of Germany.

Author Index

Index of Keywords

SpringerNeurosurgery

U. Ito, A. Baethmann, K.-A. Hossmann,
T. Kuroiwa, A. Marmarou, H.-J. Reulen,
K. Takakura (eds.)

Brain Edema IX

Proceedings of the Ninth International Symposium, Tokyo, May 16–19, 1993

1994. 281 partly coloured figures. XV, 590 pages. Cloth DM 330,–, öS 2310,–
Reduced price for subscribers to "Acta Neurochirurgica": Cloth DM 297,–, öS 2079,–
ISBN 3-211-82532-0. Acta Neurochirurgica, Supplement 60

This volume deals with (a) the blood-parenchymal cell border under normal and pathological conditions causing brain edema, (b) neuron-glial interactions and their disturbances in tissue damage, (c) formation, propagation and resolution of brain edema, and
finally (d) treatment of vasogenic and cytotoxic brain edema. In the basic science approaches emphasis is given to newly discovered molecules, such as vascular endothelial
growth factor, which might control permeability of the blood-brain barrier, e.g. in brain
tumors. The complex issue of mediator compounds of secondary brain damage is further
developed as to its manyfold involvement.

H.-J. Reulen, H.-J. Steiger (eds.)

Training in Neurosurgery

Proceedings of the Conference on Neurosurgical Training and Research, Munich, October 6–9, 1996

1997. 29 figures. VIII, 159 pages. Cloth DM 120,–, öS 840,–
Reduced price for subscribers to "Acta Neurochirurgica": Cloth DM 108,–, öS 756,–
ISBN 3-211-83002-2. Acta Neurochirurgica, Supplement 69

Experts from different countries and neurosurgical organizations have collected information on the present status of resident training in neurosurgery and the mechanisms
involved with the training. Various aspects, the recruitment process, the criteria used for
selection, the contents and structure of a program, the continuous quality control, exposi-
tion to the art of research, fellowships and subspeciality training, etc. have been covered.
The present book contains this material and thus provides a unique and comprehensive
source of information on the complex of modern neurosurgical training.

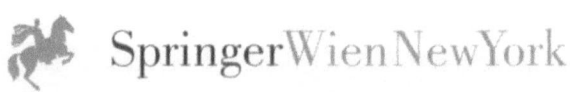 SpringerWienNewYork

Sachsenplatz 4-6, P.O.Box 89, A-1201 Wien, Fax +43-1-330 24 26, e-mail: order@springer.at, Internet: http://www.springer.at
New York, NY 10010, 175 Fifth Avenue • D-14197 Berlin, Heidelberger Platz 3 • Tokyo 113, 3-13, Hongo 3-chome, Bunkyo-ku